Davis's Pocket Clinical Drug Reference

Davis's Pocket Clinical Drug Reference

Shamim Tejani, PharmD
Pediatric Clinical Pharmacist
St. Joseph's Hospital and Medical Center
Phoenix, Arizona

Cynthia A. Sanoski, B.S., PharmD, FCCP, BCPS
Chair, Department of Pharmacy Practice
Jefferson School of Pharmacy
Thomas Jefferson University
Philadelphia, Pennsylvania

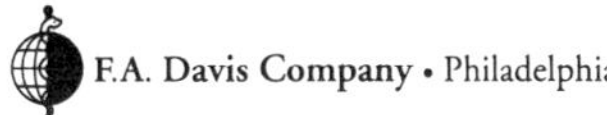
F.A. Davis Company • Philadelphia

F. A. Davis Company
1915 Arch Street
Philadelphia, PA 19103
www.fadavis.com

Printed in the United States of America

Last digit indicates print number 10 9 8 7 6 5 4 3 2 1

Director of Content Development: Darlene D. Pedersen
Senior Acquisitions Editor: Thomas A. Ciavarella
Project Editor: Meghan K. Ziegler
Design and Illustration Manager: Carolyn O'Brien

ISBN-13: 978-0-8036-2078-0

ISBN-10: 0-8036-2078-0

To my son, Cameron, the "transformer" who has changed my life forever.

To my daughter, Sierra, the "big star" without whom I could not navigate.

Your patience made this book possible.

Shamim Tejani

To my mother, Geraldine, whose continual love, support and guidance are present in all that I do. Thank you for your patience and understanding as I worked on this important project.

Cynthia Sanoski

Table of Contents

Preface

Davis's Pocket Clinical Drug Reference is a quick resource for the most commonly used drugs in clinical practice. The monographs are designed to highlight pertinent information; specifically, each monograph includes a drug's generic name, brand name, therapeutic indication, pharmacologic class, pregnancy class, contraindications, adverse drug reactions, drug interactions, dose, availability, and monitoring parameters.

To incorporate as many drugs as possible into a pocket drug guide format, only the most common adverse drug reactions and drug interactions are presented within each monograph. The table entitled **Cytochrome P450 Substrates/Inhibitors/Inducers** (page 285) provides more specific information regarding the drugs that may be involved in certain drug interactions. Additionally, within each monograph, a **Notes** section is included to highlight miscellaneous information that users should consider when initiating or monitoring drug therapy in their patients.

In the Appendix, a number of useful tables and charts, covering topics such as immunization guidelines, intravenous drugs, and narcotic equianalgesic dosing guidelines, provide additional information that is relevant to clinical practice. To obtain detailed drug information beyond what is supplied in the monographs of this pocket drug guide, the user should refer to the medical literature or the complete product information supplied by the manufacturer.

Reviewers

Naveed Ahmed, MPAS, PA-C
Drexel University
Hahnemann Physician Assistant Program
Philadelphia, Pennsylvania

Carole Berube, BSN, MSN, MA (Psychology), RN
Professor Emerita in Nursing, Instructor in Health Sciences
Bristol Community College
Fall River, Massachusetts

Mary Anne Crandall, RN, BS, MS, PhD, CLT, CCT
Doctor Therapeutic Laser and Thermal Imaging Center
Medford, Oregon

Dori Gilman, MA
LPN Coordinator, LPN & RN Instructor
North Country Community College
Saranac Lake, New York

Cheryl Gilton, RN, BSN, Med
Director, Pharmacy Technician Program
Allegany College of Maryland
Special Health Initiatives
Cumberland, Maryland

Catherine C. Goodman, PT, MBA
Faculty Affiliate, Medical Writer (Medical Multimedia Group)
University of Montana
School of Pharmacy and Allied Health
Missoula, Montana

Ellen Wruble Hakim, PT, DScPT, MS, CWS, FACCWS
Vice Chair for Professional Programs Director for Entry-Level DPT Program
University of Maryland School of Medicine
Department of Physical Therapy and Rehabilitation
Baltimore, Maryland

Ken Harbert, PhD, CHES, PA-C
Dean and Program Director
South College
Knoxville, Tennessee

Kris Hardy, CMA, RHE, CDF
Medical Assistant Program Director/Instructor
Brevard Community College
Cocoa, Florida

Marsha Hemby, ADN, CMA
Department Chair, Medical Assisting
Pitt Community College
Greenville, North Carolina

Mary Ann Laxen, PA-C, MAB
Director, Physician Assistant Program
University of North Dakota, School of Medicine and Health Sciences
Grand Forks, North Dakota

Kathy Makkar, PharmD
Clinical Pharmacy Specialist, Cardiology
Lancaster General Hospital
Lancaster, Pennsylvania

Allison A. Morgan, MPA, PA-C
Instructor
Duquesne University
John H. Rangos, Sr.
School of Health Sciences
Pittsburgh, Pennsylvania

Patti Pagels, MPAS, PA-C
Assistant Professor/Vice-Chair, Clinical Service
University of North Texas Health Science Center
Fort Worth, Texas

Karen Snipe, CPhT, Med
Pharmacy Technician Program Coordinator Department Head, Diagnostic & Imaging Services
Trident Technical College
Charleston, South Carolina

Daniel Thibodeau, MHP, PA-C
Assistant Professor, Physician Assistant Program
Eastern Virginia Medical School
Norfolk, Virginia

Marilyn M. Turner, RN, CMA
Medical Assisting Program Director
Ogeechee Technical College
Statesboro, Georgia

List of Abbreviations

↑ increase, increased
↓ decrease, decreased
A1C glycosylated hemoglobin
ABG arterial blood gas
ABW actual body weight
ac before meals
ACE angiotensin-converting enzyme
ACEI angiotensin-converting enzyme inhibitor
ACLS advanced cardiac life support
ACS acute coronary syndrome
ACT activated clotting time
AD Alzheimer's disease
ADH antidiuretic hormone
ADHD attention-deficit hyperactivity disorder
ADR adverse drug reaction
AF atrial fibrillation
AFl atrial flutter
AIDS acquired immune deficiency syndrome
alk phos alkaline phosphatase
ALL acute lymphocytic leukemia
ALT alanine aminotransferase
AML acute myelogenous leukemia
ANA antinuclear antibodies
ANC absolute neutrophil count
ANLL acute nonlymphocytic leukemia
aPTT activated partial thromboplastin time
ARB angiotensin receptor blocker
ARDS adult respiratory distress syndrome
ARF acute renal failure
ASA aspirin
ASM aggressive systemic mastocytosis
AST aspartate aminotransferase
ATP adenosine triphosphate
AV atrioventricular
Availability (G): generic availability
AVM arteriovenous malformation
BG blood glucose
bid two times a day
BMD bone mineral density
BMI body mass index
BMT bone marrow transplantation
BP blood pressure
BPH benign prostatic hyperplasia
bpm beats per minute
BSA body surface area
BUN blood urea nitrogen
BZ benzodiazepine
Ca calcium
CA cancer
CABG coronary artery bypass graft
CAD coronary artery disease
cap capsule
CAP community-acquired pneumonia
CBC complete blood count
CCB calcium channel blocker
CEL chronic eosinophilic leukemia
CK creatine kinase
CKD chronic kidney disease
CI contraindication
CML chronic myelogenous leukemia
CMV cytomegalovirus
CNS central nervous system
COMT catechol-*O*-methyltransferase
COPD chronic obstructive pulmonary disease
CP chest pain

CR controlled-release
CrCl creatinine clearance
CSF colony-stimulating factor; cerebrospinal fluid
CT computed tomography
CV cardiovascular
CVA cerebrovascular accident
CVP central venous pressure
CXR chest x-ray
CYP cytochrome P450
D5/LR 5% dextrose and lactated Ringer's solution
D5/0.9% NaCl
5% dextrose and 0.9% NaCl; 5% dextrose and normal saline
D5/0.25% NaCl
5% dextrose and 0.25% NaCl; 5% dextrose and quarter normal saline
D5/0.45% NaCl
5% dextrose and 0.45% NaCl; 5% dextrose and half normal saline
D5W 5% dextrose in water
D10W 10% dextrose in water
DBP diastolic blood pressure
derm dermatologic
DFSP dermatofibrosarcoma protuberans
DI diabetes insipidus
diff differential
DKA diabetic ketoacidosis
dl deciliter(s)
DM diabetes mellitus
DMARD disease-modifying antirheumatic drug
DNA deoxyribonucleic acid
DR delayed-release
DRE digital rectal exam
DVT deep vein thrombosis
EC enteric-coated
ECG electrocardiogram
ECMO extracorporeal membrane oxygenation
ED erectile dysfunction
EENT eye, ear, nose, and throat
EGFR epidermal growth factor receptor
endo endocrine
ENL erythema nodosum leprosum
EPS extrapyramidal symptoms
ER extended-release
ES extra-strength
esp. especially
ESRD end-stage renal disease
ET endotracheal
FAP familial adenomatous polyposis
F and E fluid and electrolyte
FQ fluoroquinolone
FSH follicle-stimulating hormone
g gram(s)
GABA gamma-aminobutyric acid
GAD generalized anxiety disorder
GERD gastroesophageal reflux disease
GFR glomerular filtration rate
GI gastrointestinal
GIST gastrointestinal stromal tumors
GNR Gram-negative rods
GnRH gonadotropin releasing hormone
G6PD glucose-6-phosphate dehydrogenase
GP glycoprotein
GPC Gram-positive cocci
gtt drop(s)
GU genitourinary
H2 histamine-2
HA headache
HBV hepatitis B virus
Hct hematocrit
HCV hepatitis C virus
HD hemodialysis
HDL high-density lipoprotein
HES hypereosinophilic syndrome
HF heart failure
Hgb hemoglobin

5-HIAA 5-hydroxyindoleacetic acid
HIT heparin-induced thrombocytopenia
HITTS heparin-induced thrombocytopenia and thrombosis syndrome
HIV human immunodeficiency virus
HMG-CoA hydroxymethyl glutaryl coenzyme A
HPA hypothalamic-pituitary-adrenal
hr hour(s)
HR heart rate
HRT hormone replacement therapy
HSV herpes simplex virus
5-HT 5-hydroxytriptamine (serotonin)
HTN hypertension
IE infective endocarditis
IA intra-articular
IBD inflammatory bowel disease
IBW ideal body weight
ICP intracranial pressure
ICU intensive care unit
IDDM insulin-dependent diabetes mellitus
IL intralesional
IM intramuscular
in. inch(es)
inhaln inhalation
inject injection
INR international normalized ratio
I/O intake and output
IOP intraocular pressure
IPPB intermittent positive-pressure breathing
IR immediate-release
IS intrasynovial
IT intrathecal
ITP immune thrombocytopenic purpura
IUD intrauterine device
IV intravenous
K potassium
KCl potassium chloride
kg kilogram(s)
KS Kaposi's sarcoma
L liter(s)
LA long-acting
LD loading dose
LDH lactic dehydrogenase
LDL low-density lipoprotein
LFT liver function test
LH luteinizing hormone
LHRH luteinizing hormone-release hormone
LMWH low molecular weight heparin
loz lozenge
LR lactated Ringer's solution
LV left ventricular
LVEF left ventricular ejection fraction
LVH left ventricular hypertrophy
M molar
MAC *Mycobacterium avium* complex; monitored anesthesia care
MAOI monoamine oxidase inhibitor
max maximum
mcg microgram(s)
MD maintenance dose
MDI metered dose inhaler
MDRSP multi-drug resistant *Streptococcus pneumoniae*
MDS myelodysplastic syndrome
meds medications
mEq milliequivalent(s)
metab metabolic
mg milligram(s)
Mg magnesium
MI myocardial infarction
min minute(s)
misc miscellaneous
ml milliliter(s)
mM millimole(s)

MMSE Mini-Mental State Examination
mo month
MPD myeloproliferative disease
MRI magnetic resonance imaging
MRSA methicillin-resistant *Staphylococcus aureus*
MS multiple sclerosis
MSSA methicillin-sensitive
MUGA multiple-gated acquisition (scan)
Na sodium
NaCl sodium chloride
$NaPO_4$ sodium phosphate
neb nebulizer
NEC necrotizing enterocolitis
neuro neurologic
ng nanogram(s)
NG nasogastric
NIDDM noninsulin-dependent diabetes mellitus
NMS neuroleptic malignant syndrome
NPO nothing by mouth
NRTI nucleoside reverse transcriptase inhibitor
NS sodium chloride, normal saline (0.9% NaCl)
NSAID nonsteroidal anti-inflammatory drug
NSTEMI non-ST-segment elevation myocardial infarction
N/V nausea and vomiting
N/V/D nausea, vomiting, and diarrhea
NYHA New York Heart Association
OA osteoarthritis
OCD obsessive-compulsive disorder
ODT orally disintegrating tablets
oint ointment
OM otitis media
ophth ophthalmic
OTC over-the-counter
oz ounce(s)
PAD peripheral arterial disease
PALS pediatric advanced life support
PAT paroxysmal atrial tachycardia
PBPC peripheral blood progenitor cell
pc after meals
PCA patient-controlled analgesia
PCI percutaneous coronary intervention
PCP *Pneumocystis carinii* pneumonia
PCWP pulmonary capillary wedge pressure
PDA patent ductus arteriosus
PDE phosphodiesterase
PE pulmonary embolism
PEA pulseless electrical activity
PFT pulmonary function test
pg picogram(s)
Ph+ Philadelphia chromosome positive
PID pelvic inflammatory disease
pkt packet
PMDD premenstrual dysphoric disorder
PNA postnatal age
PO by mouth, orally
PO_4 phosphate
PONV postoperative nausea and vomiting
PPD purified protein derivative
PPI proton pump inhibitor
Preg pregnancy category
preop preoperative, preoperatively
prn as needed
PSA prostate-specific antigen
PSE portal-systemic encephalopathy
PSVT paroxysmal supraventricular tachycardia

PT prothrombin time
PTCA percutaneous transluminal angioplasty
PTH parathyroid hormone
PTSD post-traumatic stress disorder
PUD peptic ulcer disease
PVC premature ventricular contraction
q every
qid four times a day
RA rheumatoid arthritis
RBC red blood cell
rect rectally or rectal
REM rapid eye movement
retic reticulocyte
ROM range of motion
RR respiratory rate
RSV respiratory syncytial virus
RTU ready to use
Rx prescription
SA sinoatrial
SAD social anxiety disorder
SBP systolic blood pressure
SCr serum creatinine
SDC serum digoxin concentration
sec second(s)
SIADH syndrome of inappropriate antidiuretic hormone
SJS Stevens Johnson syndrome
SL sublingual
SLE systemic lupus erythematosus
SNRI serotonin-norepinephrine reuptake inhibitor
SOB shortness of breath
soln solution
SR sustained-release
S/S signs and symptoms
SSRI selective serotonin reuptake inhibitor
stat immediately
STEMI ST-segment elevation myocardial infarction
subcut subcutaneous
supp suppository
susp suspension
SVT supraventricular tachycardia
tab tablet
TB tuberculosis
tbsp tablespoon(s)
TCA tricyclic antidepressant
temp temperature
TEN toxic epidermal necrolysis
TFT thyroid function test
TG triglyceride
TIA transient ischemic attack
TIBC total iron-binding capacity
tid three times a day
TNF tumor necrosis factor
top topical, topically
tri trimester
TSH thyroid-stimulating hormone
tsp teaspoon(s)
TT thrombin time
UA unstable angina
U/A urinalysis
UFH unfractionated heparin
ULN upper limits of normal
UO urinary output
UTI urinary tract infection
vag vaginal
VF ventricular fibrillation
VIPoma vasoactive intestinal peptide tumor
VLDL very low-density lipoprotein
VRE vancomycin-resistant *Enterococcus*
VT ventricular tachycardia
VTE venous thromboembolism
WBC white blood cell
wk week(s)
WPW Wolff-Parkinson-White (syndrome)
wt weight
× times; for
yr year(s)

abacavir (Ziagen) Uses: HIV (in combination with other antiretrovirals); **Class:** nucleoside reverse transcriptase inhibitors; **Preg:** C; **CIs:** Hypersensitivity (rechallenge may be fatal), Moderate-to-severe hepatic disease, Presence of HLA-B*5701 allele (↑ risk of hypersensitivity) Children, <3 mo (safety not established); **ADRs:** HA, HEPATOTOXICITY, N/V/D, rash, LACTIC ACIDOSIS, HYPERSENSITIVITY REACTIONS; **Interactions:** Alcohol ↑ levels, May ↓ methadone levels (↑ in methadone dose may be needed); **Dose:** *PO: Adults:* 300 mg bid or 600 mg daily; *PO: Peds:* 3 mo–16 yr 8 mg/kg bid (max: 300 mg bid); *Hepatic Impairment: PO: Adults:* ↓ dose if mild hepatic impairment; **Availability:** Tabs: 300 mg; Oral soln: 20 mg/ml; **Monitor:** S/S of hypersensitivity reactions (fever, rash, N/V/D, abdominal pain; malaise, fatigue, achiness; dyspnea, cough, pharyngitis); LFTs, TGs, viral load, CD4 count, amylase, CK; **Notes:** Not to be used as monotherapy; discontinue if S/S of hypersensitivity reaction occur (do not rechallenge). All patients should be tested for presence of HLA-B*5701 allele before starting therapy; if present, alternative therapy should be used.

acarbose (Precose) Uses: Type 2 DM (as monotherapy or with insulin or other oral hypoglycemic agent); **Class:** alpha-glucosidase inhibitors; **Preg:** B; **CIs:** Hypersensitivity, DKA, Cirrhosis, Inflammatory bowel disease, SCr >2 mg/dl; **ADRs:** abdominal pain, diarrhea, flatulence, ↑ LFTs; **Interactions:** Thiazides and loop diuretics, corticosteroids, phenothiazines, thyroid preparations, estrogens (conjugated), phenytoin, niacin, sympathomimetics, CCBs, and isoniazid may ↑ glucose, ↑ risk of hypoglycemia with sulfonylureas or insulin, May ↓ digoxin levels; **Dose:** *PO: Adults:* 25 mg tid; may ↑ q 4–8 wk prn (max: 50 mg tid if ≤60 kg or 100 mg tid if >60 kg); **Availability (G):** Tabs: 25, 50, 100 mg; **Monitor:** A1C, postprandial glucose, S/S hypoglycemia when used with oral hypoglycemic agents or insulin, LFTs; **Notes:** Does not cause hypoglycemia when taken alone while fasting; may ↑ hypoglycemia when used with hypoglycemic agents; if hypoglycemia occurs, take form of oral glucose (e.g., glucose tabs, liquid gel glucose) and not sugar (acarbose blocks sugar absorption); take with first bite of each meal tid.

acetaminophen (Acephen, APAP, Aspirin Free Anacin, Cetafen, Feverall, Genapap, Liquiprin, Mapap, Panadol, Silapap, Tylenol, Valorin) Uses: Pain, Fever; **Class:** nonopioid analgesics; **Preg:** B; **CIs:** Hypersensitivity; **ADRs:** HEPATOTOXICITY(OVERDOSE), renal failure (high doses/chronic use), anemia, leukopenia, rash, urticaria; **Interactions:** Chronic high-dose acetaminophen (>2 g/day) may ↑ risk of bleeding with warfarin, ↑ risk of hepatotoxicity with alcohol, isoniazid, rifampin, rifabutin, phenytoin, barbiturates, or carbamazepine; **Dose:** *PO: Rect: Adults and Peds:* > 12 yr 325–650 mg q 4–6 hr *or* 1 g 3–4 ×/day (max: 4 g/day [2 g/day in patients with hepatic/renal impairment]); *PO: Rect: Peds:* 1–12 yr 10–15 mg/kg/dose (up to 20 mg/kg/dose for rectal) q 4–6 hr prn (max: 2.6 g/day);

A

Availability (G): Chew tabs: 80, 160 mg[OTC]; Tabs: 325, 500 mg[OTC]; Caps: 500 mg[OTC]; ER caps: 650 mg[OTC]; Liquid: 160 mg/5 ml[OTC], 500 mg/15 ml[OTC]; Oral elixir: 160 mg/5 ml[OTC]; Oral drops: 80 mg/0.8 ml[OTC]; Oral susp: 160 mg/5 ml[OTC]; Supp: 80, 120, 325, 650 mg[OTC]; **Monitor:** Temp, pain, ROM, BUN/SCr, LFTs; **Notes:** Caution patients about using other OTC analgesics/cough and cold products (may also contain acetaminophen). Acetylcysteine is antidote in overdose.

acetaZOLAMIDE (Diamox) Uses: ↓ IOP in glaucoma, Acute altitude sickness, Edema, Seizure disorders; **Class:** carbonic anhydrase inhibitors; **Preg:** C; **CIs:** Hypersensitivity or cross-sensitivity with sulfonamides, Hyponatremia, Hypokalemia, Hyperchloremic metabolic acidosis, Severe hepatic disease, Concurrent use with ophthalmic carbonic anhydrase inhibitors (brinzolamide, dorzolamide), Chronic respiratory disease, Severe renal disease (not effective if CrCl <10 ml/min); **ADRs:** weakness, sedation, N/V, renal calculi, SJS, rash, ↑ BG, hyperchloremic acidosis, ↓ K+, APLASTIC ANEMIA, HEMOLYTIC ANEMIA, LEUKOPENIA, ↓ wt, ↑ uric acid, paresthesias, ANAPHYLAXIS; **Interactions:** May ↑ phenytoin, amphetamine, cyclosporine, and quinidine levels, May ↓ primidone and lithium levels; **Dose:** *PO: Adults: Glaucoma (open-angle)*—250–1000 mg/day in 1–4 divided doses or 500-mg ER caps bid. *Seizure disorders*—8–30 mg/kg/day in 1–4 divided doses (max: 1 g/day). *Altitude sickness*—250 mg q 8–12 hr or 500-mg ER caps q 12–24 hr; begin 24–48 hr before ascent and continue for ≥48 hr once high altitude reached. *Edema*—250–375 mg/day; *PO: Peds: Glaucoma*—8–30 mg/kg/day in 3 divided doses. *Edema*—5 mg/kg once daily. *Seizure disorders*—8–30 mg/kg/day in 1–4 divided doses (max: 1 g/day); *IV: Adults: Glaucoma (closed-angle)*—250–500 mg, may repeat in 2–4 hr to max of 1 g/day. *Edema*—250–375 mg/day; *IV: Peds: Glaucoma*—5–10 mg/kg q 6 hr (max of 1 g/day). *Edema*—5 mg/kg once daily; **Availability (G):** Tabs: 125, 250 mg; ER caps: 500 mg; Inject: 500 mg; **Monitor:** Electrolytes, IOP, neurologic status, S/S altitude sickness, CBC, glucose; **Notes:** Do not use ER caps for seizure disorders or edema; avoid IM inject. Do not chew or crush ER caps.

acyclovir (Zovirax) Uses: *PO:* Initial and recurrent genital herpes. Herpes zoster (shingles). Chickenpox (varicella). *IV:* Severe genital herpes. Mucosal or cutaneous herpes simplex. Herpes zoster (shingles). Herpes simplex encephalitis, **Top:** Cream—Recurrent herpes labialis (cold sores). Oint—Non–life-threatening herpes simplex (systemic treatment preferred); **Class:** antivirals; **Preg:** B; **CIs:** Hypersensitivity to acyclovir or valacyclovir; **ADRs:** SEIZURES, HA, N/V/D, ↑ LFTs, anorexia, RENAL FAILURE, ↑ BUN/SCr, crystalluria, hematuria, hives, rash, THROMBOTIC THROMBOCYTOPENIC PURPURA/HEMOLYTIC UREMIC SYNDROME (HIGH DOSES IN IMMUNOSUPPRESSED PATIENTS), phlebitis, local irritation; **Interactions:** Probenecid ↑ levels, Concurrent use of other nephrotoxic drugs ↑ risk of renal dysfunction; **Dose:** *PO: Adults: Herpes zoster*—800 mg q 4 hr while awake (5×/day) × 7–10 days. *Genital herpes*—Initial episode: 200 mg q 4 hr while awake (5×/day) × 10 days or 400 mg tid × 5–10 days. Recurrence: 200 mg q 4 hr while awake (5×/day) × 5 days or 400 mg tid × 5 days. Chronic suppressive therapy: 400 mg bid or 200 mg 3–5×/day for up to 12 mo. *Chickenpox*—>40 kg: 800 mg 4×/day × 5 days. Start within 24 hr of rash onset; *PO: Peds: Genital herpes (<12 yr)*—Initial episode: 40–80 mg/kg/day in 3–4 divided doses × 5–10 days (max: 1 g/day). Chronic suppressive therapy: 80 mg/kg/day in 3 divided doses for up to 12 mo (max: 1 g/day). *Genital herpes* (≥12 yr)—See adult dosing. *Chickenpox (>2 yr and <40 kg)*—20 mg/kg (max: 800 mg/dose) 4×/day × 5 days. Start within 24 hr of rash onset. *Chickenpox (≥2 yr and ≥40 kg)*—See adult dosing; *IV: Adults and Peds:* ≥12 yr *Mucosal or cutaneous herpes simplex*—5 mg/kg q 8 hr × 7 days. *Genital herpes*—5 mg/kg q 8 hr × 5 days. *Herpes simplex encephalitis*—10 mg/kg q 8 hr × 10 days. *Herpes zoster*—10 mg/kg q 8 hr × 7 days; *IV: Peds:* <12 yr *Mucosal or cutaneous herpes simplex*—10 mg/kg q 8 hr × 7 days. *Herpes simplex encephalitis*—20 mg/kg q 8 hr × 10 days. *Herpes zoster*—20 mg/kg q 8 hr × 7 days; **Top:** *Adults*: Oint—0.5-in. ribbon of 5% ointment for every 4-square-in. area q 3 hr (6×/day) × 7 days. *Cream (also for children ≥12 yr)*—Apply 5×/day × 4 days; start at first symptoms; *Renal Impairment: PO: IV: Adults and Peds:* ↓ dose if CrCl ≤ 25 ml/min (PO); ↓ dose if CrCl ≤ 50 ml/min (IV); **Availability (G):** Caps: 200 mg; Tabs: 400, 800 mg; Oral susp: 200 mg/5 ml; Powder for inject: 500 mg, 1000 mg; Soln for inject: 25 mg/ml, 50 mg/ml; Cream/Oint: 5%; **Monitor:** BUN, SCr, lesions, neuro status (for herpes encephalitis); **Notes:** Start ASAP after herpes simplex symptoms appear and within 24 hr of herpes zoster outbreak. Maintain adequate hydration (2000–3000 ml/day), especially during first 2 hr after IV infusion, to prevent crystalluria. Infuse over ≥ 1 hr to ↓ renal tubular damage. Watch for phlebitis with IV (rotate infusion site).

adalimumab (Humira) **Uses:** RA (as monotherapy or with other DMARDs), Juvenile idiopathic arthritis (as monotherapy or with methotrexate), Psoriatic arthritis (as monotherapy or with other DMARDs), Ankylosing spondylitis, Crohn's disease, Plaque psoriasis; **Class:** DMARDs, monoclonal antibodies; **Preg:** B; **CIs:** Hypersensitivity, Concurrent use of anakinra or abatacept, Active infection; **ADRs:** <u>HA</u>, HTN, abdominal pain, nausea, hematuria, <u>rash</u>, neutropenia, thrombocytopenia, <u>inject site reactions</u>, hyperlipidemia, ↑ CK, ANAPHYLAXIS, INFECTIONS (INCLUDING REACTIVATION TUBERCULOSIS), MALIGNANCY; **Interactions:** Anakinra or abatacept may ↑ risk of serious infection (contraindicated), Do not give with live vaccinations; **Dose:** *Subcut: Adults: RA, psoriatic arthritis, or ankylosing spondylitis*—40 mg every other wk; may ↑ to 40 mg once weekly, if needed, in RA patients not receiving methotrexate. *Crohn's disease*—160 mg on Day 1 (four 40-mg injects in one day or two 40-mg injects on 2 consecutive days), then 80 mg on Day 15. On Day 29, begin MD of 40 mg every other wk.

Plaque psoriasis—80 mg initially, then 40 mg every other wk (starting 1 wk after initial dose); *Subcut: Peds:* 4–17 yr *Juvenile idiopathic arthritis*—15–29 kg: 20 mg every other wk; ≥30 kg: 40 mg every other wk; **Availability:** Inject: 20 mg/0.4 ml, 40 mg/0.8 ml; **Monitor:** Pain scale, ROM, S/S infection, S/S anaphylaxis, CBC; **Notes:** Place PPD prior to initiation (may reactivate latent TB). Discontinue if serious infection develops. Use with caution in LV dysfunction (may cause or worsen HF). Needle cap of prefilled syringe contains latex.

adenosine (Adenocard, Adenoscan) Uses: PSVT, Diagnostic agent (with noninvasive techniques) to assess myocardial perfusion defects due to CAD; **Class:** Antiarrhythmics; **Preg:** C; **CIs:** Hypersensitivity, ≥ 2nd-degree AV block or sick sinus syndrome (unless pacemaker present), Asthma (may induce bronchospasm); **ADRs:** dizziness, HA, blurred vision, throat tightness, <u>SOB</u>, <u>facial flushing</u>, <u>transient arrhythmias</u>, CP, ↓ BP; **Interactions:** Dipyridamole ↑ effects, Theophylline or caffeine ↓ effects; **Dose:** *IV: Adults and Peds:* ≥50 kg *Antiarrhythmic*—6 mg over 1–2 sec; if no results in 1–2 min, repeat with 12 mg; may repeat 12-mg dose. *Diagnostic use*—140 mcg/kg/min for 6 min (0.84 mg/kg total); *IV: Peds:* <50 kg *Antiarrhythmic*—0.05–0.1 mg/kg over 1–2 sec, if no results in 1–2 min,↑ dose by 0.05–0.1 mg/kg; repeat this until sinus rhythm restored or max dose of 0.3 mg/kg used; **Availability (G):** Inject: 3 mg/ml; **Monitor:** HR, ECG (heart block or asystole may occur shortly after injection), BP, RR; **Notes:** ADRs usually transient. When used as antiarrhythmic, administer peripherally as proximal as possible to trunk and immediately follow all bolus doses with 20 ml rapid NS flush.

albumin (human) (Albuminar, Albutein, Buminate, Plasbumin) Uses: ↑ plasma volume and cardiac output in fluid volume deficits (e.g., shock, hemorrhage, burns), Hypoproteinemia (e.g., nephrotic syndrome, end-stage liver disease) (with or without edema); **Class:** blood products, colloids; **Preg:** C; **CIs:** Allergic reactions to albumin, Severe anemia, HF; **ADRs:** PULMONARY EDEMA, fluid overload, HTN, ↑ salivation, N/V, chills, fever, flushing, HYPERSENSITIVITY (urticaria, rash, hypotension); **Interactions:** None significant; **Dose:** *IV: Adults: Hypovolemia*—25 g (500 ml); may repeat within 30 min. *Hypoproteinemia*—0.5–1 g/kg/dose, may repeat q 1–2 days; *IV: Peds: Hypovolemia*—0.5–1 g/kg/dose; may repeat as needed (max: 6 g/kg/day); *IV: Infants and Neonates: Hypovolemia*—0.25–0.5 g/kg/dose; **Availability:** Inject: 5% (50 mg/mL), 25% (250 mg/mL); **Monitor:** HR, BP, temp, CVP, I/Os, edema, albumin, Hgb/Hct. If fever, tachycardia, or hypotension occurs, stop infusion; **Notes:** Administer through large-gauge (≥ 20-gauge) needle or catheter. Record lot number in patient record. 5% soln often used for hypovolemia; 25% soln often used for hypoproteinemia. Do not exceed infusion rate of 2–4 ml/min (5%) and 1 ml/min (25%).

albuterol (Accuneb, Proair HFA, Proventil HFA, Ventolin HFA, VoSpire ER) Uses: Bronchodilator for asthma or COPD, Prevents exercise-induced bronchospasm; **Class:** adrenergics; **Preg:** C; **CIs:** Hypersensitivity to adrenergic amines, Breastfeeding women and children <2 yr; **ADRs:** nervousness, restlessness, tremor, HA, insomnia, CP, palpitations, ↑ HR, angina, arrhythmias, N/V, ↑ BG, ↓ K+; **Interactions:** MAOIs or TCAs may ↑ CV effects, Beta blockers may ↓ therapeutic effect, Diuretics may ↑ risk of hypokalemia; **Dose:** *PO: Adults and Peds:* >12 yr 2–4 mg tid or qid (start with 2-mg dose in elderly) (max: 32 mg/day) or 4–8-mg ER tabs q 12 hr (max: 32 mg/day); *PO: Peds:* 6–12 yr 2 mg tid or qid (max: 24 mg/day) or 4 mg ER tabs q 12 hr (max: 24 mg/day); *PO: Peds:* 2–6 yr 0.1–0.2 mg/kg tid (max: 12 mg/day); *Inhaln: Adults: Bronchospasm*—MDI: 2 puffs q 4–6 hr prn; Neb: 1.25–5 mg q 4–8 hr prn. *Acute asthma exacerbation*—MDI: 4–8 puffs q 20 min for up to 4 hr, then q 1–4 hr prn; Neb: 2.5–5 mg q 20 min × 3 doses, then 2.5–10 mg q 1–4 hr prn. *Exercise-induced bronchospasm*—MDI: 2 puffs 5–30 min before exercise; *Inhaln: Peds: Bronchospasm*—MDI (>4 yr): 2 puffs q 4–6 hr prn; MDI (≤4 yr): 1–2 puffs q 4–6 hr prn; Neb (>4 yr): 1.25–5 mg q 4–8 hr prn; Neb (≤4 yr): 0.63–2.5 mg q 4–6 hr prn. *Acute asthma exacerbation*—MDI (≥12 yr): 4–8 puffs q 20 min for up to 4 hr, then q 1–4 hr prn; MDI (<12 yr): 4–8 puffs for up to 3 doses, then q 1–4 hr prn; Neb (≥12 yr): 2.5–5 mg q 20 min × 3 doses, then 2.5–10 mg q 1–4 hr prn; Neb (<12 yr): 0.15 mg/kg q 20 min × 3 doses, then 0.15–0.3 mg/kg (max: 10 mg) q 1–4 hr prn. *Exercise-induced bronchospasm*—MDI (>4 yr): 2 puffs 5–30 min before exercise; MDI (≤4 yr): 1–2 puffs 5 min before exercise; **Availability (G):** Tabs: 2, 4 mg; ER tabs: 4, 8 mg; Oral syrup: 2 mg/5 ml; MDI: 90 mcg/inhaln; Inhaln soln: 0.63 mg/3 ml, 1.25 mg/3 ml, 2.5 mg/3 ml, 5 mg/ml; **Monitor:** Lung sounds, HR, BP, RR, PFTs, K+ (with neb or higher doses); **Notes:** Allow 1 min between inhalns (5 min before using other inhalers). Use spacer for children. Do not chew or crush ER tabs.

alendronate (Fosamax) Uses: Treatment/prevention of postmenopausal osteoporosis, Treatment of corticosteroid-induced osteoporosis in patients receiving ≥7.5 mg of prednisone/day (or equivalent) with ↓ BMD, Treatment of osteoporosis in men, Treatment of Paget's disease; **Class:** bisphosphonates; **Preg:** C; **CIs:** Esophageal disease (that may delay emptying), Unable to stand or sit upright for ≥30 min, At risk for aspiration, Hypocalcemia, Severe renal insufficiency (CrCl <35 ml/min); **ADRs:** HA, abdominal pain, constipation, dyspepsia, dysphagia, esophagitis, flatulence, gastritis, N/V/D, musculoskeletal pain, osteonecrosis (of jaw); **Interactions:** Antacids, calcium, iron, and magnesium ↓ absorption, ↑ risk of GI effects with NSAIDs, Food, coffee, and orange juice ↓ absorption; **Dose:** *PO: Adults: Osteoporosis treatment (men or postmenopausal women)*—10 mg daily or 70 mg once weekly. *Osteoporosis prevention*—5 mg daily or 35 mg once weekly. *Paget's disease*—40 mg daily × 6 mo. May consider retreatment for relapse. *Treatment of corticosteroid-induced osteoporosis*—5 mg daily; 10 mg daily for postmenopausal women not on estrogen; **Availability (G):** Tabs: 5, 10, 35, 40, 70 mg; Oral soln: 70 mg/75 ml; **Monitor:** BMD, S/S Paget's (bone pain, HA), Ca++, Alk phos (for Paget's); **Notes:** Take first thing in AM with 6–8 oz plain water ≥30 min before other meds, beverages, or food. Remain upright for ≥30 min after dose and after eating. Calcium and vitamin D supplements recommended. Avoid dental procedures during therapy.

alfuzosin (Uroxatral) Uses: BPH; **Class:** peripherally acting antiadrenergics; **Preg:** B; **CIs:** Hypersensitivity, Moderate-to-severe hepatic impairment, Concurrent use with potent CYP3A4 inhibitors, Concurrent use with other alpha-adrenergic blockers, Severe renal impairment (CrCl <30 ml/min); **ADRs:** dizziness, fatigue, HA, postural hypotension, constipation, nausea, ED; **Interactions:** Potent CYP3A4 inhibitors (e.g., ketoconazole, itraconazole, ritonavir) significantly ↑ levels (concurrent use contraindicated), Cimetidine, atenolol, and diltiazem also ↑ levels, ↑ levels of atenolol and diltiazem, ↑ risk of hypotension with antihypertensives; **Dose:** *PO: Adults:* 10 mg daily; **Availability:** ER tabs: 10 mg; **Monitor:** BP (lying and standing), HR, S/S BPH; **Notes:** Take after same meal each day. Avoid sudden changes in position (to ↓ risk of orthostatic hypotension). Do not chew or crush.

aliskiren (Tekturna) Uses: HTN; **Class:** renin inhibitors; **Preg:** C (1st tri), D (2nd and 3rd tri); **CIs:** Hypersensitivity; **ADRs:** dizziness, cough, diarrhea, ↑ K+, ANGIOEDEMA; **Interactions:** Irbesartan ↓ levels, Atorvastatin, ketoconazole, and cyclosporine ↑ levels (use with cyclosporine not recommended), ↓ levels of furosemide, ↑ risk of hyperkalemia with ACEIs, ARBs, K+ supplements, K+ sparing diuretics, or K+ salt substitutes, High fat meals significantly ↓ absorption; **Dose:** *PO: Adults:* 150 mg daily; may be ↑ to 300 mg daily; **Availability:** Tabs: 150, 300 mg; **Monitor:** BP, HR, BUN/SCr, K+, (if symptoms); **Notes:** Correct volume depletion, advise on S/S angioedema, avoid K+ salt substitutes.

allopurinol (Aloprim, Lopurin, Zyloprim) Uses: *PO:* Prevention of attack of gouty arthritis and nephropathy, *PO: IV:* Treatment of secondary hyperuricemia, which may occur during treatment of tumors or leukemias; **Class:** xanthine oxidase inhibitors; **Preg:** C; **CIs:** Hypersensitivity; **ADRs:** ↑ LFTs, N/V, renal failure, <u>rash</u> (<u>discontinue at first sign of rash</u>), bone marrow depression, hypersensitivity reactions; **Interactions:** ↑ levels of mercaptopurine and azathioprine (↓ doses of both of these drugs), ↑ risk of rash with ampicillin or amoxicillin, ↑ effects/levels of warfarin and cyclosporine, ↑ risk of hypersensitivity reactions with thiazides or ACEIs, ↓ effects with alcohol; **Dose:** *PO: Adults and Peds:* >10 yr *Gout*—100 mg/day initially, then ↑ weekly based on uric acid levels (max: 800 mg/day) (if >300 mg/day, give in divided doses). *Secondary* *hyperuricemia*—600–800 mg/day in 2–3 divided doses given 1–2 days before chemotherapy or radiation; *PO: Peds:* 6–10 yr *Secondary hyperuricemia*—300 mg/day in 2–3 divided doses given 1–2 days before chemotherapy or radiation; *PO: Peds:* <6 yr *Secondary hyperuricemia*—150 mg/day in 3 divided doses given 1–2 days before chemotherapy or radiation; *IV: Adults and Peds:* >10 yr *Secondary hyperuricemia*—200–400 mg/m²/day (max: 600 mg/day) in divided doses q 6–24 hr given 1–2 days before chemotherapy or radiation; *IV: Peds:* <10 yr *Secondary hyperuricemia*—200 mg/m²/day initially in divided doses q 6–24 hr given 1–2 days before chemotherapy or radiation; *Renal Impairment: Adults and Peds:* ↓ dose if CrCl <50 ml/min; **Availability (G):** Tabs: 100, 300 mg; Inject: 500 mg; **Monitor:** I/Os, BUN/SCr, CBC, uric acid, LFTs, rash, joint pain/swelling; **Notes:** Ensure adequate fluid intake (≥2500–3000 ml/day) to ↓ risk of kidney stones. May need to start colchicine or NSAIDs for acute attacks (continue for 3–6 mo of therapy).

almotriptan (Axert) **Uses:** Acute treatment of migraines; **Class:** 5-HT$_1$ agonists; **Preg:** C; **CIs:** Hypersensitivity, CAD or significant CV disease, Uncontrolled HTN, Use of other 5-HT$_1$ agonists or ergot-type drugs (dihydroergotamine) within 24 hr, Basilar or hemiplegic migraine, Concurrent or recent (within 2 wk) use of MAOI, CV risk factors (use only if CV status has been determined to be safe and first dose is administered under supervision); **ADRs:** CORONARY ARTERY VASOSPASM, MI/ISCHEMIA, VT/VF, nausea; **Interactions:** MAOI ↑ levels (concurrent or recent [within 2 wk] use contraindicated), Use with other 5-HT$_1$ agonists or ergot-type compounds may ↑ risk of vasospasm (avoid use within 24 hr of each other), Use with SSRIs or SNRIs may ↑ risk of serotonin syndrome, Potent CYP3A4 inhibitors may ↑ levels; **Dose:** *PO: Adults:* 6.25–12.5 mg initially, may repeat in 2 hr (max: 2 doses in 24 hr); *Hepatic/Renal Impairment: PO: Adults:* 6.25 mg initially, may repeat in 2 hr; (max: 2 doses in 24 hr); **Availability:** Tabs: 6.25, 12.5 mg; **Monitor:** Pain/associated symptoms, **Notes:** Only aborts migraines (should not be used for prophylaxis). Administer as soon as migraine symptoms occur.

alprazolam (Niravam, Xanax, Xanax XR) **Uses:** Anxiety disorders, Panic disorder, Anxiety associated with depression; **Class:** benzodiazepines; **Preg:** D; **CIs:** Hypersensitivity (cross-sensitivity with other BZs may exist), Acute narrow-angle glaucoma, Pregnancy/lactation, Concurrent use of itraconazole or ketoconazole; **ADRs:** <u>dizziness</u>, <u>drowsiness</u>, <u>lethargy</u>, confusion, depression, blurred vision, constipation, N/V/D, ↑ wt, physical/psychological dependence, tolerance; **Interactions:** Use with alcohol, antidepressants, other BZs, antihistamines, and opioids ↑ CNS depression, CYP3A4 inhibitors may ↑ levels, CYP3A4 inducers may ↓ levels, Cigarette smoking ↓ levels; **Dose:** *PO: Adults: Anxiety disorders*—0.25–0.5 mg bid or tid (max: 4 mg/day). *Panic disorder*—0.5 mg tid; may ↑ by ≤1 mg/day q 3–4 days prn (max: 10 mg/day); ER tabs: 0.5–1 mg daily in AM; may ↑ by ≤1 mg/day q 3–4 days (usual dose); *PO: Geri:*

A

↓ starting dose; *PO: Hepatic Impairment: Adults:* ↓ starting dose; **Availability (G):** Tabs: 0.25, 0.5, 1, 2 mg; ER tabs: 0.5, 1, 2, 3 mg; Orally disintegrating tabs: 0.25, 0.5, 1, 2 mg; Oral soln: 1 mg/ml; **Monitor:** Mental status, ADRs; **Notes:** Flumazenil is antidote. When discontinuing, ↓ dose by 0.5 mg/day q 3 days to prevent withdrawal. Do not chew, crush, or break ER tabs. Schedule IV controlled substance.

alteplase (Activase, Cathflo Activase, t-PA) Uses: Acute MI, Acute ischemic stroke (within 3 hr of symptom onset), PE, Occluded central venous access devices; **Class:** plasminogen activators; **Preg:** C; **CIs:** Hypersensitivity, Active bleeding, History of CVA, Recent (within 2 mo) intracranial or intraspinal injury/trauma, Intracranial neoplasm, AVM, or aneurysm, Severe uncontrolled HTN, Recent (within 10 days) major surgery, trauma, or GI/GU bleeding, Concurrent anticoagulant therapy, Thrombocytopenia; **ADRs:** INTRACRANIAL HEMORRHAGE, BLEEDING, reperfusion arrhythmias, ALLERGIC REACTIONS INCLUDING ANAPHYLAXIS; **Interactions:** Aspirin, clopidogrel, ticlopidine, dipyridamole, NSAIDs, GP IIb/IIIa inhibitors, warfarin, heparin, and LMWHs ↑ risk of bleeding; **Dose:** *IV: Adults: MI*—15-mg bolus, then 0.75 mg/kg (up to 50 mg) over 30 min, then 0.5 mg/kg (up to 35 mg) over next 60 min (usually given with heparin). *Acute ischemic stroke*—0.9 mg/kg (not to exceed 90 mg) given over 1 hr, with 10% of dose given as bolus over 1 min. *PE*—100 mg over 2 hr (follow with heparin); *IV: Adults and Peds: Catheter clearance*— <30 kg: 110% of the lumen volume (not to exceed 2 mg/2 ml) instilled into occluded catheter; if unsuccessful after 2 hr, may repeat × 1; ≥30 kg: 2 mg/2 ml instilled into occluded catheter; if unsuccessful after 2 hr, may repeat × 1; **Availability:** Inject: 2, 50, 100 mg; **Monitor:** BP, HR, RR, ECG, cardiac enzymes, CBC, aPTT, INR, CP, bleeding, neurologic status; **Notes:** If local bleeding occurs, apply pressure to site. If severe or internal bleeding occurs, discontinue infusion. For stroke, must be administered within 3 hr of symptom onset. For catheter clearance, after 30 min dwell time, attempt to aspirate blood; if catheter remains occluded, allow 120 min dwell time; once catheter function restored, aspirate 4–5 ml of blood to remove alteplase and residual clot, then irrigate catheter with NS.

aluminum hydroxide (AlternaGel, Alu-Cap, Alu-Tab, Amphojel, Basalgel) Uses: Hyperphosphatemia, Adjunctive therapy for PUD or indigestion; **Class:** antacids, PO_4 binders; **Preg:** C; **CIs:** Hypersensitivity, Hypophosphatemia; **ADRs:** constipation, hypophosphatemia; **Interactions:** ↓ absorption of tetracyclines, iron salts, isoniazid, and FQs; **Dose:** *PO: Adults: Hyperphosphatemia*—300–600 mg tid with meals; titrate to normal serum PO_4 levels. *PUD*—600–1200 mg after meals and at bedtime; *PO: Peds: Hyperphosphatemia*—50–150 mg/kg/day in 4–6 divided doses; titrate to normal serum PO_4 levels; **Availability (G):** Caps: 475, 500 mg; Tabs: 300, 500, 600 mg; Oral susp: 320 mg/5 ml[OTC], 450 mg/5 ml[OTC], 600 mg/5 ml[OTC], 675 mg/5 ml[OTC]; **Monitor:** PO_4, Ca++,

S/S indigestion/PUD; **Notes:** Separate administration from oral medications by ≥1–2 hr. Chew tabs. Drink glass of water after each dose.

amantadine (Symmetrel) **Uses:** Parkinson's disease, Drug-induced extrapyramidal reactions; **Class:** dopamine agonists; **Preg:** C; **CIs:** Hypersensitivity, Angle-closure glaucoma; **ADRs:** dizziness, insomnia, anxiety, ataxia, confusion, depression, drowsiness, HA, nausea, anorexia, constipation, dry mouth, edema, HF, orthostatic hypotension, urinary retention, livedo reticularis; **Interactions:** Antihistamines, **phenothiazines**, and **TCAs** may ↑ anticholinergic effects; **Dose:** *PO: Adults:* 100 mg daily or bid (up to 400 mg/day); *Renal Impairment: PO: Adults:* ↓ dose if CrCl ≤50 ml/min; **Availability (G):** Caps: 100 mg; Tabs: 100 mg; Oral syrup: 50 mg/5 ml; **Monitor:** BP (sitting and standing), mental status, S/S HF, livedo reticularis (red mottling), Parkinson's symptoms, BUN/SCr; **Notes:** No longer recommended for treatment/prophylaxis of influenza A. Abrupt discontinuation can cause parkinsonian crisis (must taper).

amifostine (Ethyol) **Uses:** ↓ renal toxicity from cisplatin in advanced ovarian CA, ↓ moderate to severe xerostomia from postoperative radiation for head and neck CA where radiation port includes large portion of parotid glands; **Class:** Chemoprotectants; **Preg:** C; **CIs:** Hypersensitivity, Hypotension or dehydration, Lactation; **ADRs:** dizziness, somnolence, sneezing, ↓ BP, hiccups, N/V, flushing, hypocalcemia, ANAPHYLAXIS, SJS, TEN, ERYTHEMA MULTIFORME, EXFOLIATIVE DERMATITIS (↑ WHEN USED AS RADIOPROTECTANT), chills; **Interactions:** Antihypertensives ↑ risk of hypotension (discontinue 24 hr before treatment); **Dose:** *IV: Adults: Chemoprotectant*—910 mg/m² once daily, as a 15-min infusion, given 30 min before chemotherapy; if poorly tolerated, ↓ subsequent doses to 740 mg/m². *Radioprotectant*—200 mg/m² once daily, as a 3-min infusion, given 15–30 min before radiation therapy; **Availability:** Inject: 500 mg; **Monitor:** BP, HR, S/S anaphylaxis, dry mouth/mouth sores, Ca++; **Notes:** Correct dehydration prior to therapy. Keep in supine position during infusion. If significant ↓ BP occurs, place patient in Trendelenburg position and administer NS using separate IV line. If BP returns to normal in 5 min and patient is asymptomatic, resume infusion. Administer antiemetics before and during therapy.

amikacin (Amikin) **Uses:** Treatment of serious infections due to Gram (−) organisms (e.g., *P. aeruginosa, E. coli, Serratia, Acinetobacter*); MAC infection; **Class:** aminoglycosides; **Preg:** D; **CIs:** Hypersensitivity to aminoglycosides; **ADRs:** vertigo, ototoxicity (vestibular and cochlear), nephrotoxicity; **Interactions:** May ↑ effects of neuromuscular blockers, ↑ risk of ototoxicity with **loop diuretics**, ↑ risk of nephrotoxicity with other nephrotoxic drugs (e.g., amphotericin, vancomycin, acyclovir, cisplatin); **Dose:** *IM: IV: Adults and Peds:* 15–22.5 mg/kg/day in 1–3 divided doses (max: 1.5 g/day). *MAC infection*—10–15 mg/kg once daily; *IM: IV: Neonates: LD*—10 mg/kg. *MD*—7.5 mg/kg q 12 hr; *Renal*

Impairment: IM: IV: Adults: CrCl <60 ml/min—↓ frequency of administration or dose by levels; **Availability (G):** Inject: 50 mg/ml, 250 mg/ml; **Monitor:** HR, BP, temp, sputum, U/A, CBC, BUN/SCr, I/O's, hearing; **Notes:** Use cautiously in renal dysfunction. Monitor blood levels (traditional dosing: peak 10–20 mcg/ml; trough <10 mcg/ml; q 24 hr dosing: trough <4 mcg/ml). Keep patient well hydrated, if possible.

amiloride (Midamor) Uses: Counteracts K+ loss caused by other diuretics in HTN or HF; **Class:** potassium sparing diuretics; **Preg:** B; **CIs:** Hypersensitivity, Hyperkalemia, Concurrent use of K+ supplements or other K+ sparing agents, DM, Renal insufficiency; **ADRs:** dizziness, HA, N/V/D, ↑ K+, muscle cramps; **Interactions:** ↑ risk of hyperkalemia with ACEIs, ARBs, K+ supplements, K+ salt substitutes, NSAIDs, cyclosporine, and tacrolimus, ↑ lithium levels, NSAIDs may ↓ effectiveness; **Dose:** *PO: Adults:* 5–20 mg/day; **Availability (G):** Tabs: 5 mg; **Monitor:** BP, K+, BUN/SCr, weight, I/Os, ECG; **Notes:** Give with food or milk to ↓ GI effects.

aminophylline (Truphylline) Uses: Bronchodilator in Reversible airway obstruction caused by asthma or COPD, ↑ diaphragmatic contractility; **Class:** xanthines; **Preg:** C; **CIs:** Hypersensitivity to aminophylline or theophylline, Cardiac arrhythmias; **ADRs:** SEIZURES, anxiety, HA, insomnia, irritability, ARRHYTHMIAS, ↑ HR, angina, N/V, anorexia, tremor; **Interactions:** Additive CV and CNS side effects with adrenergics (sympathomimetic), CYP1A2 inhibitors and CYP3A4 inhibitors may ↑ levels/toxicity, CYP1A2 inducers and CYP3A4 inducers may ↓ levels/effects; **Dose: All doses expressed as aminophylline (not theophylline)** *PO: Adults and Peds:* See theophylline monograph for oral doses; *IV: Adults:* 6 mg/kg LD, then continuous infusion at the following doses: *Non-smokers*—0.7 mg/kg/hr; *Smokers*—0.9 mg/kg/hr; *Elderly or cor pulmonale*—0.6 mg/kg/hr; *HF or liver failure*—0.5 mg/kg/hr; *IV: Peds:* 6 mg/kg LD, then continuous infusion at the following doses: *12–16 yr*—0.7 mg/kg/hr; *9–12 yr*—0.9 mg/kg/hr; *1–9 yr*—1–1.2 mg/kg/hr; *6 mo-1 yr*—0.6–0.7 mg/kg/hr; *6 wk–6 mo*—0.5 mg/kg/hr; **Availability (G):** Tabs: 100, 200 mg; Inject: 25 mg/ml; **Monitor:** BP, HR, RR, ECG, lung sounds, CP, PFTs, ABGs, theophylline level; **Notes:** Peak levels should be evaluated 30 min after an IV LD, 12–24 hr after initiation of a continuous infusion and 1–2 hr after oral forms. Therapeutic levels: 10–15 mcg/ml (asthma); 6–13 mcg/ml (neonatal apnea). ↑ risk of toxicity with levels > 20 mcg/ml. Tachycardia, arrhythmias, or seizures may be first sign of toxicity.

amiodarone (Cordarone, Pacerone) Uses: Atrial or ventricular arrhythmias; **Class:** antiarrhythmics; **Preg:** D; **CIs:** Hypersensitivity to amiodarone or iodine, Cardiogenic shock, Severe sinus node dysfunction or ≥2nd-degree AV block (in absence of pacemaker), Lactation; **ADRs:** insomnia, corneal microdeposits, optic neuritis/neuropathy, PULMONARY

TOXICITY (PULMONARY FIBROSIS, PNEUMONITIS), QT prolongation, TORSADES DE POINTES, ↓ HR, ↓ BP, ↑ LFTs, anorexia, constipation, N/V, abdominal pain, photosensitivity, blue-gray discoloration, hypothyroidism, hyperthyroidism, ataxia, paresthesia, peripheral neuropathy, tremor; **Interactions:** ↑ risk of QT prolongation with FQs, macrolides, and azole antifungals (use with caution), ↑ digoxin levels (↓ digoxin dose by 50%), May ↑ levels of CYP2C9, CYP2D6, or CYP3A4 substrates, CYP3A4 inhibitors may ↑ levels, CYP3A4 inducers may ↓ levels, ↑ risk of myopathy from simvastatin or lovastatin, May ↑ levels of quinidine, mexiletine, lidocaine, flecainide, and propafenone (use concomitant antiarrhythmics with extreme caution), ↑ levels of cyclosporine and phenytoin (closely monitor levels), ↑ effects of warfarin (↓ warfarin dose by 30%), ↑ risk of AV block with beta blockers, diltiazem, and verapamil; **Dose:** *PO: Adults: Ventricular arrhythmias*—800–1600 mg/day in 1–2 doses × 1–3 wk, then 600–800 mg/day in 1–2 doses × 1 mo, then 400 mg/day. *AF*—800–1200 mg/day in 1–2 doses until 10 g total dose achieved, then ↓ to 200 mg/day; *IV: Adults: Stable VT (with pulse)*—150 mg over 10 min, followed by continuous infusion administered as 1 mg/min × 6 hr, then 0.5 mg/min × 18 hr; *Pulseless VF/VT*—300 mg IV push, may repeat with 150 mg after 3–5 min; once stable rhythm achieved, initiate continuous infusion at 1 mg/min × 6 hr, then 0.5 mg/min; *PO: Peds:* 10–20 mg/kg/day in 1–2 doses × 10 days or until response or ADR occurs, then 5 mg/kg/day for several wk, then ↓ to 2.5 mg/kg/day; *IV:* **Intraosseous:** *Peds and Infants: Pulseless VF/VT*—5 mg/kg (max: 300 mg/dose) as bolus, may repeat up to max daily dose of 15 mg/kg; *Stable VT (with pulse)*—5 mg/kg over 20–60 min; may repeat up to max daily dose of 15 mg/kg; **Availability (G):** Tabs: 200, 400 mg; Inject: 50 mg/ml; **Monitor:** BP, HR, RR, ECG, LFTs, TFTs, CXR, PFTs, ophth exam, S/S pulmonary toxicity (cough, dyspnea, ↓ breath sounds), neuro exam; **Notes:** If BP ↓ with infusion, slow rate. Titrate to lowest possible PO MD to ↓ ADRs. If neurotoxicity or ↑ LFTs, may ↓ dose. If pulmonary toxicity or visual disturbances occur, must discontinue. If hypo-/hyperthyroidism occur, treat the thyroid disorder. PO doses > 200 mg/day should be given in 2–3 divided doses (to ↓ GI effects). IV concentrations >2 mg/ml must be administered through central line. Patient should be told to wear sunscreen.

amitriptyline (Elavil) **Uses:** Depression; **Class:** tricyclic antidepressants; **Preg:** C; **CIs:** Hypersensitivity, Concurrent use with MAOIs, Post-MI, May ↑ risk of suicidal thoughts/behaviors esp. during early treatment or dose adjustment; risk may be ↑ in children or adolescents, Children ≤12 yr; **ADRs:** confusion, lethargy, sedation, blurred vision, dry mouth, ARRHYTHMIAS, ↓ BP, constipation, hepatitis, ↑ appetite, ↑ wt, urinary retention, ↓ libido, gynecomastia, blood dyscrasias, SUICIDAL THOUGHTS; **Interactions:** CYP2D6 inhibitors (e.g., phenothiazines, quinidine, cimetidine, and class Ic antiarrhythmics) may ↑ levels, ↑ risk of hypertensive crises, seizures, or death with MAOIs

A

(discontinue for ≥2 wk), ↑ risk of toxicity with SSRIs (discontinue fluoxetine for ≥5 wk), ↑ risk of arrhythmias with other drugs that prolong QT interval, ↑ CNS depression with other CNS depressants including alcohol, antihistamines, opioids, and sedative/hypnotics, ↑ risk of anticholinergic effects with other anticholinergic agents; **Dose:** *PO: Adults:* 75 mg/day in divided doses; may be ↑ up to 300 mg/day *or* 50–100 mg at bedtime, may ↑ by 25–50 mg/day up to 300 mg at bedtime; *PO: Geri and Adolescents:* 10 mg tid and 20 mg/day at bedtime *or* 25 mg at bedtime initially, slowly ↑ to 100 mg/day as a single bedtime dose or in divided doses; **Availability (G):** Tabs: 10, 25, 50, 75, 100, 150 mg; **Monitor:** BP, HR, ECG, mental status, suicidal thoughts/behaviors; **Notes:** May take 4–6 wk to see effect. May give entire dose at bedtime. Taper gradually to avoid withdrawal. Use with caution in elderly (↑ risk of sedation and anticholinergic effects).

amlodipine (Norvasc) Uses: HTN, Chronic stable angina, Vasospastic (Prinzmetal's) angina, Angiographically documented CAD (in patients without HF); **Class:** Ca channel blockers; **Preg:** C; **CIs:** Hypersensitivity; **ADRs:** HA, dizziness, peripheral edema, ↓ BP, ↑ HR, gingival hyperplasia, flushing; **Interactions:** NSAIDs may ↓ effectiveness, ↑ effects with other antihypertensives, CYP3A4 inhibitors may ↑ levels, CYP3A4 inducers may ↓ levels; **Dose:** *PO: Adults:* 2.5–10 mg/day; *PO: Peds:* ≥6 yr 2.5–5 mg/day; *Hepatic Impairment: PO: Adults: HTN*—Initiate at 2.5 mg/day, may ↑ up to 10 mg/day as needed. *Angina*—Initiate at 5 mg/day, may ↑ up to 10 mg/day as needed; **Availability (G):** Tabs: 2.5, 5, 10 mg; **Monitor:** BP, HR, ECG, peripheral edema, S/S angina; **Notes:** Avoid grapefruit juice (may ↑ effects).

amoxicillin (Amoxil) Uses: Respiratory tract infections, OM, or GU infections due to susceptible organisms (e.g., *S. pneumo, S. aureus, E. coli, H. flu, P. mirabilis*), IE prophylaxis, *H. pylori*; **Class:** aminopenicillins; **Preg:** B; **CIs:** Hypersensitivity (cross-sensitivity to other beta-lactam antibiotics may exist); **ADRs:** SEIZURES (HIGH DOSES), HA, PSEUDOMEMBRANOUS COLITIS, diarrhea, N/V, ↑ LFTs, rash, urticaria, pruritis, ANAPHYLAXIS, SERUM SICKNESS; **Interactions:** Probenecid ↓ excretion and ↑ levels, ↑ risk of rash with allopurinal; **Dose:** *PO: Adults:* 250–500 mg q 8 hr *or* 500–875 mg q 12 hr. *H. pylori*—1000 mg bid with ≥1 other antibiotic and either PPI or H_2 antagonist. *IE prophylaxis*—2 g 30–60 min before procedure; *PO: Peds:* >3 mo 20–50 mg/kg/day divided q 8 hr *or* 25–50 mg/kg/day divided q 12 hr; *Acute OM due to highly resistant S. pneumo*—80–90 mg/kg/day divided q 12 hr; *PO: Infants:* ≤3 mo and Neonates 20–30 mg/kg/day divided q 12 hr. *IE prophylaxis*—50 mg/kg 1 hr before procedure (max: 2 g/dose); *Renal Impairment: PO: Adults:* ↓ dose if CrCl ≤30 ml/min; **Availability (G):** Chew tabs: 125, 200, 250, 400 mg; Tabs: 500, 875 mg; Caps: 250, 500 mg; Oral drops: 50 mg/ml; Oral susp: 125 mg/5 ml, 200 mg/5 ml, 250 mg/5 ml, 400 mg/5 ml; **Monitor:** HR, BP, temp, sputum, U/A, CBC, LFTs, BUN/SCr; **Notes:** Use with caution in patients with beta-lactam allergy (do not use if history of anaphylaxis or hives). Refrigerate susp.

amoxicillin/clavulanate (Amoclan, Augmentin, Augmentin ES-600, Augmentin XR) **Uses:** Respiratory tract infections, OM, sinusitis, skin/skin structure infections, or urinary tract infections due to susceptible organisms (e.g., *S. pneumo*, *S. aureus*, *M. catarrhalis*, *H. flu*, *E. coli*, *Klebsiella*, *Enterobacter*); **Class:** aminopenicillins/beta lactamase inhibitors; **Preg:** B; **CIs:** Hypersensitivity (cross-sensitivity to other beta-lactam antibiotics may exist), History of amoxicillin/clavulanate-associated cholestatic jaundice or liver dysfunction; **ADRs:** SEIZURES (HIGH DOSES), HA, PSEUDOMEMBRANOUS COLITIS, diarrhea, N/V, ↑ LFTs, rash, urticaria, pruritis, ANAPHYLAXIS, SERUM SICKNESS; **Interactions:** Probenecid ↓ excretion and ↑ levels, ↑ risk of rash with allopurinol; **Dose:** *PO: Adults and Peds:* >40 kg 250 mg q 8 hr or 500 mg q 12 hr. *Severe infections or respiratory tract infections*—875 mg q 12 hr or 500 mg q 8 hr. *Acute bacterial sinusitis or CAP*—2000 mg ER tabs q 12 hr; *PO: Peds:* ≥3 mo and <40 kg 200 mg/5 ml or 400 mg/5 ml susp: 25–45 mg/kg/day divided q 12 hr; 125 mg/5 ml or 250 mg/5 ml susp: 20–40 mg/kg/day divided q 8 hr. *OM*—90 mg/kg/day divided q 12 hr (as ES formulation); *PO: Peds:* <3 mo 15 mg/kg q 12 hr (as 125 mg/ml susp); *Renal Impairment: PO: Adults:* ↓ dose if CrCl ≤30 ml/min; **Availability (G):** Tabs: 250 mg amoxicillin + 125 mg clavulanate, 500 mg amoxicillin + 125 mg clavulanate, 875 mg amoxicillin + 125 mg clavulanate; Chew tabs: 125 mg amoxicillin + 31.25 mg clavulanate, 200 mg amoxicillin + 28.5 mg clavulanate, 250 mg amoxicillin + 62.5 mg clavulanate, 400 mg amoxicillin + 57 mg clavulanate; ER tabs: 1000 mg amoxicillin + 62.5 mg clavulanate; Oral susp: 125 mg amoxicillin + 31.25 mg clavulanate/5 ml, 200 mg amoxicillin + 28.5 mg clavulanate/5 ml, 250 mg amoxicillin + 62.5 mg clavulanate/5 ml, 400 mg amoxicillin + 57 mg clavulanate/5 ml, 600 mg amoxicillin + 42.9 mg clavulanate/5 ml (ES formulation); **Monitor:** HR, BP, temp, sputum, U/A, CBC, LFTs, BUN/SCr; **Notes:** Refrigerate susp. Take with meals. Two 250-mg tabs are not bioequivalent to one 500-mg tab; 250-mg tabs and 250-mg chewable tabs are not interchangeable. Two 500-mg tabs are not interchangeable with one 1000-mg XR tab. ES susp is not interchangeable with other susps. Do not administer 250-mg chewable tabs to children <40 kg due to clavulanate content. Children <3 months should receive 125-mg/5-ml oral susp. Use with caution in patients with beta-lactam allergy (do not use if history of anaphylaxis or hives).

amphetamine mixtures (Adderall, Adderall XR) **Uses:** Narcolepsy, ADHD; **Class:** stimulants; **Preg:** C; **CIs:** Hypersensitivity, Hyperthyroidism, Current or recent (within 2 wk) use of MAOIs, Glaucoma, Serious CV disease or structural heart disease (may ↑ risk of sudden death), History of substance abuse (misuse may result in serious CV events/sudden death), HTN; **ADRs:** HA, hyperactivity, insomnia, restlessness, tremor, agitation, anxiety, dizziness, irritability, SUDDEN DEATH, ↑ BP, palpitations, ↑ HR, anorexia, dry mouth, constipation, diarrhea, N/V, ↓ wt, ED, ↓ libido, urticaria, growth inhibition (with long-term use in children), psychological dependence, tolerance; **Interactions:** ↑ risk of hypertensive crisis with MAOIs or meperidine, May ↓ effects of antihistamines and antihypertensives, Haloperidol and lithium may ↓ effects, ↑ adrenergic effects with other adrenergics or thyroid preparations, Alkalinizing agents (e.g., sodium bicarbonate, acetazolamide, antacids) ↓ excretion and ↑ effects, Acidifying agents (e.g., ammonium chloride, large doses of ascorbic acid) ↑ excretion and ↓ effects, ↑ risk of CV effects with TCAs; **Dose:** *PO: Adults: ADHD*—IR: 5 mg 1–2 times daily; ↑ by 5 mg/day at weekly intervals until optimal response (max: 40 mg/day). ER: 20 mg daily; *PO: Adults and Peds:* >12 yr *Narcolepsy*—10 mg daily initially; ↑ by 10 mg/day at weekly intervals until optimal response (max: 60 mg/day in 1–3 divided doses); *PO: Peds:* 6–12 yr *Narcolepsy*—5 mg daily; ↑ by 5 mg/day at weekly intervals until optimal response (max: 60 mg/day in 1–3 divided doses); *PO: Peds:* ≥6 yr *ADHD*—IR: 5 mg 1–2 times daily; ↑ by 5 mg/day at weekly intervals until optimal response (max: 40 mg/day). ER (for 6–12 yr): 10 mg daily; ↑ by 5–10 mg/day at weekly intervals (max: 30 mg/day). ER (for 13–17 yr): 10 mg daily; ↑ to 20 mg daily after 1 wk if adequate response not achieved; *PO: Peds:* 3–5 yr *ADHD*—IR: 2.5 mg daily in the AM; ↑ by 2.5 mg/day at weekly intervals until optimal response (max: 40 mg/day); **Availability (G):** Tabs: 5, 7.5, 10, 12.5, 15, 20, 30 mg; ER caps: 5, 10, 15, 20, 25, 30 mg; **Monitor:** BP, HR, ECG, mental status, ht/wt; **Notes:** Schedule II controlled substance. For IR tabs, give first dose upon awakening, and then subsequent doses at 4–6 hr intervals. Take last dose ≥6 hr before bedtime to minimize insomnia. If switching from IR to ER, give same total daily dose once daily. All children should have CV assessment prior to initiation. Potential for dependence/abuse with long-term use. ER caps may be swallowed whole or opened and sprinkled on applesauce.

amphotericin B cholesteryl sulfate (Amphotec) Uses: Severe fungal infections in patients who are intolerant (e.g., renal dysfunction) or refractory to amphotericin B desoxycholate; **Class:** antifungals; **Preg:** B; **CIs:** Hypersensitivity, Lactation; **ADRs:** HA, insomnia, ↓ BP, N/V/D, ↑ LFTs, NEPHROTOXICITY, ↓ K+, ↓ Mg++, anemia, pruritis, rash, phlebitis, arthralgia, myalgia, HYPERSENSITIVITY REACTIONS, chills, fever, infusion reactions; **Interactions:** ↑ risk of hypokalemia with corticosteroids, loop diuretics, or thiazide diuretics, ↑ risk of nephrotoxicity with other nephrotoxic agents such as aminoglycosides, cyclosporine, or tacrolimus; **Dose:** *IV: Adults and Peds:* 3–4 mg/kg daily (max: 7.5 mg/kg/day) (no test dose needed); **Availability:** Inject: 50, 100 mg; **Monitor:** BP, HR, temp, sputum, U/A, CBC, BUN/SCr, electrolytes, LFTs, infusion reaction; **Notes:** Premedicate with acetaminophen/NSAIDs, corticosteroids, and/or antihistamines 30–60 min before infusion to ↓ infusion reaction. Meperidine can be used to treat rigors. Lower incidence of nephrotoxicity compared to conventional amphotericin B (desoxycholate).

amphotericin B desoxycholate (No Trade) **Uses:** Severe fungal infections; **Class:** antifungals; **Preg:** B; **CIs:** Hypersensitivity, Lactation; **ADRs:** HA, insomnia, ↓ BP, N/V/D, ↑ LFTs, NEPHROTOXICITY, ↓ K+, ↓ Mg++, anemia, pruritis, rash, phlebitis, arthralgia, myalgia, HYPERSENSITIVITY REACTIONS, chills, fever, infusion reactions; **Interactions:** ↑ risk of hypokalemia with corticosteroids, loop diuretics, or thiazide diuretics, ↑ risk of nephrotoxicity with other nephrotoxic agents such as aminoglycosides, cyclosporine, or tacrolimus; **Dose:** *IV: Adults:* Test dose of 1 mg. If tolerated, give 0.25 mg/kg/day (up to 1.5 mg/kg/day may be used, depending on type of infection); *Bladder irrigation*—Instill 50 mcg/ml solution into bladder daily × 5–10 days; *IV: Peds and Infants:* Test dose of 0.1 mg/kg (max: 1 mg) or may give initial dose of 0.25–1 mg/kg/day over 6 hr (without test dose) (up to 1.5 mg/kg/day may be used); *IT: Adults:* 25–300 mcg q 48–72 hr; ↑ to 500 mcg–1 mg as tolerated (max total dose: 15 mg); *IT: Peds:* 25–100 mcg q 48–72 hr; ↑ to 500 mcg as tolerated; **Availability (G):** Inject: 50 mg; **Monitor:** BP, HR, temp, sputum, U/A, CBC, BUN/SCr, electrolytes, LFTs, infusion reaction; **Notes:** Premedicate with acetaminophen/NSAIDs, corticosteroids, and/or antihistamines 30–60 min before infusion to ↓ infusion reaction. Meperidine can be used to treat rigors. Adequate hydration and maintaining sodium balance may minimize nephrotoxicity. If BUN/SCr ↑ significantly, may need to discontinue or consider switching to cholesteryl sulfate, lipid complex, or liposomal formulation. IT route used for cryptococcal meningitis.

amphotericin B lipid complex (Abelcet) **Uses:** Severe fungal infections in patients who are intolerant (e.g., renal dysfunction) or refractory to amphotericin B desoxycholate; **Class:** antifungals; **Preg:** B; **CIs:** Hypersensitivity, Lactation; **ADRs:** HA, insomnia, ↓ BP, N/V/D, ↑ LFTs, NEPHROTOXICITY, ↓ K+, ↓ Mg++, anemia, pruritis, rash, phlebitis, arthralgia, myalgia, HYPERSENSITIVITY REACTIONS, chills, fever, infusion reactions; **Interactions:** ↑ risk of hypokalemia with corticosteroids, loop diuretics, or thiazide diuretics, ↑ risk of nephrotoxicity with other nephrotoxic agents such as aminoglycosides, cyclosporine, or tacrolimus; **Dose:** *IV: Adults and Peds:* 2.5–5 mg/kg daily (no test dose needed); **Availability:** Inject: 100 mg; **Monitor:** BP, HR, temp, sputum, U/A, CBC, BUN/SCr, electrolytes, LFTs, infusion reaction; **Notes:** Premedicate with acetaminophen/NSAIDs, corticosteroids, and/or antihistamines 30–60 min before infusion to ↓ infusion reaction. Meperidine can be used to treat rigors. Lower incidence of nephrotoxicity and infusion reactions compared to conventional amphotericin B (desoxycholate).

A

amphotericin B liposome (AmBisome) **Uses:** Severe fungal infections in patients who are intolerant (e.g., renal dysfunction) or refractory to amphotericin B desoxycholate, Suspected fungal infections in febrile neutropenic patients, Visceral leishmaniasis, Cryptococcal meningitis in HIV patients; **Class:** antifungals; **Preg:** B; **CIs:** Hypersensitivity, Lactation; **ADRs:** HA, insomnia, ↓ BP, N/V/D, ↑ LFTs, NEPHROTOXICITY, ↓ K+, ↓ Mg++, anemia, pruritis, rash, phlebitis, arthralgia, myalgia, HYPERSENSITIVITY REACTIONS, chills, fever, infusion reactions; **Interactions:** ↑ risk of hypokalemia with corticosteroids, loop diuretics, or thiazide diuretics, ↑ risk of nephrotoxicity with other nephrotoxic agents such as aminoglycosides, cyclosporine, or tacrolimus; **Dose:** *IV: Adults and Peds: Empiric therapy*—3 mg/kg daily; *Documented infections*—3–5 mg/kg daily; *Visceral leishmaniasis (immunocompetent)*—3 mg/kg daily on Days 1–5, then 3 mg/kg daily on Days 14 and 21; *Visceral leishmaniasis (immunosuppressed)*—4 mg/kg daily on Days 1–5, then 4 mg/kg daily on Days 10, 17, 24, 31, and 38; *Cryptococcal meningitis in HIV patients*—6 mg/kg daily; **Availability:** Inject: 50 mg; **Monitor:** BP, HR, temp, sputum, U/A, CBC, BUN/SCr, electrolytes, infusion reaction; **Notes:** No test dose needed. Premedicate with acetaminophen/NSAIDs, corticosteroids, and/or antihistamines 30–60 min before infusion to ↓ infusion reaction. Meperidine can be used to treat rigors. Lower incidence of nephrotoxicity and infusion reactions compared to conventional amphotericin B (desoxycholate).

ampicillin (Omnipen, Principen) **Uses:** Skin/skin structure infections, respiratory tract infections, OM, sinusitis, GU infections, meningitis, or septicemia due to susceptible organisms (e.g., *S. aureus*, *H. flu*, *Listeria*, *Salmonella*, *Shigella*, *E. coli*, *Enterobacter*, *Klebsiella*), IE prophylaxis; **Class:** aminopenicillins; **Preg:** B; **CIs:** Hypersensitivity (cross-sensitivity to other beta-lactams); **ADRs:** SEIZURES (HIGH DOSES), HA, PSEUDOMEMBRANOUS COLITIS, diarrhea, N/V, ↑ LFTs, rash, urticaria, pruritis, pain at IM or IV site, ALLERGIC REACTIONS INCLUDING ANAPHYLAXIS, SERUM SICKNESS; **Interactions:** Probenecid ↓ excretion and ↑ levels, ↑ risk of rash with allopurinol; **Dose:** *PO: Adults and Peds:* ≥ 20 kg 250–500 mg q 6 hr; *PO: Peds:* <20 kg 50–100 mg/kg/day divided q 6 hr (max: 4 g/day); *IM: IV: Adults and Peds:* ≥40 kg 250–500 mg q 6 hr (max: 12 g/day). *IE prophylaxis*—2 g 30–60 min before procedure. *Meningitis*—150–250 mg/kg/day divided q 3–4 hr (max: 12 g/day); *IM: IV: Peds:* <40 kg 100–150 mg/kg/day divided q 6 hr (max: 4 g/day). *IE prophylaxis*—50 mg/kg (not to exceed 2 g) 30–60 min before procedure. *Meningitis*—200–400 mg/kg/day divided q 6 hr (max: 12 g/day); *PO: IM: IV: Adults and Peds:* ↓ dose if CrCl ≤50 ml/min; **Availability (G):** Caps: 250, 500 mg; Oral susp: 125 mg/5 ml, 250 mg/5 ml; Inject: 125, 250, 500 mg, 1, 2, 10 g; **Monitor:** HR, BP, temp, sputum, U/A, CBC, LFTs, BUN/SCr; **Notes:** Give on empty stomach ≥1 hr before or 2 hr after meals with full glass of water. Use with caution in patients with beta-lactam allergy (do not use if history of anaphylaxis or hives).

ampicillin/sulbactam (Unasyn) **Uses:** Skin/skin structure infections, intra-abdominal infections, or gynecological infections due to susceptible organisms (e.g., *S. aureus*, *E. coli*, *Klebsiella*, *P. mirabilis*, *Enterobacter*, *B. fragilis*); **Class:** aminopenicillins/beta lactamase inhibitors; **Preg:** B; **CIs:** Hypersensitivity (cross-sensitivity to other beta-lactam antibiotics may exist); **ADRs:** SEIZURES (HIGH DOSES), HA, PSEUDOMEMBRANOUS COLITIS, diarrhea, N/V, ↑ LFTs, rash, urticaria, pruritis, pain at IM or IV site, ANAPHYLAXIS, SERUM SICKNESS; **Interactions:** Probenecid ↓ excretion and ↑ levels, ↑ risk of rash with allopurinol; **Dose:** **Dose expressed as ampicillin/sulbactam** *IM: IV: Adults and Peds:* ≥40 kg 1.5–3 g q 6 hr; *IM: IV: Peds:* ≥1 yr 75 mg/kg q 6 hr (max: 12 g/day); *Renal Impairment: IM: IV: Adults and Peds:* ↓ dose if CrCl <30 ml/min; **Availability (G):** Inject: 1.5 g (1 g ampicillin + 500 mg sulbactam), 3 g (2 g ampicillin + 1 g sulbactam), 15 g (10 g ampicillin + 5 g sulbactam); **Monitor:** HR, BP, temp, sputum, U/A, CBC, LFTs, BUN/SCr; **Notes:** Use with caution in patients with beta-lactam allergy (do not use if history of anaphylaxis or hives).

anakinra (Kineret) **Uses:** RA (in patients who have failed other DMARDs) (may be used with other DMARDs except for TNF blockers); **Class:** interleukin antagonists; **Preg:** B; **CIs:** Hypersensitivity, Active infection, Concurrent use of TNF blockers (e.g., adalimumab, etanercept, infliximab); **ADRs:** HA, diarrhea, nausea, neutropenia, injection site reactions, INFECTIONS, MALIGNANCY; **Interactions:** ↑ risk of serious infection with TNF blockers, including adalimumab, etanercept, and infliximab (contraindicated). Do not give with live vaccinations; **Dose:** *Subcut: Adults:* 100 mg daily; *Renal Impairment: Subcut: Adults:* ↓ dose if CrCl <30 ml/min; **Availability:** Inject: 100 mg/0.67 ml; **Monitor:** Pain scale, ROM, S/S infection, CBC; **Notes:** Discontinue if serious infection develops. Needle cap of prefilled syringe contains latex.

anastrazole (Arimidex) **Uses:** Postmenopausal hormone receptor—positive early breast CA, Postmenopausal hormone receptor—positive or unknown, locally advanced, or metastatic breast CA, Advanced postmenopausal breast CA with disease progression despite tamoxifen; **Class:** aromatase inhibitors; **Preg:** D; **CIs:** Pregnancy (potential harm to fetus or spontaneous abortion), Premenopausal women; **ADRs:** HA, weakness, dizziness, dyspnea, cough, edema, ↑ BP, nausea, abdominal pain, anorexia, constipation, diarrhea, dry mouth, vomiting, ↑ LFTs, pelvic pain, vaginal bleeding, rash, sweating, ↑ wt, hypercholesterolemia, bone pain, osteoporosis, paresthesia, hot flashes; **Interactions:** Estrogen-containing therapies ↓ effects.; Dose: *PO: Adults:* 1 mg daily; **Availability:** Tabs: 1 mg; **Monitor:** LFTs, lipid panel, BMD; **Notes:** Vaginal bleeding may occur during first few wk after changing over from other hormonal therapy.

A

anidulafungin (Eraxis) Uses: Candidemia and other candidal infections (intra-abdominal abscesses, peritonitis), Esophageal candidiasis; **Class:** echinocandins; **Preg:** C; **CIs:** Hypersensitivity, Children (safety not established); **ADRs:** dyspnea, ↓ BP, diarrhea, ↑ LFTs, flushing, rash, urticaria, ↓ K+; **Interactions:** None noted; **Dose:** *IV: Adults: Esophageal candidiasis*—100 mg on Day 1, then 50 mg daily. *Candidemia and other candidal infections*—200 mg on Day 1, then 100 mg daily; **Availability:** Inject: 50 mg, 100 mg; **Monitor:** HR, BP, temp, sputum, U/A, CBC, LFTs, K+; **Notes:** Administer at a rate ≤ 1.1 mg/min to ↓ infusion reactions.

apomorphine (Apokyn) Uses: Acute, intermittent treatment of hypomotility, "off" episodes due to advanced Parkinson's disease; **Class:** dopamine agonists; **Preg:** C; **CIs:** Hypersensitivity to apomorphine or bisulfites, Concurrent use of 5-HT_3 antagonists (granisetron, ondansetron, palonosetron, alosetron, dolasetron), Lactation, Conditions predisposing to QT prolongation (↑ risk of arrhythmias); **ADRs:** dizziness, hallucinations, somnolence, confusion, rhinorrhea, CP, orthostatic hypotension, HF, edema, QT prolongation, N/V, priapism, flushing, pallor, sweating, injection site pain, dyskinesia, yawning; **Interactions:** ↑ risk of severe ↓ BP and loss of consciousness with 5-HT_3 antagonists (contraindicated), ↑ risk of ↓ BP with alcohol, antihypertensives, or vasodilators, Dopamine antagonists may ↓ effects, ↑ risk of QT prolongation with other QT-prolonging drugs; **Dose:** *Subcut: Adults:* Give test dose of 0.2 mL (2 mg); if tolerates and responds to test dose, start with 0.2 ml (2 mg) prn to treat "off" episodes; may ↑ dose by 0.1 mL (1 mg) every few days as an outpatient. If tolerates, but does not respond to 2 mg test dose, give 0.4 ml (4 mg) at next "off" period but no sooner than 2 hr after initial test dose; if tolerates and responds, start with 0.3 ml (3 mg) prn to treat "off" episodes; may ↑ dose by 0.1 mL (1 mg) every few days as an outpatient. Only single doses should be used during a particular "off" period. If >1 wk passes between doses, titration should be restarted at the 0.2-mL (2-mg) level. Doses should not exceed 0.6 mL (6 mg); **Availability:** Inject: 10 mg/mL; **Monitor:** BP (supine and standing), N/V, drowsiness, S/S Parkinson's; **Notes:** Give trimethobenzamide 300 mg PO tid 3 days before therapy and continue for at least the first 2 mo of therapy (do not use 5-HT_3 antagonists). Prime the pen before every injection and after loading new cartridge. Inject subcut into stomach, upper arm, or upper leg. Store at room temp. Should be dosed in mL (not mg). Should not be used to prevent "off" episodes.

aprepitant (Emend) Uses: Prevention of acute and delayed N/V caused by highly or moderately emetogenic chemotherapy (with other antiemetics), Prevention of postoperative N/V; **Class:** neurokinin antagonists; **Preg:** B; **CIs:** Hypersensitivity, Concurrent use with pimozide; **ADRs:** dizziness, fatigue, HA, weakness, constipation, diarrhea, hiccups; **Interactions:** Inhibits, induces, and is a substrate of CYP3A4; also induces CYP2C9. May ↑ effects/toxicity of other CYP3A4 substrates including docetaxel, paclitaxel, etoposide, irinotecan, ifosfamide, imatinib, vinorelbine, vinblastine, vincristine, and midazolam (use with caution), CYP3A4 inhibitors may ↑ levels/effects, CYP3A4 inducers may ↓ levels/effects, ↑ levels of dexamethasone (regimen below in Dose section reflects 50% dose ↓); similar effect occurs with methylprednisolone (↓ IV dose by 25%, ↓ PO dose by 50%), May ↓ the effects of warfarin, oral contraceptives, and phenytoin; **Dose:** *PO: Adults: Chemotherapy*—125 mg 1 hr before chemo, then 80 mg daily × 2 days (for highly emetogenic chemo, use with dexamethasone 12 mg PO 30 min before chemo, then 8 mg PO daily × 3 days and ondansetron 32 mg IV 30 min before chemo; for moderately emetogenic chemo, use with dexamethasone 12 mg PO 30 min before chemo and ondansetron 8 mg PO 30–60 min before chemo and 8 hr later); *Postoperative*—40 mg within 3 hr before induction of anesthesia; **Availability:** Caps: 40, 80, 125 mg; **Monitor:** N/V, I/Os, INR (for 2 wk after tx in patients on warfarin); **Notes:** Use alternative method of contraception during and for 1 mo after therapy in patients taking oral contraceptives. Should not be used for treatment of N/V. Not to be used chronically.

argatroban (Argatroban) **Uses:** Prophylaxis or treatment of thrombosis in HIT, Anticoagulant in patients with HIT undergoing PCI; **Class:** thrombin inhibitors; **Preg:** B; **CIs:** Major bleeding, Hypersensitivity, Lactation; **ADRs:** ↓ BP, N/V/D, BLEEDING, ANAPHYLAXIS, fever; **Interactions:** ↑ risk of bleeding with antiplatelets, thrombolytics, or other anticoagulants; **Dose:** *IV: Adults: HIT*—2 mcg/kg/min continuous infusion; adjust infusion rate (max: 10 mcg/min) based on aPTT (target: 1.5–3 × baseline). *Patients undergoing PCI*—350 mcg/kg bolus, then 25 mcg/kg/min continuous infusion (monitor ACT 5–10 min after bolus); if ACT 300–450 sec, start PCI; if ACT <300 sec, give bolus of 150 mcg/kg and ↑ infusion rate to 30 mcg/kg/min (monitor ACT 5–10 min after bolus); if ACT >450 sec, ↓ infusion rate to 15 mcg/kg/min and check ACT 5–10 min later. Once therapeutic ACT achieved (300–450 sec), continue at current infusion rate; *Hepatic Impairment: IV: Adults: Moderate hepatic impairment for HIT*—0.5 mcg/kg/min continuous infusion; adjust infusion rate based on aPTT; **Availability:** Inject: 100 mg/ml; **Monitor:** BP, HR, CBC, aPTT (for HIT), ACT (for PCI), INR (if initiating warfarin), bleeding; **Notes:** For HIT, check aPTT 2 hr after starting infusion, and then daily once therapeutic. Start warfarin before discontinuing argatroban (combination causes ↑ INR). If on argatroban 2 mcg/kg/min, discontinue argatroban when INR >4 on combined therapy, and then recheck INR in 4–6 hr; if INR less than goal, resume argatroban until desired INR achieved. If on argatroban >2 mcg/kg/min, ↓ to 2 mcg/kg/min and recheck INR in 4–6 hr; then follow process above. No antidote available.

aripiprazole (Abilify) **Uses:** Schizophrenia, Bipolar disorder, Depression (as adjunct to antidepressants), Agitation associated with

A

schizophrenia or bipolar mania; **Class:** atypical antipsychotics; **Preg:** C; **CIs:** Hypersensitivity, Lactation, Elderly patients with dementia-related psychosis have ↑ mortality risk; **ADRs:** akathisia, anxiety, dizziness, drowsiness, extrapyramidal reactions, HA, insomnia, restlessness, confusion, depression, impaired cognitive function, SEIZURES, SUICIDAL THOUGHTS, tardive dyskinesia, orthostatic hypotension, blurred vision, constipation, N/V, anorexia, dysphagia, ↑ wt, tremor, NMS, ↑ BG; **Interactions:** CYP3A4 inhibitors (e.g., ketoconazole) may ↑ levels (↓ aripiprazole dose by 50%), CYP3A4 inducers (e.g., carbamazepine) may ↓ levels (double aripiprazole dose), CYP2D6 inhibitors (e.g., fluoxetine, paroxetine) may ↑ levels (↓ aripiprazole dose by 50%); **Dose:** *PO: Adults: Schizophrenia*—10–15 mg daily; may ↑ after ≥2 wk to 30 mg daily, if needed. *Bipolar disorder*—15–30 mg daily. *Depression (adjunctive therapy)*—2–5 mg daily; may further ↑ dose in 5-mg increments, if needed (max: 15 mg/day); *PO: Peds:* 13–17 yr. *Schizophrenia*—2 mg daily, then ↑ to 5 mg daily after 2 days, then ↑ to 10 mg daily after 2 days; may further ↑ dose in 5-mg increments, if needed (max: 30 mg/day); *PO: Peds:* 10–17 yr. *Bipolar disorder*—2 mg daily, then ↑ to 5 mg daily after 2 days, then ↑ to 10 mg daily after another 2 days; may further ↑ dose in 5-mg increments, if needed (max: 30 mg/day); *IM: Adults: Agitation*—5.25–9.75 mg as single dose, may repeat dose at ≥2-hr intervals (max: 30 mg/day); if ongoing therapy needed, switch to PO; **Availability:** Tabs: 2, 5, 10, 15, 20, 30 mg; Orally disintegrating tabs: 10, 15 mg; Oral soln: 1 mg/ml; Inject: 7.5 mg/ml; **Monitor:** Mental status, suicidal thoughts/behaviors (esp. in patients with depression), wt, BG, lipids, BP (sitting, standing), EPS, tardive dyskinesia, NMS; **Notes:** If CYP3A4 or CYP2D6 inhibitor is discontinued, ↑ aripiprazole dose; if CYP3A4 inducer is discontinued, ↓ aripiprazole dose. Can use soln instead of tabs (same dose up to 25 mg; if receiving 30 mg in tabs, should receive 25-mg dose of soln).

asparaginase (Elspar) **Uses:** ALL; **Class:** antineoplastics; **Preg:** C; **CIs:** Previous hypersensitivity, Pancreatitis with previous therapy, History of thrombosis or bleeding with previous therapy; **ADRs:** SEIZURES, agitation, coma, confusion, depression, fatigue, hallucinations, somnolence, N/V, anorexia, cramps, ↑ LFTs, ↑ bilirubin, PANCREATITIS, azotemia, rash, urticaria, ↑ BG, THROMBOSIS, bone marrow depression, fever, ANAPHYLAXIS; **Interactions:** May ↓ effects of methotrexate, When given IV, may ↑ toxicity of vincristine and prednisone; **Dose:** *IM: IV: Adults and Peds:* Give intradermal test dose (see below for dose) prior to first dose. 6000 units/m^2 3 ×/week for 6–9 doses; *Intradermal: Adults and Peds: Test dose*—2 units; **Availability:** Inject: 10,000 units; **Monitor:** BP, HR, BUN/SCr, BG, LFTs, bilirubin, CBC (with diff), aPTT, PT/INR; **Notes:** **High Alert:** Fatalities have occurred with chemotherapeutic agents. Before administering, clarify all ambiguous orders; double-check single, daily, and course-of-therapy dose limits; have second practitioner independently double-check original order and dose calculations. Do not confuse asparaginase with pegaspargase. For IM, administer no more than 2 ml per injection site. Observe for 1 hr after test dose for reaction (wheal or erythema).

aspirin (Ascriptin, Aspergum, Aspirtab, Bayer Aspirin, Bufferin, Easprin, Ecotrin, Halfprin, St. Joseph Adult Chewable Aspirin, ZORprin) **Uses:** Inflammatory disorders including RA, OA, and gout, Mild-to-moderate pain, Fever, Primary and secondary prevention of stroke, TIA, and MI; **Class:** salicylates; **Preg:** D; **CIs:** Hypersensitivity to aspirin, other salicylates, or NSAIDs, Bleeding disorders or thrombocytopenia, Children <16 yr with viral infection (may ↑ risk of Reye's syndrome), Pregnancy (may have adverse effects on fetus and mother and should be avoided esp. during 3rd tri); **ADRs:** tinnitus, GI BLEEDING,<u>dyspepsia</u>, HEPATOTOXICITY,<u>N/V</u>, abdominal pain, anorexia, anemia, rash, urticaria, ANAPHYLAXIS, LARYNGEAL EDEMA; **Interactions:** May ↑ risk of bleeding with other antiplatelet drugs, warfarin, heparin, LMWHs, NSAIDs, or thrombolytics, although these agents are frequently used safely in combination, Ibuprofen may negate the cardioprotective effects of low-dose aspirin, ↑ risk of GI irritation with NSAIDs and alcohol, May ↑ methotrexate and valproic acid levels, **Urinary acidification** ↑ reabsorption and may ↑ salicylate levels, **Alkalinization of the urine** or the ingestion of large amounts of **antacids** ↑ excretion and ↓ salicylate levels; **Dose:** *PO: Rect: Adults: Pain/fever*—325–650 mg q 4–6 hr (max: 4 g/day); *Inflammation*—2.4–3.6 g/day in divided doses (usual maintenance: 3.6–5.4 g/day in divided doses); *MI prevention*—75–162 mg/day (may require 325 mg/day for limited period of time in patients with stents) (160–325 mg/day should be used for treatment of MI); *Stroke/TIA prevention*—30–325 mg daily; *PO: Rect: Peds: Pain/fever*—2–11 yr: 10–15 mg/kg q 4–6 hr (max: 4 g/day); *Inflammation*—60–90 mg/kg/day in divided doses (usual maintenance: 80–100 mg/kg/day in divided doses); **Availability (G):** Tabs: 81, 325 mg; Chew tabs: 81 mg; Chewing gum: 227 mg; Buffered tabs: 325, 500 mg; EC tabs: 81, 162, 325, 500, 650, 975 mg; ER tabs: 800 mg; Supp: 300, 600 mg; **Monitor:** Temp, pain, bleeding, S/S hypersensitivity, CBC, LFTs (high-dose); **Notes:** Do not crush or chew EC tabs.Do not take antacids within 1–2 hr of EC tabs. Give non–EC tab if MI suspected (should be chewed). Discard if tabs have vinegar-like odor.

atazanavir (Reyataz) **Uses:** HIV (with other antiretrovirals); **Class:** protease inhibitors; **Preg:** B; **CIs:** Hypersensitivity, Severe hepatic impairment, Concurrent use of ergot derivatives, midazolam, triazolam, pimozide, rifampin, irinotecan, lovastatin, simvastatin, indinavir, nevirapine, or St. John's wort, Infants <3 mo (↑ risk of kernicterus); **ADRs:** HA, insomnia, cough, ↑ PR interval, abdominal pain, ↑ <u>bilirubin</u>, diarrhea, jaundice, ↑ LFTs, N/V, <u>rash</u>, ↑ BG, ↑ cholesterol, nephrolithiasis, fat redistribution, myalgia, fever; **Interactions:** Inhibits the CYP3A and UGT1A1 enzyme systems. It is also a substrate of CYP3A, CYP3A4 inhibitors may

A

↑ levels, CYP3A4 inducers may ↓ levels, May ↑ levels of CYP3A4 substrates, May ↑ levels of UGT1A1 substrates, ↑ levels of ergot derivatives, midazolam, triazolam, pimozide, lovastatin, simvastatin, and irinotecan (contraindicated), Tenofovir and efavirenz ↓ levels (when used together, add ritonavir 100 mg/day and ↓ atazanavir dose), Rifampin, nevirapine, and St. John's wort ↓ levels (contraindicated), ↑ risk of hyperbilirubinemia with indinavir (contraindicated), Didanosine-buffered tabs or antacids may ↓ levels (give atazanavir 2 hr before or 1 hr after these drugs), ↑ saquinavir levels, Ritonavir ↑ levels (↓ atazanavir dose to 300 mg/day), ↑ risk of bleeding with warfarin, ↑ levels of rifabutin; ↓ rifabutin dose by 75%, ↑ levels of CCBs; ↓ diltiazem dose by 50% and monitor ECG, ↑ levels of fluticasone; consider alternative therapy; should not be used when ritonavir also used, ↑ levels of sildenafil, vardenafil, and tadalafil; ↓ dose of these agents, ↑ risk of myopathy with atorvastatin or rosuvastatin, H_2 antagonists and PPIs may ↓ levels (separate doses by at least 10 hr and add ritonavir 100 mg/day) (do not use PPIs in treatment-experienced patients), ↑ levels of clarithromycin; ↓ clarithromycin dose by 50% or consider alternative therapy, May ↓ levels of hormonal contraceptives; use alternative non-hormonal contraceptive; **Dose:** *PO: Adults: Therapy-naive*—300 mg daily with ritonavir 100 mg daily or 400 mg daily if unable to tolerate ritonavir. If on efavirenz, give atazanavir 400 mg daily and ritonavir 100 mg daily with efavirenz 600 mg daily (all as single daily dose). If on tenofovir, give atazanavir 300 mg daily and ritonavir 100 mg daily with tenofovir 300 mg (all as single daily dose). *Therapy-experienced with prior virologic failure*—300 mg daily with ritonavir 100 mg daily; *PO: Peds:* 6–17 yr *Therapy-naive*—15–24 kg: 150 mg daily with ritonavir 80 mg daily. 25–31 kg: 200 mg daily with ritonavir 100 mg daily. 32–38 kg: 250 mg daily with ritonavir 100 mg daily. ≥39 kg: 300 mg daily with ritonavir 100 mg daily. *Therapy-experienced with prior virologic failure*—25–31 kg: 200 mg daily with ritonavir 100 mg daily. 32–38 kg: 250 mg daily with ritonavir 100 mg daily. ≥39 kg: 300 mg daily with ritonavir 100 mg daily; *Renal Impairment: PO: Adults:* If therapy-naive on HD, give 300 mg daily with ritonavir 100 mg daily; *Hepatic Impairment: PO: Adults:* If therapy-naive, ↓ dose to 300 mg daily; **Availability:** Caps: 100, 150, 200, 300 mg; **Monitor:** Viral load, CD4 count, BG, LFTs, bilirubin, lipids, ECG; **Notes:** Not to be used as monotherapy. Use with caution in patients with cardiac conduction disorders. Take with food. Rash can occur within first 8 wk and usually resolves within 2 wk.

atenolol (Tenormin) **Uses:** HTN, Angina/MI; **Class:** beta blockers; **Preg:** D; **CIs:** Hypersensitivity, Decompensated HF, Pulmonary edema, Cardiogenic shock, Bradycardia, ≥2nd-degree AV block (in absence of pacemaker); **ADRs:** <u>fatigue</u>, <u>weakness</u>, depression, dizziness, drowsiness, nightmares, blurred vision, bronchospasm, ↓ HR, HF, PULMONARY EDEMA, ↓ BP, N/V/D, <u>ED</u>, ↓ libido, ↑ BG, ↓ BG; **Interactions:** ↑ risk of bradycardia with digoxin, diltiazem, verapamil, or clonidine, ↑ effects with other antihypertensives, ↑ risk of hypertensive crisis if concurrent clonidine discontinued, May alter the effectiveness of insulins or oral hypoglycemic agents, May ↓ the effects of $beta_1$ agonists (e.g., dopamine or dobutamine); **Dose:** *PO: Adults: Angina/post-MI*—50–200 mg daily. *HTN*—25–100 mg; *Renal Impairment: PO: Adults:* ↓ dose if CrCl ≤35 ml/min; **Availability (G):** Tabs: 25, 50, 100 mg; **Monitor:** HR, BP, ECG, S/S HF, edema, wt, S/S angina, BG (in DM); **Notes:** Abrupt withdrawal may cause life-threatening arrhythmias, hypertensive crises, or myocardial ischemia. May mask S/S of hypoglycemia (esp. tachycardia) in DM.

atomoxetine (Strattera) Uses: ADHD; **Class:** selective norepinephrine reuptake inhibitors; **Preg:** C; **CIs:** Hypersensitivity, Current or recent (within 2 wk) use of MAOIs, Narrow-angle glaucoma, Serious CV disease or structural heart disease (may ↑ risk of sudden death), May ↑ risk of suicidal thoughts/behaviors esp. during early treatment or dose adjustment; risk may be ↑ in children or adolescents; **ADRs:** <u>fatigue</u>, <u>HA</u>, <u>insomnia</u>, irritability, <u>sedation</u>, dizziness, ↑ BP, HEPATOTOXICITY, <u>abdominal pain</u>, <u>constipation</u>, <u>dry mouth</u>, <u>N/V</u>, <u>dysmenorrhea</u>, hot flashes, ↓ <u>libido</u>, <u>ED</u>, urinary retention, ↓ <u>appetite</u>, ↓ wt/growth, ANGIOEDEMA; **Interactions:** Concurrent use with MAOIs may result in serious, potentially fatal reactions (do not use within 2 wk of each other), ↑ risk of CV effects with albuterol or vasopressors (use cautiously), CYP2D6 inhibitors (e.g., quinidine, paroxetine, fluoxetine) may ↑ levels (↓ dose of atomoxetine); **Dose:** *PO: Peds and Adolescents:* <70 kg 0.5 mg/kg/day initially, may be ↑ after ≥3 days to target dose of 1.2 mg/kg/day, given as single dose in AM or in divided doses in AM and late afternoon/early evening (max: 1.4 mg/kg/day or 100 mg/day, whichever is less). *If taking concurrent CYP2D6 inhibitor (quinidine, fluoxetine, paroxetine)*—0.5 mg/kg/day initially, may ↑ if needed to 1.2 mg/kg/day after 4 wk; *PO: Adults, Adolescents and Peds:* >70 kg 40 mg/day initially, may be ↑ after ≥3 days to target dose of 80 mg/day given as single dose in the AM or divided doses in AM and late afternoon/early evening; may be further ↑ after 2–4 wk up to 100 mg/day. *If taking concurrent CYP2D6 inhibitor (quinidine, fluoxetine, paroxetine)*—40 mg/day initially, may ↑ if needed to 80 mg/day after 4 wk; *Hepatic Impairment: PO: Adults and Peds:* ↓ dose for moderate or severe hepatic impairment; **Availability:** Caps: 10, 18, 25, 40, 60, 80, 100 mg; **Monitor:** BP, HR, ECG, mental status, suicidal thoughts/behaviors, ht/wt, jaundice, LFTs; **Notes:** All children should have CV assessment prior to initiation.

atorvastatin (Lipitor) Uses: Hypercholesterolemia, Primary and secondary prevention of CV disease; **Class:** HMG-CoA reductase inhibitors; **Preg:** X; **CIs:** Hypersensitivity, Liver disease, Pregnancy/lactation; **ADRs:** HA, abdominal cramps, constipation, diarrhea, dyspepsia, flatulence, ↑ LFTs, nausea, rash, RHABDOMYOLYSIS, myalgia; **Interactions:** CYP3A4 inhibitors may ↑ levels/toxicity, CYP3A4 inducers may ↓ levels/effects, ↑ risk of myopathy with cyclosporine, gemfibrozil, erythromycin, clarithromycin, protease inhibitors, niacin (≥1 g/day), and azole antifungals (consider ↓ doses of atorvastatin), May ↑ digoxin levels, May ↑ effects of warfarin; **Dose:** *PO: Adults:* 10–80 mg daily; *PO: Peds:* 10–17 yr 10–20 mg/day; **Availability:** Tabs: 10, 20, 40, 80 mg; **Monitor:** Lipid profile, LFTs, CK (if symptoms); **Notes:** Avoid grapefruit juice.

atovaquone (Mepron) Uses: Treatment/prevention of PCP in patients unable to tolerate trimethoprim/sulfamethoxazole; **Class:** Antiprotozoals; **Preg:** C; **CIs:** Hypersensitivity; **ADRs:** anxiety, depression, HA, insomnia, cough, N/V/D, ↑ LFTs, rash, fever; **Interactions:** Highly protein-bound drugs may ↑ levels, Rifampin ↓ levels; **Dose:** *PO: Adults and Adolescents:* 13–16 yr *Prevention*—1500 mg once daily with meal. *Treatment*—750 mg bid with a meal × 21 days; **Availability:** Oral susp: 750 mg/5 ml; **Monitor:** BP, HR, lung sounds, sputum, CBC, LFTs; **Notes:** Give with food (↑ absorption).

atropine (Atro-Pen) Uses: *IM: IV: PO:* ↓ salivation and secretions, *IV:* Asystole or bradycardia, *IM: IV:* Antidote for anticholinesterase (organophosphate pesticide) poisoning, *Ophth:* Produces mydriasis and cycloplegia for examination of retina and optic disc; **Class:** anticholinergics; **Preg:** C; **CIs:** Hypersensitivity, Narrow-angle glaucoma, Tachycardia, Mobitz type II heart block, Obstructive disease of GI tract, Severe ulcerative colitis, Myasthenia gravis, BPH, Hepatic disease; **ADRs:** blurred vision, drowsiness, confusion, cycloplegia, photophobia, dry eyes, mydriasis, ↑ HR, arrhythmias, palpitations, dry mouth, constipation, impaired GI motility, urinary hesitancy, dyspnea, flushing, ↓ sweating; **Interactions:** ↑ effects with other anticholinergics, including antihistamines, TCAs, phenothiazines, and disopyramide, Anticholinergics may alter absorption of other orally administered drugs by ↓ GI motility; **Dose:** *IM: IV: Subcut: PO: Adults: Inhibit salivation and secretions*—0.4–0.6 mg 30–60 min preoperatively and repeat q 4–6 hr prn; *IV: Adults: Asystole*—1 mg q 3–5 min (max total cumulative dose: 3 mg). *Bradycardia*—0.5–1 mg q 5 min (max cumulative dose: 3 mg; Endotracheal: *Adults: Asystole*—2–2.5 mg (diluted in 10 ml of NSS or distilled water) administered down ET tube q 3–5 min; *IM: Adults: Organophosphate poisoning*—2 mg initially, then 2 mg q 10 min prn up to 3 ×/total; *IV: Adults: Organophosphate poisoning*—1–5 mg initially; double dose q 5 min until muscarinic S/S diminish; may also be given as continuous infusion at 0.5–1 mg/hr; *Ophth: Adults: Mydriasis/cycloplegia*—Instill 1–2 drops of 1% soln 1 hr before procedure; *IM: IV: Subcut: PO: Peds: Inhibit salivation and secretions*—>5 kg: 0.01–0.02 mg/kg/dose (min: 0.1 mg/dose; max: 0.4 mg/dose) 30–60 min preop; <5 kg: 0.02 mg/kg/dose 30–60 min preop then q 4–6 hr prn; *IV: Peds: Bradycardia*— 0.02 mg/kg; may repeat q 5 min (max total cumulative dose: 1 mg in children (2 mg in adolescents)); Endotracheal: *Peds: Bradycardia*—Use the IV dose and dilute in 1–5 ml NSS before administering down ET tube; *IM: Peds: Organophosphate* *poisoning*—>90 lbs: 2 mg initially, then 2 mg q 10 min prn up to 3 ×/total; 40–90 lbs: 1 mg initially, then 1 mg q 10 min prn up to 3 ×/total; 15–40 lbs: 0.5 mg initially, then 0.5 mg q 10 min prn up to 3 ×/total; *IV: Peds: Organophosphate poisoning*—0.03–0.05 mg/kg q 10–20 min until atropinic effects observed, then q 1–4 hr for ≥24 hr; **Availability (G):** Tabs: 0.4 mg; Inject: 0.05 mg/ml, 0.1 mg/ml, 0.4 mg/0.5 ml, 0.4 mg/ml, 1 mg/ml; Inject (auto-injector): 0.25 mg/0.3 ml, 0.5 mg/0.7 ml, 1 mg/0.7 ml, 2 mg/0.7 ml; Ophth soln: 1%; **Monitor:** HR, BP, RR, ECG, bowel sounds, I/Os; **Notes:** Physostigmine is antidote. Give undiluted via rapid IV injection. Slow IV administration (over >1 min) and IV doses <0.5 mg may cause paradoxical bradycardia.

azathioprine (Azasan, Imuran) Uses: Adjunct in prevention of renal transplant rejection, RA; **Class:** purine antagonists; **Preg:** D; **CIs:** Hypersensitivity, Pregnancy/lactation, Patients previously treated with alkylating agents (e.g., cyclophosphamide, melphalan, etc.) (↑ risk of malignancy); **ADRs:** anorexia, HEPATOTOXICITY, N/V/D, anemia, leukopenia, pancytopenia, thrombocytopenia, INFECTION, MALIGNANCY; **Interactions:** ↑ risk of myelosuppression with antineoplastics, ACEIs, and other myelosuppressive agents, Allopurinol inhibits metabolism and may ↑ risk of toxicity (↓ azathioprine dose by 25–33%), Aminosalicylates (e.g., sulfasalazine, mesalamine, olsalazine) may ↑ risk of toxicity, May ↓ effects of warfarin; **Dose:** *PO: IV: Adults and Peds: Renal transplant*—3–5 mg/kg daily initially; MD: 1–3 mg/kg/day; *PO: Adults and Peds: RA*—1 mg/kg/day in 1–2 divided doses for 6–8 wk; may then ↑ by 0.5 mg/kg/day q 4 wk until response or up to 2.5 mg/kg/day, then ↓ by 0.5 mg/kg/day q 4–8 wk to minimal effective dose; **Availability (G):** Tabs: 50, 75, 100 mg; Inject: 100 mg; **Monitor:** S/S infection, BUN/SCr, CBC (with diff), LFTs, wt, ROM/pain/joint swelling (for RA); **Notes:** If WBC <3000 or platelets <100,000, may need to ↓ dose or temporarily discontinue. For RA, if no improvement by 12 wk, consider refractory.

azithromycin (AzaSite, Zithromax, Zmax) Uses: Respiratory tract infections, pharyngitis/tonsillitis, OM, skin/skin structure infections, urethritis/cervicitis/chancroid, or PID due to susceptible organisms (e.g., *S. pneumo*, *S. pyogenes*, *S. aureus*, *M. catarrhalis*, *H. flu*, *Chlamydia*, *Mycoplasma*, *N. gonorrhoeae*), Prevention or treatment of MAC infection in patients with advanced HIV, Bacterial conjunctivitis; **Class:** macrolides; **Preg:** B; **CIs:** Hypersensitivity to macrolides or ketolides; **ADRs:** PSEUDOMEMBRANOUS COLITIS, abdominal pain, N/V/D, ↑ LFTs, rash; **Interactions:** Antacids may ↓ levels, Nelfinavir may ↑ levels, May ↑ effects of warfarin, May ↑ levels of CYP3A4 substrates, May ↑ digoxin levels; **Dose:** *PO: Adults: CAP, pharyngitis/tonsillitis, skin/skin structure infections*—500 mg on Day 1, then 250 mg daily × 4 days. For CAP, may also use single 2-g dose of ER susp (Zmax). *Acute bacterial exacerbations of COPD*—500 mg on Day 1, then 250 mg daily × 4 days or 500 mg daily × 3 days. *Acute bacterial sinusitis*—500 mg daily × 3 days or single 2-g dose of ER susp (Zmax). *Chancroid/nongonococcal urethritis or cervicitis*—1-g single dose. *Gonococcal urethritis/cervicitis*—2-g single dose. *MAC*—Prophylaxis: 1200 mg once weekly (alone or with rifabutin); Treatment: 600 mg daily (with ethambutol); *PO: Peds:* ≥6 months *OM*—30-mg/kg single dose (max: 1.5 g), or 10 mg/kg daily × 3 days (max: 500 mg/day), or 10 mg/kg (max: 500 mg/day) on Day 1, then 5 mg/kg (max: 250 mg/day) daily × 4 days. *CAP*—10 mg/kg (max: 500 mg/day) on Day 1, then 5 mg/kg (max: 250 mg/day) daily × 4 days. *Pharyngitis/tonsillitis*—12 mg/kg daily × 5 days (max: 500 mg/day). *Acute bacterial sinusitis*—10 mg/kg daily × 3 days (max: 500 mg/day). *MAC*—5 mg/kg daily (max: 250 mg/day) or 20 mg/kg (max: 1200 mg/dose) once weekly (alone or with rifabutin); *IV: PO: Adults: CAP*—500 mg IV daily for ≥ 2 days, then 500 mg PO daily for total of 7–10 days; *PID*—500 mg IV daily for 1–2 days, then 250 mg PO daily for total of 7 days; *Ophth: Adults and Peds:* ≥1 yr 1 drop bid × 2 days, then 1 drop daily × 5 days; **Availability (G):** Tabs: 250, 500, 600 mg; Oral susp: 100 mg/5 ml, 200 mg/5 ml, 1 g/pkt; ER oral susp (Zmax): 2 g; Inject: 500 mg; Ophth soln: 1%; **Monitor:** HR, BP, temp, sputum, U/A, CBC, LFTs; **Notes:** ER susp is not interchangeable with other susp. Give ER susp 1 hr before or 2 hr after meals. Do not use 1-g packet for children.

baclofen (Kemstro, Lioresal) **Uses:** *PO:* Muscle spasms due to MS or spinal cord disorders, *IT:* Treatment of severe spasticity originating in the spinal cord; **Class:** skeletal muscle relaxants; **Preg:** C; **CIs:** Hypersensitivity; **ADRs:** SEIZURES (IT), confusion, dizziness, drowsiness, fatigue, weakness, HA, ↓ BP, nausea, constipation, urinary frequency, rash, ataxia, hypersensitivity reactions, hypotonia; **Interactions:** ↑ CNS depression with other CNS depressants including alcohol, antihistamines, opioids, and sedative/hypnotics; **Dose:** *PO: Adults:* 5 mg tid; may ↑ q 3 days by 5 mg/dose (max: 80 mg/day) (may also give qid); *IT: Adults: Screening dose*—50–100 mcg (if >50 mcg, give in 25-mcg increments separated by 24 hr). If patient does not respond to 100-mcg test dose, should not be considered candidate for pump. *MD*—Double the screening dose that patient responded to and infuse over 24 hr; can be titrated to effect after first 24 hr; *IT: Peds: Screening dose*—25–100 mcg (if >50 mcg, give in 25-mcg increments separated by 24 hr). If patient does not respond to 100-mcg test dose, should not be considered candidate for pump. *MD*—Double screening dose that patient responded to and infuse over 24 hr; can be titrated to effect after first 24 hr; **Availability (G):** Tabs: 10, 20 mg; Orally disintegrating tabs (Kemstro): 10, 20 mg; IT inject: 50 mcg/ml, 500 mcg/ml, 2000 mcg/ml; **Monitor:** Muscle spasticity, neuro status; **Notes:** Discontinue gradually over ≥2 wk (do not discontinue abruptly). For IT, resuscitative equipment should be immediately available for life-threatening or intolerable side effects. IT delivered by implantable IT pump.

beclomethasone (QVAR, Beconase AQ) **Uses:** *Inhaln:* Maintenance treatment of asthma (prophylactic therapy), *Intranasal:* Seasonal or perennial allergic or nonallergic rhinitis or prevention of recurrence of nasal polyps after surgical removal; **Class:** corticosteroids; **Preg:** C; **CIs:** Hypersensitivity, Acute asthma attack/status asthmaticus; **ADRs:** HA, dizziness, cataracts, dysphonia, epistaxis, nasal irritation, nasal stuffiness, oropharyngeal fungal infections, pharyngitis, rhinorrhea, sinusitis, sneezing, tearing eyes, nausea, bronchospasm, cough, wheezing, adrenal suppression (with ↑ dose, long-term therapy only), ↓ growth (children); **Interactions:** None noted; **Dose:** *Inhaln: Adults and Peds:* ≥12 yr. *Previously on bronchodilators alone*—40–80 mcg bid (max: 320 mcg bid). *Previously on inhaled corticosteroids*—40–160 mcg bid (max: 320 mcg bid); *Inhaln: Peds:* 5–11 yr *Previously on bronchodilators alone*—40 mcg bid (max: 80 mcg bid). *Previously on inhaled corticosteroids*—40 mcg bid (max: 80 mcg bid); *Intranasal: Adults and Peds:* ≥6 yr 1–2 sprays in each nostril bid (max: 2 sprays in each nostril bid); **Availability:** Inhaln aerosol (QVAR): 40 mcg/metered inhaln, 80 mcg/metered inhaln; Nasal spray (Beconase AQ): 42 mcg/metered spray; **Monitor:** RR, lung sounds, PFTs, growth rate (in children), S/S asthma/allergies; **Notes:** After desired effect achieved, ↓ dose to lowest amount required to control symptoms (if possible). For asthma, use bronchodilator first and allow 5 min to elapse before using beclomethasone. Allow ≥1 min between oral inhalns of aerosol. Inhaler should not be used to treat acute asthma attack. When using inhaler, rinse mouth with water or mouthwash after each use to minimize fungal infections, dry mouth, and hoarseness.

benazepril (Lotensin) **Uses:** HTN; **Class:** ACEIs; **Preg:** C (first tri), D (2nd and 3rd tri); **CIs:** Previous sensitivity/intolerance to ACEIs, CrCl <30 ml/min (children only), Children <6 yr (safety not established), Pregnancy/lactation; **ADRs:** dizziness, cough, ↓ BP, ↑ SCr, ↑ K+, rash, ANGIOEDEMA; **Interactions:** ↑ effects with other antihypertensives, ↑ risk of hyperkalemia with ARBs, K+ supplements, K+ salt substitutes, K+ sparing diuretics, or NSAIDs, NSAIDs may ↓ effectiveness, ↑ lithium levels; **Dose:** *PO: Adults:* 5–10 mg daily (5 mg if receiving diuretic); may ↑ gradually to 20–40 mg/day in 1–2 divided doses; *PO: Peds:* ≥6 yr 0.2 mg/kg daily; may ↑ up to 0.6 mg/kg/day (or 40 mg/day); *Renal Impairment: PO: Adults:* ↓ dose if CrCl <30 ml/min; **Availability (G):** Tabs: 5, 10, 20, 40 mg; **Monitor:** BP, HR, BUN/SCr, K+; **Notes:** Correct volume depletion. Advise on S/S angioedema. Avoid K+ salt substitutes.

benzonatate (Tessalon) **Uses:** Cough (nonproductive); **Class:** antitussives; **Preg:** C; **CIs:** Hypersensitivity (cross-sensitivity with other ester-type local anesthetics (tetracaine, procaine, etc.) may occur); **ADRs:** dizziness, HA, sedation, burning sensation in eyes, nasal congestion, constipation, GI upset, nausea, pruritus, skin eruptions, bronchospasm;

B

Interactions: Additive CNS depression may occur with antihistamines, alcohol, opioids, and sedative/hypnotics; **Dose:** *PO: Adults and Peds:* ≥10 yr 100–200 mg tid; **Availability (G):** Caps: 100, 200 mg; **Monitor:** Cough, lung sounds; **Notes:** Swallow caps whole. Do not chew (may cause local anesthetic effect and choking).

benztropine (Cogentin) Uses: Adjunctive treatment of Parkinson's disease, including drug-induced EPS and acute dystonic reactions; **Class:** anticholinergics; **Preg:** C; **CIs:** Hypersensitivity, Children <3 yr, Angle-closure glaucoma, Tardive dyskinesia; **ADRs:** confusion, depression, hallucinations, sedation, weakness, <u>blurred vision</u>, <u>dry eyes</u>, mydriasis, ↓ BP, ↑ HR, <u>constipation</u>, <u>dry mouth</u>, ileus, N/V, urinary retention, ↓ sweating; **Interactions:** ↑ risk of anticholinergic effects with other anticholinergic agents, Counteracts cholinergic effects of bethanechol; **Dose:** *PO: Adults: Parkinsonism*—0.5–6 mg/day in 1–2 divided doses; *IM: IV: Adults: Acute dystonia*—1–2 mg; *PO: IM: IV: Adults: Drug-induced EPS*—1–4 mg daily or bid; **Availability (G):** Tabs: 0.5, 1, 2 mg; Inject: 1 mg/ml; **Monitor:** S/S Parkinson's, EPS, bowel function, I/Os, mental status, BP/HR (with IM/IV); **Notes:** IV route rarely used because onset is same as IM.

betamethasone (Beta-Val, Celestone, Diprolene, Diprolene AF, Luxiq) Uses: *PO: IM:* Wide variety of chronic diseases including inflammatory, allergic, hemat, neoplastic, autoimmune disorders, *IM:* Antepartum therapy for fetal maturation in pregnant women (24–34 wk gestation) with preterm labor, **Top:** Inflammation and pruritis associated with various allergic/immunologic skin problems; **Class:** corticosteroids; **Preg:** C; **CIs:** Hypersensitivity, Active untreated infections; **ADRs:** <u>depression</u>, <u>euphoria</u>, personality changes, restlessness, cataracts, ↑ <u>BP</u>, PEPTIC ULCERATION, <u>anorexia</u>, <u>N/V</u>, <u>acne</u>, <u>hirsutism</u>, <u>petechiae</u>, allergic contact dermatitis, atrophy, burning, dryness, folliculitis, hypertrichosis, irritation, ↓ <u>wound healing</u>, <u>adrenal suppression</u>, ↑ BG, edema (long-term high doses), ↓ K+, THROMBOEMBOLISM, ↑ wt, <u>muscle wasting</u>, <u>osteoporosis</u>, muscle pain, <u>cushingoid appearance</u>, infection; **Interactions:** Additive hypokalemia with thiazide and loop diuretics, or amphotericin B, May ↑ requirement for insulins or oral hypoglycemic agents, Phenytoin, phenobarbital, and rifampin may ↓ levels, ↑ risk of adverse GI effects with NSAIDs; **Dose:** *PO: Adults and Peds:* ≥13 yr *Inflammatory conditions*—0.6–7.2 mg/day in 2–4 divided doses; *IM: Adults and Peds:* ≥13 yr *Inflammatory conditions*—0.5–9 mg/day in 1–2 divided doses; *IM: Adults: Antepartum therapy for fetal maturation*—12 mg q 24 hr × 2 doses; **Top:** *Adults and Peds:* ≥12 yr Apply to affected area(s) 1–3 times daily (depends on preparation and condition being treated); *PO: Peds:* ≤12 yr *Inflammatory conditions*—17.5–250 mcg/kg/day in 3–4 divided doses; *IM: Peds:* ≤12 yr *Inflammatory conditions*—17.5–125 mcg/kg/day in 2–4 divided doses; **Top:** *Peds:* Apply to affected area(s) daily; **Availability (G):** Oral soln: 0.6 mg/5 ml; Susp for inject (sodium phosphate and acetate): 6 mg (total)/ml; Aerosol foam:

0.12%; Cream: 0.05%, 0.1%; Gel: 0.05%; Lotion: 0.05%, 0.1%; Oint: 0.05%, 0.1%; **Monitor:** Systemic therapy: S/S adrenal insufficiency, wt/ht (children), edema, electrolytes, BG, pain; **Top:** skin condition (inflammation, erythema, pruritis); **Notes:** Do not administer susp IV. Oints are more occlusive and preferred for dry, scaly lesions. Creams should be used on oozing or intertriginous areas (may cause more skin drying than ointments). Gels, aerosols, and lotions are useful in hairy areas.

bevacizumab (Avastin) Uses: Metastatic colorectal CA (with IV 5-fluorouracil), Unresectable, locally advanced, recurrent or metastatic non-squamous, non-small cell lung CA (with carboplatin and paclitaxel), Patients who have not received chemotherapy for metastatic HER2-negative breast CA (with paclitaxel); **Class:** monoclonal antibodies; **Preg:** C; **CIs:** Hypersensitivity, First 28 days after major surgery, Recent hemoptysis or other serious recent bleeding; **ADRs:** RPLS,THROMBOEMBOLIC EVENTS (E.G., STROKE/TIA, MI, VTE), HF, ↑ BP, non-GI fistulas, GI PERFORATION, anorexia, N/V/D, nephrotic syndrome, proteinuria, BLEEDING, neutropenia, WOUND DEHISCENCE, impaired wound healing, infection, infusion reactions; **Interactions:** ↑ blood levels of the active metabolite of irinotecan; **Dose:** *IV: Adults: Colorectal CA*—5–10 mg/kg infusion q 14 days (with 5-fluorouracil-based chemotherapy). *Non-small cell lung CA*—15 mg/kg infusion q 3 wk. *Breast CA*—10 mg/kg infusion q 14 days; **Availability:** Inject: 25 mg/ml; **Monitor:** BP, CBC, U/A, S/S GI perforation/fistula/wound dehiscence/bleeding/thromboembolic events/infusion reactions/HF/RPLS; **Notes:** Discontinue if GI perforation, fistula, wound healing complications, serious bleeding, thromboembolic events, hypertensive crises, or nephrotic syndrome develops. Do not administer as IV push or bolus.

bisacodyl (Correctol, Dulcolax, Fleet Laxative) Uses: Constipation, Bowel evacuation before radiologic studies or surgery; **Class:** stimulant laxatives; **Preg:** C; **CIs:** Hypersensitivity, Abdominal pain or obstruction, N/V; **ADRs:** abdominal cramps, nausea, diarrhea, rectal burning; **Interactions:** May ↓ the absorption of other orally administered drugs because of ↑ motility, Milk or antacids may ↓ effects; **Dose:** *PO: Adults:* 5–15 mg as single dose (may use up to 30 mg when complete bowel evacuation needed); *PO: Peds:* >6 yr 5–10 mg as single dose; *Rect: Adults and Peds:* >2 yr 10-mg single dose; *Rect: Peds:* <2 yr 5-mg single dose; **Availability (G):** EC tabs: 5 mg^OTC; Supp: 10 mg^OTC; Rectal susp: 10 mg/30 ml^OTC; **Monitor:** Bowel sounds, bowel movements; **Notes:** May be administered at bedtime for AM results. For tabs, taking on empty stomach will produce more rapid results; do not take within 1 hr of milk or antacids. Retain the supp or enema 15–30 min before expelling.

bismuth subsalicylate (Bismatrol, Kaopectate, Kapectolin, Pepto-Bismol) Uses: Mild-to-moderate diarrhea or traveler's diarrhea (due to *E. coli*), Treatment of PUD associated with

H. pylori (with anti-infectives); **Class:** adsorbents; **Preg:** C (1st and 2nd tri), D (3rd tri); **CIs:** Hypersensitivity to bismuth or aspirin, chickenpox or flu-like illness (contains salicylate, which can cause Reye's syndrome), GI bleeding, Pregnancy (3rd tri); **ADRs:** tinnitus, constipation, gray-black stools, impaction (infants, debilitated patients), tongue discoloration; **Interactions:** ↑ risk of toxicity with aspirin or other salicylates, May ↓ absorption of tetracycline; **Dose:** *PO: Adults and Peds:* >12 yr *Antidiarrheal*—2 tabs or 30 ml (15 ml of extra/maximum strength) q 30–60 min prn (max: 8 doses/24 hr). *H. pylori (adults only)*— 524 mg qid (as 2 tabs, 30 ml of regular strength susp, or 15 ml of extra/maximum strength susp); *PO: Peds:* 9–12 yr *Antidiarrheal*—1 tab or 15 ml (7.5 ml of extra/maximum strength) q 30–60 min prn (max: 8 doses/24 hr); *PO: Peds:* 6–9 yr *Antidiarrheal*—10 ml (5 ml of extra/maximum strength) q 30–60 min prn (max: 8 doses/24 hr); *PO: Peds:* 3–6 yr *Antidiarrheal*—5 ml (2.5 ml of extra/maximum strength) q 30–60 min prn (max: 8 doses/24 hr); **Availability (G):** Tabs: 262 mg; Chew tabs: 262 mg; Oral liquid: 262 mg/15 ml, 525 mg/15 ml; **Monitor:** Bowel sounds, bowel movements, I/Os, S/S dehydration, abdominal pain; **Notes:** May temporarily cause stools and tongue to appear gray-black. Contains salicylate (caution when also using aspirin).

bisoprolol (Zebeta) **Uses:** HTN; **Class:** beta blockers; **Preg:** C; **CIs:** Hypersensitivity, Decompensated HF, Pulmonary edema, Cardiogenic shock, Bradycardia, ≥2nd-degree AV block, or sick-sinus syndrome (in absence of pacemaker); **ADRs:** fatigue, weakness, depression, dizziness, drowsiness, nightmares, blurred vision, bronchospasm, BRADYCARDIA, HF, PULMONARY EDEMA, ↓ BP, N/V/D, ED, ↓ libido, ↑ BG, ↓ BG; **Interactions:** ↑ risk of bradycardia with digoxin, diltiazem, verapamil, or clonidine, ↑ effects with other antihypertensives, ↑ risk of hypertensive crisis if concurrent clonidine discontinued, May alter the effectiveness of insulins or oral hypoglycemic agents, May ↓ the effects of $beta_1$ agonists (e.g., dopamine or dobutamine); **Dose:** *PO: Adults:* 2.5–5 mg daily; may be ↑ up to 10 mg daily (max: 20 mg/day); *Renal Impairment: Hepatic Impairment: PO: Adults:* ↓ dose if CrCl <40 ml/min or with hepatitis or cirrhosis; **Availability (G):** Tabs: 5, 10 mg; **Monitor:** HR, BP, ECG, S/S HF, edema, wt, BG (in DM); **Notes:** Abrupt withdrawal may cause life-threatening arrhythmias, hypertensive crises, or myocardial ischemia. May mask S/S of hypoglycemia (esp. tachycardia) in DM.

bivalirudin (Angiomax) **Uses:** Patients with unstable angina who are undergoing PTCA, Patients undergoing PCI (with GP IIb/IIIa inhibitor), Patients with or at risk of HIT and HITTS who are undergoing PCI; Moderate-to-high risk patients with acute coronary syndrome undergoing PCI; **Class:** thrombin inhibitors; **Preg:** B; **CIs:** Major bleeding, Hypersensitivity; **ADRs:** HA, ↓ BP, ↓ HR, HTN, N/V, abdominal pain, dyspepsia, BLEEDING, inject site pain, back pain, fever;

Interactions: ↑ risk of bleeding with antiplatelets, thrombolytics, or other anticoagulants; **Dose:** *IV: Adults:* 0.75 mg/kg bolus, then infusion of 1.75 mg/kg/hr for duration of PCI; monitor ACT 5 min after bolus and give additional 0.3 mg/kg bolus if needed. Continuing infusion (at rate of 1.75 mg/kg/hr) for up to 4 hr post-procedure is optional. If needed, infusion may be continued beyond this initial 4 hr at a rate of 0.2 mg/kg/hr for up to 20 hr; *IV: Adults:* Acute coronary syndrome: 0.1 mg/kg bolus, then infusion of 0.25 mg/kg/hr. Prior to PCI, give additional bolus of 0.5 mg/kg and ↑ infusion rate to 1.75 mg/kg/hr. Infusion should be discontinued at end of PCI, with option to continue at 0.25 mg/kg/hr if GP IIb/IIIa inhibitor not used. *Renal Impairment: IV: Adults:* ↓ infusion rate if CrCl <30 ml/min (do not need to ↓ bolus dose); **Availability:** Inject: 250 mg; **Monitor:** BP, HR, CBC, ACT, bleeding; **Notes:** Initiate before PCI and give with aspirin. No antidote available.

bleomycin (Blenoxane) Uses: Squamous cell carcinoma, lymphomas, or testicular CA, Malignant pleural effusions (via intrapleural administration); **Class:** antitumor antibiotics; **Preg:** D; **CIs:** Hypersensitivity; **ADRs:** PULMONARY FIBROSIS, pneumonitis, stomatitis, anorexia, hyperpigmentation, mucocutaneous toxicity, alopecia, erythema, rash, urticaria, vesiculation, phlebitis, ↓ wt, ANAPHYLACTOID REACTIONS, chills, fever; **Interactions:** Cisplatin or other nephrotoxic drugs may ↑ toxicity; **Dose:** *IV: IM: Subcut: Adults and Peds: For lymphoma,* give test dose of 1–2 units before first 2 doses (wait ≥1 hr before administering remainder of dose; if no reaction, follow regular dosing schedule). Dose – 0.25–0.5 units/kg (10–20 units/m^2) 1–2 ×/wk. *For Hodgkin's lymphoma,* if favorable response occurs, may ↓ MD to 1 unit/day or 5 units/wk IM or IV. May also be given as continuous IV infusion at 15 units/m^2/day for 4 days; **Intrapleural:** *Adults:* 60 units instilled for 4 hr, then removed; *Renal Impairment: Adults and Peds:* ↓ dose if CrCl <50 ml/min; **Availability (G):** Inject: 15 units, 30 units; **Monitor:** BP, HR, RR, temp, lung sounds, CXR, PFTs, wt, BUN/SCr, CBC; **Notes: High Alert:** Fatalities have occurred with chemotherapeutic agents. Before administering, clarify all ambiguous orders; double-check single, daily, and course-of-therapy dose limits; have second practitioner independently double-check original order and dose calculations. Max cumulative lifetime dose: 400 units (↑ risk of pulmonary toxicity). Discontinue if pulmonary toxicity occurs. For intrapleural use, administer through thoracostomy tube.

budesonide (Entocort EC, Pulmicort Respules, Pulmicort Flexhaler, Rhinocort Aqua) Uses: *Inhaln:* Maintenance treatment of asthma (prophylactic therapy), *Intranasal:* Seasonal or perennial allergic rhinitis, *PO:* Mild-to-moderate Crohn's disease; **Class:** corticosteroids; **Preg:** B (inhaln, intranasal), C (PO); **CIs:** Hypersensitivity, Acute asthma attack/status asthmaticus; **ADRs:** HA, agitation, confusion, dizziness, drowsiness, insomnia,

B

vertigo, cataracts, dysphonia, epistaxis, nasal irritation, nasal stuffiness, oropharyngeal fungal infections, pharyngitis, rhinorrhea, sinusitis, sneezing, tearing eyes, edema, ↑ BP, ↑ appetite, nausea, dyspepsia, bronchospasm, cough, wheezing, easy bruising, hirsutism, alopecia, striae, adrenal suppression (↑ dose, long-term therapy only), ↓ K+, ↑ BG, ↑ wt, ↓ growth (children), cushingoid appearance; **Interactions:** CYP3A4 inhibitors may ↑ levels, CYP3A4 inducers may ↓ levels; **Dose:** *Inhaln: Adults:* 180–360 mcg bid (max: 720 mcg bid); *Inhaln: Peds:* ≥6 yr 180–360 mcg bid (max: 360 mcg bid); *Inhaln: Peds:* 1–8 yr (Respules) *Previously on bronchodilators alone*—0.5 mg daily or 0.25 mg bid (max: 0.5 mg/day); *Previously on other inhaled corticosteroids*—0.5 mg daily or 0.25 mg bid (max: 1 mg/day); *Previously on PO corticosteroids*—1 mg daily or 0.5 mg bid (max: 1 mg/day); *Intranasal: Adults and Peds:* >6 yr 1 spray in each nostril daily (max: peds <12 yr = 2 sprays in each nostril daily; adults and peds ≥12 yr = 4 sprays in each nostril daily); *PO: Adults: Active Crohn's disease*—9 mg daily in AM for up to 8 wk; may repeat 8-wk course for recurring episodes; *Maintenance of remission*—6 mg daily for up to 3 mo; once symptoms controlled, taper off; **Availability:** Inhaln powder (Flexhaler): 90 mcg/metered inhaln, 180 mcg/metered inhaln; Inhaln susp (Respules): 0.25 mg/2 mL, 0.5 mg/2 mL, 1 mg/2 mL; EC caps (Entocort EC): 3 mg; Nasal susp (Rhinocort Aqua): 32 mcg/spray; **Monitor:** BP, HR, RR, lung sounds, PFTs, growth rate (in children), S/S asthma/allergies/Crohn's disease, S/S adrenal insufficiency (PO); **Notes:** After desired effect achieved, ↓ dose to lowest amount required to control symptoms (if possible). For asthma, use bronchodilator first and allow 5 min to elapse before using budesonide. Inhaler should not be used to treat acute asthma attack. When using inhaler, rinse mouth with water or mouthwash after each use to minimize fungal infections, dry mouth, and hoarseness.Do not break, crush, or chew caps.

bumetanide (Bumex) Uses: Edema due to HF, hepatic disease, or renal impairment; **Class:** loop diuretics; **Preg:** C; **CIs:** Hypersensitivity (cross-sensitivity with thiazides and sulfonamides may occur), Hepatic coma, Anuria, Severe electrolyte depletion, Critically ill or jaundiced neonates (↑ risk of kernicterus); **ADRs:** dizziness, HA, hearing loss, tinnitus, ↓ BP, N/V/D, photosensitivity, rash, ↑ BG, ↑ uric acid, dehydration, ↓ Ca++, ↓ K+, ↓ Mg++, ↓ Na+, hypovolemia, metabolic alkalosis, muscle cramps, azotemia; **Interactions:** ↑ effects with other antihypertensives, May ↑ lithium levels, ↑ risk of ototoxicity with aminoglycosides, NSAIDs may ↓ effectiveness, **Dose:** *PO: Adults:* 0.5–2 mg/day in 1–2 doses; titrate to response (max: 10 mg/day); *IM: IV: Adults:* 0.5–1 mg/dose, may repeat q 2–3 hr prn (max: 10 mg/day); *PO: IM: IV: Peds:* >6 mo 0.015–0.1 mg/kg q 24–48 hr (max: 10 mg/day); **Availability (G):** Tabs: 0.5, 1, 2 mg; Inject: 0.25 mg/ml; **Monitor:** BP, HR, electrolytes, BUN/SCr, BG, uric acid, wt, I/Os, edema, **Notes:** 1 mg bumetanide =

40 mg furosemide. If giving bid, give last dose no later than 5 PM. Advise patient to wear sunscreen.

bupivacaine (Marcaine, Sensorcaine) **Uses:** Local or regional anesthesia or analgesia for surgical, obstetric, or diagnostic procedures; **Class:** local anesthetics; **Preg:** C; **CIs:** Hypersensitivity (cross-sensitivity with other amide local anesthetics [ropivacaine, lidocaine, mepivacaine, prilocaine]) may occur, Obstetrical paracervical block anesthesia; **ADRs:** SEIZURES, anxiety, dizziness, HA, blurred vision, tinnitus, CARDIAC ARREST, arrhythmias, ↓ HR, ↓ BP, N/V, pruritus, circumoral tingling/numbness, allergic reactions; **Interactions:** Additive toxicity may occur with concurrent use of other amide local anesthetics; **Dose:** *Epidural: Adults and Peds:* >12 yr 10–20 ml of 0.25% (partial-to-moderate block), 0.5% (moderate-to-complete block), or 0.75% (complete block) solution. Administer in increments of 3–5 ml allowing sufficient time to detect toxic S/S of inadvertent IV or IT administration. A test dose of 2–3 ml of 0.5% with epinephrine solution is recommended prior to epidural blocks; Caudal block: *Adults and Peds:* >12 yr 15–30 ml of 0.25% or 0.5% solution. A test dose of 2–3 ml of 0.5% with epinephrine solution is recommended prior to caudal blocks; Peripheral nerve block: *Adults and Peds:* >12 yr 5 ml of 0.25% or 0.5% solution (max dose: 400 mg); Sympathetic nerve block: *Adults and Peds:* >12 yr 20–50 ml of 0.25% solution; Dental block: *Adults and Peds:* >12 yr 1.8-3.6 ml per site of 0.5% with epinephrine solution; Local Infiltration: *Adults and Peds:* >12 yr 0.25% soln infiltrated locally (max dose: 175 mg); **Availability (G):** Inject (with and without preservatives): 0.25%, 0.5%, 0.75%; **Monitor:** BP, HR, RR, S/S systemic toxicity (circumoral tingling/numbness, tinnitus, metallic taste, dizziness, blurred vision, tremor, slow speech, irritability, twitching, seizures, arrhythmias); **Notes:** Solns containing preservatives should not be used for epidural or caudal blocks.

buPROPion (Budeprion SR, Budeprion XL, Buproban, Wellbutrin, Wellbutrin SR, Wellbutrin XL, Zyban) **Uses:** Depression, Prevention of depression in patients with SAD (XL only), Smoking cessation (Zyban only); **Class:** dopamine reuptake inhibitors; **Preg:** C; **CIs:** Hypersensitivity, Seizure disorder or receiving meds that ↓ seizure threshold (theophylline, antipsychotics, antidepressants, corticosteroids), History of bulimia or anorexia nervosa (↑ risk of seizures), Undergoing abrupt withdrawal of alcohol or sedatives, Concurrent use with MAOIs, Lactation, May ↑ risk of suicidal thoughts/behaviors esp. during early treatment or dose adjustment; risk may be ↑ in children or adolescents; **ADRs:** SEIZURES, agitation, dizziness, HA, insomnia, ↑ HR, anorexia, dry mouth, N/V/D, ↑ wt, ↓ wt, rash, tremor, ↑ sweating; **Interactions:** ↑ risk of toxicity with MAOIs (discontinue for ≥2 wk), amantadine, or levodopa, May ↑ levels of CYP2D6 substrates, including TCAs, SSRIs, antipsychotics, beta-blockers, class Ic antiarrhythmics,

B

↑ risk of seizures with phenothiazines, antidepressants, theophylline, corticosteroids, or cessation of alcohol or BZs, Carbamazepine, phenytoin, or phenobarbital may ↓ levels/effects, Concurrent use with nicotine replacement may cause HTN; **Dose:** *PO: Adults: IR*—100 mg bid; after 3 days, may ↑ to 100 mg tid (max: 450 mg/day). *SR*—150 mg daily in AM; after 3 days, may ↑ to 150 mg bid (max: 400 mg/day). *XL*—Depression: 150 mg daily in AM; after 3 days, may ↑ to 300 mg daily (max: 450 mg/day). SAD: 150 mg daily in AM; after 1 wk, may ↑ to 300 mg daily. Taper dose to 150 mg/day for 2 wk before discontinuing. *Zyban*—150 mg daily × 3 days, then 150 mg bid for 7–12 wk (doses should be ≥8 hr apart) (initiate while smoking; discontinue smoking during 2nd wk of therapy); *Hepatic Impairment: PO: Adults:* ↓ dose in hepatic impairment; **Availability (G):** Tabs: 75, 100 mg; SR tabs: 100, 150, 200 mg; Zyban: 150 mg; ER tabs (XL): 150, 300 mg; **Monitor:** BP, HR, mental status, suicidal thoughts/behaviors; **Notes:** Do not confuse bupropion with buspirone. Administer doses in equally spaced time increments to minimize risk of seizures. Risk of seizures ↑ in doses >450 mg/day. Avoid giving at bedtime to ↓ insomnia. For SAD, begin therapy in autumn and continue through winter; begin to taper and discontinue in early spring. For depression, may require ≥4 wk to see effect. Do not break, crush, or chew SR tabs, ER tabs, or Zyban.

busPIRone (BuSpar) Uses: Anxiety disorders; **Class:** antianxiety agents; **Preg:** B; **CIs:** Hypersensitivity, Severe hepatic or renal impairment, Concurrent use with MAOIs; **ADRs:** dizziness, drowsiness, excitement, fatigue, HA, nervousness, blurred vision, insomnia, nausea, abdominal pain, diarrhea, dry mouth; **Interactions:** ↑ risk of HTN with MAOIs, CYP3A4 inhibitors may ↑ levels/toxicity, CYP3A4 inducers may ↓ levels/effects, Avoid concurrent use with alcohol; **Dose:** *PO: Adults:* 7.5 mg bid; may ↑ by 5 mg/day q 2–3 days prn (max: 60 mg/day). *If taking potent CYP3A4 inhibitor*—2.5 mg bid (daily with nefazodone); any ↑ should be based on clinical assessment; **Availability (G):** Tabs: 5, 7.5, 10, 15, 30 mg; **Monitor:** Mental status, S/S anxiety; **Notes:** Does not cause physical or psychological dependence/tolerance. Do not confuse with bupropion.

busulfan (Busulfex, Myleran) Uses: *PO:* CML, *IV:* With cyclophosphamide as conditioning regimen before allogeneic hematopoietic progenitor cell transplantation for CML; **Class:** alkylating agents; **Preg:** D; **CIs:** Hypersensitivity; **ADRs:** SEIZURES, anxiety, confusion, depression, dizziness, HA, insomnia, epistaxis, pharyngitis, PULMONARY FIBROSIS, cough, dyspnea, asthma, rhinitis, CARDIAC TAMPONADE (WITH HIGH-DOSE CYCLOPHOSPHAMIDE), CP, edema, ↑ BP, ↓ BP, ↑ HR, thrombosis, arrhythmias, HEPATIC VENO-OCCLUSIVE DISEASE, abdominal pain, anorexia, constipation, dry mouth, dyspepsia, hematemesis, ↑ bilirubin, ↑ LFTs, N/V/D, rectal discomfort, stomatitis, hepatomegaly, oliguria, ↑ SCr, dysuria, hematuria, hemorrhagic cystitis, itching, rash, acne, alopecia, hyperpigmentation, sterility, ↓ Ca++, ↓ K+, ↓ Mg++, ↓ PO_4, BONE MARROW DEPRESSION, inflammation/pain at inject site, ↑ BG, arthralgia, myalgia, allergic reactions, chills, fever, infection; **Interactions:** Concurrent or previous (within 72 hr) use of acetaminophen may ↑ levels/toxicity, Itraconazole may ↑ levels/toxicity, Phenytoin may ↓ levels/effects, ↑ bone marrow suppression with other antineoplastics or radiation therapy; **Dose:** *PO: Adults: Induction*—1.8 mg/m^2/day or 0.06 mg/kg/day until WBCs <15,000. Usual dose is 4–8 mg/day (range: 1–12 mg/day). *Maintenance*—1–3 mg/day; *PO: Peds:* 0.06–0.12 mg/kg/day or 1.8–4.6 mg/day. Titrate dose to maintain WBCs to >40,000; ↓ dose by 50% if WBCs = 30,000–40,000. Discontinue when WBCs ≤20,000; *IV: Adults:* 0.8 mg/kg q 6 hr (dose based on IBW or ABW, whichever is less; in obese patients, base dosage on adjusted IBW) × 4 days (total of 16 doses); given in combination with cyclophosphamide; **Availability:** Tabs: 2 mg; Inject: 6 mg/ml; **Monitor:** BP, HR, LFTs, bilirubin, BUN/SCr, CBC (with diff), CXR, bleeding, S/S infection, I/Os, lung sounds; **Notes: High Alert:** Fatalities have occurred with chemotherapeutic agents. Before administering, clarify all ambiguous orders; double-check single, daily, and course-of-therapy dose limits; have second practitioner independently double-check original order, calculations, and infusion pump settings. Administer IV through central venous catheter; premedicate with phenytoin to ↓ risk of seizures. Recovery of neutropenia at ~13 days; onset of thrombocytopenia ~5 days.

butorphanol (Stadol, Stadol NS) **Uses:** Pain (including migraine for nasal spray), Analgesia during labor, Sedation before surgery; **Class:** opioid agonists/antagonists; **Preg:** C; **CIs:** Hypersensitivity, Opioid dependence (may precipitate withdrawal); **ADRs:** confusion, dizziness, insomnia, sedation, euphoria, HA, unusual dreams, blurred vision, nasal congestion, respiratory depression, ↓ BP, palpitations, N/V, constipation, dry mouth, physical/psychological dependence, tolerance; **Interactions:** Use with extreme caution in patients receiving MAOIs (may produce severe, potentially fatal reactions), ↑ CNS depression with other CNS depressants, alcohol, antihistamines, opioids, and sedative/hypnotics, May precipitate withdrawal in patients physically dependent on opioids, May ↓ effects of concurrently administered opioids; **Dose:** *IM: Adults:* 2 mg q 3–4 hr prn (range: 1–4 mg). *Preop*—2 mg 60–90 min before surgery; *IV: Adults:* 1 mg q 3–4 hr prn (range: 0.5–2 mg); *IM: IV: Adults: Labor*—1–2 mg; may repeat after 4 hr; *Intranasal: Adults:* 1 mg (1 spray in 1 nostril); an additional dose may be given 60–90 min later. This sequence may be repeated in 3–4 hr. If pain is severe, an initial dose of 2 mg (1 spray in each nostril) may be given; may be repeated in 3–4 hr; **Availability (G):** Inject: 1 mg/ml, 2 mg/ml; Nasal spray: 10 mg/ml (1 mg/spray); **Monitor:** BP, HR, RR, pain (assess before and 30–60 min after IM, 5 min after IV, and 60–90 min after intranasal administration); **Notes: High Alert:** Accidental overdosage of opioid analgesics has resulted in fatalities. Before administering, clarify all ambiguous orders; have second practitioner independently check original order, dose calculations, route of administration, and infusion pump programming. Potential for dependence/abuse with long-term use. Naloxone can be used as antidote. Schedule IV controlled substance.

calcitonin (Fortical, Miacalcin) Uses: *IM: Subcut:* Paget's disease of bone, Hypercalcemia, *IM: Subcut: Intranasal:* Treatment of postmenopausal osteoporosis; **Class:** hormones; **Preg:** C; **CIs:** Hypersensitivity to calcitonin or salmon, Pregnancy/lactation; **ADRs:** HA, rhinitis, epistaxis, nasal irritation, N/V, urinary frequency, rash, inject site reactions, arthralgia, back pain, ANAPHYLAXIS, facial flushing, swelling; **Interactions:** Previous bisphosphonate therapy may ↓ response to calcitonin; **Dose:** *IM: Subcut: Adults: Postmenopausal osteoporosis*—100 units every other day. *Paget's disease*—100 units/day initially; MD is usually 50 units/day or every other day. *Hypercalcemia*—4 units/kg q 12 hr; if adequate response not achieved, may ↑ after 1–2 days to 8 units/kg q 12 hr, and then to 8 units/kg q 6 hr after 2 more days, if needed; *Intranasal: Adults: Postmenopausal osteoporosis*—1 spray/day in alternating nostrils; **Availability:** Inject (Miacalcin): 200 units/ml; Nasal spray (Miacalcin and Fortical): 200 units/spray; **Monitor:** BMD, Ca++, alk phos, S/S hypersensitivity, nasal mucosa/septum; **Notes:** Consider test dose in patients with suspected hypersensitivity. Subcut is preferred parenteral route (use IM if volume > 2 ml). Refrigerate nasal spray.

calcitriol (Calcijex, Rocaltrol) Uses: Treatment of hypocalcemia in patients undergoing chronic renal dialysis (IV and PO), Treatment of hypocalcemia in patients with hypoparathyroidism (PO), Treatment of secondary hyperparathyroidism in predialysis patients with moderate-to-severe CKD (PO); **Class:** fat-soluble vitamins; **Preg:** C; **CIs:** Hypersensitivity, Hypercalcemia, Vitamin D toxicity, Concurrent use of Mg++-containing antacids or other vitamin D supplements; **ADRs:** HA, sedation, weakness, photophobia, arrhythmias, HTN, abdominal pain, anorexia, constipation, dry mouth, ↑ LFTs, N/V, PANCREATITIS, polydipsia, ↓ wt, azotemia, polyuria, pruritus, ↑ Ca++, pain at inject site, hyperthermia, bone pain, metastatic calcification, muscle pain, allergic reactions (pruritis, rash, urticaria); **Interactions:** Cholestyramine, colestipol, or mineral oil ↓ absorption, Phenytoin or phenobarbital may ↓ levels/effects, ↑ risk of hypercalcemia with thiazide diuretics, Ca++-containing drugs, and vitamin D supplements, Corticosteroids may ↓ effectiveness, ↑ risk of arrhythmias with digoxin, ↑ risk of hypermagnesemia with Mg++-containing drugs; **Dose:** *PO: Adults: Dialysis patients*—0.25 mcg daily or every other day; if needed, may ↑ by 0.25 mcg/day q 4–8 wk (range: 0.5–1 mcg/day). *Hypoparathyroidism*—0.25 mcg daily; if needed, may ↑ by 0.25 mcg/day q 2–4 wk (range: 0.5–2 mcg/day). *Predialysis*—0.25 mcg daily; if needed, may ↑ up to 0.5 mcg/day; *PO: Peds: Dialysis patients*—0.25–1 mcg/day. *Hypoparathyroidism*—≥6 yr: 0.5–2 mcg/day; 1–5 yr: 0.25–0.75 mcg/day; <1 yr: 0.04–0.08 mcg/kg/day. *Vitamin-D dependent rickets*—1 mcg daily; *Familial hypophosphatemia*—0.015–0.06 mcg/kg daily (max: 2 mcg/day); *Hypocalcemia in CKD* >10 kg: 0.1–0.25 mcg daily. *Hypocalcemia in prematurity*—1 mcg daily for the first 5 days of life; *IV: Adults:* 1–2 mcg (0.02 mcg/kg) 3× weekly during dialysis; may ↑ by 0.5–1 mcg/dose q 2–4 wk (range: 0.5–4 mcg 3× weekly); *IV: Peds: Dialysis patients*—0.0075–0.025 mcg/kg 3× weekly during dialysis. *Hypocalcemic tetany in prematurity*—0.05 mcg/kg daily × 5–12 days; **Availability (G):** Caps: 0.25, 0.5 mcg; Oral soln: 1 mcg/ml; Inject: 1 mcg/ml; **Monitor:** Ca++, PO_4, Mg++, alk phos, PTH, bone pain; **Notes:** Ca × PO_4 product should be <70 (or patients at ↑ risk of calcification). Toxicity manifested as ↑ Ca++, ↑ PO_4, and hypercalciuria.

C

calcium carbonate (Calci-Chew, Caltrate, Maalox Antacid Caplets, Os-Cal, Oyst-Cal, Oystercal, Rolaids Calcium Rich, Titralac, Tums) **Uses:** Treatment and prevention of hypocalcemia, Adjunct in the prevention of postmenopausal osteoporosis, Indigestion/heartburn, Treatment of hyperphosphatemia in CKD; **Class:** minerals/electrolytes; **Preg:** C; **CIs:** Hypercalcemia, Renal calculi, Hypophosphatemia, Digoxin toxicity; **ADRs:** HA, constipation, N/V, renal calculi, ↑ Ca++, ↓ PO_4; **Interactions:** Hypercalcemia ↑ risk of digoxin toxicity, ↓ absorption of tetracyclines, FQs, iron salts, zinc, thyroid hormones and bisphosphonates, ↑ risk of ↑ hypercalcemia with thiazide diuretics; **Dose:** *PO: Adults: Prevention/treatment of hypocalcemia, osteoporosis*—1–2 g/day in 3–4 divided doses. *Antacid*—0.5–1.5 g prn. *Hyperphosphatemia in CKD*—1 g with each meal, ↑ to 4–7 g as needed; *PO: Peds: Supplementation*—45–65 mg/kg/day in 4 divided doses; **Availability (G):** Tabs: 364 mg (146 mg Ca)^{OTC}, 600 mg (240 mg Ca)^{OTC}, 1.25 g (500 mg Ca)^{OTC}, 1.5 g (600 mg Ca)^{OTC}; Chew tabs: 400 mg (161 mg Ca)^{OTC}, 420 mg (168 mg Ca)^{OTC}, 500 mg (200 mg Ca)^{OTC}, 600 mg (222 mg Ca)^{OTC}, 650 mg (260 mg Ca)^{OTC}, 750 mg (300 mg Ca)^{OTC}, 850 mg (340 mg Ca)^{OTC}, 1 g (400 mg Ca)^{OTC}, 1.177 g (471 mg Ca)^{OTC}, 1.25 g (500 mg Ca)^{OTC}; Gum: 250 mg (100 mg Ca) ^{OTC}, 500 mg (200 mg Ca)^{OTC}; Caps: 364 mg (146 mg Ca)^{OTC}, 1.25 g (500 mg Ca)^{OTC}; Oral susp: 1.25 g (500 mg Ca)/5 ml^{OTC}; Oral powder: 4 g (1.6 g Ca)/tsp^{OTC}; **Monitor:** S/S hypo-/hypercalcemia and hypo-/hyperphosphatemia, heartburn, abdominal pain, bowel sounds, electrolytes, PTH (for CKD); **Notes:** Do not take within 1–2 hr of other medications, if possible.

calcium chloride (No Trade) **Uses:** Treatment of hypocalcemia, hyperkalemia and hypermagnesemia, CCB toxicity; **Class:** minerals/electrolytes; **Preg:** C; **CIs:** Hypercalcemia, Digoxin toxicity; **ADRs:** HA, tingling, syncope,CARDIAC ARREST, arrhythmias, ↓ HR, constipation, N/V, renal calculi, ↑ Ca++, phlebitis; **Interactions:** Hypercalcemia

↑ risk of digoxin toxicity, ↑ risk of hypercalcemia with thiazide diuretics; **Dose:** *IV: Adults: Hypocalcemia, hyperkalemia, or hypermagnesemia*—500–1000 mg; may repeat prn. *CCB toxicity*—1 g q 10–20 min × 4 doses or 1 g q 2–3 min until desired effect; if favorable response, start continuous infusion of 20–50 mg/kg/hr. *Hypocalcemic tetany*—1 g over 10–30 min, may repeat after 6 hr; *IV: Peds: Hypocalcemia, hyperkalemia, or hypermagnesemia*—20 mg/kg/dose, may repeat prn. *CCB toxicity*—20 mg/kg (max: 1 g/dose), if favorable response, start continuous infusion of 20–50 mg/kg/hr. *Hypocalcemic tetany*—10 mg/kg over 5–10 min, may repeat after 6–8 hr or start continuous infusion up to 200 mg/kg/day; **Availability (G):** Inject: 10% (100 mg/ml); **Monitor:** BP, HR, ECG, S/S hypo-/hypercalcemia, Ca++ (or ionized Ca++), K+, Mg++, extravasation/phlebitis; **Notes:** 1 g CaCl = 270 mg elemental Ca. Has 3× more elemental Ca than Ca gluconate. Used to stabilize myocardium in hyperkalemia.

calcium gluconate (No Trade) Uses: *PO: IV:* Hypocalcemia, *PO:* Adjunct in the prevention of postmenopausal osteoporosis, *IV:* Hyperkalemia, hypermagnesemia, and CCB toxicity; **Class:** minerals/electrolytes; **Preg:** C; **CIs:** Hypercalcemia, Digoxin toxicity; **ADRs:** HA, tingling, syncope, CARDIAC ARREST, arrhythmias, ↓ HR, constipation, N/V, renal calculi, ↑ Ca++, phlebitis; **Interactions:** Hypercalcemia ↑ risk of digoxin toxicity, ↓ absorption of tetracyclines, FQs, iron salts, zinc, thyroid hormones and bisphosphonates, ↑ risk of hypercalcemia with thiazide diuretics; **Dose:** *PO: Adults: Hypocalcemia*—500–2000 mg 2–4 times/day; *PO: Peds: Hypocalcemia*—200–500 mg/kg/day in 4 divided doses; *IV: Adults: Hypocalcemia*—2–15 g/day as continuous infusion or in divided doses. *Hypocalcemic tetany*—1–3 g may be administered until response occurs. *Hyperkalemia or hypermagnesemia*—500–1000 mg; may repeat prn. *CCB toxicity*—1 g q 1–10 min until desired effect; can start continuous infusion of 0.6–1.2 ml/kg/hr; *IV: Peds and Infants: Hypocalcemia*—200–500 mg/kg/day as continuous infusion or in 4 divided doses (max: 2–3 g/dose). *Hypocalcemic tetany*—100–200 mg/kg/dose over 5–10 min; may repeat q 6–8 hr or follow with continuous infusion of 500 mg/kg/day. *Hyperkalemia or hypermagnesemia*—60–100 mg/kg/dose (max: 3 g/dose); *IV: Neonates: Hypocalcemia*—200–800 mg/kg/day as continuous infusion or in 4 divided doses (max: 1 g/dose); **Availability (G):** Caps: 515 mg (50 mg Ca); Tabs: 500 mg (45 mg Ca)[OTC], 650 mg (58.5 mg Ca)[OTC], 975 mg (87.75 mg Ca)[OTC]; Oral powder: 347 mg (31.23 mg Ca)/tablespoonful; Inject: 10% (100 mg/mL); **Monitor:** BP, HR, ECG, S/S hypo-/hypercalcemia, Ca++ (or ionized Ca++), K+, Mg++, extravasation/phlebitis; **Notes:** 1 g Ca gluconate = 90 mg elemental Ca. Ca chloride has 3× more elemental Ca than Ca gluconate. Used to stabilize myocardium in hyperkalemia.

candesartan (Atacand) Uses: HTN, HF (NYHA class II-IV); **Class**: angiotensin II receptor antagonists; **Preg:** C (1st tri), D (2nd and

3rd tri); **CIs:** Hypersensitivity, Pregnancy, Lactation; **ADRs:** dizziness, ↓ BP, ↑ SCr, ↑ K+, ANGIOEDEMA; **Interactions:** ↑ effects with other antihypertensives, ↑ risk of hyperkalemia with ACEIs, K+ supplements, K+ salt substitutes, K+ sparing diuretics, or NSAIDs, NSAIDs may ↓ effectiveness, ↑ lithium levels; **Dose:** *PO: Adults:* 4–32 mg/day in 1–2 divided doses; **Availability:** Tabs: 4, 8, 16, 32 mg; **Monitor:** BP, HR, wt, edema, BUN/SCr, K+; **Notes:** Can be used in patients intolerant to ACEI (due to cough); just as likely as ACEI to cause ↑ K+ and ↑ SCr.

C

capecitabine (Xeloda) **Uses:** Metastatic colorectal CA, Adjuvant treatment for Dukes' C colon CA following primary resection, Metastatic breast CA resistant/intolerant to prior therapy; **Class:** antimetabolites; **Preg:** D; **CIs:** Hypersensitivity to capecitabine or 5-fluorouracil, Dihydropyrimidine dehydrogenase deficiency (enzyme metabolizes 5-fluorouracil to nontoxic compounds), Severe renal impairment (CrCl <30 ml/min); **ADRs:** fatigue, HA, dizziness, insomnia, DIARRHEA, NECROTIZING ENTEROCOLITIS, abdominal pain, anorexia, dysgeusia, ↑ bilirubin, N/V, stomatitis, constipation, dyspepsia, xerostomia, dermatitis, hand-and-foot syndrome, alopecia, erythema, rash, anemia, leukopenia, thrombocytopenia, peripheral neuropathy, fever; **Interactions:** May ↑ risk of bleeding with warfarin (frequently monitor PT/INR), Toxicity ↑ by concurrent leucovorin, Antacids may ↑ absorption, May ↑ levels/toxicity of phenytoin (may need to ↓ phenytoin dose); **Dose:** *PO: Adults:* 1250 mg/m^2 bid × 14 days, followed by 7-day rest period; given as 3-wk cycles; *Renal Impairment: PO: Adults:* ↓ dose if CrCl 30-50 ml/min; **Availability:** Tabs: 150, 500 mg; **Monitor:** Bowel function, S/S infection/bleeding/hand-and-foot syndrome, CBC (with diff), LFTs, bilirubin, BUN/SCr, INR (if on warfarin); **Notes: High Alert:** Notify physician if symptoms of toxicity (stomatitis, uncontrollable vomiting, diarrhea, fever) occur; drug may need to be discontinued or dose ↓. Give fluids and electrolyte replacement if patients have severe diarrhea with dehydration. Metabolized to 5-fluorouracil. Dose modifications based on degree of toxicity encountered. Once dose has been ↓ because of toxicity, it should not be ↑ later. Give within 30 min after meal.

captopril (Capoten) **Uses:** HTN, HF, Post-MI, Diabetic nephropathy in patients with Type 1 DM and retinopathy; **Class:** ACEIs; **Preg:** C (1st tri), D (2nd and 3rd tri); **CIs:** Previous sensitivity/intolerance to ACEIs, Pregnancy/lactation; **ADRs:** dizziness, cough, ↓ BP, taste disturbances, ↑ SCr, ↑ K+, rash, AGRANULOCYTOSIS, neutropenia, ANGIOEDEMA; **Interactions:** ↑ effects with other antihypertensives, ↑ risk of hyperkalemia with ARBs, K+ supplements, K+ salt substitutes, K+ sparing diuretics, or NSAIDs, NSAIDs may ↓ effectiveness, ↑ lithium levels; **Dose:** *PO: Adults and Adolescents: HTN*—12.5–25 mg bid or tid; may ↑ q 1–2 wk up to 150 mg tid (initiate with 6.25–12.5 mg bid or tid if receiving diuretics); *PO: Adults: HF*—25 mg tid (6.25–12.5 mg tid if vigorously diuresed); titrate up to target dose of 50 mg tid (max: 450 mg/day).

Post-MI—6.25 mg × 1, then 12.5 mg tid; may ↑ up to 50 mg tid. *Diabetic nephropathy*—25 mg tid; *PO: Peds:* 0.5 mg/kg tid; may titrate up to a max of 6 mg/kg/day in 2–4 divided doses. *Older Children:* 6.25–12.5 mg q 12–24 hr; may titrate up to a max of 6 mg/kg/day in 2–4 divided doses; *PO: Infants:* 0.15–0.3 mg/kg/dose; may titrate up to a max of 6 mg/kg/day in 1–4 divided doses; *Renal Impairment: PO: Adults:* ↓ dose if CrCl ≤ 50 ml/min; **Availability (G):** Tabs: 12.5, 25, 50, 100 mg; **Monitor:** BP, HR, wt, edema, BUN/SCr, K+, CBC, U/A; **Notes:** Correct volume depletion. Advise on S/S angioedema. Avoid K+ salt substitutes. Give 1 hr before or 2 hr after meals (food ↓ absorption).

carbamazepine (Carbatrol, Epitol, Equetro, Tegretol, Tegretol-XR) **Uses:** Tonic-clonic, mixed, and complex-partial seizures, Management of pain in trigeminal neuralgia, **Equetro only:** Acute mania and mixed mania in Bipolar I disorder; **Class:** anticonvulsants; **Preg:** D; **CIs:** Hypersensitivity to carbamazepine or TCAs, Bone marrow suppression, Concurrent use with MAOIs, History of porphyria, Use only during pregnancy if potential benefits outweigh risks to the fetus, Lactation; **ADRs:** <u>ataxia</u>, <u>dizziness</u>, <u>drowsiness</u>, <u>HA</u>, fatigue, vertigo, blurred vision, nystagmus, <u>N/V</u>, ↑ LFTs, hepatitis, SJS, TEN, photosensitivity, pruritis, rash, urticaria, SIADH, ↓ Na+, AGRANULOCYTOSIS, APLASTIC ANEMIA, THROMBOCYTOPENIA; **Interactions:** CYP3A4 inhibitors may ↑ levels/toxicity, CYP3A4 inducers may ↓ levels/effects, May ↓ levels/effects of CYP1A2, CYP2C9, CYP2C19, and CYP3A4 substrates, May ↑ risk of CNS toxicity from lithium, ↑ risk of hyperpyrexia, HTN, seizures, or death with MAOIs (discontinue for ≥2 wk); **Dose:** *PO: Adults and Peds:* >12 yr *Anticonvulsant*—200 mg bid (tabs) *or* 100 mg qid (susp); ↑ by 200 mg/day q 7 days until therapeutic levels achieved (max: 1 g/day in children 12–15 yr, 1200 mg/day in patients >15 yr). *Trigeminal neuralgia*—100 mg bid (tabs) *or* 50 mg qid (susp); ↑ by up to 200 mg/day until pain relieved (max: 1200 mg/day); *PO: Adults: Bipolar disorder*—200 mg bid (tabs or ER tabs/caps) or 100 mg qid (susp); may ↑ by 200 mg/day until desired response (max: 600 mg/day); *PO: Peds:* 6–12 yr *Anticonvulsant*—100 mg bid (tabs *or* ER tabs) *or* 50 mg qid (susp); ↑ by 100 mg weekly until therapeutic levels achieved (max: 1000 mg/day); *PO: Peds:* <6 yr *Anticonvulsant*—10–20 mg/kg/day in 2–3 divided doses; may ↑ at weekly intervals until optimal response and therapeutic levels achieved (max: 35 mg/kg/day); **Availability (G):** Tabs: 200 mg; Chew tabs: 100 mg; ER caps: 100, 200, 300 mg; ER tabs: 100, 200, 400 mg; Oral susp: 100 mg/5 ml; **Monitor:** Seizure activity, facial pain, mental status, CBC, electrolytes, LFTs, serum blood levels (therapeutic: 4–12 mcg/ml); **Notes:** Asian patients have higher risk of SJS or TEN (should be genetically screened for HLA-B*1502 before starting therapy). ER products are given bid. Susp given 3–4 × daily. Do not crush, chew, or break ER tabs. Do not crush or chew ER caps; may be opened and sprinkled on applesauce.

carbidopa/levodopa (Parcopa, Sinemet, Sinemet CR) Uses: Parkinson's disease; **Class:** dopamine agonists; **Preg:** C; **CIs:** Hypersensitivity, Narrow-angle glaucoma, Concurrent MAOI therapy (in previous 14 days), Malignant melanoma, Undiagnosed skin lesions; **ADRs:** involuntary movements, anxiety, dizziness, hallucinations, memory loss, psychiatric problems, blurred vision, mydriasis, N/V, anorexia, dry mouth, HEPATOTOXICITY, melanoma, hemolytic anemia, leukopenia, darkening of urine or sweat; **Interactions:** Use with MAOIs may result in severe orthostatic hypotension (contraindicated), Phenothiazines, haloperidol, papaverine, metoclopramide, risperidone, and phenytoin may ↓ effects, ↑ risk of hypotension with concurrent antihypertensives; **Dose:** *PO: Adults: IR*—25 mg carbidopa/100 mg levodopa tid initially; may ↑ q 2 days until desired effect is achieved; *ER*—50 mg carbidopa/200 mg levodopa bid (minimum of 6 hr apart) initially; may ↑ q 3 days until desired effect is achieved; **Availability (G):** Tabs: 10 mg carbidopa/100 mg levodopa, 25 mg carbidopa/100 mg levodopa, 25 mg carbidopa/250 mg levodopa; Orally disintegrating tabs: 10 mg carbidopa/100 mg levodopa, 25 mg carbidopa/100 mg levodopa, 25 mg carbidopa/250 mg levodopa; ER tabs: 25 mg carbidopa/100 mg levodopa, 50 mg carbidopa/200 mg levodopa; **Monitor:** BP, HR, LFTs, parkinsonian symptoms, mental status; **Notes:** ER tabs may be broken in half, but should not be crushed or chewed.

carboplatin (Paraplatin) Uses: Advanced ovarian CA (with other agents), Palliative treatment of ovarian CA unresponsive to other chemotherapy (monotherapy); **Class:** alkylating agents; **Preg:** D; **CIs:** Hypersensitivity to carboplatin, cisplatin, or platinum-containing drugs, Severe bone marrow depression, Significant bleeding, Pregnancy or lactation; **ADRs:** hearing loss, ↑ LFTs, N/V/D, ↑ bilirubin, constipation, stomatitis, ↑ BUN/SCr, alopecia, rash, ↓ Ca++, ↓ K+, ↓ Mg++, ↓ Na+, ANEMIA, LEUKOPENIA, THROMBOCYTOPENIA, peripheral neuropathy, ANAPHYLACTIC-LIKE REACTIONS; **Interactions:** ↑ risk of nephrotoxicity and ototoxicity with other nephrotoxic and ototoxic drugs (e.g., aminoglycosides, loop diuretics), ↑ bone marrow suppression with other antineoplastics or radiation therapy; **Dose:** *IV: Adults: With other agents*—300 mg/m^2 with cyclophosphamide q 4 wk for 6 cycles. *Monotherapy*—360 mg/m^2; may be repeated q 4 wk, depending on response. *Renal Impairment: IV: Adults:* ↓ dose if CrCl <60 ml/min; **Availability (G):** Powder for inject: 50, 150, 450 mg; Soln for inject: 10 mg/ml; **Monitor:** BP, HR, temp, neuro exam, N/V, bleeding, S/S infection/anaphylaxis, BUN/SCr, electrolytes, CBC (with diff), LFTs, bilirubin; **Notes: High Alert:** Fatalities have occurred with chemotherapeutic agents. Before administering, clarify all ambiguous orders; double-check single, daily, and course-of-therapy dose limits; have second practitioner independently double-check original order, calculations, and infusion pump settings. Do not confuse carboplatin with cisplatin. Use prophylactic antiemetics. Median nadir = 21 days. Neutrophil count should be ≥2000 and platelets ≥100,000 to give subsequent doses. Adjust subsequent doses if neutropenia or thrombocytopenia develop.

C

carisoprodol (Soma) Uses: Short-term relief of acute painful musculoskeletal conditions; **Class:** skeletal muscle relaxants; **Preg:** C; **CIs:** Hypersensitivity to carisoprodol or meprobamate, Porphyria; **ADRs:** dizziness, drowsiness, HA; **Interactions:** ↑ CNS depression with other CNS depressants, alcohol, antihistamines, opioids, and sedative/hypnotics, CYP2C19 inhibitors may ↑ levels of carisoprodol, CYP2C19 inducers may ↓ levels of carisoprodol and ↑ levels of meprobamate; **Dose:** *PO: Adults and Adolescents:* ≥16 yr 250–350 mg qid (use no longer than 2–3 wk); **Availability (G):** Tabs: 250, 350 mg; **Monitor:** Pain, ROM; **Notes:** Metabolized to meprobamate (anxiolytic). Soma compound also contains aspirin 325 mg (also available with codeine). Give last dose at bedtime. Potential for dependence/abuse with long-term use (use with caution in patients at risk for addiction).

carmustine (BiCNU, Gliadel) Uses: Brain tumors, multiple myeloma, or Hodgkin's/Non-Hodgkin's lymphomas; **Class:** alkylating agents; **Preg:** D; **CIs:** Hypersensitivity, Pregnancy/lactation; **ADRs:** PULMONARY FIBROSIS, pulmonary infiltrates, N/V, anorexia, constipation, ↑ LFTs, ↑ BUN/SCr, BONE MARROW DEPRESSION (DELAYED), pain at IV site, secondary malignancy; **Interactions:** ↑ bone marrow suppression with other antineoplastics or radiation therapy; **Dose:** *IV: Adults:* 150–200 mg/m^2 as single dose q 6 wk *or* 75–100 mg/m^2/day × 2 days q 6 wk; Intracavitary: *Adults:* Up to 61.6 mg (8 implants) placed in cavity created during surgical resection of brain tumor; **Availability:** Inject: 100 mg; Intracavitary wafer: 7.7 mg/wafer; **Monitor:** BP, HR, RR, temp, BUN/SCr, LFTs, CBC (with diff), CXR, PFTs, S/S infection/bleeding, lung sounds, N/V; **Notes: High Alert:** Fatalities have occurred with chemotherapeutic agents. Before administering, clarify all ambiguous orders; double-check single, daily, and course-of-therapy dose limits; have second practitioner independently double-check original order, calculations, and infusion pump settings. Bone marrow toxicity is delayed (4–6 wk after treatment) and cumulative. Thrombocytopenia and leukopenia may persist for 1–2 wk. Recovery usually occurs in 6–7 wk but may take 10–12 wk after prolonged therapy. ↑ risk of pulmonary toxicity when cumulative dose >1400 mg/m^2. Use prophylactic antiemetics. Neutrophil count should be >4000 and platelets >100,000 to give subsequent doses. Adjust subsequent doses if neutropenia or thrombocytopenia develops.

carvedilol (Coreg, Coreg CR) Uses: HTN, Chronic HF, LV dysfunction post-MI; **Class:** beta blockers; **Preg:** C; **CIs:** Hypersensitivity, Pulmonary edema, Bradycardia, ≥2nd-degree AV block, or sick sinus syndrome (in absence of pacemaker), Cardiogenic shock, Decompensated HF, Severe hepatic impairment, Asthma or other bronchospastic disorders; **ADRs:** dizziness, fatigue, weakness, depression, drowsiness, nightmares, blurred vision, bronchospasm, BRADYCARDIA, HF, PULMONARY EDEMA, ↓ BP, N/V/D, ED, ↓ libido, ↑ BG; ↓ BG; **Interactions:** ↑ risk of bradycardia with digoxin, diltiazem, verapamil, or clonidine, ↑ effects with other antihypertensives, ↑ risk of hypertensive crisis if concurrent clonidine discontinued, May alter the effectiveness of insulins or oral hypoglycemic agents, May ↓ the effects of $beta_1$ agonists (e.g., dopamine or dobutamine), May ↑ levels of cyclosporine or digoxin, Rifampin may ↓ levels, Cimetidine may ↑ levels; **Dose:** *PO: Adults: HTN*—6.25–25 mg bid; ER: 20–80 mg daily; *HF*—3.125–50 mg bid (can double dose ≥ q 2 wk, as tolerated) (max: <85 kg—25 mg bid; >85 kg—50 mg bid). ER: 10–80 mg daily (can double dose ≥ q 2 wk, as tolerated); *LV dysfunction post-MI*—3.125–25 mg bid (can double dose q 3–10 days, as tolerated). ER: 20–80 mg daily (can double dose q 3–10 days, as tolerated); **Availability (G):** Tabs: 3.125, 6.25, 12.5, 25 mg; ER caps: 10, 20, 40, 80 mg; **Monitor:** HR, BP, ECG, S/S HF, edema, wt, S/S angina, BG (in DM); **Notes:** Abrupt withdrawal may cause worsening HF, life-threatening arrhythmias, hypertensive crises, or myocardial ischemia. May mask S/S of hypoglycemia (esp. tachycardia) in DM. Give with food to minimize orthostatic hypotension. To convert from IR to ER: 3.125 mg bid → 10 mg daily; 6.25 mg bid → 20 mg daily; 12.5 mg bid → 40 mg daily; 25 mg bid → 80 mg daily. Do not crush or chew ER caps; may be opened and sprinkled on applesauce.

caspofungin (Cancidas) **Uses:** Invasive aspergillosis, Candidemia and other candidal infections (intra-abdominal abscesses, peritonitis, pleural space infections), Esophageal candidiasis, Suspected fungal infections in febrile neutropenia; **Class:** echinocandins; **Preg:** C; **CIs:** Hypersensitivity; **ADRs:** HA, N/V/D, ↑ LFTs, ↓ K+, flushing, phlebitis, ALLERGIC REACTIONS INCLUDING ANAPHYLAXIS, fever; **Interactions:** ↑ risk of hepatotoxicity when used with cyclosporine, May ↓ tacrolimus levels, Rifampin may ↓ levels (↑ dose of caspofungin to 70 mg/day), Efavirenz, nelfinavir, nevirapine, phenytoin, dexamethasone, or carbamazepine may also ↓ levels (consider ↑ caspofungin dose to 70 mg/day); **Dose:** *IV: Adults:* 70 mg on Day 1, then 50 mg daily. *Esophageal candidiasis*—50 mg daily; *IV: Peds:* ≥3 mo 70 mg/m² on day 1 (max: 70 mg/dose) then 50 mg/m² daily (max: 70 mg/dose). *Hepatic Impairment: IV: Adults: Moderate hepatic impairment*—70 mg on Day 1, then 35 mg daily; **Availability:** Inject: 50, 70 mg; **Monitor:** HR, BP, temp, sputum, U/A, CBC, LFTs, S/S anaphylaxis, K+; **Notes:** ↑ MD in patients on CYP450 enzyme inducers.

cefadroxil (Duricef) **Uses:** Skin/skin structure infections, pharyngitis/tonsillitis, or UTIs due to susceptible organisms (e.g., *E.coli*, *P. mirabilis*, *Klebsiella*, *S. aureus*, *S. pyogenes*); **Class:** first-generation

C

cephalosporins; **Preg:** B; **CIs:** Hypersensitivity (cross-sensitivity to other beta-lactam antibiotics may exist); **ADRs:** SEIZURES (VERY HIGH DOSES), PSEUDOMEMBRANOUS COLITIS, diarrhea, rash, urticaria, pruritis, ANAPHYLAXIS; **Interactions:** Probenecid ↓ excretion and ↑ levels; **Dose:** *PO: Adults: Skin/soft tissue infections, pharyngitis/tonisillitis*—500 mg q 12 hr *or* 1 g daily. *UTIs*—1–2 g in 1–2 divided doses; *PO: Peds: Pharyngitis/tonsillitis or impetigo*—15 mg/kg q 12 hr *or* 30 mg/kg daily. *Skin/soft tissue infections, UTIs*—15 mg/kg q 12 hr; *Renal Impairment: PO: Adults and Peds:* ↓ dose if CrCl ≤50 ml/min; **Availability (G):** Caps: 500 mg; Tabs: 1 g; Oral susp: 250 mg/5 ml, 500 mg/5 ml; **Monitor:** HR, BP, temp, sputum, U/A, CBC; **Notes:** Refrigerate susp. Use with caution in patients with beta-lactam allergy (do not use if history of anaphylaxis or hives).

cefazolin (Ancef, Kefzol) **Uses:** Respiratory tract infections, UTIs, skin/skin structure infections, biliary tract infections, bone/joint infections, genital infections, septicemia, or IE due to susceptible organisms (e.g., *S. pneumo, S. pyogenes, S. aureus, E. coli, H. flu, Klebsiella, P. mirabilis*), Perioperative prophylaxis; **Class:** first-generation cephalosporins; **Preg:** B; **CIs:** Hypersensitivity (cross-sensitivity to other beta-lactam antibiotics may exist); **ADRs:** SEIZURES (HIGH DOSES), PSEUDOMEMBRANOUS COLITIS, diarrhea, rash, urticaria, pruritis, SJS, neutropenia, thrombocytopenia, phlebitis, ANAPHYLAXIS; **Interactions:** Probenecid ↓ excretion and ↑ levels; **Dose:** *IM: IV: Adults: Moderate-to-severe infections*—500 mg–1 g q 6–8 hr. *Mild infections with GPC*—250–500 mg q 8 hr. *Uncomplicated UTIs*—1 g q 12 hr. *Pneumococcal pneumonia*—500 mg q 12 hr. *IE or septicemia*—1–1.5 g q 6 hr. *Perioperative prophylaxis*—1 g within 30–60 min prior to incision (an additional 500 mg–1 g if surgery ≥ 2 hr), then 500 mg–1 g q 6–8 hr × 24 hr after surgery; *IM: IV: Peds and Infants:* >1 mo 25–100 mg/kg/day divided q 6–8 hr (max: 6 g/day); *Renal Impairment: IM: IV: Adults: CrCl ≤10–30 ml/min*—Give q 12 hr. *CrCl ≤10 ml/min*—Give q 24 hr; **Availability (G):** Inject: 500 mg, 1, 10, 20 g; **Monitor:** HR, BP, temp, sputum, U/A, CBC; **Notes:** Use with caution in patients with beta-lactam allergy (do not use if history of anaphylaxis or hives).

cefdinir (Omnicef) **Uses:** Respiratory tract infections, pharyngitis/tonsillitis, skin/skin structure infections, or OM due to susceptible organisms (e.g., *S. pneumo, S. pyogenes, S. aureus, M. catarrhalis, H. flu*); **Class:** third-generation cephalosporins; **Preg:** B; **CIs:** Hypersensitivity (cross-sensitivity to other beta-lactam antibiotics may exist); **ADRs:** SEIZURES (HIGH DOSES), HA, PSEUDOMEMBRANOUS COLITIS, diarrhea, nausea, rash, urticaria, pruritis, ANAPHYLAXIS; **Interactions:** Antacids and iron supplements ↓ absorption, Probenecid ↓ excretion and ↑ levels; **Dose:** *PO: Adults and Peds:* ≥13 yr 300 mg q 12 hr *or* 600 mg daily (q 12 hr for CAP or skin/skin structure infections); *PO: Peds:* 6 mo–12 yr

7 mg/kg q 12 hr *or* 14 mg/kg q 24 hr (max: 600 mg/day) (q 12 hr for skin/skin structure infections); *Renal Impairment: PO: Adults and Peds:* ↓ dose if CrCl <30 ml/min;**Availability (G):** Oral susp: 125 mg/5 ml, 250 mg/5 ml; Caps: 300 mg; **Monitor:** HR, BP, temp, sputum, U/A, CBC; **Notes:** Use with caution in patients with beta-lactam allergy (do not use if history of anaphylaxis or hives). Give ≥2 hr before or after iron supplements or antacids.

C

cefepime (Maxipime) Uses: Pneumonia, UTIs, skin/skin structure infections, or intra-abdominal infections (with metronidazole) due to susceptible organisms (e.g., *S. pneumo, S. aureus, E. coli, Klebsiella, P. mirabilis, Enterobacter, P. aeruginosa, B. fragilis*), Empiric treatment of febrile neutropenia; **Class:** fourth-generation cephalosporins; **Preg:** B; **CIs:** Hypersensitivity (cross-sensitivity to other beta-lactam antibiotics may exist); **ADRs:** SEIZURES (HIGH DOSES IN RENAL DYSFUNCTION), PSEUDOMEMBRANOUS COLITIS,<u>diarrhea</u>, <u>rash</u>, urticaria, pruritis, <u>phlebitis</u>, <u>pain at IM site</u>, ANAPHYLAXIS;**Interactions:** Probenecid ↓ excretion and ↑ levels, ↑ risk of nephrotoxicity with loop diuretics or aminoglycosides; **Dose:** *IM: Adults: Mild-to-moderate UTIs due to E. coli*—500 mg–1 g q 12 hr; *IV: Adults: Most infections*—500 mg–2 g q 12 hr. *Febrile neutropenia*—2 g q 8 hr; *IV: Peds:* 2 mo–16 yr *Most infections*—50 mg/kg q 12 hr (max: 2 g/dose). *Febrile neutropenia*—50 mg/kg q 8 hr (max: 2 g/dose); *Renal Impairment: IM: IV: Adults:* ↓ dose if CrCl ≤60 ml/min; **Availability (G):** Inject: 500 mg, 1, 2 g; **Monitor:** HR, BP, temp, sputum, U/A, CBC; **Notes:** Use with caution in patients with beta-lactam allergy (do not use if history of anaphylaxis or hives).

cefixime (Suprax) Uses: UTIs, pharyngitis/tonsillitis, bronchitis, gonorrhea, or OM due to susceptible organisms (e.g., *S. pneumo, S. pyogenes, E. coli, H. flu, P. mirabilis, N. gonorrhoeae*); **Class:** third-generation cephalosporins; **Preg:** B; **CIs:** Hypersensitivity (cross-sensitivity to other beta-lactam antibiotics may exist); **ADRs:** SEIZURES (HIGH DOSES), PSEUDOMEMBRANOUS COLITIS, diarrhea, nausea, rash, urticaria, pruritis, ANAPHYLAXIS;**Interactions:** Probenecid ↓ excretion and ↑ levels, May ↑ carbamazepine levels, May ↑ effects of warfarin; **Dose:** *PO: Adults and Peds:* >12 yr or >50 kg *Most infections*—400 mg daily. *Gonorrhea*—400 mg single dose; *PO: Peds:* ≥6 mo–12 yr or ≤50 kg 8 mg/kg daily *or* 4 mg/kg q 12 hr; *Renal Impairment: PO: Adults:* ↓ dose if CrCl ≤60 ml/min;**Availability:** Oral susp: 100 mg/5 ml; Tabs: 400 mg; **Monitor:** HR, BP, temp, sputum, U/A, CBC; **Notes:** Use susp for OM. Use with caution in patients with beta-lactam allergy (do not use if history of anaphylaxis or hives).

cefotaxime (Claforan) Uses: Pneumonia, UTIs, gonorrhea, gynecological infections, septicemia, skin/skin structure infections, intra-abdominal infections, bone/joint infections, or meningitis caused by susceptible organisms (e.g., *S. pneumo, S. pyogenes, S. aureus, E. coli, H. flu,*

Klebsiella, P. mirabilis, Serratia, Enterobacter, N. meningitidis, N. gonorrhoeae, B. fragilis), Perioperative prophylaxis; **Class:** third-generation cephalosporins; **Preg:** B; **CIs:** Hypersensitivity (cross-sensitivity to other beta-lactam antibiotics may exist); **ADRs:** SEIZURES (HIGH DOSES), PSEUDOMEMBRANOUS COLITIS, diarrhea, rash, urticaria, pruritis, phlebitis, pain at IM site, ANAPHYLAXIS; **Interactions:** Probenecid ↓ excretion and ↑ levels, ↑ risk of nephrotoxicity with aminoglycosides; **Dose:** *IM: IV: Adults and Peds:* >12 yr or ≥50 kg. *Most uncomplicated infections*—1 g q 12 hr. *Moderate-to-severe infections*—1–2 g q 6–8 hr. *Life-threatening infections*—2 g q IV hr. *Gonococcal urethritis/cervicitis (males or females) or rectal gonorrhea (females)*—500 mg IM single dose. *Rectal gonorrhea (males)*—1 g IM single dose. *Perioperative prophylaxis*—1 g 30–90 min before initial incision (single dose); *IM: IV: Peds:* 1 mo–12 yr *<50 kg*—50–200 mg/kg/day divided q 6–8 hr. *Meningitis*—50 mg/kg q 6 hr. *Invasive pneumococcal meningitis*—225–300 mg/kg/day divided q 6–8 hr; *IV: Neonates: ≤1 wk*—50 mg/kg q 12 hr. *1–4 wk*—50 mg/kg q 8 hr; *Renal Impairment: IM: IV: Adults:* ↓ dose if CrCl <20 ml/min; **Availability (G):** Inject: 500 mg, 1, 2, 10, 20 g; **Monitor:** HR, BP, temp, sputum, U/A, CBC; **Notes:** Use with caution in patients with beta-lactam allergy (do not use if history of anaphylaxis or hives).

cefoxitin (Mefoxin) Uses: Lower respiratory tract infections, skin/skin structure infections, bone/joint infections, UTIs, gynecological infections, intra-abdominal infections, or septicemia due to susceptible organisms (e.g., *E. coli, Klebsiella, Proteus, B. fragilis*), Perioperative prophylaxis; **Class:** second-generation cephalosporins; **Preg:** B; **CIs:** Hypersensitivity (cross-sensitivity to other beta-lactam antibiotics may exist); **ADRs:** SEIZURES (HIGH DOSES IN RENAL DYSFUNCTION), PSEUDOMEMBRANOUS COLITIS, diarrhea, rash, urticaria, pruritis, phlebitis, pain at IM site, ANAPHYLAXIS; **Interactions:** Probenecid ↓ excretion and ↑ levels, ↑ risk of nephrotoxicity with loop diuretics or aminoglycosides; **Dose:** *IM: IV: Adults: Most infections*—1–2 g q 6–8 hr. *Perioperative prophylaxis*—1–2 g 30–60 min before initial incision, then 1–2 g q 6 hr × 24 hr after surgery; *IM: IV: Peds and Infants:* >3 mo *Most infections*—80–160 mg/kg/day divided q 6 hr. *Perioperative prophylaxis*—30–40 mg/kg 30–60 min before initial incision, then 30–40 mg/kg q 6 hr × 24 hr after surgery; *Renal Impairment: IM: IV: Adults:* ↓ dose if CrCl ≤50 ml/min; **Availability (G):** Inject: 1, 2, 10 g; **Monitor:** HR, BP, temp, sputum, U/A, CBC; **Notes:** Use with caution in patients with beta-lactam allergy (do not use if history of anaphylaxis or hives). Anaerobic coverage.

cefpodoxime (Vantin) Uses: Respiratory tract infections, gonorrhea, skin/skin structure infections, or UTIs due to susceptible organisms (e.g., *S. pneumo, S. pyogenes, S. aureus, M. catarrhalis, H. flu, N. gonorrhoeae, E. coli, Klebsiella, P. mirabilis*); **Class:** third-generation cephalosporins;

Preg: B; **CIs:** Hypersensitivity (cross-sensitivity to other beta-lactam antibiotics may exist); **ADRs:** SEIZURES (HIGH DOSES), HA, PSEUDOMEMBRANOUS COLITIS, diarrhea, nausea, rash, urticaria, pruritis, ANAPHYLAXIS; **Interactions:** Probenecid ↓ excretion and ↑ levels, ↑ risk of nephrotoxicity with loop diuretics or aminoglycosides, Antacids or H_2 antagonists ↓ absorption; **Dose:** *PO: Adults and Peds:* ≥12 yr *Most infections*—200 mg q 12 hr. *Skin/skin structure infections*—400 mg q 12 hr. *UTIs/pharyngitis/tonsillitis*—100 mg q 12 hr. *Gonorrhea*—200 mg single dose; *PO: Peds:* 2 mo–11 yr *Pharyngitis/tonsillitis/OM/acute maxillary sinusitis*—5 mg/kg q 12 hr (max: 200 mg/dose); *Renal Impairment: PO: Adults:* ↑ dosing interval to q 24 hr if CrCl <30 ml/min; **Availability (G):** Tabs: 100, 200 mg; Oral susp: 50 mg/5 ml, 100 mg/5 ml; **Monitor:** HR, BP, temp, sputum, U/A, CBC; **Notes:** Give tabs with food (↑ absorption). Refrigerate susp. Use with caution in patients with beta-lactam allergy (do not use if history of anaphylaxis or hives). Give ≥2 hr before or after antacids or H_2 antagonists.

cefprozil (Cefzil) Uses: Respiratory tract infections or skin/skin structure infections due to susceptible organisms (e.g., *S. pneumo*, *S. pyogenes*, *S. aureus*, *M. catarrhalis*, *H. flu*); **Class:** second-generation cephalosporins; **Preg:** B; **CIs:** Hypersensitivity (cross-sensitivity to other beta-lactam antibiotics may exist); **ADRs:** SEIZURES (HIGH DOSES), HA, PSEUDOMEMBRANOUS COLITIS, diarrhea, nausea, rash, urticaria, pruritis, ANAPHYLAXIS; **Interactions:** Probenecid ↓ excretion and ↑ levels, ↑ risk of nephrotoxicity with aminoglycosides; **Dose:** *PO: Adults and Peds:* ≥13 yr *Pharyngitis/tonsillitis*—500 mg daily. *Sinusitis*—250–500 mg q 12 hr. *Bronchitis*—500 mg q 12 hr. *Skin/skin structure infections*—250–500 mg q 12 hr *or* 500 mg daily; *PO: Peds:* 6 mo–12 yr *OM*—15 mg/kg q 12 hr. *Sinusitis*—7.5–15 mg/kg q 12 hr; *PO: Peds:* 2–12 yr *Pharyngitis/tonsillitis*—7.5 mg/kg q 12 hr. *Skin/skin structure infections*—20 mg/kg daily; *Renal Impairment: Adults and Peds:* ≥6 mo ↓ dose if CrCl <30 ml/min; **Availability (G):** Tabs: 250, 500 mg; Oral susp: 125 mg/5 ml, 250 mg/5 ml; **Monitor:** HR, BP, temp, sputum, U/A, CBC; **Notes:** Refrigerate susp. Use with caution in patients with beta-lactam allergy (do not use if history of anaphylaxis or hives).

ceftazidime (Fortaz, Tazicef) Uses: Pneumonia, skin/skin structure infections, UTIs, septicemia, bone/joint infections, gynecological infections, intra-abdominal infections, or meningitis due to susceptible organisms (e.g., *S. pneumo*, *S. aureus*, *E. coli*, *H. flu*, *Klebsiella*, *P. mirabilis*, *Enterobacter*, *Serratia*, *P. aeruginosa*, *N. meningitidis*, *B. fragilis*), Empiric treatment of febrile neutropenia; **Class:** third-generation cephalosporins; **Preg:** B; **CIs:** Hypersensitivity (cross-sensitivity to other beta-lactam antibiotics may exist); **ADRs:** SEIZURES (HIGH DOSES IN RENAL DYSFUNCTION), PSEUDOMEMBRANOUS COLITIS, diarrhea, rash, urticaria, pruritis, phlebitis, pain at IM site, ANAPHYLAXIS; **Interactions:**

Probenecid ↓ excretion and ↑ levels, ↑ risk of nephrotoxicity with loop diuretics or aminoglycosides; **Dose:** *IM: IV: Adults and Peds:* ≥12 yr *Most infections*—500 mg–1 g q 8–12 hr. *Bone/joint infections*—2 g IV q 12 hr. *Severe and life-threatening infections/meningitis/febrile neutropenia*—2 g IV q 8 hr. *Uncomplicated UTIs*—250 mg q 12 hr. *Cystic fibrosis lung infection due to P. aeruginosa*—30–50 mg/kg IV q 8 hr (max: 6 g/day); *IV: Peds:* 1 mo–12 yr 30–50 mg/kg q 8 hr (max: 6 g/day); *IM: IV: Neonates:* ≤4 wk 30 mg/kg q 12 hr; *Renal Impairment: IM: IV: Adults:* ↓ dose if CrCl ≤50 ml/min; **Availability:** Inject: 500 mg, 1, 2, 6 g; **Monitor:** HR, BP, temp, sputum, U/A, CBC; **Notes:** Use with caution in patients with beta-lactam allergy (do not use if history of anaphylaxis or hives).

ceftriaxone (Rocephin) Uses: Lower respiratory tract infections, OM, skin/skin structure infections, UTIs, gonorrhea, PID, septicemia, bone/joint infections, intra-abdominal infections, or meningitis due to susceptible organisms (e.g., *S. pneumo*, *S. pyogenes*, *S. aureus*, *E. coli*, *H. flu*, *M.catarrhalis*, *Klebsiella*, *Proteus*, *Serratia*, *Enterobacter*, *N. meningitidis*, *N. gonorrhoeae*, *B. fragilis*), Perioperative prophylaxis; **Class:** third-generation cephalosporins; **Preg:** B; **CIs:** Hypersensitivity (cross-sensitivity to other beta-lactam antibiotics may exist), Hyperbilirubinemic neonates (may lead to kernicterus), Use with solutions containing Ca (may form dangerous precipitate); **ADRs:** SEIZURES (HIGH DOSES), PSEUDOMEMBRANOUS COLITIS, <u>diarrhea</u>, cholelithiasis, <u>rash</u>, <u>urticaria</u>, pruritis, phlebitis, <u>pain at IM site</u>, ANAPHYLAXIS; **Interactions:** Probenecid ↓ excretion and ↑ levels; **Dose:** *IM: IV: Adults: Most infections*—1–2 g q 12–24 hr. *Gonorrhea*—250 mg IM single dose. *Meningitis*—2 g IV q 12 hr. *Perioperative prophylaxis*—1 g IV 0.5–2 hr before surgery (single dose); *IM: IV: Peds: Most infections*—50–75 mg/kg/day divided q 12–24 hr (max: 2 g/day). *Meningitis*—100 mg/kg/day divided q 12–24 hr (max: 4 g/day). *Uncomplicated gonorrhea*—125 mg IM single dose. *Acute OM*—50 mg/kg (max: 1 g) IM single dose; **Availability (G):** Inject: 250, 500 mg, 1, 2, 10 g; **Monitor:** HR, BP, temp, sputum, U/A, CBC, bilirubin, jaundice (newborns); **Notes:** Use with caution in patients with beta-lactam allergy (do not use if history of anaphylaxis or hives).

cefuroxime (Ceftin, Zinacef) Uses: Respiratory tract infections, UTIs, skin/skin structure infections, septicemia, meningitis, gonorrhea, bone/joint infections, or Lyme disease due to susceptible organisms (e.g., *S. pneumo*, *S. pyogenes*, *S. aureus*, *E. coli*, *H. flu*, *Klebsiella*, *N. meningitidis*, *N. gonorrhoeae*), Perioperative prophylaxis; **Class:** second-generation cephalosporins; **Preg:** B; **CIs:** Hypersensitivity (cross-sensitivity to other beta-lactam antibiotics may exist); **ADRs:** SEIZURES (HIGH DOSES), PSEUDOMEMBRANOUS COLITIS, <u>diarrhea</u>, N/V, <u>rash</u>, <u>urticaria</u>, pruritis, phlebitis, <u>pain at IM site</u>, ANAPHYLAXIS; **Interactions:** Probenecid ↓ excretion and ↑ levels, Antacids or H_2 antagonists may ↓ absorption; **Dose:** *PO: Adults and Peds:* >12 yr *Most infections*—250–500 mg q 12 hr. *Gonorrhea*—1 g single dose; *PO: Peds:* 3 mo–12 yr *OM,* *acute bacterial maxillary sinusitis, impetigo*—15 mg/kg q 12 hr (susp) (max: 1 g/day) *or* 250 mg q 12 hr (tabs). *Pharyngitis/tonsillitis*—10 mg/kg q 12 hr (susp) (max: 500 mg/day); *IM: IV: Adults: Most infections*—750 mg–1.5 g q 8 hr. *Life-threatening infections*—1.5 g q 6 hr. *Perioperative prophylaxis*—1.5 g IV 30–60 min before initial incision; 750 mg IM/IV q 8 hr can be given if procedure is prolonged. *Prophylaxis during open-heart surgery*—1.5 g IV at induction of anesthesia and then q 12 hr for 3 additional doses. *Gonorrhea*—1.5 g IM (750 mg in two sites) with 1 g probenecid; *IM: IV: Peds and Infants:* >3 mo *Most infections*—50–100 mg/kg/day divided q 6–8 hr (max: 6 g/day). *Bone and joint infections*—150 mg/kg/day divided q 8 hr (max: 6 g/day); *Renal Impairment: IM: IV: Adults:* ↓ dose if CrCl ≤20 ml/min; **Availability (G):** Tabs: 250, 500 mg; Oral susp: 125 mg/5 ml, 250 mg/5 ml; Inject: 750 mg, 1.5, 7.5 g; **Monitor:** HR, BP, temp, sputum, U/A, CBC; **Notes:** Give susp with food. Refrigerate susp. Use with caution in patients with beta-lactam allergy (do not use if history of anaphylaxis or hives). Give ≥2 hr before or after antacids or H_2 antagonists. Tabs and susp are not interchangeable.

celecoxib (Celebrex) **Uses:** OA, RA, ankylosing spondylitis, and juvenile RA, Acute pain, Primary dysmenorrhea, ↓ number of adenomatous colorectal polyps in FAP as adjunct to usual care (endoscopic surveillance, surgery); **Class:** COX-2 inhibitors; **Preg:** C; **CIs:** Hypersensitivity (cross-sensitivity may exist with other NSAIDs, including aspirin), Allergy to sulfonamides, Severe renal dysfunction, Perioperative pain from CABG surgery, Pregnancy (3rd tri) (may cause premature closure of the PDA), Lactation, CV disease or risk factors for CV disease (may ↑ risk of serious CV thrombotic events, MI, and stroke, esp. with prolonged use), HTN, HF, Safety not established in children <2 yr or for longer than 6 mo, History of PUD or GI bleeding; **ADRs:** dizziness, HA, insomnia, edema, GI BLEEDING, abdominal pain, diarrhea, dyspepsia, flatulence, nausea, ↑ LFTs, HEPATOTOXICITY, ↑ BP, EXFOLIATIVE DERMATITIS, SJS, TEN, rash; **Interactions:** CYP2C9 inhibitors may ↑ levels, CYP2C9 inducers may ↓ levels, May ↓ effectiveness of antihypertensives and diuretics, May ↑ risk of bleeding with warfarin or aspirin, May ↑ lithium levels; **Dose:** *PO: Adults: OA*—200 mg daily *or* 100 mg bid. *RA*—100–200 mg bid. *Ankylosing spondylitis*—200 mg daily *or* 100 mg bid; if no effect after 6 wk, may ↑ to 400 mg daily. *FAP*—400 mg bid. *Acute pain, primary dysmenorrhea*—400 mg initially, then a 200-mg dose if needed on the first day; then 200 mg bid prn; *PO: Peds:* ≥2 yr *Juvenile RA*—10–25 kg: 50 mg bid; >25 kg: 100 mg bid; **Availability:** Caps: 50, 100, 200, 400 mg; **Monitor:** ROM, pain, BUN/SCr, LFTs, CBC; **Notes:** Do not give if patient has allergy to sulfonamides, NSAIDs, or aspirin. Discontinue if rash develops. Do not confuse with Celexa (citalopram), Cerebyx (fosphenytoin), or Zyprexa (olanzapine).

cephalexin (Keflex) **Uses:** Respiratory tract infections, OM, skin/skin structure infections, bone infections, or GU infections due to susceptible organisms (e.g., *S. pneumo, S. pyogenes, S. aureus, M. catarrhalis, H. flu, P. mirabilis, Klebsiella, E. coli*); **Class:** first-generation cephalosporins; **Preg:** B; **CIs:** Hypersensitivity (cross-sensitivity to other beta-lactam antibiotics may exist); **ADRs:** SEIZURES (HIGH DOSES), HA, PSEUDOMEMBRANOUS COLITIS, diarrhea, nausea, rash, urticaria, pruritis, ANAPHYLAXIS; **Interactions:** Probenecid ↓ excretion and ↑ levels; **Dose:** *PO: Adults: Most infections*—250–500 mg q 6 hr. *Uncomplicated cystitis, skin/skin structure infections, Streptococcal pharyngitis*—500 mg q 12 hr; *PO: Peds: Most infections*—25–50 mg/kg/day divided q 6–8 hr (can be administered q 12 hr in skin/skin structure infections or Streptococcal pharyngitis). *OM*—18.75–25 mg/kg q 6 hr (max: 4 g/day); **Availability (G):** Caps: 250, 500, 750 mg; Tabs: 250, 500 mg; Oral susp: 125 mg/5 ml, 250 mg/5 ml; **Monitor:** HR, BP, temp, sputum, U/A, CBC; **Notes:** Refrigerate susp. Use with caution in patients with beta-lactam allergy (do not use if history of anaphylaxis or hives).

cetirizine (Zyrtec) **Uses:** Seasonal and perennial allergic rhinitis, Chronic urticaria; **Class:** antihistamines; **Preg:** B; **CIs:** Hypersensitivity to cetirizine or hydroxyzine, Lactation, CrCl <11 ml/min (not on dialysis); **ADRs:** dizziness, drowsiness, fatigue, HA, insomnia, N/V/D, pharyngitis, dry mouth; **Interactions**: ↑ risk of CNS depression with other CNS depressants, including alcohol, antidepressants, sedatives/hypnotics, and opioid analgesics; **Dose:** *PO: Adults and Peds:* >6 yr 5–10 mg daily; *PO: Peds:* 2–5 yr 2.5 mg daily; may ↑ to 5 mg daily or 2.5 mg q 12 hr; *PO: Peds:* 1– <2 yr 2.5 mg daily; may ↑ to 2.5 mg q 12 hr; *PO: Peds:* 6–12 mo 2.5 mg daily; *Hepatic/Renal Impairment: PO: Adults and Children:* ≥12 yr *CrCl <11–31 ml/min, hepatic impairment, or HD*—5 mg daily. *CrCl <11 ml/min (not on HD)*—use not recommended; *PO: Peds:* 6–11 yr <2.5 mg/day; *PO: Peds:* <6 yr use not recommended; **Availability (G):** Tabs: 5, 10 mg; Chew tabs: 5, 10 mg; Oral syrup: 1 mg/ml; **Monitor:** Allergy symptoms (rhinitis, conjunctivitis, hives); **Notes:** Also available OTC.

cetuximab (Erbitux) **Uses:** Advanced squamous cell carcinoma of the head and neck (with radiation), Recurrent or metastatic squamous cell carcinoma of the head and neck progressing after platinum-based therapy (as monotherapy), EGFR-expressing metastatic colorectal CA in patients who have not responded to irinotecan and oxaliplatin or are intolerant to irinotecan (as monotherapy), EGFR-expressing metastatic colorectal CA that has not responded to irinotecan (with irinotecan); **Class:** monoclonal antibodies; **Preg:** C; **CIs:** Hypersensitivity, Pregnancy or lactation; **ADRs:** anxiety, depression, HA, fatigue, insomnia, INTERSTITIAL LUNG DISEASE, PULMONARY EMBOLISM, cough, dyspnea, SUDDEN DEATH, abdominal pain, constipation, N/V/D, stomatitis, anorexia, acneform rash, nail disorder, pruritus, skin desquamation, dehydration, ↓ Mg++, ↓ wt, INFUSION REACTIONS, chills, fever, infection; **Interactions:** None noted; **Dose:** *IV: Adults: Head/neck CA*—With radiation: 400 mg/m^2 1 wk prior to initiation of radiation therapy, then 250 mg/m^2 weekly for the duration of radiation therapy. Complete infusion 1 hr prior to radiation therapy. Monotherapy: 400 mg/m^2 initially, then 250 mg/m^2 weekly until disease progression or intolerance. *Colorectal CA*—400 mg/m^2 initially, then 250 mg/m^2 weekly until disease progression or intolerance; **Availability:** Inject: 2 mg/ml; **Monitor:** BP, HR, temp, lung sounds, infusion reactions (monitor for ≥1 hr after infusion), derm toxicity, wt, BUN/SCr, electrolytes, CBC; **Notes:** Premedicate with diphenhydramine 50 mg 30–60 min before first dose; base subsequent administration on presence and severity of infusion reactions. ↓ dose for derm toxicity and infusion reactions. Most infusion reactions occur during first dose, but may also occur with later doses. For severe reactions, immediately stop infusion and discontinue permanently. Epinephrine, corticosteroids, IV antihistamines, bronchodilators, and O_2 should be available for severe reactions. Mild-to-moderate reactions may be managed by ↓ infusion rate and giving antihistamines. Caution patient to limit sun exposure during therapy.

chloral hydrate (Aquachloral) **Uses:** Short-term sedative and hypnotic (effectiveness ↓ after 2 wk of use), Sedation/hypnotic prior to diagnostic procedures; **Class:** hypnotics; **Preg:** C; **CIs:** Hypersensitivity, Severe cardiac disease, Hepatic or renal impairment (CrCl <50 ml/min), Esophagitis, gastritis, or ulcer disease; **ADRs:** <u>sedation</u>, ataxia, disorientation, dizziness, hallucinations, HA, paradoxical excitation (children), respiratory depression, <u>N/V/D</u>, flatulence, rash, <u>tolerance</u>, physical dependence, psychological dependence; **Interactions:** ↑ CNS depression with other CNS depressants, including alcohol, antihistamines, opioids, and sedative/hypnotics, May ↑ effects of warfarin, May cause diaphoresis, ↑ BP, and flushing when given within 24 hr of IV furosemide; **Dose:** *PO: Rect: Adults: Hypnotic*—500–1000 mg 15–30 min before bedtime. *Preop sedation*—500–1000 mg 30 min before surgery. *Sedation/anxiety*—250 mg tid; *PO: Rect: Peds:* >1 month *Pre-EEG sedation*—20–25 mg/kg 30–60 min prior to EEG; may repeat in 30 min (max cumulative dose: 2 g). *Sedation prior to dental/medical procedures*—50–75 mg/kg 30–60 min prior to procedure; may repeat in 30 min if needed (max cumulative dose: 1 g). *Hypnotic*—20–40 mg/kg (max: 2 g/day). *Sedation/anxiety*—5–15 mg/kg q 8 hr (max: 500 mg/dose); **Availability (G):** Caps: 500 mg; Oral syrup: 500 mg/5 ml; Supp: 325, 500 mg; **Monitor:** Mental status; **Notes:** **High Alert:** Pedi: Chloral hydrate overdosage has resulted in fatalities in children. Orders should be written in milligrams (mg), not volume (tsp.) or concentration. Chloral hydrate should be administered to children only by trained staff in the health care setting. When administered to children for sedation before outpatient procedures, administer at the facility where procedure is to be performed. Continue monitoring until level of consciousness is safe for discharge. Schedule IV controlled substance. Do not discontinue abruptly (may cause delirium); taper over 2 wk. Potential for dependence/abuse with long-term use. Should not be used for >2 wk.

C

chlordiazepoxide (Librium) Uses: Anxiety (including preop), Alcohol withdrawal; **Class:** benzodiazepines; **Preg:** D; **CIs:** Hypersensitivity, Pregnancy/lactation, Narrow-angle glaucoma; **ADRs:** dizziness, drowsiness, ataxia, paradoxical excitation, blurred vision, ↓ BP, constipation, nausea, ↑ wt, rash, pain at IM site, physical/psychological dependence, tolerance; **Interactions:** ↑ CNS depression with other CNS depressants, including alcohol, antihistamines, opioids, and sedative/hypnotics, CYP3A4 inhibitors may ↑ levels/toxicity, CYP3A4 inducers may ↓ levels/effects; **Dose:** *PO: Adults: Alcohol withdrawal*—50–100 mg, repeat until agitation is controlled (max: 300 mg/day). *Anxiety*—5–25 mg 3–4 × daily. *Preop*—5–10 mg 3–4 × on the day before surgery; *PO: Geri: Anxiety*—5 mg 2–4 × daily; may ↑ prn; *PO: Peds:* >6 yr *Anxiety*—5 mg 2–4 × daily; may ↑ up to 10 mg bid or tid; *IM: IV: Adults: Alcohol withdrawal*—50–100 mg initially; may repeat in 2–4 hr (max: 300 mg/day). *Anxiety*—50–100 mg initially, then 25–50 mg 3–4 × daily prn. *Preop*—50–100 mg 1 hr preop; *IM: IV: Geri: Anxiety/sedation*—25–50 mg/dose; **Availability (G):** Caps: 5, 10, 25 mg; Inject: 100 mg; **Monitor:** BP, HR, RR, mental status, S/S alcohol withdrawal (esp. seizures); **Notes:** Schedule IV controlled substance. Potential for dependence/abuse with long-term use (use with caution in patients at risk for addiction). Flumazenil is antidote. IV is preferred over IM (erratic absorption). Do not discontinue abruptly; taper by 10 mg q 3 days to ↓ risk of withdrawal.

chlorothiazide (Diuril) Uses: HTN, Edema due to HF, renal dysfunction, cirrhosis, glucocorticoids, or estrogens; **Class:** thiazide diuretics; **Preg:** C; **CIs:** Hypersensitivity (cross-sensitivity with other thiazides or sulfonamides may exist), Anuria, Lactation; **ADRs:** dizziness, weakness, ↓ BP, anorexia, cramping, N/V, photosensitivity, rash, ↑ BG, ↓ K+, dehydration, ↑ Ca++, metabolic alkalosis, ↓ Mg++, ↓ Na+, ↑ uric acid, muscle cramps; **Interactions:** ↑ effects with other antihypertensives, May ↑ lithium levels, Cholestyramine or colestipol may ↓ absorption, NSAIDs may ↓ effectiveness; **Dose:** *PO: Adults:* 125–2000 mg/day in 1–2 divided doses; *PO: Peds:* >6 mo 10–20 mg/kg/day in 1–2 divided doses; max dose: 375 mg/day (<2 yr); 1000 mg/day (2–12 yr); *PO: Infants:* <6 mo 10–30 mg/kg/day in 2 divided doses (max: 375 mg/day); *IV: Adults: Edema*—500–1000 mg daily or bid; *IV: Peds:* >6 mo 4 mg/kg/day in 1–2 divided doses (max: 20 mg/kg/day); *IV: Infants:* <6 mo 2–8 mg/kg/day in 2 divided doses (max: 20 mg/kg/day); *Renal Impairment: PO: Adults: CrCl <30 ml/min*—Ineffective; **Availability (G):** Tabs: 250, 500 mg; Oral susp: 250 mg/5 ml; Inject: 500 mg; **Monitor:** BP, electrolytes, BUN/SCr, BG, uric acid, wt, I/Os, edema; **Notes:** Administer in AM. Advise patient to use sunscreen.

chlorthalidone (Thalitone) **Uses:** HTN, Edema due to HF, renal dysfunction, cirrhosis, glucocorticoids, or estrogens; **Class:** thiazide diuretics; **Preg:** B; **CIs:** Hypersensitivity (cross-sensitivity with other thiazides or sulfonamides may exist), Anuria, Lactation; **ADRs:** dizziness, weakness, ↓ BP, anorexia, cramping, N/V, photosensitivity, rash, ↑ BG, ↓ K+, dehydration, ↑ Ca++, metabolic alkalosis, ↓ Mg++, ↓ Na+, ↑ uric acid, muscle cramps; **Interactions:** ↑ effects with other antihypertensives, May ↑ lithium levels, Cholestyramine or colestipol may ↓ absorption, NSAIDs may ↓ effectiveness; **Dose:** *PO: Adults:* 12.5–100 mg daily; *Renal Impairment: PO: Adults: CrCl <30 ml/min*—Ineffective; **Availability (G):** Tabs: 15, 25, 50, 100 mg; **Monitor:** BP, electrolytes, BUN/SCr, BG, uric acid, wt, I/Os, edema; **Notes:** Administer in AM. Advise patient to use sunscreen.

chlorzoxazone (Parafon Forte DSC) **Uses:** Muscle spasms; **Class:** skeletal muscle relaxants; **Preg:** C; **CIs:** Hypersensitivity, Liver disease; **ADRs:** <u>dizziness</u>, <u>drowsiness</u>, GI BLEEDING, N/V, HEPATOTOXICITY, rash, ANGIOEDEMA; **Interactions:** ↑ risk of CNS depression with other CNS depressants, including alcohol, antihistamines, antidepressants, sedative/hypnotics, and opioid analgesics; **Dose:** *PO: Adults:* 250–750 mg tid or qid; *PO: Peds:* 20 mg/kg/day in 3–4 divided doses; **Availability (G):** Tabs: 250 mg, 500 mg; **Monitor:** Pain, ROM, muscle stiffness, LFTs; **Notes:** May give with meals to ↓ GI irritation. Beers drug (potentially inappropriate for use in elderly).

cholestyramine (LoCHOLEST, LoCHOLEST Light, Prevalite, Questran, Questran Light) **Uses:** Primary hypercholesterolemia, Pruritus associated with ↑ bile acids; **Class:** bile acid sequestrants; **Preg:** C; **CIs:** Hypersensitivity, Complete biliary obstruction; T6 >500 mg/dl; **ADRs:** <u>abdominal discomfort</u>, <u>constipation</u>, <u>N/V</u>, flatulence, hemorrhoids, perianal irritation, steatorrhea, rash, vitamin A, D, E, and K deficiency, ↑ TGs; **Interactions:** May ↓ absorption/effects of numerous medications (e.g., digoxin, diuretics, glipizide, corticosteroids, NSAIDs, penicillin, phenytoin, propranolol, tetracyclines, thyroid preparations, warfarin, and fat-soluble vitamins (A, D, E, and K)); **Dose:** *PO: Adults:* 4 g daily-bid; may ↑ up to 24 g/day as needed in 2–6 divided doses; *PO: Peds:* 240 mg/kg/day in 3 divided doses; **Availability (G):** Powder for oral susp with aspartame (LoCHOLEST Light, Prevalite, Questran Light): 4 g/packet or scoop; Powder for oral susp (LoCHOLEST, Questran): 4 g/packet or scoop; **Monitor:** Lipid panel; **Notes:** Give other meds either 1 hr before or 4–6 hr after cholestyramine. Mix with 4–6 oz water, milk, fruit juice, or other noncarbonated beverages. Give with meals. May need to give multivitamin. Consider ↑ in fluids, fiber, exercise, stool softeners, and laxatives to manage constipation.

cidofovir (Vistide) **Uses:** CMV retinitis in patients with AIDS (to be used with probenecid); **Class:** Antivirals; **Preg:** C; **CIs:** Hypersensitivity to cidofovir, probenecid, or sulfonamides, SCr >1.5 mg/dl,

CrCl ≤55 ml/min, or urine protein ≥100 mg/dl (≥2+ proteinuria), Concurrent use of nephrotoxic medications, Lactation; **ADRs:** HA, ↓ IOP, iritis, ocular hypotony, uveitis, dyspnea, pneumonia, N/V/D, anorexia, NEPHROTOXICITY, proteinuria, alopecia, rash, neutropenia, anemia, METABOLIC ACIDOSIS, chills, fever, infection; **Interactions:** ↑ risk of nephrotoxicity with aminoglycosides, amphotericin B, foscarnet, vancomycin, NSAIDs, and pentamidine (avoid concurrent use; discontinue for ≥7 days before starting cidofovir); **Dose:** *IV: Adults:* 5 mg/kg once weekly × 2 wk, then 5 mg/kg q 2 wk (give probenecid 2 g 3 hr before cidofovir, then 1 g at 2 and 8 hr after infusion; also give 1 L of IV NS before and after [or with] infusion); *Renal Impairment: IV: Adults:* ↑ *SCr of 0.3–0.4 mg/dl over baseline*—↓ dose to 3 mg/kg; discontinue if SCr ↑ by ≥0.5 mg/dl over baseline; **Availability:** Inject: 75 mg/ml; **Monitor:** Visual acuity, IOP, ocular symptoms, BP, HR, temp, S/S infection, BUN/SCr, urine protein, CBC (with diff); **Notes:** Give with probenecid and IV NS to ↓ nephrotoxicity. Give probenecid with meals or antiemetic to ↓ N/V. Not a cure for CMV retinitis. ↓ zidovudine dose by 50% on day of infusion (due to interaction with probenecid). Contraception needed for 1 mo (women) and 3 mo (men) after treatment.

cilostazol (Pletal) Uses: ↓ symptoms of intermittent claudication; **Class:** platelet aggregation inhibitors; **Preg:** C; **CIs:** Hypersensitivity, HF, Active bleeding, Lactation; **ADRs:** HA, dizziness, palpitations, ↑ HR, diarrhea; **Interactions:** CYP2C19 inhibitors and CYP3A4 inhibitors may ↑ levels/toxicity (↓ dose of cilostazol); CYP3A4 inducers may ↓ levels/effect; **Dose:** *PO: Adults:* 100 mg bid (50 mg bid if receiving CYP2C19 inhibitors or CYP3A4 inihibitors); **Availability (G):** Tabs: 50, 100 mg; **Monitor:** S/S intermittent claudication; **Notes:** Administer on empty stomach (1 hr before or 2 hr after meals). May take 12 wk to see benefit.

cimetidine (Tagamet, Tagamet HB 200) Uses: Short-term treatment of duodenal and gastric ulcers, Maintenance therapy for duodenal ulcers, GERD, Heartburn (OTC use), Gastric hypersecretory states (Zollinger-Ellison syndrome), Stress-induced upper GI bleeding in critically ill patients; **Class:** histamine H_2 antagonists; **Preg:** B; **CIs:** Hypersensitivity; **ADRs:** confusion, HA, diarrhea, hepatitis, nausea, gynecomastia, AGRANULOCYTOSIS, APLASTIC ANEMIA, anemia, neutropenia, thrombocytopenia, pain at IM site, hypersensitivity reactions; **Interactions:** May ↑ levels/toxicity of CYP1A2 substrates, CYP2C19 substrates, CYP2D6 substrates, or CYP3A4 substrates, May ↑ effects of warfarin, ↓ absorption of ketoconazole and itraconazole; **Dose:** *PO: Adults: Short-term treatment of active ulcers*—300 mg qid or 800 mg at bedtime or 400 mg bid (duration: up to 8 wk). *Duodenal ulcer prophylaxis*—400 mg at bedtime. *GERD*—400 mg qid or 800 mg bid (duration: 12 wk). *Gastric hypersecretory conditions*—300–600 mg q 6 hr. *OTC use*—200 mg bid; *IV: IM: PO: Peds: Short-term treatment of active* *ulcers*—20–40 mg/kg/day in 4 divided doses; *IM: IV: Adults: Short-term treatment of active ulcers*—300 mg q 6 hr or 37.5 mg/hr as continuous infusion. *Gastric hypersecretory conditions*—300–600 mg q 6 hr. *Prevention of upper GI bleeding in critically ill patients*—50 mg/hr by continuous infusion; *Renal Impairment: PO: IV: Adults:* ↓ dose if CrCl <50 ml/min; **Availability (G):** Tabs: 200, 300, 400, 800 mg; Oral soln: 300 mg/5 ml; Inject: 150 mg/ml; **Monitor:** S/S GERD/PUD, bleeding, BUN/SCr, CBC, LFTs; **Notes:** Should not take OTC for >2 wk. Has most drug interactions of all the H_2 antagonists.

ciprofloxacin (Ciloxan, Cipro, Cipro XR, Proquin XR)

Uses: Respiratory tract infections, UTIs, prostatitis, gonorrhea, skin/skin structure infections, bone/joint infections, intra-abdominal infections, infectious diarrhea, or typhoid fever due to susceptible organisms (e.g., *S. pneumo*, *S. pyogenes*, *S. epidermidis*, *S. saprophyticus*, *E. faecalis*, *E. coli*, *Klebsiella*, *H. flu*, *M. catarrhalis*, *Enterobacter*, *Serratia*, *Proteus*, *Providencia*, *Morganella*, *Citrobacter*, *N. gonorrhoeae*, *P. aeruginosa*, *Shigella*, *Salmonella*), Empiric treatment of febrile neutropenia, Post-exposure prophylaxis of inhalational anthrax, Conjunctivitis/corneal ulcers; **Class:** FQs; **Preg:** C; **CIs:** Hypersensitivity (cross-sensitivity within class may exist), Concurrent use of tizanidine, QT prolongation, Do not use during pregnancy unless potential benefit outweighs potential fetal risk, Use only for treatment of anthrax and complicated UTIs in children 1–17 yr due to possible arthropathy; **ADRs:** SEIZURES, agitation, dizziness, drowsiness, HA, insomnia, QT prolongation, PSEUDOMEMBRANOUS COLITIS, abdominal pain, diarrhea, nausea, vaginitis, photosensitivity, rash, SJS, ↑ BG, ↓ BG, phlebitis at IV site, tendonitis, tendon rupture, peripheral neuropathy, ANAPHYLAXIS; **Interactions:** May ↑ tizanidine levels (contraindicated), May ↑ levels/toxicity of CYP1A2 substrates, ↑ risk of QT prolongation with other QT-prolonging drugs, May ↑ theophylline levels/toxicity; if concurrent use cannot be avoided, monitor theophylline levels, Antacids, Ca^{++} supplements, iron salts, dairy products, zinc, aluminum, didanosine, or sucralfate may ↓ absorption, May ↑ the effects of warfarin, May ↑ or ↓ phenytoin levels, May ↑ risk of hypoglycemia with sulfonylureas, May ↑ methotrexate levels/toxicity, May ↑ risk of nephrotoxicity from cyclosporine, May ↑ risk of seizures when used with NSAIDs, ↑ risk of tendon rupture with corticosteroids; **Dose:** *PO: Adults: Gonorrhea*—250 mg single dose. *Uncomplicated UTIs*—250 mg q 12 hr × 3 days *or* 500 mg daily × 3 days (as ER tabs). *Complicated UTIs*—500 mg q 12 hr × 7–14 days *or* 1000 mg daily × 7–14 days (as ER tabs). *Other infections*—500–750 mg q 12 hr; *IV: Adults: UTIs*—200–400 mg q 12 hr. *Other infections*—400 mg q 12 hr (may be given q 8 hr for severe infections or in febrile neutropenia); *Ophth: Adults and Peds:* >1 yr for soln, >2 yr for oint. *Soln*—Instill 1–2 gtt in eye q 2 hr while awake × 2 days, then 1–2 gtt q 4 hr while awake × 5 days. *Oint*—Apply 1/2-in. ribbon to conjunctival sac tid × 2 days, then bid × 5 days; *PO: Peds:* 1–17 yr.

Complicated UTIs—10–20 mg/kg q 12 hr (max: 750 mg/dose). *Anthrax*—15 mg/kg q 12 hr (max: 500 mg/dose); *IV: Peds:* 1–17 yr *Complicated UTIs*—6–10 mg/kg q 8 hr (max: 400 mg/dose). *Anthrax*—10 mg/kg q 12 hr (max: 400 mg/dose); *Renal Impairment: Adults:* ↓ dose if CrCl ≤50 ml/min (<30 ml/min for ER tabs and IV); **Availability (G):** Tabs: 100, 250, 500, 750 mg; ER tabs: 500, 1000 mg; Oral susp: 250 mg/5 ml, 500 mg/5 ml; Ophth oint: 0.3%; Ophth soln: 0.3%; Inject: 10 mg/ml; **Monitor:** HR, BP, temp, sputum, U/A, CBC, BG (in patients with DM); **Notes:** Give ≥2 hr before (≥4 hr for Proquin XR) or ≥6 hr after products/foods containing Ca++, Mg++, aluminum, iron, or zinc. Do not give susp through feeding tube (can crush IR tabs and dilute in H_2O). Do not split, crush, or chew ER tabs. Advise patient to wear sunscreen.

cisplatin (Platinol-AQ) Uses: Metastatic testicular and ovarian CA, Advanced bladder CA; **Class:** alkylating agents; **Preg:** D; **CIs:** Hypersensitivity to cisplatin, carboplatin, or platinum-containing drugs, Renal impairment, Bone marrow depression, Hearing impairment, Pregnancy or lactation; **ADRs:** hearing loss, ↑ LFTs, N/V, ↑ bilirubin, constipation, diarrhea, stomatitis, nephrotoxicity, alopecia, rash, ↓ Ca++, ↓ K+, ↓ Mg++, ↓ Na+, ANEMIA, LEUKOPENIA, THROMBOCYTOPENIA, hyperuricemia, peripheral neuropathy, ANAPHYLACTIC-LIKE REACTIONS; **Interactions:** ↑ risk of nephrotoxicity and ototoxicity with other nephrotoxic and ototoxic drugs (e.g., aminoglycosides, loop diuretics), ↑ risk of hypokalemia and hypomagnesemia with loop diuretics and amphotericin B, ↑ bone marrow suppression with other antineoplastics or radiation therapy; **Dose:** *IV: Adults: Testicular CA*—20 mg/m^2 daily × 5 days repeat q 3–4 wk. *Ovarian CA*—75–100 mg/m^2, repeat q 4 wk in combination with cyclophosphamide *or* 100 mg/m^2 q 3 wk if used as single agent. *Bladder CA*—50–70 mg/m^2 q 3–4 wk as single agent; *IV: Peds:* 15–20 mg/m^2/daily × 5 days q 3–4 wk *or* 37–75 mg/m^2 q 2–3 wk *or* 50–100 mg/m^2 over 4–6 hr q 3–4 wk (refer to individual protocols); **Availability (G):** Inject: 1 mg/ml; **Monitor:** BP, HR, temp, neuro exam, hearing, N/V, bleeding, S/S infection/anaphylaxis, I/Os, BUN/SCr, electrolytes, CBC (with diff), LFTs, bilirubin; **Notes: High Alert:** Fatalities have occurred with chemotherapeutic agents. Before administering, clarify all ambiguous orders; double-check single, daily, and course-of-therapy dose limits; have second practitioner independently double-check original order, calculations, and infusion pump settings. Do not confuse carboplatin with cisplatin. Renal function must normalize (SCr <1.5 mg/dl and/or BUN <25 mg/dl) before giving subsequent doses. Nadir for platelets and WBCs = 18–23 days; recovery usually occurs by Day 39. WBCs should be ≥4000 and platelets ≥100,000 to give subsequent doses. Hydrate patient with at least 1–2 L of IV fluid 8–12 hr before initiating therapy. To ↓ risk of nephrotoxicity, maintain a urinary output of ≥100 ml/hr × 4 hr before and ≥24 hr after administration.

Amifostine may be administered to minimize nephrotoxicity. Severe and protracted N/V usually occur 1–4 hr after dose and may last for 24 hr. Administer parenteral antiemetic agents 30–45 min before therapy and routinely for next 24 hr.

citalopram (Celexa) Uses: Depression; **Class:** SSRIs; **Preg:** C; **CIs:** Hypersensitivity, Concurrent MAOI or pimozide therapy, May ↑ risk of suicidal thoughts/behaviors, esp. during early treatment or dose adjustment; risk may be ↑ in children or adolescents; **ADRs:** SUICIDAL THOUGHTS, drowsiness, insomnia, agitation, anxiety, fatigue, migraines, cough, postural hypotension, ↑ HR, abdominal pain, dry mouth, N/V/D, anorexia, flatulence, ↑ appetite, ↑ saliva, amenorrhea, dysmenorrhea, ejaculatory delay, ED, ↓ libido, ↑ sweating, pruritus, rash, arthralgia, myalgia, paresthesia, tremor, yawning; **Interactions:** ↑ risk of toxicity with MAOIs (discontinue for ≥2 wk), ↑ risk of QT prolongation with pimozide (contraindicated), Use cautiously with other centrally acting drugs (including antihistamines, opioid analgesics, and sedative/hypnotics; use with alcohol not recommended), Cimetidine may ↑ levels, ↑ risk of serotonin syndrome with lithium $5HT_1$ agonists, linezolid, tramadol, or St. John's wort, May ↑ levels of metoprolol, May ↑ risk of bleeding with antiplatelets, NSAIDs, or warfarin; **Dose:** *PO: Adults:* 20 mg daily initially; may ↑ by 20 mg/day at weekly intervals, up to 40 mg/day (max: 60 mg/day); *Hepatic Impairment: PO: Adults:* 20 mg daily initially; may ↑ to 40 mg/day only in nonresponding patients; **Availability (G):** Tabs: 10, 20, 40 mg; Oral soln: 10 mg/5 ml; **Monitor:** Mental status, suicidal thoughts/behaviors, sexual dysfunction; **Notes:** Do not confuse with Celebrex (celecoxib), Cerebyx (fosphenytoin), or Zyprexa (olanzapine).

clarithromycin (Biaxin, Biaxin XL) Uses: Respiratory tract infections, pharyngitis/tonsillitis, OM, and skin/skin structure infections due to susceptible organisms (e.g., *S. pneumo*, *S. pyogenes*, *S. aureus*, *M. catarrhalis*, *H. flu*, *Chlamydia pneumoniae*, *Mycoplasma*), Prevention or treatment of disseminated MAC infection, Part of a combination regimen for *H. pylori*; **Class:** macrolides; **Preg:** C; **CIs:** Hypersensitivity to macrolides or ketolides, Concurrent use of pimozide or ergot derivatives, Avoid use during pregnancy unless no alternatives are available; **ADRs:** HA, pruritus, rash, SJS, PSEUDOMEMBRANOUS COLITIS, abdominal pain, abnormal taste, dyspepsia, N/V/D; **Interactions:** May ↑ levels of CYP3A4 substrates, CYP3A4 inhibitors may ↑ levels/effects, CYP3A4 inducers may ↓ levels/effects, ↑ risk of QT prolongation and arrhythmias with pimozide (contraindicated), May ↑ risk of ergot toxicity with ergotamine or dihydroergotamine (contraindicated, Use caution when using with other drugs that prolong the QT interval, May ↑ effects of warfarin, May ↑ risk of digoxin toxicity, May ↑ or ↓ effects of zidovudine, ↑ risk of colchicine toxicity, esp. in the elderly; **Dose:** *PO: Adults:*

Pharyngitis/tonsillitis—250 mg q 12 hr × 10 days. *Acute maxillary sinusitis*—500 mg q 12 hr × 14 days *or* 1000 mg daily × 14 days as ER tabs. *Acute exacerbation of chronic bronchitis*—250–500 mg q 12 hr × 7–14 days *or* 1000 mg daily × 7 days as ER tabs. *CAP*—250 mg q 12 hr × 7–14 days or 1000 mg daily × 7 days as ER tabs; *Skin/skin structure infections*—250 mg q 12 hr × 7–14 days. *H. pylori*—500 mg bid-tid with a PPI or ranitidine with or without amoxicillin × 10–14 days. *MAC prophylaxis/treatment*—500 mg bid (use with another antimycobacterial for treatment); *PO: Peds: Most infections*—7.5 mg/kg q 12 hr × 10 days (up to 500 mg/dose for MAC); *Renal Impairment: Adults and Peds:* ↓ dose if CrCl <30 ml/min; **Availability (G):** Tabs: 250, 500 mg; ER tabs: 500 mg; Oral susp: 125 mg/5 ml, 250 mg/5 ml; **Monitor:** BP, HR, temp, sputum, U/A, CBC; **Notes:** Administer ER tabs with food or milk. Do not crush, chew, or break ER tabs.

clindamycin (Cleocin, Cleocin T, Clinda-Derm, Clindagel, Clindesse, Clindamax, Clindets, Evoclin) **Uses:** *PO: IM: IV:* Respiratory tract infections, skin/skin structure infections, gynecological infections, intra-abdominal infections, septicemia, bone/joint infections caused by susceptible anaerobic organisms and GPC, **Top:** Acne, *Vag:* Bacterial vaginosis; **Class:** lincosamides; **Preg:** B; **CIs:** Hypersensitivity, Previous pseudomembranous colitis; **ADRs:** ↓ BP (with rapid IV administration), PSEUDOMEMBRANOUS COLITIS, bitter taste (IV only), ↑ LFTs, N/V/D, burning/itching/dry skin (topical), rash, phlebitis at IV site; **Interactions:** May ↑ effects of neuromuscular blocking agents, **Top:** ↑ risk of irritation with irritants, abrasives, or desquamating agents; **Dose:** *PO: Adults:* 150–450 mg q 6 hr; *PO: Peds:* >1 mo 8–25 mg/kg/day in 3–4 divided doses; *IM: IV: Adults:* 1200–2700 mg/day in 2–4 divided doses (max: 4.8 g/day); *IM: IV: Peds:* 1 mo–16 yr 20–40 mg/kg/day in 3–4 divided doses; *IM: IV: Infants:* <1 mo 15–20 mg/kg/day in 3–4 divided doses; *Vag: Adults and Adolescents: Cleocin, Clindamax*—1 applicatorful (5 g) at bedtime × 3 or 7 days (7 days in pregnant patients). *Clindesse*—1 applicatorful (5 g) single dose. *Cleocin*—1 supp (100 mg) at bedtime × 3 nights; **Top:** *Adults and Adolescents: Lotion, gel, soln*—Apply bid. *Foam*—Apply daily; **Availability (G):** Caps: 75, 150, 300 mg; Oral susp: 75 mg/5 ml; Inject: 150 mg/ml, 300 mg/50 ml, 600 mg/50 ml, 900 mg/50 ml; **Top:** 1% lotion, gel, foam, solution, single-use applicators; Vag cream: 2%; Vag supp: 100 mg; **Monitor:** BP, HR, temp, sputum, U/A, CBC, LFTs, bowel movements (diarrhea), stool for blood; **Notes:** ↑ risk of C. diff. Vag cream contains mineral oil (may weaken condoms; do not use within 72 hr of cream).

clobetasol (Clobex, Cormax, Olux, Olux E, Temovate, Temovate E) **Uses:** Management of inflammation and pruritis associated with various dermatoses; **Class:** corticosteroids; **Preg:** C;

CIs: Hypersensitivity, Children <12 yr (safety not established); **ADRs:** burning, dryness, folliculitis, hypersensitivity reactions, hypopigmentation, irritation, secondary infection, striae, adrenal suppression (with use of occlusive dressings or long-term therapy); **Interactions:** None significant; **Dose: Top:** *Adults and Peds:* ≥12 yr Apply bid for up to 2 wk; **Availability (G):** Cream/Oint/Gel/Lotion/Foam/Spray: 0.05%; Scalp soln/ Shampoo: 0.05%; **Monitor:** Skin condition (inflammation, erythema, pruritis); **Notes:** Oints are more occlusive and preferred for dry, scaly lesions. Creams should be used on oozing or intertriginous areas (may cause more skin drying than oints). Soln, spray, and shampoo are useful in hairy areas.

clocortolone (Cloderm) Uses: Management of inflammation and pruritis associated with various dermatoses; **Class:** corticosteroids; **Preg:** C; **CIs:** Hypersensitivity; **ADRs:** burning, dryness, folliculitis, hypersensitivity reactions, hypertrichosis, hypopigmentation, irritation, secondary infection, striae, adrenal suppression (with use of occlusive dressings or long-term therapy); **Interactions:** None significant; **Dose: Top:** *Adults:* Apply tid; **Availability:** Cream: 0.1%; **Monitor:** Skin condition (inflammation, erythema, pruritis); **Notes:** Creams should be used on oozing or intertriginous areas.

clonazepam (Klonopin) Uses: Petit mal, petit mal variant, akinetic, or myoclonic seizures, Panic disorder with or without agoraphobia; **Class:** benzodiazepines; **Preg:** D; **CIs:** Hypersensitivity to clonazepam or other BZs, Severe liver disease, Narrow-angle glaucoma, Pregnancy/ lactation; **ADRs:** ataxia, behavioral changes, depression, dizziness, drowsiness, diplopia, nystagmus, ↑ secretions, ↑ LFTs, hypotonia, psychological/ physical dependence, tolerance; **Interactions:** ↑ CNS depression with other CNS depressants, including alcohol, antihistamines, opioids, and sedative/hypnotics, CYP3A4 inhibitors may ↑ levels/toxicity, CYP3A4 inducers may ↓ levels/effects; **Dose:** *PO: Adults: Seizure disorders*—0.5 mg tid; may ↑ by 0.5–1 mg q 3 days (max: 20 mg/day). *Panic disorder*—0.25 mg bid; may ↑ after 3 days to target dose of 1 mg/day (max: 4 mg/day); *PO: Peds:* <10 yr or ≤30 kg. *Seizure disorders*—0.01–0.03 mg/kg/day in 2–3 divided doses; may ↑ by 0.25–0.5 mg q 3 days until seizures controlled (max: 0.2 mg/kg/day); **Availability (G):** Tabs: 0.5, 1, 2 mg; Orally-disintegrating tabs: 0.125, 0.25, 0.5, 1, 2 mg; **Monitor:** Neuro exam, mental status, seizure activity, LFTs; **Notes:** Schedule IV controlled substance. Do not discontinue abruptly (may cause withdrawal); taper by 0.25 mg q 3 days (some patients may require longer taper period [several mo]). Potential for dependence/abuse with long-term use (use with caution in patients at risk for addiction). Do not confuse with clonidine. Flumazenil is antidote.

clonidine (Catapres, Catapres-TTS, Duraclon) Uses: *PO: Transdermal:* HTN, *Epidural:* CA pain unresponsive to opioids alone; **Class:** adrenergics; **Preg:** C; **CIs:** Hypersensitivity, Recent MI, CVA,

C

or chronic renal insufficiency, *Epidural*—inject site infection, anticoagulant therapy, bleeding problems, or hemodynamic instability; **ADRs:** confusion, dizziness, drowsiness, weakness, depression, insomnia, nightmares, ↓ HR, ↓ BP (↑ with epidural), palpitations, constipation, dry mouth, N/V, ↓ libido, erythema/pruritis (with transdermal), rash, withdrawal phenomenon; **Interactions:** ↑ sedation with CNS depressants, including alcohol, antihistamines, opioid analgesics, and sedative/hypnotics, ↑ risk of hypotension with other antihypertensives, ↑ risk of bradycardia with beta blockers, digoxin, diltiazem, or verapamil, TCAs may ↑ antihypertensive effect, ↑ risk of hypertensive crisis if concurrent beta blocker discontinued, Epidural clonidine prolongs the effects of epidurally administered local anesthetics; **Dose:** *PO: Adults: HTN*—0.1 mg bid; may ↑ by 0.1–0.2 mg/day q 2–4 days; usual MD is 0.2–0.8 mg/day in 2–3 divided doses (max: 2.4 mg/day). *Hypertensive urgency*—0.1–0.2 mg × 1, then 0.1 mg q hr until BP controlled or 0.6 mg total has been administered; *PO: Peds: HTN*—5–10 mcg/kg/day in 2–3 divided doses; may ↑ gradually q 5–7 days to 25 mcg/kg/day (max: 0.9 mg/day); *Transdermal: Adults: HTN*—Transdermal system delivering 0.1 mg/24 hr applied q 7 days; may ↑ by 0.1 mg q 1–2 wk (max: 0.6 mg/24 hr); *Epidural: Adults:* 30 mcg/hr initially; titrate according to need (max: 40 mcg/hr); *Renal Impairment: Adults and Peds:* ↓ dose for CrCl <10 ml/min; **Availability (G): Tabs:** 0.1, 0.2, 0.3 mg; Transdermal: 0.1 mg/24 hr, 0.2 mg/24 hr, 0.3 mg/24 hr; Soln for epidural inject: 100 mcg/ml, 500 mcg/ml; **Monitor:** BP, HR; Epidural: pain, S/S infection; **Notes:** Do not discontinue abruptly (may cause hypertensive crises); taper over 2–4 days. Change patch q 7 days. When changing from PO to patch, overlap for 3 days, then discontinue PO. Patch cannot be worn in MRI. Do not confuse with clonazepam.

clopidogrel (Plavix) Uses: ↓ atherosclerotic events (MI, stroke, vascular death) in patients at risk for such events including recent MI/stroke or established PAD, ACS (UA/NSTEMI or STEMI); **Class:** platelet aggregation inhibitors; **Preg:** B; **CIs:** Hypersensitivity, Pathologic bleeding (PUD, intracranial hemorrhage), Lactation; **ADRs:** abdominal pain, diarrhea, dyspepsia, gastritis, nausea, pruritus, purpura, rash, BLEEDING, THROMBOTIC THROMBOCYTOPENIC PURPURA; **Interactions:** ↑ risk of bleeding with GpIIb/IIIa inhibitors, aspirin, NSAIDs, heparin, LMWHs, direct thrombin inhibitors, thrombolytic agents, and warfarin; **Dose:** *PO: Adults: Recent MI/stroke or established PAD*—75 mg daily. *ACS*—LD of 300 mg × 1 (LD is optional for STEMI), then 75 mg daily; aspirin 75–325 mg daily should be given concurrently; **Availability:** Tabs: 75, 300 mg; **Monitor:** Bleeding, S/S MI/stroke/PAD, CBC; **Notes:** May also be used after stent implantation (clopidogrel + aspirin should be used for ≥1 mo for bare-metal stents, and for ≥12 mo for drug-eluting stents). Discontinue for 5 days before surgery.

clotrimazole (Cruex, Gyne-Lotrimin-3, Gyne-Lotrimin-7, Lotrimin AF, Mycelex) **Uses:** Treatment of a variety of fungal infections, including cutaneous candidiasis, oropharyngeal candidiasis, vulvovaginal candidiasis, tinea pedis (athlete's foot), tinea cruris (jock itch), tinea corporis (ringworm), and tinea versicolor; **Class:** azole antifungals; **Preg:** B (topical), C (troches); **CIs:** Hypersensitivity; **ADRs:** ↑ LFTs (troches), N/V (troches), burning, itching, local hypersensitivity reactions, redness, stinging; **Interactions:** May ↑ levels of CYP3A4 substrates (troches); **Dose:** *PO: Adults and Peds:* >3 yr *Prophylaxis*—10 mg tid for duration of chemotherapy or until steroid dose ↓ to maintenance. *Treatment*—10 mg 5 ×/day × 14 days; **Top:** *Adults and Peds:* >12 yr Apply cream or soln bid × 1–4 wk; *Vag: Adults and Peds:* >12 yr 1 applicatorful (5 g) of 1% cream at bedtime × 7 days *or* 1 applicatorful (5 g) of 2% cream at bedtime × 3 days; **Availability (G):** Cream/Soln: 1%; Troches: 10 mg; Vag cream: 1%, 2%; **Monitor:** Skin condition, LFTs (with troche); **Notes:** Do not swallow troche; dissolve in mouth for 15–30 min. Patient should complete full course of therapy, even if feeling better. Therapy for vag infection should be continued during menstrual period; patient should remain recumbent for ≥30 min after insertion.

clozapine (Clozaril, FazaClo) **Uses:** Refractory schizophrenia, To ↓ recurrent suicidal behavior in schizophrenic patients; **Class:** antipsychotics; **Preg:** B; **CIs:** Hypersensitivity, Myeloproliferative disorder, Paralytic ileus, Severe CNS depression/coma, Uncontrolled seizure disorder, Granulocytopenia, Concurrent use of drugs that cause bone marrow depression, Lactation; **ADRs:** NMS, SEIZURES, dizziness, sedation, HA, tremor, visual disturbances, orthostatic hypotension, ↓ BP, ↑ HR, constipation, dry mouth, ↑ salivation, hepatitis, N/V, ↑ wt, sweating, ↑ BG, AGRANULOCYTOSIS, LEUKOPENIA, fever; **Interactions:** CYP1A2 inhibitors, CYP2D6 inhibitors, and CYP3A4 inhibitors may ↑ levels/toxicity, CYP1A2 inducers and CYP3A4 inducers may ↓ levels/effects, May ↑ effects/toxicity of CYP2D6 substrates, ↑ anticholinergic effects with other agents having anticholinergic properties, including antihistamines, quinidine, disopyramide, and antidepressants, ↑ CNS depression with other CNS depressants, including alcohol, antihistamines, opioids, and sedative/hypnotics, ↑ risk of hypotension with antihypertensives, ↑ risk of bone marrow suppression with antineoplastics or radiation therapy; **Dose:** *PO: Adults:* 12.5 mg daily-bid initially; may ↑ by 25–50 mg/day over a period of 2 wk up to target dose of 300–450 mg/day. May subsequently ↑ by up to 100 mg/day by no more than once or twice weekly (max: 900 mg/day). Treatment should be continued for ≥2 yr in patients with suicidal behavior; **Availability (G):** Tabs: 25, 50, 100, 200 mg; Orally-disintegrating tabs: 12.5, 25, 100 mg; **Monitor:** Mental status, suicidal thoughts/behaviors, wt, CBC (with diff), BG, BP (sitting, standing), HR, S/S NMS, seizure activity; **Notes:** Monitor WBC (with diff) and ANC before initiation of therapy, then q wk for first 6 mo; if these counts remain acceptable (WBC ≥3500 and ANC ≥2000), then check q 2 wk during next 6 mo; if these counts still remain acceptable, can then perform q 4 wk; if discontinued, monitor weekly for ≥4 wk or until counts acceptable. Available in a 1-wk supply through Clozaril Patient Management System. Do not discontinue abruptly (taper over 1–2 wk). Minimal risk of EPS/tardive dyskinesia.

codeine (No Trade) Uses: Mild-to-moderate pain, Antitussive (in smaller doses); **Class:** opioid agonists; **Preg:** C; **CIs:** Hypersensitivity, Pregnancy or lactation (avoid chronic use); **ADRs:** confusion, sedation, euphoria, hallucinations, blurred vision, diplopia, miosis, respiratory depression, ↓ BP, constipation, N/V, urinary retention, physical/psychological dependence, tolerance; **Interactions:** Use with extreme caution in patients receiving MAOIs (↓ initial dose to 25% of usual dose), ↑ CNS depression with other CNS depressants including alcohol, antihistamines, and sedative/hypnotics, Use of partial antagonists (e.g., buprenorphine, butorphanol, nalbuphine, pentazocine) may precipitate opioid withdrawal in physically dependent patients; **Dose:** *PO: Adults: Analgesic*—15–120 mg q 4–6 hr prn. *Antitussive*—10–20 mg q 4–6 hr prn (max: 120 mg/day); *PO: Peds: Analgesic*—0.5–1 mg/kg q 4–6 hr (up to 4 × daily) prn. *Antitussive*—1–1.5 mg/kg/day divided q 4–6 hr prn (max: 30 mg/day for patients <6 yr or 60 mg/day for those 6–12 yr); *IM: IV: Subcut: Adults: Analgesic*—15–120 mg q 4–6 hr prn; *IM: IV: Subcut: Infants and Peds: Analgesic*—0.5–1 mg/kg q 4–6 hr prn; **Availability (G):** Tabs: 15, 30, 60 mg; Inject: 15 mg/ml, 30 mg/ml; **Monitor:** BP, HR, RR, bowel function, pain; **Notes:** Schedule II controlled substance. When combined with other drugs, tablet form is Schedule III, liquid is Schedule IV, and elixir/cough suppressant is Schedule V. Metabolized to morphine. Bowel regimen needed if using >2–3 days. Use equianalgesic chart when changing routes or when changing from one opioid to another. Potential for dependence/abuse with long-term use (should not prevent patients from receiving adequate analgesia). Naloxone is antidote.

colchicine (No Trade) Uses: Treatment and prevention of gouty attacks; **Class:** none assigned; **Preg:** D; **CIs:** Hypersensitivity, Pregnancy, Severe renal (CrCl <10 ml/min), hepatic, or GI disease, Bone marrow depression; **ADRs:** abdominal pain, N/V/D, alopecia, AGRANULOCYTOSIS, APLASTIC ANEMIA, leukopenia, thrombocytopenia, phlebitis at IV site, peripheral neuritis; **Interactions:** CYP3A4 inhibitors may ↑ levels/toxicity, CYP3A4 inducers may ↓ levels/effects, ↑ bone marrow suppression with antineoplastics or radiation therapy, Additive adverse GI effects with NSAIDs; **Dose:** *PO: Adults: Treatment*—0.6–1.2 mg, then 0.6 mg q 1–2 hr until symptoms subside or side effects occur (max total dose: 6 mg). *Prophylaxis*—0.6 mg daily (may be used up to tid or as little as 1–4 × weekly); *IV: Adults: Treatment*—1–2 mg initially, then 0.5 mg q 6 hr until symptoms subside or side effects occur (max total dose: 4 mg); *Renal Impairment: Adults:* ↓ dose if CrCl <50 ml/min; **Availability (G):** Tabs: 0.6 mg; Inject: 0.5 mg/ml; **Monitor:** Pain, S/S toxicity (weakness, abdominal discomfort, N/V/D), BUN/SCr, CBC; **Notes:** Do not administer additional doses for ≥7 days after full course of IV therapy.

C

colesevelam (Welchol) **Uses:** Primary hypercholesterolemia, Improving glycemic control in adults with type 2 DM (with diet and exercise); **Class:** bile acid sequestrants; **Preg:** B; **CIs:** Hypersensitivity, History of bowel obstruction, TGs >500 mg/dl; **ADRs:** dyspepsia, constipation, nausea, ↓ BG, vitamin A, D, E, and K deficiency, ↑ TGs; **Interactions:** May ↓ absorption/effects of thyroid hormones, glyburide, phenytoin, warfarin, oral contraceptives containing ethinyl estradiol and norethindrone and fat soluble vitamins (A, D, E, and K); **Dose:** *PO: Adults:* 3 tabs bid or 6 tabs daily; **Availability:** Tabs: 625 mg; **Monitor:** Lipid panel, BG, A1C; **Notes:** Interacting drugs should be administered ≥4 hr before colesevelam. Take with a meal and liquid.

cortisone (No Trade) **Uses:** Replacement therapy in adrenal insufficiency; **Class:** corticosteroids; **Preg:** C; **CIs:** Active fungal infections, Lactation (avoid chronic use); **ADRs:** depression, euphoria, hallucinations, HA, insomnia, psychoses, restlessness, cataracts, ↑ IOP, ↑ BP, edema, PEPTIC ULCER, nausea, ↑ appetite, ↓ wound healing, hirsutism, adrenal suppression, ↑ BG, amenorrhea, ↓ K+, ↑ wt, muscle wasting, tendon rupture, osteoporosis, cushingoid appearance (moon face, buffalo hump), infection; **Interactions:** CYP3A4 inhibitors may ↑ levels, CYP3A4 inducers may ↓ levels, ↑ risk of hypokalemia with thiazide and loop diuretics, or amphotericin B, May ↑ requirement for insulin or oral hypoglycemic agents, ↑ risk of adverse GI effects with NSAIDs (including aspirin) and alcohol, At chronic doses that suppress adrenal function, may ↓ the antibody response to and ↑ risk of ADRs from live-virus vaccines, May ↑ or ↓ the effects of warfarin, May ↑ risk of tendon rupture when used with FQs; **Dose:** *PO: Adults:* 25–300 mg/day divided q 12–24 hr; *PO: Peds:* 0.5–0.75 mg/kg/day (20–25 mg/m²/day) divided q 8 hr; **Availability (G):** Tabs: 25 mg; **Monitor:** BP, HR, edema, wt, electrolytes, BG, S/S of adrenal insufficiency; **Notes:** Give in AM. Chronic treatment will lead to adrenal suppression; use lowest possible dose for shortest period of time. Need to taper therapy (abrupt discontinuation may lead to adrenal insufficiency).

cromolyn (Crolom, Intal, Gastrocrom, NasalCrom) **Uses:** *Inhaln:* Asthma, Prevention of exercise-induced bronchospasm, *Intranasal:* Prevention/treatment of seasonal and perennial allergic rhinitis, *PO:* Mastocytosis, *Ophth:* Vernal conjunctivitis/keratitis; **Class:** mast cell stabilizers; **Preg:** B; **CIs:** Hypersensitivity, Acute asthma attacks (inhaln products), Children <2 yr (safety not established);

ADRs: ANGIOEDEMA, nasal irritation, nasal congestion, sneezing, throat/tracheal irritation, cough, wheezing, bronchospasm, nausea, unpleasant taste, ANAPHYLAXIS; **Interactions:** None known; **Dose:** *Inhaln: Adults and Peds:* >2 yr *Nebulized soln*—Asthma: 20 mg qid; Prevention of bronchospasm: 20 mg 10–15 min before exercise or allergen exposure; *Inhaler (for adults and children ≥5 yr)*—Asthma: 2 inhaln qid (can taper to lowest effective dose); Prevention of bronchospasm: 2 inhaln 10–15 min before exercise or allergen exposure; *Intranasal: Adults and Peds:* ≥2 yr 1 spray in each nostril 3–4 ×/day; *PO: Adults and Peds:* >12 yr 200 mg qid; if symptoms persist after 2–3 wk, may ↑ dose (max: 40 mg/kg/day); *PO: Peds:* 2–12 yr 100 mg qid; if symptoms persist after 2–3 wk, may ↑ dose (max: 40 mg/kg/day); *Ophth: Adults:* Instill 1–2 drops in each eye 4–6 ×/day; **Availability:** Inhaln soln: 10 mg/ml; Inhaln aerosol: 800 mcg/inhaln; Nasal soln: 40 mg/ml (5.2 mg/spray)^OTC; Ophth soln: 4%; Oral soln: 100 mg/5 ml; **Monitor:** Lung sounds, S/S rhinitis/asthma; **Notes:** For PO, give 30 min before meals and at bedtime. Inhaler is for prophylactic use (may take 2–4 wk to see effect). For intranasal, start using product up to 1 wk before coming into contact with allergen and then daily while in contact with allergen.

cyanocobalamin (Calomist, Nascobal) **Uses:** Vitamin B_{12} deficiency (parenteral products or nasal spray should be used when deficiency due to malabsorption), Pernicious anemia (parenteral products should be used for initial therapy; nasal or PO products not indicated until patient has achieved hematologic remission following parenteral therapy and has no signs of CNS involvement), Part of the Schilling test (vitamin B_{12} absorption test) (diagnostic); **Class:** water-soluble vitamins; **Preg:** C; **CIs:** Hypersensitivity; **ADRs:** dizziness, HA, rhinorrhea, diarrhea, pain at IM site, ANAPHYLAXIS; **Interactions:** Chloramphenicol may ↓ hematologic response to vitamin B_{12}, Excessive intake of alcohol may ↓ absorption/effectiveness; **Dose:** *PO: Adults: Vitamin B_{12} deficiency*—250 mcg/day. *Pernicious anemia (for hematologic remission only)*—1000–2000 mcg/day; *IM: Subcut: Adults: Vitamin B_{12} deficiency*—30 mcg/day × 5–10 days, then 100–200 mcg/mo. *Pernicious anemia*—100 mcg/day × 6–7 days; if improvement, give same dose every other day × 7 doses, then q 3–4 days × 2–3 wk; once in remission, give 100 mcg/month. *Schilling test*—Flushing dose = 1000 mcg; *IM: Subcut: Peds: Vitamin B_{12} deficiency*—0.2 mcg/kg × 2 days, then 1000 mcg/day × 2–7 days, then 100 mcg/wk × 1 mo. *Pernicious anemia*—30–50 mcg/day × ≥2 wk (to total dose of 1000–5000 mcg), then 100 mcg/mo; *Intranasal: Adults: Calomist (for hematologic remission only)*—1 spray in each nostril daily; may be ↑ to bid if inadequate response. *Nascobal (for treatment and remission)*—1 spray in one nostril once weekly; **Availability (G):** Tabs: 50, 100, 250, 500, 1000 mcg; ER tabs: 1000, 1500 mcg; SL tabs: 1000, 2500, 5000 mcg; Loz: 50, 100, 250, 500 mcg; Nasal spray:

25 mcg/0.1 ml spray (Calomist), 500 mcg/0.1 ml spray (Nascobal); Inject: 1000 mcg/ml; **Monitor:** S/S vitamin B_{12} deficiency, folate/vitamin B_{12}/iron levels, Hgb/Hct, reticulocyte count; **Notes:** PO usually not recommended due to poor absorption (should be used only if patient refuses IM, deep subcut, or intranasal route of administration). If subcut, deep subcut administration preferred. IV route not recommended. For intranasal, do not give dose within 1 hr of hot foods or liquids.

cyclobenzaprine (Amrix, Fexmid, Flexeril) **Uses:** Short-term relief of acute painful musculoskeletal conditions associated with muscle spasm; **Class:** skeletal muscle relaxants; **Preg:** B; **CIs:** Hypersensitivity, Current or recent (within 2 wk) use of MAOIs, Post-MI, Arrhythmias or conduction disorders, HF, Hyperthyroidism, Children <15 yr (safety not established); **ADRs:** dizziness, drowsiness, confusion, HA, dry mouth, blurred vision, ARRHYTHMIAS, constipation, nausea, unpleasant taste, urinary retention; **Interactions:** ↑ CNS depression with other CNS depressants, including alcohol, antihistamines, opioids, and sedative/hypnotics, ↑ risk of anticholinergic effects with other anticholinergic agents, Avoid use within 14 days of MAOIs (hyperpyretic crisis, seizures, and death may occur); **Dose:** *PO: Adults and Peds:* >15 yr *IR*—5 mg tid; may ↑ to 7.5–10 mg tid, if needed. *ER (not for peds)*—15–30 mg daily; **Availability (G):** Tabs: 5, 7.5, 10 mg; ER caps: 15, 30 mg; **Monitor:** Pain, ROM; **Notes:** Should not be used for >2–3 wk. Do not crush or chew ER caps.

cyclophosphamide (Cytoxan) **Uses:** Lymphomas, Multiple myeloma, Leukemias, Mycosis fungoides, Neuroblastoma, Retinoblastoma, Breast CA, Minimal change nephrotic syndrome in children; **Class:** alkylating agents; **Preg:** D; **CIs:** Hypersensitivity, Pregnancy/lactation, Bone marrow depression; **ADRs:** PULMONARY FIBROSIS, HF, N/V, HEMORRHAGIC CYSTITIS, hematuria, alopecia, rash, ↓ fertility, SIADH, LEUKOPENIA, thrombocytopenia, anemia, ↑ uric acid; **Interactions:** ↑ risk of toxicity with phenobarbital, phenytoin, carbamazepine, or rifampin, Cardiotoxicity may be additive with other cardiotoxic agents (e.g., daunorubicin, doxorubicin), May ↓ digoxin levels, ↑ bone marrow suppression with other antineoplastics or radiation therapy; **Dose:** *PO: Adults and Peds: Malignancy*—1–5 mg/kg/day; *PO: Peds: Nephrotic syndrome*—2.5-3 mg/kg daily × 60–90 days; *IV: Adults and Peds:* 40–50 mg/kg in divided doses over 2–5 days *or* 10–15 mg/kg q 7–10 days *or* 3–5 mg/kg twice weekly *or* 1.5–3 mg/kg/day. Other regimens may use larger doses; **Availability (G):** Tabs: 25, 50 mg; Inject: 500 mg, 1, 2 g; **Monitor:** BP, HR, temp, BUN/SCr, CBC (with diff), uric acid, U/A, LFTs, CXR, S/S infection, S/S HF, bleeding, I/Os, lung sounds; **Notes: High Alert:** Fatalities have occurred with chemotherapeutic agents. Before administering, clarify all ambiguous orders; double-check single, daily, and course-of-therapy dose limits; have second practitioner independently double-check original order, calculations, and infusion pump settings. To ↓ risk of hemorrhagic cystitis, fluid intake should be at least 3000 ml/day for adults and 1000–2000 ml/day for children; mesna can also be used. Give antiemetics. Leukopenia nadir = 7–12 days (recovery in 17–21 days). Maintain WBCs at 2500–4000. Give oral dose in AM.

cycloSPORINE (Neoral, Sandimmune, Gengraf, Restasis) Uses: *PO: IV:* Prevention and treatment of rejection in renal, cardiac, and hepatic transplantation (with corticosteroids), *PO:* Treatment of severe RA (not responsive to methotrexate) (Gengraf or Neoral), Severe recalcitrant psoriasis (Gengraf or Neoral), *Ophth:* ↑ lacrimation in ocular inflammatory disorders; **Class:** immunosuppressants; **Preg:** C; **CIs:** Hypersensitivity, Pregnancy/lactation (unless benefits outweigh risks), Renal dysfunction, uncontrolled HTN, or malignancy (for RA or psoriasis), Concurrent immunosuppressant or radiation therapy (for psoriasis), Active ocular infection (for ophth); **ADRs:** SEIZURES, tremor, flushing, HA, ocular burning (ophth), blurred vision (ophth), HTN, N/V/D, ↑ LFTs, PANCREATITIS, ↑ BUN/SCr, hirsutism, acne, ↑ K+, ↓ Mg++, anemia, leukopenia, thrombocytopenia, ↑ lipids, ↑ uric acid, paresthesia, gingival hyperplasia, hypersensitivity reactions, malignancy, infections; **Interactions:** CYP3A4 inhibitors may ↑ levels/toxicity, CYP3A4 inducers may ↓ levels/effects, May ↑ levels/toxicity of CYP3A4 substrates, ↑ risk of nephrotoxicity with other nephrotoxic drugs (e.g., amphotericin, aminoglycosides, FQs, trimethoprim/sulfamethoxazole, vancomycin, acyclovir, cisplatin, NSAIDs), ↑ immunosuppression with other immunosuppressants (e.g., cyclophosphamide, azathioprine, corticosteroids), ↑ risk of hyperkalemia with K+ sparing diuretics, K+ supplements, ACEIs, or ARBs, May ↑ digoxin and methotrexate levels, May ↓ antibody response to live-virus vaccines and ↑ risk of ADRs, ↑ risk of rhabdomyolysis with HMG-CoA reductase inhibitors; **Dose:** *PO: Adults and Peds: Transplant rejection prevention*-Sandimmune: 14–18 mg/kg 4–12 hr before transplant then 5–15 mg/kg/day divided q 12–24 hr postoperatively; taper by 5% weekly to MD of 3–10 mg/kg/day; Neoral/Gengraf: 4–12 mg/kg/day divided q 12 hr (dose varies depending on organ transplanted). *RA (Neoral/Gengraf only)*—1.25 mg/kg bid; may ↑ by 0.5–0.75 mg/kg/day after 8 and 12 wk (max: 4 mg/kg/day); *PO: Adults: Psoriasis (Neoral/Gengraf only)*—1.25 mg/kg bid; if no improvement after 4 wk, may ↑ by 0.5 mg/kg/day q 2 wk (max: 4 mg/kg/day); *IV: Adults and Peds: Transplant rejection prevention (Sandimmune only)*—5–6 mg/kg 4–12 hr before transplant, then 2–10 mg/kg/day in divided doses q 8–24 hr; change to PO as soon as possible; *PO: Ophth: Adults and Peds:* ≥16 yr Instill 1 drop in each eye q 12 hr; **Availability (G):** Caps, modified (Gengraf, Neoral): 25, 50, 100 mg; Oral soln, modified (Gengraf, Neoral): 100 mg/ml; Caps, non-modified (Sandimmune): 25, 100 mg; Oral soln, non-modified (Sandimmune): 100 mg/ml; Inject (Sandimmune): 50 mg/ml; Ophth emulsion (Restasis): 0.05%; **Monitor:** BP, S/S infection, BUN/SCr, electrolytes, uric acid, lipid panel, CBC,

LFTs, bilirubin, cyclosporine levels, wt, S/S organ rejection, ROM/ pain/joint swelling (for RA), skin lesions (for psoriasis); **Notes:** Neoral = Gengraf; Neoral/Gengraf ≠ Sandimmune. Doses are adjusted based on serum levels. Mix oral soln with milk or apple/orange juice. In RA and psoriasis, ↓ dose by 25–50% if ADRs occur. Therapeutic range: 100–400 ng/ml (varies by indication/organ transplanted).

cytarabine (Cytosar-U, DepoCyt) **Uses:** *IV:* Leukemias and non-Hodgkin's lymphomas, *IT:* Lymphomatous meningitis; **Class:** antimetabolites; **Preg:** D; **CIs:** Hypersensitivity, Pregnancy/lactation, Active meningeal infection (IT only); **ADRs:** CNS dysfunction (high dose), confusion, drowsiness, HA, corneal toxicity (high dose), hemorrhagic conjunctivitis (high dose), PULMONARY EDEMA (HIGH DOSE), N/V/D, ↑ LFTs, severe GI ulceration (high dose), stomatitis, alopecia, rash, sterility, LEUKOPENIA, anemia, thrombocytopenia, ↑ uric acid, CHEMICAL ARACHNOIDITIS, abnormal gait, cytarabine syndrome (fever, myalgia, bone pain, rash), ANAPHYLAXIS, fever; **Interactions:** ↑ bone marrow depression with other antineoplastics or radiation therapy, ↑ risk of cardiomyopathy when used in high-dose regimens with cyclophosphamide, May ↓ absorption of digoxin, Recent treatment with asparaginase may ↑ risk of pancreatitis, ↑ neurotoxicity with concurrently administered IT antineoplastics (IT only); **Dose:** *IV: Adults: Induction dose*—100–200 mg/m²/day × 5–10 days *or* 100 mg/m²/day × 7 days *or* 100 mg/m²/dose q 12 hr × 7 days. *MD*—70–200 mg/m²/day × 2–5 days/mo; *Subcut, IM: Adults: MD*—1–1.5 mg/kg q 1–4 wk; *IT: Adults: DepoCyt Induction* —50 mg (intraventricular or lumbar puncture) q 14 days × 2 doses (Wk 1 and 3); *Consolidation*—50 mg (intraventricular or lumbar puncture) q 14 days × 3 doses (Wk 5, 7, and 9), followed by one additional dose at Wk 13; *MD*—50 mg (intraventricular or lumbar puncture) q 28 days × 4 doses (Wk 17, 21, 25, and 29); *IT: Peds:* <1 yr: 20 mg; 1–2 yrs: 30 mg; 2–3 yrs: 50 mg; >3 yrs: 75 mg; *Renal Impairment: Adults and Peds:* ↓ dose if CrCl <60 ml/min; **Availability: (G):** Inject: 100, 500 mg, 1, 2 g; Liposome inject for IT use: 50 mg; **Monitor:** BP, HR, RR, temp, neuro exam (S/S neurotoxicity with IT), lung sounds, N/V, bleeding, S/S infection, S/S cytarabine syndrome (occurs 6–12 hr after administration), CBC (with diff), BUN/SCr, LFTs, bilirubin, uric acid, BM biopsy; **Notes:** **High Alert:** Fatalities have occurred with chemotherapeutic agents. Before administering, clarify all ambiguous orders; double-check single, daily, and course-of-therapy dose limits; have second practitioner independently double-check original order, calculations, and infusion pump settings. Start dexamethasone 4 mg PO/IV q 12 hr × 5 days beginning on first day of IT cytarabine therapy. Treat cytarabine syndrome with corticosteroids. Initial neutropenia nadir occurs in 7–9 days; after small ↑, a second, deeper nadir occurs 15–24 days after administration. Patient should lie flat for 1 hr after IT administration.

dalteparin (Fragmin) Uses: Prevention of DVT/PE in surgical (hip, abdominal) or medical patients; Extended treatment of symptomatic DVT/PE in CA patients to ↓ risk of recurrent DVT/PE; Prevention of ischemic complications (with aspirin) in UA/NSTEMI; **Class:** antithrombotics, heparins (low molecular weight); **Preg:** B; **CIs:** Hypersensitivity to dalteparin, heparin, or pork products; Active bleeding; Thrombocytopenia related to previous dalteparin or heparin therapy; Severe renal or hepatic impairment; Spinal or epidural anesthesia; Peds (safety not established); **ADRs:** BLEEDING, thrombocytopenia, pain at inject site; **Interactions:** ↑ risk of bleeding with antiplatelets, thrombolytics, or other anticoagulants; **Dose:** *Subcut: Adults: Abdominal surgery*—2500 units 1–2 hr before surgery, then daily × 5–10 days; for high-risk patients, give 5000 units the evening before surgery, then daily × 5–10 days *or* 2500 units 1–2 hr before surgery, another 2500 units 12 hr later, then 5000 units daily × 5–10 days. *Hip replacement surgery*—2500 units 4–8 hr after surgery, then 5000 units daily (start ≥6 hr after postoperative dose) × 5–10 days *or* 2500 units within 2 hr before surgery, another 2500 units 4–8 hr after surgery, then 5000 units daily (start ≥6 hr after postoperative dose) × 5–10 days *or* 5000 units 10–14 hr before surgery, another 5000 units 4–8 hr after surgery, then 5000 units daily × 5–10 days. *Medically ill patients*—5000 units × 12–14 days. *Extended VTE treatment in CA patients:* —200 units/kg daily (max: 18,000 units/day) × 1 mo, then 150 units/kg daily (max: 18,000 units/day) × 5 mo; *UA/NSTEMI*—120 units/kg (max: 10,000 units/dose) q 12 hr (with aspirin); **Availability:** *Inject:* 2500 units/0.2 ml, 5000 units/0.2 ml, 7500 units/0.3 ml, 10,000 units/ml, 12,500 units/0.5 ml, 15,000 units/0.6 ml, 18,000 units/0.72 ml, 25,000 units/ml; **Monitor:** BUN/SCr, CBC, anti-Xa (if renal dysfunction or obese), bleeding; **Notes:** Anti-Xa levels can be monitored after 3 or 4 doses; obtain 4–6 hr after a dose (target anti-Xa level = 0.5–1.5 units/ml).

dantrolene (Dantrium) Uses: PO: Spasticity associated with: Spinal cord injury, Stroke, Cerebral palsy, MS; Prophylaxis of malignant hyperthermia; **IV:** Treatment of malignant hyperthermia; **Class:** skeletal muscle relaxants; **Preg:** C; **CIs:** Liver disease; Lactation; Situations in which spasticity is used to maintain posture or balance; **ADRs:** dizziness, drowsiness, muscle weakness, confusion, HA, insomnia, nervousness, ↑ lacrimation, visual disturbances, PULMONARY EDEMA (IV), changes in BP, ↑ HR, HEPATOTOXICITY, diarrhea, anorexia, cramps, dysphagia, GI bleeding, vomiting, crystalluria, dysuria, ED, incontinence, nocturia, pruritus, sweating, urticaria, eosinophilia, irritation at IV site, phlebitis (IV), myalgia, chills, fever; **Interactions:** ↑ CNS depression with alcohol, antidepressants, other BZs, antihistamines, and opioids; ↑ risk of hepatotoxicity with other hepatotoxic agents or estrogens, ↑ risk of CV collapse with CCBs; **Dose:** *PO: Adults: Spasticity*—25 mg/day × 7 days, then 25 mg tid × 7 days, then 50 mg tid × 7 days, then 100 mg tid (max: 400 mg/day). *PO: Adults and Peds: >5 yr Prevention of malignant* *hyperthermia (preop)*—4–8 mg/kg/day in 3–4 divided doses × 1–2 days before procedure, last dose 3–4 hr preop. *Post-malignant hyperthermia*—4–8 mg/kg/day in 4 divided doses × 1–3 days after IV treatment. *PO: Peds: >5 yr Spasticity*—0.5 mg/kg/day × 7 days, then 0.5 mg/kg tid × 7 days, then 1 mg/kg tid × 7 days, then 2 mg/kg tid (max: 400 mg/day). *IV: Adults and Peds: Treatment of malignant hyperthermia*—at least 1 mg/kg (up to 2.5 mg/kg), continued until symptoms ↓ or a cumulative dose of 10 mg/kg has been given; if symptoms reappear, repeat. *Prevention of malignant hyperthermia (preop)*—2.5 mg/kg 1.25 hr before anesthesia; **Availability: (G):** *Caps*: 25, 50, 100 mg. *Inject:* 20 mg; **Monitor:** BP, HR, RR, temp, ECG, electrolytes, LFTs, UO, bowel function, neuromuscular status, muscle spasms; **Notes:** ↑ risk of hepatotoxicity in females and in patients >35 yr. Discontinue if no improvement in spasticity after 45 days.

daptomycin (Cubicin) Uses: Complicated skin and skin structure infections and bacteremia (including patients with right-sided endocarditis) caused by Gram (+) bacteria (including MRSA); **Class:** cyclic lipopeptide antibacterial agents; **Preg:** B; **CIs:** Hypersensitivity, Peds <18 yr (safety not established); **ADRs:** dizziness, HA, insomnia, dyspnea, ↓ BP, PSEUDOMEMBRANOUS COLITIS, constipation, N/V/D, ↑ LFTs, renal failure, pruritus, rash, anemia, inject site reactions, ↑ CK; **Interactions:** ↑ risk of myopathy with HMG-CoA reductase inhibitors; **Dose:** *IV: Adults: Skin/skin structure infections*—4 mg/kg q 24 hr. *Bacteremia*—6 mg/kg q 24 hr. *Renal Impairment IV: Adults:* ↓ dose if CrCl <30 ml/min; **Availability:** *Inject:* 500 mg; **Monitor:** BP, HR, temp, sputum, U/A, CBC, LFTs, BUN/SCr, CK (at least weekly), muscle pain; **Notes:** Discontinue if CK >1000 units/L and S/S of myopathy occur (or if CK >2000 units/L in absence of S/S).

darbepoetin (Aranesp) Uses: Anemia in chronic renal failure; Chemotherapy-induced anemia in non-myeloid malignancies; **Class:** colony-stimulating factors; **Preg:** C; **CIs:** Hypersensitivity; Uncontrolled HTN; **ADRs:** SEIZURES, HA, dizziness, fatigue, dyspnea, cough, ARRHYTHMIAS, HF, MI, STROKE, THROMBOTIC EVENTS (esp with Hgb >12 g/dL), edema, ↑↓ BP, CP, abdominal pain, N/V/D, constipation, pruritus, arthralgia, myalgia, allergic reactions, fever, ↑ MORTALITY (esp with Hgb >12 g/dL), TUMOR GROWTH (esp with Hgb >12 g/dL); **Interactions:** None reported; **Dose:** *IV, Subcut: Adults: Chronic renal failure*—0.45 mcg/kg once weekly; adjust dose to attain target Hgb of 10–12 g/dl; if Hgb ↑ by >1.0 g/dl in 2 wk or if the Hgb is ↑ and nearing 12 g/dl, ↓ dose by 25%; if Hgb ↑ by <1.0 g/dl after 4 wk of therapy (with adequate iron stores), ↑ dose by 25%; do not ↑ dose more frequently than q 4 wk. Some patients may be dosed q 2 wk. If patient previously on epoetin, see package insert for equivalent darbepoetin dose. *Subcut: Adults: CA patients on chemotherapy*—2.25 mcg/kg weekly *or* 500 mcg q 3 wk; target Hgb should not exceed 12 g/dl. If Hgb

↑ by >1.0 g/dl in 2 wk or if the Hgb >12 g/dL or Hgb reaches level to avoid transfusion, ↓ dose by 40%; if Hgb ↑ by <1.0 g/dl after 6 wk of therapy, ↑ dose to 4.5 mcg/kg; discontinue after chemotherapy completed; **Availability:** *Single-dose vials*: 25 mcg/ml, 40 mcg/ml, 60 mcg/ml, 100 mcg/ml, 150 mcg/ml, 200 mcg/ml, 300 mcg/ml, 500 mcg/ml. *Prefilled syringes*: 25 mcg/0.42 ml, 40 mcg/0.4 ml, 60 mcg/0.3 ml, 100 mcg/0.5 ml, 150 mcg/0.3 ml, 200 mcg/0.4 ml, 300 mcg/0.6 ml, 500 mcg/ml; **Monitor:** BP, S/S thrombosis, Hgb/Hct, serum ferritin, transferrin, and iron levels; **Notes:** IV route recommended for HD patients. Most patients require supplemental iron during therapy. Correct folate and vitamin B_{12} deficiencies before therapy.

D

darunavir (Prezista) Uses: HIV (with ritonavir and other antiretrovirals) in adults who have already received and progressed on other antiretroviral combinations; **Class:** protease inhibitors; **Preg:** B; **CIs:** Sulfa allergy; Severe hepatic impairment; Concurrent use of ergot derivatives, midazolam, triazolam, pimozide, phenytoin, phenobarbital, carbamazepine, rifampin, lovastatin, simvastatin, or St. John's wort; Pregnancy (use only if maternal benefit outweighs fetal risk); Lactation; Peds (safety not established); Infants <3 mo (↑ risk of kernicterus); **ADRs:** HA, HEPATOTOXICITY, ↑ amylase/lipase, diarrhea, nausea, vomiting, neutropenia, fat redistribution, ↑ BG, ↑ lipids, rash; **Interactions:** CYP3A4 inhibitors may ↑ levels; CYP3A4 inducers may ↓ levels; May ↑ levels of CYP3A4 substrates; ↑ levels of ergot derivatives, midazolam, triazolam, pimozide, lovastatin, or simvastatin (contraindicated); Rifampin, phenytoin, phenobarbital, carbamazepine, and St. John's wort ↓ levels (contraindicated); Concurrent use with efavirenz ↓ darunavir levels and ↑ efavirenz levels (use cautiously); Lopinavir/ritonavir and saquinavir may ↓ levels/effects and may ↓ antiretroviral effectiveness (concurrent use not recommended); May ↑ digoxin levels; May ↓ effects of warfarin; ↑ levels of clarithromycin (↓ dose of clarithromycin for CrCl <60 ml/min); ↓ effects of voriconazole (avoid concurrent use if possible); Concurrent use with rifabutin ↑ rifabutin levels and ↓ darunavir levels (↓ rifabutin dose); May ↓ methadone levels; ↑ levels of sildenafil, vardenafil, and tadalafil (↓ dose of these agents); May ↓ levels/effects of sertraline and paroxetine; **Dose:** *PO: Adults:* 600 mg with ritonavir 100 mg bid; **Availability:** *Tabs:* 300, 600 mg; **Monitor:** Viral load, CD4 count, BG, LFTs, bilirubin, amylase/lipase, lipid panel; **Notes:** Must be used with ritonavir. Take with food. Sulfa drug.

DAUNOrubicin citrate liposome (DaunoXome) Uses: Advanced Kaposi's sarcoma in HIV-infected patients; **Class:** anthracyclines; **Preg:** D; **CIs:** Hypersensitivity; Bone marrow depression; Pregnancy/lactation; **ADRs:** fatigue, HA, depression, dizziness, insomnia, malaise, rhinitis, sinusitis, cough, dyspnea, CARDIOTOXICITY, edema, CP, ↑ BP, abdominal pain, N/V/D, anorexia, constipation, stomatitis, red urine, infertility, alopecia, sweating, pruritus, LEUKOPENIA, anemia, thrombocytopenia, phlebitis, ↑ uric acid, arthralgia, myalgia, neuropathy, allergic reactions, chills, fever, flushing, flu-like symptoms; **Interactions:** ↑ bone marrow suppression with other antineoplastics or radiation therapy; Cardiotoxicity may be additive with other cardiotoxic agents (cyclophosphamide, doxorubicin); **Dose:** *IV: Adults:* 40 mg/m² q 2 wk. *Renal Impairment IV: Adults:* ↓ dose if SCr ≥1.2 mg/dl. *Hepatic Impairment IV: Adults:* ↓ dose if serum bilirubin ≥1.2 mg/dl; **Availability:** *Inject:* 2 mg/ml; **Monitor:** BP, HR, temp, BUN/SCr, CBC (with diff), uric acid, LFTs, S/S infection, S/S HF, bleeding, echo (LVEF), ECG; **Notes: High Alert:** Fatalities have occurred with chemotherapeutic agents. Before administering, clarify all ambiguous orders; double-check single, daily, and course-of-therapy dose limits; have second practitioner independently double-check original order, calculations, and infusion pump settings. Do not confuse with daunorubicin hydrochloride (Cerubidine), doxorubicin (Adriamycin), or doxorubicin hydrochloride liposome (Doxil). To prevent confusion, orders should include generic and brand name. 30% ↓ in QRS voltage and ↓ in LVEF are early signs of cardiotoxicity. ↑ risk of cardiotoxicity with cumulative doses >550 mg/m² and mediastinal radiation. Leukocyte count nadir = 10–14 days (recovery in 21 days after administration).

DAUNOrubicin hydrochloride (Cerubidine) **Uses:** In combination with other antineoplastics for leukemias; **Class:** anthracyclines; **Preg:** D; **CIs:** Hypersensitivity; Bone marrow depression; Pregnancy/lactation; **ADRs:** rhinitis, CARDIOTOXICITY, N/V, diarrhea, stomatitis, red urine, infertility, alopecia, LEUKOPENIA, anemia, thrombocytopenia, phlebitis, ↑ uric acid, chills, fever; **Interactions:** ↑ bone marrow suppression with other antineoplastics or radiation therapy; Cardiotoxicity may be additive with other cardiotoxic agents (cyclophosphamide, doxorubicin); ↑ risk of toxicity with hepatotoxic agents; **Dose:** *IV: Adults: AML induction (as part of combination regimen)*— <60 yr: 45 mg/m²/day for Days 1, 2, and 3 in first course, then on Days 1 and 2 of 2nd course; ≥60 yr: 30 mg/m²/day for Days 1, 2, and 3 in 1st course, then on Days 1 and 2 of 2nd course. *ALL induction (as part of combination regimen)*—45 mg/m²/day for Days 1, 2, and 3; *IV: Peds: ALL induction (as part of combination regimen)*—>2 yr: 25 mg/m² once weekly; ≤2 yr or BSA <0.5 m²: 1 mg/kg/dose per protocol; **Availability (G):** *Inject:* 20 mg (powder), 5 mg/ml (soln); **Monitor:** BP, HR, temp, BUN/SCr, CBC (with diff), uric acid, LFTs, S/S infection, S/S HF, bleeding, echo (LVEF), ECG, infusion site; **Notes: High Alert:** Fatalities have occurred with chemotherapeutic agents. Before administering, clarify all ambiguous orders; double-check single, daily, and course-of-therapy dose limits; have second practitioner independently double-check original order, calculations, and infusion pump settings. Do not confuse with daunorubicin citrate liposome (DaunoXome), doxorubicin (Adriamycin), or doxorubicin hydrochloride liposome (Doxil). To prevent confusion, orders should include generic and brand name. 30% ↓ in QRS voltage and ↓ in

LVEF are early signs of cardiotoxicity. ↑ risk of cardiotoxicity with cumulative doses >550 mg/m² and mediastinal radiation. Leukocyte count nadir = 10–14 days (recovery in 21 days after administration). Potent vesicant.

deferoxamine (Desferal) Uses: Acute iron toxicity; Chronic iron overload due to multiple transfusions; **Class:** heavy metal antagonists; **Preg:** C; **CIs:** Severe renal disease; Anuria; Peds <3 yr (safety not established); **ADRs:** blurred vision, cataracts, hearing loss, tinnitus, ↓ BP, ↑ HR, N/V/D, red urine, erythema, flushing, urticaria, pain at inject site, leg cramps, allergic reactions, fever, shock (after rapid IV); **Interactions:** ↑ risk of HF with ascorbic acid; **Dose:** *IM, IV: Adults and Peds: ≥3 yr Acute iron toxicity*—1000 mg, then 500 mg q 4 hr × 2 doses; additional doses of 500 mg q 4–12 hr may be needed (max: 6 g/24 hr). *Chronic iron overload*—500–1000 mg/day; additional doses of 2 g should be given IV for each unit of blood transfused. *Subcut: Adults and Peds: ≥3 yr Chronic iron overload*—1–2 g/day (20–40 mg/kg/day) infused (via infusion pump) over 8–24 hr; **Availability (G):** *Inject:* 500 mg, 2 g; **Monitor:** BP, HR, S/S iron toxicity (early acute: abdominal pain, bloody diarrhea, emesis; late acute: ↓ consciousness, shock, metabolic acidosis), audiovisual exam, I/Os, BUN/SCr, LFTs, serum iron, TIBC, ferritin, and urinary iron excretion; **Notes:** IM preferred unless patient in shock (then use IV). Avoid rapid IV infusion (may cause ↓ BP, ↑ HR, erythema, urticaria, wheezing, convulsions, or shock; do not exceed infusion rate of 15 mg/kg/hr).

desipramine (Norpramin) Uses: Depression; **Class:** tricyclic antidepressants; **Preg:** C; **CIs:** Hypersensitivity; Current or recent (within 2 wk) use of MAOIs; Post-MI; May ↑ risk of suicidal thoughts/behaviors esp. during early treatment or dose adjustment (risk may be ↑ in children or adolescents); Peds ≤12 yr (safety not established); **ADRs:** confusion, lethargy, sedation, blurred vision, dry mouth, ARRHYTHMIAS, ↓ BP, constipation, hepatitis, ↑ appetite, ↑ wt, urinary retention, ↓ libido, gynecomastia, blood dyscrasias, SUICIDAL THOUGHTS; **Interactions:** CYP2D6 inhibitors may ↑ levels; ↑ risk of hypertensive crises, seizures, or death with MAOIs (discontinue for ≥2 wk); ↑ risk of toxicity with SSRIs (discontinue fluoxetine for ≥5 wk); ↑ risk of arrhythmias with other drugs that prolong QTc interval; ↑ CNS depression with other CNS depressants, alcohol, antihistamines, opioids, and sedative/hypnotics; ↑ risk of anticholinergic effects with other anticholinergic agents; **Dose:** *PO: Adults:* 100–200 mg/day as single dose or in divided doses (max: 300 mg/day). *PO: Geriatric Patients and Adolescents:* 25–100 mg/day in divided doses (max: 150 mg/day); **Availability (G):** *Tabs:* 10, 25, 50, 75, 100, 150 mg; **Monitor:** BP, HR, ECG, mental status, suicidal thoughts/behaviors; **Notes:** May take 4–6 wk to see effect. May give entire dose at bedtime. Taper to avoid withdrawal. Use with caution in elderly (↑ risk of sedation and anticholinergic effects).

desloratadine (Clarinex) **Uses:** Seasonal or perennial allergic rhinitis; Chronic idiopathic urticaria; **Class:** antihistamines; **Preg:** C; **CIs:** Hypersensitivity; Lactation; Peds <6 mo (safety not established); **ADRs:** HA, drowsiness, pharyngitis, dry mouth, nausea; **Interactions:** ↑ CNS depression may occur with other CNS depressants, alcohol, antidepressants, opioids, and sedative/hypnotics; **Dose:** *PO: Adults and Peds: ≥12 yr:* 5 mg/day. *PO: Peds:* 6–11 yr: 2.5 mg/day; 1–5 yr: 1.25 mg/day; 6–11 mo: 1 mg/day. *Hepatic/Renal Impairment Adults:* ↓ dose to 5 mg every other day; **Availability:** *Tabs:* 5 mg. *ODT (RediTabs):* 2.5, 5 mg. Syrup: 0.5 mg/ml; **Monitor:** Allergy symptoms, lung sounds; **Notes:** Maintain fluid intake of 1500–2000 ml/day to ↓ secretion viscosity. Rarely causes drowsiness.

desmopressin (DDAVP, Stimate) **Uses: PO:** Primary nocturnal enuresis; Central DI; **PO, Subcut, IV, Intranasal:** (DDAVP only) Central DI; **IV, Intranasal** (Stimate only) Hemophilia A and von Willebrand's disease; **Class:** antidiuretic hormones; **Preg:** B; **CIs:** Hypersensitivity; Renal impairment (CrCl <50 ml/min); Hyponatremia (currently or history of); Nephrogenic DI; **ADRs:** SEIZURES, HA, nasal congestion, epistaxis, rhinitis, ↑ BP, nausea, HYPONATREMIA/WATER INTOXICATION, flushing, phlebitis at IV site; **Interactions:** ↑ risk of hyponatremia with chlorpropamide, TCAs, SSRIs (e.g., chlorpromazine, lamotrigine, or carbamazepine); Demeclocycline or lithium, or norepinephrine may ↓ effects; Large doses may ↑ effects of vasopressors; **Dose:** *PO: Adults and Peds: DI*—0.05 mg bid; adjusted as needed (usual range: 0.1–1.2 mg/day in 2–3 divided doses); *Nocturnal enuresis*—≥6 yr: 0.2 mg at bedtime (max: 0.6 mg at bedtime). *Intranasal: Adults: DI (DDAVP only)*—10–40 mcg/day in 1–3 divided doses. *Intranasal: Peds: 3 mo–12 yr DI (DDAVP only)*—5–30 mcg/day in 1–2 divided doses. *Intranasal: Adults and Peds: ≥50 kg Hemophilia A/von Willebrand's disease (Stimate only)*—≥50 kg: 1 spray (150 mcg) in each nostril; <50 kg: 1 spray (150 mcg) in one nostril. *Subcut: IV: Adults: DI*—2–4 mcg/day in 2 divided doses. *IV: Adults and Peds: >3 mo Hemophilia A/von Willebrand's disease*—0.3 mcg/kg, repeated prn; **Availability (G):** *Tabs:* 0.1, 0.2 mg. *Nasal spray (DDAVP):* 10 mcg/spray. *Nasal spray (Stimate):* 150 mcg/spray. *Rhinal tube nasal soln:* 0.1 mg/ml. *Inject:* 4 mcg/ml; **Monitor:** BP, HR, Na+, S/S hyponatremia (HA, N/V, ↑ wt, restlessness, lethargy, disorientation, ↓ reflexes, ↓ appetite, irritability, muscle weakness/spasms/cramps, hallucinations, ↓ consciousness, confusion, seizures), I/Os, S/S dehydration, urine and plasma osmolality, urine volume, wt, enuresis frequency, plasma factor VIII coagulant, factor VIII antigen, ristocetin cofactor, aPTT, bleeding; **Notes:** Fluid restriction (esp. in peds and elderly). Begin PO 12 hr after last intranasal dose.

desonide (Desonate, DesOwen, LoKara, Verdeso) **Uses:** Management of inflammation and pruritis associated with various dermatoses; **Class:** corticosteroids; **Preg:** C; **CIs:** Hypersensitivity; **ADRs:** burning sensation, dryness, folliculitis, hypersensitivity reactions, hypopigmentation, irritation, secondary infection, striae, adrenal suppression (with use of occlusive dressings or long-term therapy); **Interactions:** None significant; **Dose:** *Topical: Adults and Peds: ≥3 mo:* Apply 2–4 times/day for up to 2 wk (depends on preparation and condition being treated); **Availability (G):** *Cream/Gel/Oint/Lotion/Foam:* 0.05%; **Monitor:** Skin condition (inflammation, erythema, pruritis); **Notes:** Oints are more occlusive and preferred for dry, scaly lesions. Creams should be used on oozing or intertriginous areas (may cause more skin drying than ointments). Lotion is useful in hairy areas.

desoximetasone (Topicort, Topicort LP) **Uses:** Management of inflammation and pruritis associated with various dermatoses; **Class:** corticosteroids; **Preg:** C; **CIs:** Hypersensitivity; **ADRs:** burning sensation, dryness, folliculitis, hypersensitivity reactions, hypopigmentation, irritation, secondary infection, striae, adrenal suppression (with use of occlusive dressings or long-term therapy); **Interactions:** None significant; **Dose:** *Topical: Adults and Peds: ≥10 yr:* Apply bid; **Availability (G):** *Cream:* 0.05%, 0.25%. *Gel:* 0.05%. *Oint:* 0.25%; **Monitor:** Skin condition (inflammation, erythema, pruritis); **Notes:** Oints are more occlusive and preferred for dry, scaly lesions. Creams should be used on oozing or intertriginous areas (may cause more skin drying than ointments). Gel is useful in hairy areas.

dexamethasone (DexPak) **Uses:** Used systemically and locally in a wide variety of chronic diseases including: Inflammatory, Allergic, Hematologic, Endocrine, Rheumatic, Neoplastic, Respiratory, Dermatologic; Management of cerebral edema; Diagnostic agent in adrenal disorders; **Class:** corticosteroids; **Preg:** C; **CIs:** Active fungal infections; Lactation (avoid chronic use); **ADRs:** <u>depression</u>, <u>euphoria</u>, hallucinations, HA, insomnia, psychoses, restlessness, cataracts, ↑ IOP, ↑ <u>BP</u>, edema, PUD, nausea, ↑ appetite, ↓ <u>wound healing</u>, <u>hirsutism</u>, <u>adrenal suppression</u>, ↑ BG, amenorrhea, ↓ K+, ↑ wt, <u>muscle wasting</u>, tendon rupture, <u>osteoporosis</u>, <u>cushingoid appearance</u> (<u>moon face</u>, <u>buffalo hump</u>), infection; **Interactions:** CYP3A4 inhibitors may ↑ levels; CYP3A4 inducers may ↓ levels; May ↓ levels of CYP3A4 substrates; ↑ risk of hypokalemia with thiazide and loop diuretics, or amphotericin B; May ↑ requirement for insulin or oral hypoglycemic agents; ↑ risk of adverse GI effects with NSAIDs (including aspirin) or alcohol; At chronic doses that suppress adrenal function, may ↓ the antibody response to and ↑ risk of ADRs from live-virus vaccines; May ↑ or ↓ the effects of warfarin; May ↑ risk of tendon rupture when used with fluoroquinolones; **Dose:** *PO, IM, IV: Adults: Anti-inflammatory*—0.75–9 mg/day divided q 6–12 hr. *Airway edema or extubation*—0.5–2 mg/kg/day divided q 6 hr; begin 24 hr prior to extubation and continue for 24 hr post-extubation. *Cerebral edema*—10 mg IV, then 4 mg IM or IV q 6 hr until max response, then switch to PO and taper over 5–7 days. *Chemotherapy-induced emesis*—10–20 mg IV/PO given 15–30 min before each treatment *or* 10 mg IV/PO q 12 hr on each treatment day. *Delayed N/V*—4–10 mg PO 1–2 ×/day × 2–4 days *or* 8 mg PO q 12 hr × 2 days, then 4 mg PO q 12 hr × 2 days. *Suppression test*—1 mg PO at 11 PM *or* 0.5 mg PO q 6 hr × 48 hr. *Intrasinovial Adults:* 0.4–6 mg/day. *PO, IM, IV: Peds: Airway edema or extubation*—0.5–2 mg/kg/day divided q 6 hr; begin 24 hr prior to extubation and continue for 24 hr post-extubation. *Anti-inflammatory*—0.08–0.3 mg/kg/day divided q 6–12 hr. *Physiologic replacement*—0.03–0.15 mg/kg/day divided q 6–12 hr. *Chemotherapy-induced emesis*—5–20 mg IV given 15–30 min before chemotherapy. *Cerebral edema*—1–2 mg/kg IV, then 1–1.5 mg/kg/day divided q 4–6 hr × 5 days (max: 16 mg/day); then taper over 1–6 wk; **Availability (G):** *Tabs:* 0.5, 0.75, 1, 1.5, 2, 4, 6 mg. *Elixir:* 0.5 mg/5 ml. *Oral soln:* 0.5 mg/5 ml, 1 mg/ml. *Inject (sodium phosphate):* 4 mg/ml, 10 mg/ml; **Monitor:** BP, HR, edema, wt, electrolytes, glucose, signs of adrenal insufficiency; **Notes:** Give in AM. Chronic treatment will lead to adrenal suppression; use lowest possible dose for shortest period of time. For dexamethasone suppression test (to diagnose Cushing's syndrome), obtain baseline cortisol level; administer dexamethasone at 11 PM and obtain cortisol levels at 8 AM the next day (normal response is ↓ cortisol level). Need to taper therapy (abrupt discontinuation may lead to adrenal insufficiency).

dexmethylphenidate (Focalin, Focalin XR) **Uses:** ADHD; **Class:** central nervous system stimulants; **Preg:** C; **CIs:** Hypersensitivity; Marked anxiety, agitation, or tension; Motor tics, family history or diagnosis of Tourette's; Current or recent (within 2 wk) use of MAOIs; Glaucoma; Serious CV disease or structural heart disease (may ↑ risk of sudden death); History of substance abuse; HTN, Peds <6 yr (safety not established); **ADRs:** HA, anxiety, insomnia, visual disturbances, SUDDEN DEATH, ↑ BP, ↑ HR, abdominal pain, anorexia, nausea, growth suppression (with long-term use in peds), ↓ wt, twitching, fever, psychological dependence, tolerance; **Interactions:** Use with MAOIs can result in hypertensive crisis (contraindicated); May ↓ effects of antihypertensives; ↑ risk of serious ADRs with clonidine; May ↑ effects of warfarin, phenobarbital, phenytoin, TCAs, or SSRIs; **Dose:** *PO: Adults and Peds: ≥6 yr Not previously taking methylphenidate*—IR tabs: 2.5 mg bid; may ↑ by 2.5–5 mg q wk (max: 10 mg bid). ER caps: 5 mg/day for peds, 10 mg/day for adults; may ↑ by 5 mg (peds) or 10 mg (adults) q wk (max: 20 mg/day). *Currently taking methylphenidate*—IR tabs or ER caps: starting dose is 50% of the methylphenidate dose; may titrate up to 10 mg bid (IR) or 20 mg/day (ER); **Availability (G):** *Tabs:* 2.5, 5, 10 mg. *ER caps:* 5, 10, 15, 20 mg; **Monitor:** BP, HR, ECG, mental status, ht/wt; **Notes:** Schedule II controlled substance. For IR, administer bid ≥4 hr apart. For ER, take dose in AM (caps should be swallowed whole; if difficulty swallowing, open caps and sprinkle on a spoonful of applesauce).

Do not crush or chew ER caps. If switching from IR to ER, give same total daily dose once daily. All peds should have CV assessment prior to initiation. Potential for dependence/abuse with long-term use.

dextroamphetamine (Dexedrine, Dextrostat) **Uses:** Narcolepsy; ADHD; **Class:** amphetamines; **Preg:** C; **CIs:** Hypersensitivity; Hyperthyroidism; Current or recent (within 2 wk) use of MAOIs; Glaucoma; Serious CV disease or structural heart disease (may ↑ risk of sudden death); History of substance abuse (misuse may result in serious CV events/sudden death); HTN; Peds <3 yr (safety not established); **ADRs:** hyperactivity, insomnia, restlessness, tremor, agitation, dizziness, SUDDEN DEATH, ↑ BP, palpitations, ↑ HR, anorexia, dry mouth, constipation, N/V/D, ↓ wt, ED, ↓ libido, urticaria, growth inhibition (with long-term use in peds), psychological dependence, tolerance; **Interactions:** Use with MAOIs can result in hypertensive crisis; May ↓ effects of antihistamines and antihypertensives; Haloperidol and lithium may ↓ effects; ↑ adrenergic effects with other adrenergics or thyroid preparations; Alkalinizing agents (e.g., sodium bicarbonate, acetazolamide, antacids) ↓ excretion and ↑ effects; Acidifying agents (e.g., ammonium chloride, large doses of ascorbic acid) ↑ excretion and ↓ effects, ↑ risk of CV effects with TCAs; **Dose:** *PO: Adults: ADHD*—5 mg 1–2 times daily; ↑ by 5 mg/day q wk until optimal response (max: 40 mg/day). *PO: Adults and Peds: ≥12 yr Narcolepsy*—10 mg/day initially; ↑ by 10 mg/day q wk until optimal response (max: 60 mg/day in 1–3 divided doses). *PO: Peds: 6–12 yr Narcolepsy*—5 mg/day; ↑ by 5 mg/day q wk until optimal response (max: 60 mg/day in 1–3 divided doses). *PO: Peds: ≥6 yr ADHD*—5 mg 1–2 ×/day; ↑ by 5 mg/day q wk until optimal response (max: 40 mg/day). *PO: Peds: 3–5 yr ADHD*—2.5 mg/day; ↑ by 2.5 mg/day q wk until optimal response (max: 40 mg/day); **Availability (G):** *Tabs:* 5, 10 mg. *SR caps:* 5, 10, 15 mg; **Monitor:** BP, HR, ECG, mental status, ht/wt; **Notes:** Schedule II controlled substance. Give 1st dose upon awakening, and then any subsequent doses at 4–6 hr intervals. Take last dose ≥6 hr before bedtime to minimize insomnia. SR caps can be given once daily (should be swallowed whole; do not break, crush, or chew). All peds should have CV assessment prior to initiation. Potential for dependence/abuse with long-term use.

diazepam (Diastat, Valium) **Uses:** Anxiety disorders; Alcohol withdrawal; Muscle spasms; Status epilepticus/uncontrolled seizures (inject or rectal); **Class:** benzodiazepines; **Preg:** D; **CIs:** Hypersensitivity (cross-sensitivity with other BZs may exist); Acute narrow-angle glaucoma; Myasthenia gravis; Severe hepatic disease; Severe pulmonary impairment; Sleep apnea; Pregnancy/lactation; Peds <6 mo (oral); **ADRs:** ataxia, dizziness, drowsiness, lethargy, confusion, depression, blurred vision, respiratory depression, ↓ BP (IV only), constipation, N/V/D, ↑ wt, pain (at IM site), phlebitis (IV), physical/psychological dependence, tolerance; **Interactions:** ↑ CNS depression with alcohol, antidepressants, other

BZs, antihistamines, and opioids; CYP2C19 inhibitors and CYP3A4 inhibitors may ↑ levels; CYP2C19 inducers and CYP3A4 inducers may ↓ levels; **Dose:** *PO: Adults: Anxiety or muscle spasms*—2–10 mg 2–4 ×/day. *Alcohol withdrawal*—10 mg 3–4 × for 24 hr, then 5 mg 3–4 ×/day. *IM, IV: Adults: Anxiety or muscle spasms*—2–10 mg; may repeat in 3–4 hr prn. *Status epilepticus*—5–10 mg IV; may repeat q 10–15 min to total of 30 mg; may repeat regimen again in 2–4 hr. *Alcohol withdrawal*—10 mg initially, then 5–10 mg in 3–4 hr prn. *PO: Peds: >1 mo Anxiety or muscle spasms*—0.12–0.8 mg/kg/day in 3–4 divided doses. *IM, IV: Peds: Anxiety*—0.04–0.3 mg/kg q 2–4 hr prn (max total dose: 0.6 mg/kg within 8-hr period). *Status epilepticus*—1 mo–5 yr: 0.05–0.3 mg/kg q 15–30 min (max total dose: 5 mg); repeat in 2–4 hr if needed. ≥5 yr: 0.05–0.3 mg/kg q 15–30 min (max total dose: 10 mg); repeat in 2–4 hr if needed. *Rect: Adults and Peds: ≥12 yr Status epilepticus*—0.2 mg/kg; may repeat 4–12 hr later. *Rect Peds: <12 yr Status epilepticus*—2–5 yr: 0.5 mg/kg; may repeat 4–12 hr later. 6–11 yr: 0.3 mg/kg; may repeat 4–12 hr later; **Availability (G):** *Tabs:* 2, 5, 10 mg. *Oral soln:* 5 mg/ml, 1 mg/ml. *Inject:* 5 mg/ml. *Rect: gel:* 2.5, 5, 10, 20 mg; **Monitor:** BP, HR, RR, mental status, S/S alcohol withdrawal, seizure activity, pain, LFTs, BUN/SCr; **Notes:** Schedule IV controlled substance. Potential for dependence/abuse with long-term use (use with caution in patients at risk for addiction). Flumazenil is antidote. Do not discontinue abruptly; taper by 2 mg q 3 days to ↓ risk of withdrawal. IM injections are painful and erratically absorbed. Do not administer as continuous infusion.

diclofenac (Cataflam, Flector, Solaraze, Voltaren, Voltaren-XR) **Uses: PO:** Inflammatory disorders including: RA, OA, Ankylosing spondylitis; Primary dysmenorrhea; Mild-to-moderate pain; **Topical** OA (1% gel). Actinic keratoses (3% gel). Acute pain due to minor strains/sprains/contusions (transdermal patch); **Ophth:** Postoperative inflammation after cataract surgery. Relief of pain and photophobia from corneal refractive surgery; **Class:** NSAIDs; **Preg:** B (topical gel 3%), **C** (oral, topical gel 1%, transdermal patch), **D** (3rd tri); **CIs:** Hypersensitivity to aspirin or NSAIDs; Active GI bleeding/PUD; Perioperative pain after CABG surgery; Non-intact or damaged skin (topical); **ADRs:** dizziness, HA, tinnitus, edema, ↑ BP, GI BLEEDING, abdominal pain, constipation, diarrhea, dyspepsia, flatulence, heartburn, ↑ LFTs, N/V, acute renal failure, EXFOLIATIVE DERMATITIS, SJS, TEN; Top—pruritis, rash, eczema, photosensitivity, anemia, contact dermatitis, dry skin, exfoliation, ANAPHYLAXIS; **Interactions:** ↑ adverse GI effects with aspirin or corticosteroids; May ↓ effectiveness of diuretics or other antihypertensives; May ↑ levels/toxicity of cyclosporine, lithium, and methotrexate; ↑ risk of bleeding with antiplatelet agents or warfarin; **Dose:** Different formulations of PO: diclofenac (diclofenac Na EC tabs, diclofenac Na ER tabs, and diclofenac K IR tabs are not bioequivalent and should not be substituted on a mg-to-mg basis) *PO: Adults:*

D

(Diclofenac K) Analgesic/antidysmenorrheal—100 mg initially, then 50 mg tid prn; *RA* —50 mg tid–qid; after initial response ↓ to lowest dose that controls symptoms. *OA*—50 mg bid–tid; after initial response ↓ to lowest dose that controls symptoms. *PO: Adults: (Diclofenac Na) RA (EC tabs)*—50 mg tid–qid *or* 75 mg bid; after initial response, ↓ to lowest dose that controls symptoms. *RA (ER tabs)*—100 mg/day; may be ↑ to 100 mg bid. *OA (EC tabs)*—50 mg bid–tid *or* 75 mg bid; after initial response, ↓ to lowest dose that controls symptoms. *OA (ER tabs)*—100 mg/day. *Ankylosing spondylitis (EC tabs)*—25 mg qid, with an additional 25 mg given at bedtime, if needed. *Topical: Adults: 3% gel*—Apply to lesions bid × 60–90 days. *1% gel*—Lower extremities: Apply 4 g qid (max: 16 g/joint/day); Upper extremities: Apply 2 g qid (max: 8 g/joint/day) (max total body dose: 32 g/day). *Transdermal patch*—1 patch applied to most painful area bid. *Ophth Adults: Cataract surgery*—1 gtt in affected eye qid beginning 24 hr after surgery and continuing for 2 wk. *Corneal refractive surgery*—1–2 gtt in affected eye within hr before and then 15 min after surgery, then continue qid for up to 3 days; **Availability (G):** *Diclofenac K IR tabs (Cataflam):* 50 mg. *Diclofenac Na EC tabs (Voltaren):* 50, 75 mg. *Diclofenac Na ER tabs (Voltaren-XR):* 100 mg. *Gel:* 1% (Voltaren), 3% (Solaraze); *Transdermal patch (Flector):* 180 mg; **Monitor:** BP, BUN/SCr, CBC, LFTs, pain, ROM, skin lesions; **Notes:** Give with food or milk to ↓ GI irritation. Use of PO NSAIDs during topical therapy should be minimized. Do not crush, chew, or break EC or ER tabs. With gel, avoid covering lesion with occlusive dressing and avoid applying sunscreen or cosmetics to the affected area.

dicloxacillin (Dycill, Dynapen, Pathocil) **Uses:** Sinusitis, osteomyelitis, and skin/skin structure infections due to penicillinase-producing staphylococci; **Class:** penicillinase resistant penicillins; **Preg:** B; **CIs:** Hypersensitivity (cross-sensitivity to other beta-lactam antibiotics may exist); **ADRs:** SEIZURES, PSEUDOMEMBRANOUS COLITIS, <u>N/V/D</u>, ↑ LFTs, interstitial nephritis, <u>rash</u>, urticaria, eosinophilia, leukopenia, ANAPHYLAXIS and SERUM SICKNESS, superinfection; **Interactions:** Probenecid ↓ excretion and ↑ levels; **Dose:** *PO: Adults:* 125–500 mg q 6 hr. *PO: Peds: ≥40 kg:* 125–250 mg q 6 hr. *PO: Peds: <40 kg:* 12.5–25 mg/kg/day divided q 6 hr (up to 50–100 mg/kg/day divided q 6 hr has been used for osteomyelitis); **Availability (G):** *Caps:* 250, 500 mg; **Monitor:** HR, BP, temp, sputum, U/A, CBC, LFTs; **Notes:** Use with caution in patients with beta-lactam allergy (do not use if history of anaphylaxis or hives). Give 1 hr ac or 2 hr pc.

dicyclomine (Bentyl) **Uses:** Irritable bowel syndrome; **Class:** anticholinergics; **Preg:** B; **CIs:** Hypersensitivity, Obstruction of the GI or GU tract; Reflux esophagitis; Severe ulcerative colitis; Unstable CV status in acute hemorrhage; Glaucoma; Myasthenia gravis; Infants <6 mo; Lactation; **ADRs:** confusion (↑ in geriatric patients), drowsiness, lightheadedness, blurred vision, diplopia, mydriasis, ↑ IOP, palpitations, ↑ HR, PARALYTIC ILEUS, constipation, dry mouth, N/V, urinary retention, ↓ sweating, pain/redness at IM site, ANAPHYLAXIS; **Interactions:** ↑ risk of anticholinergic effects with other anticholinergic agents; May alter the absorption of other orally administered drugs by slowing motility of the GI tract; Antacids may ↓ absorption; **Dose:** *PO: Adults:* 20 mg qid (max: 160 mg/day). *IM: Adults:* 20 mg q 6 hr, adjusted as tolerated; **Availability (G):** *Tabs:* 20 mg. *Caps:* 10 mg. *Syrup:* 10 mg/5 ml. *Inject:* 10 mg/ml; **Monitor:** S/S irritable bowel syndrome (cramping, alternating constipation/diarrhea, mucus in stool), bowel sounds, I/Os; **Notes:** IM should only be used when NPO. Physostigmine or neostigmine are antidotes. Give 30–60 min ac. Caution patients to avoid heat (could cause heat stroke because of ↓ sweating).

D

difenoxin/atropine (Motofen) **Uses:** Diarrhea; **Class:** anticholinergics; **Preg:** C; **CIs:** Hypersensitivity; Severe liver disease; Infectious diarrhea; Diarrhea associated with pseudomembranous colitis; Peds <2 yr; **ADRs:** dizziness, drowsiness, HA, blurred vision, dry eyes, ↑ HR, dry mouth, N/V, urinary retention; **Interactions:** ↑ CNS depression with other CNS depressants including alcohol, antihistamines, opioids, and sedative/hypnotics; ↑ risk of anticholinergic effects with other anticholinergic agents; Use with MAOIs may result in hypertensive crisis; **Dose:** *PO: Adults:* 2 tabs initially, then 1 tab after each loose stool or q 3–4 hr prn (max 8 tabs/day); **Availability:** *Tabs:* 1 mg difenoxin/0.025 mg atropine; **Monitor:** stool frequency, I/Os, electrolytes; **Notes:** Schedule IV controlled substance. Risk of dependence ↑ with high-dose, long-term use. Atropine added to the formulation to discourage abuse. Do not use if suspect *C. diff.* Difenoxin is active metabolite of diphenoxylate (in Lomotil).

diflorasone (ApexiCon, ApexiCon E, Psorcon) **Uses:** Management of inflammation and pruritis associated with various dermatoses; **Class:** corticosteroids; **Preg:** C; **CIs:** Hypersensitivity; **ADRs:** burning sensation, dryness, folliculitis, hypersensitivity reactions, hirsutism, hypopigmentation, irritation, secondary infection, striae, adrenal suppression (with use of occlusive dressings or long-term therapy); **Interactions:** None significant; **Dose:** *Topical: Adults:* Apply 1–3 ×/day (depends on condition being treated); **Availability: (G):** *Cream/Oint:* 0.05%; **Monitor:** Skin condition (inflammation, erythema, pruritis); **Notes:** Oints are more occlusive and preferred for dry, scaly lesions. Creams should be used on oozing or intertriginous areas (may cause more skin drying than oint).

digoxin (Digitek, Lanoxicaps, Lanoxin) **Uses:** HF; AF (to control ventricular rate); **Class:** digitalis glycosides; **Preg:** C; **CIs:** Hypersensitivity; Ventricular arrhythmias; ≥2nd-degree heart block or sick sinus syndrome (in absence of pacemaker); Arrhythmia associated with bypass tract (e.g., WPW); **ADRs:** blurred vision, yellow or green vision,

ARRHYTHMIAS, ↓ HR, ECG changes, heart block, anorexia, N/V, diarrhea; **Interactions:** Diuretics, amphotericin B, and corticosteroids may cause hypokalemia (may ↑ risk of toxicity); Amiodarone, carvedilol, cyclosporine, propafenone, quinidine, spironolactone, clarithromycin, azithromycin, diltiazem, and verapamil may ↑ levels; Cholestyramine, colestipol, antacids, or rifampin may ↓ levels; ↑ risk of bradycardia with diltiazem, verapamil, beta blockers, or clonidine; **Dose:** *IV: Adults: LD*—0.5–1 mg; give 50% of the dose initially and 25% of the initial dose in each of 2 subsequent doses at 6–8 hr intervals. *IV: Peds: >10 yr LD*—8–12 mcg/kg (>10 yr); 15–30 mcg/kg (5–10 yr); 25–35 mcg/kg (2–5 yr); 30–50 mcg/kg (1–24 mo); give 50% of the dose initially and 25% of the initial dose in each of 2 subsequent doses at 6–12 hr intervals. *PO: Adults: LD*—0.75–1.5 mg; give 50% of the dose initially and 25% of the initial dose in each of 2 subsequent doses at 6–8 hr intervals. *MD*—0.125–0.5 mg/day, depending on patient's IBW, renal function, and serum level. *PO: Geriatric Patients:* Daily dosage should not exceed 0.125 mg (AF may be exception). *PO: Peds: LD*—10–15 mcg/kg (>10 yr); 20–35 mcg/kg (5–10 yr); 30–40 mcg/kg (2–5 yr); 35–60 mcg/kg (1–24 mo); give 50% of the dose initially and 25% of the initial dose in each of 2 subsequent doses at 6–8 hr intervals. *MD*—2.5–5 mcg/kg (>10 yr); 5–10 mcg/kg (5–10 yr); 7.5–10 mcg/kg (2–5 yr); 10–15 mcg/kg (1–24 mo); given daily as single dose (for >10 yr) or in 2 divided doses (other age groups). *Renal Impairment Adults:* ↓ dose if CrCl <50 ml/min; **Availability (G):** *Tabs:* 0.125, 0.25 mg. *Caps:* 0.1, 0.2 mg. *Oral soln:* 0.05 mg/ml. *Inject:* 0.25 mg/ml. *Pediatric inject:* 0.1 mg/ml; **Monitor:** BP, HR, ECG, S/S HF, BUN/SCr, electrolytes, digoxin level (therapeutic: 0.8–2 ng/ml (AF); 0.5–1 ng/ml (HF)), S/S toxicity (N/V, anorexia, visual disturbances, arrhythmias); **Notes:** ↓ dose by 50% when starting amiodarone. LD usually reserved for AF (not for HF). Digoxin immune Fab is antidote.

digoxin immune Fab (Digibind, DigiFab) **Uses:** Potentially life-threatening digoxin toxicity; **Class:** antibody fragments; **Preg:** C; **CIs:** None known; **ADRs:** re-emergence of AF, re-emergence of HF, ↓ K+, ANAPHYLAXIS; **Interactions:** None known; **Dose:** *IV: Adults and Peds: Known amount of digoxin ingested*—Dose (# vials) = dose of digoxin ingested (mg)/0.5 mg of digitalis bound/vial *or* Dose (# vials) = [SDC (ng/ml) × wt (kg)]/100. *Unknown amount ingested/SDCs unavailable*—20 vials [760 mg (Digibind); 800 mg (DigiFab)]. *Toxicity during chronic digoxin therapy/SDCs unavailable*—6 vials [228 mg (Digibind); 240 mg (DigiFab)]; **Availability:** *Inject:* 38 mg/vial (Digibind), 40 mg/vial (DigiFab); **Monitor:** HR, ECG, digoxin levels (before administration, if possible), S/S HF, K+; **Notes:** For Digibind, each vial (38 mg) will bind 0.5 mg of digoxin; for DigiFab, each vial (40 mg) will bind 0.5 mg of digoxin. Free serum digoxin levels fall rapidly after administration. Total serum concentrations ↑ suddenly after administration but are bound to Fab molecule and are inactive. Digoxin levels will not be valid for 5–7 days after administration.

dihydroergotamine (D.H.E. 45, Migranal) **Uses:** Migraine or cluster HAs; **Class:** ergot alkaloids; **Preg:** X; **CIs:** PAD; Ischemic heart disease; Uncontrolled HTN; Severe renal or liver disease; Pregnancy/lactation; Concurrent use of potent CYP3A4 enzyme inhibitors (macrolides, azole antifungals, and protease inhibitors); Concurrent use with other vasoconstrictors (including 5–HT_3 agonists); Peds (safety not established); **ADRs:** dizziness, PULMONARY FIBROSIS, rhinitis, MI, ↑ BP, angina pectoris, intermittent claudication, VALVULAR HEART DISEASE, nausea, altered taste, diarrhea, vomiting, muscle pain, leg weakness, numbness or tingling in fingers or toes; **Interactions:** ↑ risk of life-threatening ischemia with potent CYP3A4 inhibitors, including macrolides, azole antifungals, and protease inhibitors (contraindicated); ↑ risk of peripheral vasoconstriction with beta blockers, oral contraceptives, and nicotine; ↑ risk of HTN with other use with vasoconstrictors (contraindicated); ↑ risk of prolonged vasoconstriction with $5HT_3$ agonists (allow 24 hr between use); **Dose:** *IM, IV, Subcut: Adults:* 1 mg; may repeat q 1 hr to a max total dose of 3 mg (2 mg for IV) (max: 3 mg/day or 6 mg/wk). *Intranasal: Adults:* 1 spray (0.5 mg) in each nostril, repeat in 15 min with 1 spray (0.5 mg) in each nostril (max total dose: 2 mg/day); **Availability (G):** *Inject:* 1 mg/ml. *Nasal spray:* 4 mg/1 ml; **Monitor:** BP, peripheral pulses, pain, signs of ergotism (cold/numb fingers/toes, N/V, HA, muscle pain, weakness); **Notes:** May give metoclopramide to minimize N/V. Administer as soon as patient reports prodromal symptoms or HA. Not for chronic use.

diltiazem (Cardizem, Cardizem CD, Cardizem LA, Cartia XT, Dilacor XR, Dilt-CD, Diltia XT, Taztia XT, Tiazac) **Uses:** HTN; Angina (chronic stable or vasospastic); Supraventricular tachyarrhythmias (AF, AFl, or PSVT) (to control ventricular rate); **Class:** Calcium channel blockers; **Preg:** C; **CIs:** Hypersensitivity; ≥2nd-degree heart block or sick sinus syndrome (in absence of pacemaker); BP <90 mmHg; Recent MI or pulmonary congestion; Arrhythmia associated with a bypass tract (e.g., WPW); Ventricular arrhythmias; Lactation or peds (safety not established); **ADRs:** dizziness, HA, weakness, dyspnea, HF, ↓ HR, edema, ↓ BP, syncope, constipation, nausea, flushing, gingival hyperplasia; **Interactions:** ↑ effects with other antihypertensives; CYP3A4 inhibitors may ↑ levels/toxicity; CYP3A4 inducers may ↓ levels/effects; May ↑ levels/toxicity of CYP3A4 substrates; NSAIDs may ↓ effectiveness; May ↑ digoxin levels/toxicity; ↑ risk of bradycardia with digoxin, beta blockers, or clonidine; **Dose:** *PO: Adults: HTN*—120–540 mg/day (as ER tabs/caps) *or* 60–180 mg bid (as SR caps). *Angina*—30–90 mg qid (as IR) *or* 120–480 mg/day (as ER tabs/caps). *IV: Adults:* 0.25 mg/kg; may repeat in 15 min with 0.35 mg/kg. May follow with continuous infusion at 10 mg/hr (range: 5–15 mg/hr); **Availability (G):** *Tabs:* 30, 60, 90, 120 mg. *SR caps:* 60, 90, 120 mg. *ER caps (Cardizem CD, Dilacor XR, Dilt-CD, Diltia XT, Tiazac, Cartia XT, Taztia XT):* 120, 180,

240, 300, 360, 420 mg. *ER tabs (Cardizem LA):* 120, 180, 240, 300, 360, 420 mg. *Inject:* 5 mg/ml; **Monitor:** BP, HR, ECG, wt, S/S angina, S/S HF; **Notes:** Do not open, crush, break, or chew SR/ER caps/tabs.

diphenhydrAMINE (Benadryl Allergy, Benadryl, Diphenhist, Genahist, Nytol, Sominex, Unisom) **Uses:** Seasonal and perennial allergic rhinitis; Allergic dermatosis; Itching due to insect bites or poison ivy/oak/sumac; Parkinson's disease and drug-induced EPS; Insomnia; Motion sickness; Antitussive (syrup only); **Class:** antihistamines; **Preg:** B; **CIs:** Hypersensitivity; Acute attacks of asthma; Lactation; Peds <2 yr; **ADRs:** drowsiness, dizziness, HA, paradoxical excitation (↑ in peds), blurred vision, ↓ BP, dry mouth, constipation, nausea, urinary retention, thickened bronchial secretions, wheezing, pain at IM site; **Interactions:** ↑ CNS depression with other CNS depressants including alcohol, other antihistamines, opioids, and sedative/hypnotics; May ↑ levels/effects of CYP2D6 substrates; ↑ risk of anticholinergic effects with other anticholinergic agents; **Dose:** *PO: Adults and Peds: ≥12 yr Allergic reactions or motion sickness*—25–50 mg q 4–6 hr prn (max: 300 mg/day). *Antitussive*—25 mg q 4 hr prn (max: 150 mg/day). *Dystonic reaction*—25–50 mg q 4 hr (max: 400 mg/day). *Sedative/hypnotic*—50 mg 20–30 min before bedtime. *PO: Peds: 6–11 yr Allergic reactions or motion sickness*—12.5–25 mg q 4–6 hr prn (max: 150 mg/day). *Antidyskinetic*—0.5–1 mg/kg q 6–8 hr prn (max: 300 mg/day). *Antitussive*—12.5 mg q 4 hr prn (max: 75 mg/day). *PO: Peds: 2–5 yr Allergic reactions or motion sickness*—6.25 mg q 4–6 hr prn (max: 37.5 mg/day). *Antidyskinetic*—0.5–1 mg/kg q 4–6 hr prn (max: 300 mg/day). *Antitussive*—6.25 mg q 4 hr prn (max: 37.5 mg/day). *IM, IV: Adults:* 25–50 mg q 4 hr prn (max: 400 mg/day). *IM, IV: Peds:* 1.25 mg/kg q 6 hr prn (max: 300 mg/day). *Topical: Adults and Peds: ≥2 yr* Apply 3–4 times/day; **Availability (G):** *Caps/Tabs:* 25, 50 mg ^{OTC}. *Chew tabs:* 12.5, 25 mg ^{OTC}. *ODT:* 19 mg, 25 mg ^{OTC}. *Oral strips:* 12.5, 25 mg ^{OTC}. *Elixir:* 12.5 mg/5 ml ^{OTC}. *Syrup:* 12.5 mg/5 ml ^{OTC}. *Susp:* 25 mg/5 ml ^{OTC}. *Inject:* 50 mg/ml. *Cream/Gel/Top soln:* 2%^{OTC}; **Monitor:** Allergy symptoms, S/S EPS, sleep patterns, N/V, cough, skin condition; **Notes:** Use with caution in elderly (may ↑ anticholinergic effects and fall risk).

diphenoxylate/atropine (Lomotil, Lonox) **Uses:** Diarrhea; **Class:** anticholinergics; **Preg:** C; **CIs:** Hypersensitivity; Severe liver disease; Infectious diarrhea; Diarrhea associated with pseudomembranous colitis; Children <2 yr; **ADRs:** dizziness, drowsiness, HA, blurred vision, dry eyes, ↑ HR, dry mouth, N/V, urinary retention; **Interactions:** ↑ CNS depression with other CNS depressants, alcohol, antihistamines, opioids, and sedative/hypnotics; ↑ risk of anticholinergic effects with other anticholinergic agents; Use with MAOIs may result in hypertensive crisis; **Dose:** *PO: Adults:* 2 tabs (or 10 ml of liquid) qid until diarrhea controlled, then may continue with 2 tabs (or 10 ml of liquid) daily (max: 20 mg/day). *PO: Peds: >2 yr:* 0.3–0.4 mg/kg/day qid (use liquid only); **Availability (G):** *Tabs:* 2.5 mg diphenoxylate/0.025 mg atropine. *Liquid:* 2.5 mg diphenoxylate/0.025 mg atropine per 5 ml; **Monitor:** stool frequency, I/Os, electrolytes; **Notes:** Schedule V controlled substance. Risk of dependence ↑ with high-dose, long-term use. Atropine added to the formulation to discourage abuse. Do not use if suspect *C. diff.*

D

disopyramide (Norpace, Norpace CR) Uses: VT; AF; **Class:** antiarrhythmics; **Preg:** C; **CIs:** Hypersensitivity; Cardiogenic shock; ≥2nd-degree heart block or sick sinus syndrome (in absence of pacemaker); QT interval prolongation; HF; Hypotension; Glaucoma; Myasthenia gravis; Lactation; Peds (safety not established); **ADRs:** dizziness, fatigue, HA, blurred vision, dry eyes, HF, ARRHYTHMIAS, AV block, edema, ↓ BP, constipation, dry mouth, nausea, urinary retention; **Interactions:** ↑ risk of anticholinergic effects with other anticholinergic agents; CYP3A4 inhibitors may ↑ levels; CYP3A4 inducers may ↓ levels; ↑ risk of QT prolongation with other QT-prolonging drugs; May have additive toxic cardiac effects when used with other antiarrhythmics (↑ QRS or QT interval); **Dose:** *PO: Adults: IR (<50 kg or hepatic impairment)*—100 mg q 6 hr. *IR (>50 kg)*—150 mg q 6 hr (max: 800 mg/day). *CR (<50 kg or hepatic impairment)*—200 mg q 12 hr. *CR (>50 kg)*—300 mg q 12 hr. *PO: Peds: <1 yr*—10–30 mg/kg/day divided q 6 hr. *1–4 yr*—10–20 mg/kg/day divided q 6 hr. *4–12 yr*—10–15 mg/kg/day divided q 6 hr. *12–18 yr*—6–15 mg/kg/day divided q 6 hr. *Renal Impairment PO: Adults:* ↓ dose if CrCl ≤40 ml/min; **Availability (G):** *Caps:* 100, 150 mg. *ER caps:* 100, 150 mg; **Monitor:** BP, HR, ECG, wt, S/S HF, BUN/SCr, LFTs, electrolytes; **Notes:** When changing from IR to ER, give 1st dose of ER form 6 hr after last IR dose. Do not break open, crush, or chew ER form.

DOBUTamine (Dobutrex) Uses: Short-term (<48 hr) treatment of decompensated HF; **Class:** adrenergics; **Preg:** B; **CIs:** Hypersensitivity to dobutamine or bisulfites; Idiopathic hypertrophic subaortic stenosis; **ADRs:** ARRHYTHMIAS, ↑↓ BP, ↑ HR, angina, palpitations, N/V, phlebitis; **Interactions:** ↓ effect with beta blockers; ↑ risk of arrhythmias with some anesthetics or dopamine; **Dose:** *IV: Adults and Peds:* 2.5 mcg/kg/min; titrate to response (usual range: 2.5–20 mcg/kg/min; max: 40 mcg/kg/min); **Availability (G):** *Inject:* 12.5 mg/ml. *Premixed infusion:* 250 mg/250 ml, 500 mg/500 ml, 500 mg/250 ml, 1000 mg/250 ml; **Monitor:** BP, HR, ECG, cardiac index, PCWP, CVP, I/Os, peripheral pulses, BUN/SCr, electrolytes, S/S HF; **Notes: High Alert:** IV vasoactive meds are potentially dangerous. Have second practitioner independently check original order, dosage calculations, and infusion pump settings. Correct electrolyte abnormalities (↑ risk of arrhythmias with ↓ K+ or ↓ Mg++). Administer into large vein and assess IV site frequently. Dose should be titrated so HR does not ↑ by >10% of baseline.

docetaxel (Taxotere) Uses: Breast CA; Non–small-cell lung CA; Advanced metastatic hormone-refractory prostate CA; Squamous cell carcinoma of head and neck; Advanced gastric adenocarcinoma; **Class:** taxoids; **Preg:** D; **CIs:** Hypersensitivity to docetaxel or polysorbate 80; Neutrophils <1500; Hepatic impairment; Pregnancy or lactation; **ADRs:** fatigue, weakness, CARDIAC TAMPONADE, PERICARDIAL EFFUSION, PULMONARY EDEMA, peripheral edema, ↑ bilirubin, ↑ LFTs, N/V/D, stomatitis, alopecia, nail disorders, rash, dermatitis, erythema, anemia, neutropenia, thrombocytopenia, inject site reactions, myalgia, arthralgia, peripheral neuropathy, ANAPHYLAXIS; **Interactions:** ↑ bone marrow depression may occur with other antineoplastics or radiation therapy; CYP3A4 inhibitors may ↑ levels/toxicity; CYP3A4 inducers may ↓ levels/effects; **Dose:** *IV: Adults: Breast CA*—60–100 mg/m^2 q 3 wk. *Breast CA adjuvant therapy*—75 mg/m^2 q 3 wk for 6 cycles (with doxorubicin and cyclophosphamide). *Non–small-cell lung CA*—75 mg/m^2 q 3 wk (alone or with platinum). *Prostate CA*—75 mg/m^2 q 3 wk (with PO prednisone). *Gastric adenocarcinoma*—75 mg/m^2 q 3 wk (with cisplatin and fluorouracil). *Head/neck CA*—75 mg/m^2 q 3 wk for 4 cycles (with cisplatin and fluorouracil); **Availability:** *Inject:* 20 mg/0.5 ml, 80 mg/2 ml; **Monitor:** BP, HR, RR, temp, BUN/SCr, LFTs, CBC (with diff), N/V, S/S infection, rash, hypersensitivity reactions (most common after 1st and 2nd doses; bronchospasm, ↓ BP and/or erythema), edema; **Notes: High Alert:** Fatalities have occurred with chemotherapeutic agents. Before administering, clarify all ambiguous orders; double-check single, daily, and course-of-therapy dose limits; have second practitioner independently double-check original order, calculations, and infusion pump settings. Do not confuse Taxotere (docetaxel) with Taxol (paclitaxel). Premedicate with dexamethasone 8 mg PO bid to ↓ risk of edema and hypersensitivity reactions (start day before receiving docetaxel and continue for 2 more days; for prostate CA, dose of dexamethasone is 8 mg given 12 hr, 3 hr, and 1 hr before docetaxel, and then discontinue). Neutrophil nadir = 8 days with duration of 7 days. Neutrophil count should be >1500 and platelets >100,000 to give subsequent doses. Adjust subsequent doses if severe neutropenia develops. Discontinue and do not rechallenge if severe hypersensitivity reaction occurs.

docusate (Colace, Diocto, Docusoft S, DOK, DOS Softgels, DSS, Dulcolax Stool Softener, Fleet Sof-Lax, Genasoft, Phillips' Stool Softener, Silace, Surfak) Uses: PO: Prevention of constipation; **Rect:** Used as enema to soften fecal impaction; **Class:** stool softeners; **Preg:** C; **CIs:** Hypersensitivity; Abdominal pain or N/V, esp. when associated with fever or other signs of acute abdomen; **ADRs:** diarrhea, mild cramps, rash; **Interactions:** None significant; **Dose:** *PO: Adults and Peds: >12 yr:* 50–500 mg/day in 1–4 divided doses. *Rect: Adults:* 50–100 mg. *PO: Peds: 6–12 yr:* 40–150 mg/day in 1–4 divided doses. *PO: Peds: 3–6 yr:* 20–60 mg/day in 1–4 divided doses. *PO: Peds: <3 yr* 10–40 mg/day in 1–4 divided doses; **Availability (G):** *Caps:* 50, 100, 240, 250 mg. *Tabs:* 100 mg. *Syrup:* 20 mg/5 ml. *Liquid:* 150 mg/15 ml. *Enema:* 283 mg/5 ml; **Monitor:** Bowel sounds/function; **Notes:** Stool softener, not a stimulant laxative. May dilute oral soln in milk or fruit juice to ↓ bitter taste.

D

dofetilide (Tikosyn) Uses: Maintenance of sinus rhythm in patients with AF/AFl; Conversion of AF/AFl to sinus rhythm; **Class:** antiarrhythmics; **Preg:** C; **CIs:** Hypersensitivity; Congenital or acquired prolonged QT syndromes; Baseline QT_C interval >440 msec (500 msec in ventricular conduction abnormalities); CrCl <20 ml/min; Concurrent use of verapamil, cimetidine, ketoconazole, trimethoprim, megestrol, hydrochlorothiazide, prochlorperazine, or drugs that cause QT interval prolongation; Pregnancy (use only when benefit to patient outweighs potential risk to fetus); Lactation; Peds <18 yr (safety not established); **ADRs:** HA, dizziness, VENTRICULAR ARRHYTHMIAS, QT_C interval prolongation, nausea; **Interactions:** ↑ risk of QT prolongation with other QT-prolonging drugs; Verapamil, cimetidine, ketoconazole, trimethoprim, megestrol, hydrochlorothiazide, and prochlorperazine may ↑ levels (contraindicated); ↓ K+ or ↓ Mg++ from K^+- or Mg^{++}-depleting agents (e.g., diuretics, amphotericin, aminoglycosides, or cyclosporine) ↑ risk of arrhythmias (correct prior to administration); Amiloride, metformin, triamterene, and CYP3A4 inhibitors may also ↑ levels (use with caution); **Dose:** *PO: Adults:* 500 mcg bid (dosage adjustments may be required based on CrCl and QT_C interval); if QTc interval 2–3 hr after 1st dose is >15% of baseline or is >500 msec, ↓ dose [if 500 mcg bid (starting), ↓ to 250 mcg bid; if 250 mcg bid (starting), ↓ to 125 mcg bid; if 125 mcg bid (starting), ↓ to 125 mcg daily]. If QT_C >500 msec at any time after 2nd dose, discontinue dofetilide. *Renal Impairment PO: Adults:* ↓ dose if CrCl ≤60 ml/min; **Availability:** *Caps:* 125, 250, 500 mcg; **Monitor:** HR, ECG (QT_C interval), BUN/SCr, electrolytes; **Notes:** Patients must be hospitalized for ≥3 days when initiating therapy. Patients should not be discharged from the hospital within 12 hr of electrical or pharmacological conversion to sinus rhythm. Hospitals/prescribers must receive education before prescribing. Prescriptions can only be filled at certain pharmacies.

dolasetron (Anzemet) Uses: Prevention of N/V associated with emetogenic chemotherapy; Prevention and treatment of PONV (IV only for treatment); **Class:** 5–HT_3 antagonists; **Preg:** B; **CIs:** Hypersensitivity; QT interval prolongation; **ADRs:** HA, dizziness, sedation, ↑ BP, QT prolongation, diarrhea, fever; **Interactions:** ↑ risk of QT prolongation with other QT-prolonging drugs; Atenolol and cimetidine may ↑ hydrodolasetron (active metabolite) levels; Rifampin may ↓ levels of hydrodolasetron; **Dose:** *PO: Adults: Prevention of chemotherapy-induced N/V*—100 mg given ~1 hr before chemotherapy. *Prevention of PONV*—100 mg given ~2 hr before surgery. *PO: Peds: 2–16 yr*

Prevention of chemotherapy-induced N/V—1.8 mg/kg (max: 100 mg) given ~1 hr before chemotherapy. *Prevention of PONV*—1.2 mg/kg (max: 100 mg) given ~2 hr before surgery. *IV: Adults: Prevention of chemotherapy-induced N/V*—1.8 mg/kg (or 100 mg) given ~30 min before chemotherapy. *Prevention/treatment of PONV*—12.5 mg given ~15 min before discontinuation of anesthesia or as soon as N/V begins. *IV: Peds: 2–16 yr Prevention of chemotherapy-induced N/V*—1.8 mg/kg (max: 100 mg) given ~30 min before chemotherapy. *Prevention/treatment of PONV*—0.35 mg/kg (max: 12.5 mg) given ~15 min before discontinuation of anesthesia or as soon as N/V begins; **Availability:** *Tabs:* 50, 100 mg. *Inject:* 12.5 mg/0.625 ml, 20 mg/ml; **Monitor:** BP, HR, N/V, I/Os, ECG; **Notes:** Injectable dolasetron may be mixed in apple or apple-grape juice for PO dosing for peds.

D

donepezil (Aricept, Aricept ODT) **Uses:** Dementia associated with AD; **Class:** cholinergics; **Preg:** C; **CIs:** Hypersensitivity; Lactation; **ADRs:** HA, abnormal dreams, depression, dizziness, drowsiness, fatigue, insomnia, ↓ HR, ↑ BP, diarrhea, nausea, anorexia, vomiting, polyuria, ecchymoses, ↓ wt, arthritis, muscle cramps; **Interactions:** ↓ effects of anticholinergics; ↑ cholinergic effects of other cholinergic agonists; May ↑ risk of GI bleeding from NSAIDs; Ketoconazole may ↑ levels/toxicity; Rifampin, carbamazepine, dexamethasone, phenobarbital, and phenytoin may ↓ levels/effects; **Dose:** *PO: Adults:* 5 mg/day; may ↑ to 10 mg/day after 4–6 wk; **Availability:** *Tabs:* 5, 10 mg. *ODT:* 5, 10 mg; **Monitor:** BP, HR, MMSE, cognitive function; **Notes:** Administer in PM at bedtime. Allow ODTs to dissolve on tongue, and follow with water.

DOPamine (Intropin) **Uses:** Adjunct to standard measures to improve: BP, Cardiac output, Urine output; **Class:** adrenergics; **Preg:** C; **CIs:** Ventricular arrhythmias; Pheochromocytoma; **ADRs:** ARRHYTHMIAS, ↓ BP, angina, ECG changes, palpitations, ↑ HR, N/V, phlebitis; **Interactions:** MAOIs, ergot alkaloids, and some antidepressants result in severe HTN; IV phenytoin may cause hypotension and bradycardia; Beta blockers may antagonize effects; **Dose:** *IV: Adults: Dopaminergic (renal vasodilation) effects*—0.5–3 mcg/kg/min. *Beta-adrenergic (cardiac stimulation) effects*—3–10 mcg/kg/min. *Alpha-adrenergic (↑ peripheral vascular resistance) effects*—10–20 mcg/kg/min. *IV: Peds:* 1–20 mcg/kg/min, depending on desired response; **Availability (G):** *Inject:* 40 mg/ml, 80 mg/ml, 160 mg/ml. *Premixed inject:* 200 mg/250 ml, 400 mg/250 ml, 800 mg/250 ml, 400 mg/500 ml, 800 mg/500 ml; **Monitor:** BP, HR, ECG, cardiac index, PCWP, CVP, I/Os, peripheral pulses, BUN/SCr, electrolytes, S/S HF; **Notes:** **High Alert:** IV vasoactive meds are potentially dangerous. Have second practitioner independently check original order, dosage calculations, and infusion pump settings. Correct electrolyte abnormalities (↑ risk of arrhythmias with ↓ K+ or ↓ Mg++). Administer into large vein and assess IV site frequently. Correct hypovolemia before administering. Use phentolamine if infiltration occurs.

doxazosin (Cardura, Cardura XL) **Uses:** HTN (IR only); BPH (IR and ER); **Class:** peripherally acting antiadrenergics; **Preg:** C; **CIs:** Hypersensitivity; Peds (safety not established); **ADRs:** dizziness, HA, drowsiness, blurred vision, first-dose orthostatic hypotension, edema, ↑ HR, diarrhea, dry mouth, nausea; **Interactions:** ↑ effects with other antihypertensives; **Dose:** *PO: Adults: HTN*—IR: 1 mg/day in AM or PM, may be gradually ↑ q 2 wk to 2–16 mg/day (↑ risk of postural hypotension at doses >4 mg/day). *BPH*—IR: 1 mg/day in AM or PM; may be gradually ↑ q 2 wk to 2–8 mg/day; ER: 4 mg/day in AM; may be ↑ in 3–4 wk to 8 mg/day; **Availability (G):** *Tabs:* 1, 2, 4, 8 mg. *ER tabs:* 4, 8 mg; **Monitor:** BP (sitting, standing), HR, PSA, S/S BPH, I/Os, wt, edema; **Notes:** Preferable to administer daily dose at bedtime. In HTN, should not be used as monotherapy. ER tabs should be swallowed whole; do not split, crush, or chew.

D

DOXOrubicin hydrochloride (Adriamycin) **Uses:** Treatment of various malignancies including: Breast CA, Ovarian CA, Bladder CA, Gastric CA, Soft tissue and bone sarcomas, Thyroid CA, Neuroblastoma, Bronchogenic carcinoma, Malignant lymphomas, and leukemias; **Class:** anthracyclines; **Preg:** D; **CIs:** Hypersensitivity; Bone marrow depression; Pregnancy/lactation; History of CV disease or high cumulative doses of anthracyclines; Severe hepatic impairment; **ADRs:** CARDIOMYOPATHY, ECG changes, esophagitis, N/V, stomatitis, diarrhea, red urine, alopecia, photosensitivity, sterility, LEUKOPENIA, anemia, thrombocytopenia, secondary leukemia, phlebitis at IV site, ↑ uric acid, hypersensitivity reactions; **Interactions:** ↑ bone marrow suppression with other antineoplastics or radiation therapy; Cardiotoxicity may be additive with other cardiotoxic agents (e.g., cyclophosphamide, daunorubicin, paclitaxel); ↑ risk of toxicity with hepatotoxic agents; Cyclosporine may ↑ effects/toxicity; May ↑ risk of hemorrhagic cystitis from cyclophosphamide; Phenobarbital may ↓ levels/effects; May ↓ levels/effects of phenytoin; **Dose:** *IV: Adults:* 60–75 mg/m^2/dose, repeat q 21 days *or* 20–30 mg/m^2 daily for 2–3 days, repeat q 4 wk *or* 20 mg/m^2/dose once weekly. Total cumulative dose should not exceed 550 mg/m^2 without monitoring of cardiac function or 400 mg/m^2 in patients with previous chest radiation or other cardiotoxic chemotherapy. *IV: Peds:* 35–75 mg/m^2/dose, repeat q 21 days *or* 20–30 mg/m^2/dose once weekly. *Hepatic Impairment IV: Adults:* ↓ dose if serum bilirubin ≥1.2 mg/dl; **Availability (G):** *Powder for inject:* 10 mg, 20 mg, 50 mg. *Inject:* 2 mg/ml; **Monitor:** BP, HR, RR, temp, BUN/SCr, CBC (with diff), uric acid, LFTs, S/S infection, S/S HF, bleeding, echo (LVEF), ECG, CXR, infusion site; **Notes: High Alert:** Fatalities have occurred with incorrect administration of chemotherapeutic agents. Before administering, clarify all ambiguous orders; double-check single, daily, and course-of-therapy dose limits; have second practitioner independently double-check original order, calculations, and infusion pump settings. Do not confuse with doxorubicin hydrochloride liposome (Doxil), daunorubicin hydrochloride (Cerubidine), or daunorubicin citrate liposome (Dauno Xome). Clarify orders that do not include generic and brand names. Dexrazoxane may be used to prevent cardiotoxicity if receiving cumulative doses of >300 mg/m². Leukocyte count nadir = 10–14 days (recovery in 21 days after administration). Do not give next dose unless ANC ≥1000 and platelets ≥100,000. Potent vesicant.

DOXOrubicin hydrochloride liposome (Doxil) Uses: AIDS-related KS in patients who are intolerant or fail conventional therapy; Ovarian CA; Multiple myeloma (with bortezomib); **Class:** anthracyclines; **Preg:** D; **CIs:** Hypersensitivity; Pregnancy/lactation; History of cardiac disease or high cumulative doses of anthracyclines; Bone marrow depression; **ADRs:** HA, CARDIOMYOPATHY, ECG changes, esophagitis, N/V/D, stomatitis, red urine, alopecia, hand-foot syndrome, photosensitivity, sterility, LEUKOPENIA, anemia, thrombocytopenia, secondary leukemia, phlebitis at IV site, ↑ uric acid, inject site reactions, fever, hypersensitivity reactions; **Interactions:** ↑ bone marrow suppression with other antineoplastics or radiation therapy; Cardiotoxicity may be additive with other cardiotoxic agents (e.g., cyclophosphamide, daunorubicin, paclitaxel); ↑ risk of toxicity with hepatotoxic agents; Cyclosporine may ↑ effects/toxicity; May ↑ risk of hemorrhagic cystitis from cyclophosphamide; Phenobarbital may ↓ levels/effects; May ↓ levels/effects of phenytoin; **Dose:** *IV: Adults: AIDS-related KS*—20 mg/m² q 3 wk. *Ovarian CA*—50 mg/m² q 4 wk. *Multiple myeloma*—30 mg/m² on Day 4 after following bortezomib for up to 8 cycles. *Hepatic Impairment IV: Adults:* ↓ dose if bilirubin ≥1.2 mg/dl; **Availability:** *Inject:* 2 mg/ml; **Monitor:** BP, HR, RR, temp, CBC (with diff), uric acid, LFTs, S/S infection, S/S HF, bleeding, echo (LVEF), ECG, CXR, infusion site, infusion reactions; **Notes: High Alert:** Fatalities have occurred with incorrect administration of chemotherapeutic agents. Before administering, clarify all ambiguous orders; double-check single, daily, and course-of-therapy dose limits; have second practitioner independently double-check original order, calculations, and infusion pump settings. Do not confuse with doxorubicin hydrochloride (Adriamycin), daunorubicin hydrochloride (Cerubidine), or daunorubicin citrate liposome (Dauno Xome). Clarify orders that do not include generic and brand names. Leukocyte count nadir = 10–14 days (recovery in 21–28 days after administration). Do not give next dose unless ANC ≥1500 and platelets ≥75,000.

doxycycline (Doryx, Doxy, Monodox, Periostat, Vibramycin, Vibra-Tabs) Uses: Various infections caused by unusual organisms, including *Mycoplasma*, *Chlamydia*, *Rickettsia*, and *Borrelia burgdorferi*; Inhalational anthrax (postexposure); Gonorrhea and syphilis in penicillin-allergic patients; Respiratory tract infections caused by *S. pneumo*, *H. flu*, or *Klebsiella*; Acne; Prevention of malaria due to

Plasmodium falciparum in short-term travelers (<4 months) to areas with chloroquine and/or pyrimethamine/sulfadoxine-resistant strains; Periodontitis; **Class:** tetracyclines; **Preg:** D; **CIs:** Hypersensitivity; Pregnancy, lactation, or peds <8 yr—risk of permanent staining of teeth in infants/peds (for pregnancy, risk is ↑ during last half of pregnancy); Nephrogenic DI; **ADRs:** PSEUDOMEMBRANOUS COLITIS, N/V/D, esophagitis, ↑ LFTs, photosensitivity, rash, neutropenia, thrombocytopenia, phlebitis at IV site, hypersensitivity reactions; **Interactions:** Use with antacids, bismuth subsalicylate, or drugs containing Ca^{++}, aluminum, Mg^{++}, iron, or zinc may ↓ absorption; May ↑ effects of warfarin; May ↓ effectiveness of estrogen-containing oral contraceptives; Phenobarbital, carbamazepine, and phenytoin may ↓ levels/effects, Ca^{++} in foods or dairy products may ↓ absorption; **Dose:** *PO, IV: Adults and Peds: >45 kg Most infections*—100–200 mg/day in 1–2 divided doses. *Gonorrhea*—100 mg q 12 hr × 7 days *or* 300 mg followed 1 hr later by another 300-mg dose. *Malaria prophylaxis*—100 mg/day. *Periodontitis*—20 mg PO bid for up to 9 mo. *Acne*—40 mg/day. *Inhalational anthrax*—100 mg q 12 hr × 60 days. *PO, IV: Peds: >8 yr and <45 kg Most infections*—2–5 mg/kg/day in 1–2 divided doses (max: 200 mg/day). *Inhalational anthrax*—2.2 mg/kg q 12 hr × 60 days; **Availability (G):** *Tabs:* 20, 50, 75, 100, 150 mg. *Caps:* 50, 100 mg. *ER caps:* 100 mg. *ER tabs:* 75, 100 mg. *Variable-release caps (Oracea):* 40 mg. *Oral susp:* 25 mg/5 ml. *Syrup:* 50 mg/5 ml. *Inject:* 100 mg; **Monitor:** BP, HR, temp, sputum, U/A, CBC, LFTs, acne lesions; **Notes:** Do not administer within 1–3 hr of other meds. Give with ≥8 oz of liquid, ≥ 1 hr before bedtime, and have patient sit up for ≥30 min after dose to ↓ esophageal irritation. Give ≥1 hr ac or ≥2 hr pc (may be taken with food if GI irritation occurs). Instruct patient to use sunscreen. Do not crush or chew ER tabs/caps.

droperidol (Inapsine) **Uses:** Treatment of N/V associated with surgical/diagnostic procedures; **Class:** butyrophenones; **Preg:** C; **CIs:** Hypersensitivity; QT interval prolongation (>440 msec); N/V outside of perioperative/periprocedural setting; Concurrent use of drugs that cause QT interval prolongation; Peds <2 yr (safety not established); **ADRs:** EPS, anxiety, dizziness, hallucinations, hyperactivity, restlessness, sedation, tardive dyskinesia, VENTRICULAR ARRHYTHMIAS, ↓ BP, ↑ HR, QT prolongation, NMS, chills, shivering; **Interactions:** ↑ risk of QT prolongation with other QT-prolonging drugs; ↓ K+ or ↓ Mg++ from K- or Mg-depleting agents (e.g., diuretics, amphotericin, aminoglycosides, or cyclosporine) ↑ risk of arrhythmias (correct prior to administration); ↑ CNS depression with other CNS depressants including alcohol, antihistamines, opioids, and sedative/hypnotics; Additive hypotension with antihypertensives or nitrates; **Dose:** *IV, IM: Adults:* 2.5 mg initially; additional doses of 1.25 mg may be needed, but should be undertaken with caution. *IM, IV: Peds: 2–12 yr:* 0.1 mg/kg; additional doses should be given with caution; **Availability (G):** *Inject:* 2.5 mg/ml; **Monitor:** BP,

HR, ECG (QT_C interval), electrolytes, EPS, N/V, I/Os; **Notes:** If ↓ BP occurs, avoid use of epinephrine as droperidol reverses its pressor effects and may cause paradoxical hypotension.

D

drotrecogin (Xigris) **Uses:** Adult patients with sepsis who have high risk of death; **Class:** activated protein C, human; **Preg:** C; **CIs:** Hypersensitivity; High risk of bleeding, including: Active internal bleeding, Recent (within 3 mo) hemorrhagic stroke, Recent (within 2 mo) intracranial or intraspinal injury or severe head trauma, Trauma associated with ↑ risk of life-threatening bleeding, Epidural catheter, Intracranial neoplasm/mass lesion/cerebral herniation; Patients not expected to survive due to pre-existing medical condition(s); HIV+ patients with CD4 counts ≤50/mm³; Chronic dialysis; Bone marrow, lung, liver, pancreas, or small bowel transplantation; Lactation; Peds; **ADRs:** BLEEDING; **Interactions:** Risk of serious bleeding may be ↑ by antiplatelet agents, anticoagulants, thrombolytic agents, or other agents that may affect coagulation; **Dose:** *IV: Adults:* 24 mcg/kg/hr × 96 hr; **Availability:** *Inject:* 5 mg, 20 mg; **Monitor:** BP, HR, temp, sputum, U/A, blood cultures, CBC, bleeding, PT; **Notes:** May prolong aPTT; monitor PT to assess coagulation status; discontinue 2 hr before invasive surgical procedures or procedures with risk of bleeding; once hemostasis achieved, may be restarted 12 hr after procedure. Should be started within 24 hr of the onset of at least 3 signs of systemic inflammation and evidence of at least 1 organ/system dysfunction.

duloxetine (Cymbalta) **Uses:** Depression; Diabetic peripheral neuropathy; GAD; **Class:** selective serotonin/norepinephrine reuptake inhibitors; **Preg:** C; **CIs:** Hypersensitivity; Concurrent use with MAOIs; Uncontrolled narrow-angle glaucoma; May ↑ risk of suicidal thoughts/behaviors, esp. during early treatment or dose adjustment (risk may be ↑ in peds and adolescents); Significant alcohol use; Severe renal impairment (CrCl <30 ml/min); Liver dysfunction; Lactation; May cause neonatal serotonin syndrome during 3rd tri of pregnancy; **ADRs:** SEIZURES, fatigue, drowsiness, insomnia, activation of mania, agitation, dizziness, ↑ BP, orthostatic hypotension, HEPATOTOXICITY, ↓ appetite, constipation, diarrhea, dry mouth, nausea, vomiting, ED, ↓ libido, ↑ sweating, tremor, SEROTONIN SYNDROME; **Interactions:** ↑ risk of potentially fatal reactions with MAOIs (discontinue for ≥2 wk); ↑ risk of hepatotoxicity with chronic alcohol abuse; CYP1A2 inhibitors and CYP2D6 inhibitors may ↑ effects/toxicity; May ↑ levels of CYP2D6 substrates; ↑ risk of bleeding with antiplatelets or anticoagulants; ↑ risk of serotonin syndrome with linezolid, tramadol, lithium, St. John's wort, and triptans; **Dose:** *PO: Adults: Depression*—20–30 mg bid *or* 60 mg/day (max: 120 mg/day). *Neuropathic pain or GAD*—60 mg/day; **Availability:** *Caps:* 20, 30, 60 mg; **Monitor:** BP, mental status, suicidal thoughts/behaviors, sexual dysfunction, pain, LFTs; **Notes:** Do not crush, chew, or open caps; may affect enteric coating.

dutasteride (Avodart) **Uses:** Symptomatic BPH; **Class:** androgen inhibitors; **Preg:** X; **CIs:** Hypersensitivity (cross-sensitivity to other 5-alpha-reductase inhibitors may occur); Women; Peds; **ADRs:** ↓ libido, ejaculation disorders, ED, gynecomastia, allergic reactions (angioedema); **Interactions:** CYP3A4 inhibitors may ↑ levels/effects; **Dose:** *PO: Adults:* 0.5 mg/day; **Availability:** *Caps:* 0.5 mg; **Monitor:** Rect exam, PSA, S/S BPH; **Notes:** PSA ↓ by about 50% after 6, 12, and 24 mo of therapy; new baseline PSA concentrations should be established after 3–6 mo of therapy. Patients should avoid donating blood for ≥ 6 mo after discontinuation of therapy. Do not crush, break, or chew caps.

efavirenz (Sustiva) **Uses:** HIV (with other antiretrovirals); **Class:** non-nucleoside reverse transcriptase inhibitors; **Preg:** D; **CIs:** Hypersensitivity; Concurrent use of midazolam, pimozide, triazolam, ergot derivatives, or standard doses of voriconazole; Pregnancy/lactation (use in pregnancy only if other options have been exhausted); **ADRs:** anxiety, dizziness, insomnia, abnormal dreams, depression, drowsiness, hallucinations, HA, impaired concentration, nervousness, suicidal thoughts, nausea, anorexia, diarrhea, dyspepsia, ↑ LFTs, ↑ cholesterol, ↑ TGs, rash, pruritus; **Interactions:** CYP3A4 inhibitors may ↑ levels; May ↑ levels of CYP2C9 substrates, CYP2C19 substrates, and CYP3A4 substrates; May ↓ levels of CYP3A4 substrates; ↑ levels of midazolam, triazolam, pimozide, or ergot alkaloids (contraindicated); ↓ voriconazole levels; voriconazole also ↑ efavirenz levels (use of standard doses of both agents is contraindicated; when used concurrently, ↓ efavirenz dose to 300 mg/day and ↑ voriconazole dose to 400 mg q 12 hr); ↑ risk of side effects (esp. hepatotoxicity) with ritonavir; ↓ indinavir levels (↑ indinavir dose); ↓ fosamprenavir levels (if used concurrently with fosamprenavir/ritonavir once daily regimen, an additional 100 mg of ritonavir [total of 300 mg] should be given); ↓ lopinavir levels (↑ lopinavir dose); ↓ saquinavir levels (avoid using saquinavir as the only protease inhibitor with efavirenz); ↓ atazanavir levels (if used concurrently in treatment-naive patients, add ritonavir 100 mg/day and ↓ atazanavir dose); May alter the effects of warfarin; Use with St. John's wort may ↓ levels and effectiveness (avoid concurrent use); ↓ levels of itraconazole and ketoconazole (consider alternative antifungals); ↓ rifabutin levels (↑ rifabutin dose by 50%); ↓ levels of clarithromycin, CCBs, atorvastatin, simvastatin, pravastatin, or methadone; May alter the effectiveness of hormonal contraceptives (use additional method of non-hormonal contraception); **Dose:** *PO: Adults and Peds:* $\geq$*3 yr and* $\geq$*40 kg:* 600 mg/day. *PO: Peds:* $\geq$*3 yr* 32.5–39 kg: 400 mg/day; 25–<32.5 kg: 350 mg/day; 20–<25 kg: 300 mg/day; 15–<20 kg: 250 mg/day; 10–<15 kg: 200 mg/day; **Availability:** *Caps:* 50, 200 mg. *Tabs:* 600 mg; **Monitor:** Viral load, CD4 count, LFTs, lipid panel, mental status; **Notes:** Take on empty stomach, preferably at bedtime (absorption ↑ with high-fat foods; bedtime dosing may ↓ CNS side effects). Do not break tabs. Onset of rash is usually within 1st 2 wk of therapy and resolves with continued therapy within 1 mo. CNS symptoms usually begin during 1st or 2nd day of therapy and resolve after 2–4 wk.

eletriptan (Relpax) Uses: Acute treatment of migraines; **Class:** 5-HT_1 agonists; **Preg:** C; **CIs:** Hypersensitivity; CAD or significant CV disease; Uncontrolled HTN; Use of other 5-HT_1 agonists or ergot-derivatives within 24 hr; Basilar or hemiplegic migraine; Severe hepatic impairment; CV risk factors (use only if CV status has been determined to be safe and 1st dose is administered under supervision); Use of potent CYP3A4 inhibitors (e.g., ketoconazole, itraconazole, nefazodone, clarithromycin, ritonavir, and nelfinavir) within 72 hr; Peds <18 yr (safety not established); **ADRs:** dizziness, drowsiness, weakness, CORONARY ARTERY VASOSPASM, MI/ISCHEMIA, VT/VF, chest tightness/pressure, abdominal pain, dry mouth, nausea; **Interactions:** Use with other 5-HT_1 agonists or ergot derivatives compounds may ↑ risk of vasospasm (use within 24 hr is contraindicated); Use with SSRIs or SNRIs may ↑ risk of serotonin syndrome; Potent CYP3A4 inhibitors may ↑ levels/toxicity (use within 72 hr is contraindicated); **Dose:** *PO: Adults:* 20 or 40 mg (max single dose: 40 mg); may be repeated in 2 hr if ineffective (max dose: 80 mg/24 hr or treatment of 3 HAs/mo); **Availability:** *Tabs:* 20, 40 mg; **Monitor:** Pain and associated symptoms; **Notes:** Only aborts migraines (should not be used for prophylaxis). Administer as soon as migraine symptoms occur.

emtricitabine (Emtriva) Uses: HIV (with other antiretrovirals); **Class:** nucleoside reverse transcriptase inhibitors; **Preg:** B; **CIs:** Hypersensitivity; HBV infection (may exacerbate following discontinuation); **ADRs:** depression, dizziness, HA, insomnia, weakness, nightmares, cough, abdominal pain, N/V/D, SEVERE HEPATOMEGALY WITH STEATOSIS, dyspepsia, rash, skin discoloration, LACTIC ACIDOSIS, arthralgia, myalgia, neuropathy, paresthesia, fat redistribution, ↑ TGs; **Interactions:** None noted; **Dose:** *PO: Adults: ≥18 yr Caps*—200 mg/day. *Oral soln*—240 mg/day. *PO: Peds: 3 mo–17 yr and >33 kg Caps*—200 mg/day. *PO: Peds: 3 mo–17 yr and ≤33 kg Oral soln*—6 mg/kg/day (max: 240 mg/day). *PO: Peds: 0–3 mo Oral soln*—3 mg/kg/day. *Renal Impairment PO: Adults: ≥18 yr* ↓ dose if CrCl <50 ml/min; **Availability:** *Caps:* 200 mg. *Oral soln:* 10 mg/ml; **Monitor:** Viral load, CD4 count, TGs, LFTs, CK; **Notes:** Not to be used as monotherapy. Component of Truvada and Atripla. Test for HBV before starting therapy.

enalapril, enalaprilat (Vasotec, Vasotec IV) Uses: HTN; HF; **Uses:** HTN; **Class:** ACEIs; **Preg:** C (1st tri), D (2nd and 3rd tri); **CIs:** Previous sensitivity/intolerance to ACEIs; Pregnancy/lactation; CrCl <30 ml/min (peds only); **ADRs:** dizziness, cough, ↓ BP, ↑ SCr, ↑ K+, rash, ANGIOEDEMA; **Interactions:** ↑ effects with other antihypertensives; ↑ risk of hyperkalemia with ARBs, K+ supplements, K+ salt substitutes, K+ sparing diuretics, or NSAIDs; NSAIDs may

↓ effectiveness; ↑ lithium levels; **Dose:** *PO: Adults: HTN*—2.5–5 mg/day (2.5 mg if receiving diuretic or has hyponatremia); may be ↑ q 1–2 wk (max: 40 mg/day in 1–2 divided doses). *HF*—2.5 mg bid; titrate up to target dose of 10 mg bid. *PO: Peds and Neonates:* 0.08 mg/kg/day in 1–2 divided doses (max: 5 mg/day); may be slowly titrated up to a max of 0.5 mg/kg/day (40 mg/day). *IV: Adults:* 0.625–1.25 mg (0.625 mg if receiving diuretics) q 6 hr; can be titrated up to 5 mg q 6 hr. *IV: Peds and Neonates:* 5–10 mcg/kg q 8–24 hr. *Renal Impairment PO, IV: Adults:* ↓ dose if CrCl <30 ml/min (HTN) or SCr >1.6 mg/dl (HF); **Availability (G):** *Tabs (Enalapril):* 2.5, 5, 10, 20 mg. *Inject (Enalaprilat):* 1.25 mg/ml; **Monitor:** BP, HR, wt, edema, BUN/SCr, K+; **Notes:** Correct volume depletion. Advise on S/S angioedema. Avoid K+ salt substitutes. Do not use IV in post-MI patients.

enfuvirtide (Fuzeon) **Uses:** HIV (with other antiretrovirals) in patients with evidence of progressive HIV-1 replication despite ongoing treatment; **Class:** fusion inhibitors; **Preg:** B; **CIs:** Hypersensitivity; Lactation; Pregnancy (use only if clearly indicated); Peds <6 yr (safety not established); **ADRs:** <u>fatigue</u>, conjunctivitis, cough, pneumonia, sinusitis, <u>diarrhea</u>, <u>nausea</u>, abdominal pain, anorexia, dry mouth, pancreatitis, ↓ wt, <u>inject site reactions</u>, myalgia, limb pain, hypersensitivity reactions, herpes simplex; **Interactions:** None noted; **Dose:** *Subcut: Adults:* 90 mg bid. *Subcut: Peds: 6–16 yr:* 2 mg/kg bid (max: 90 mg/dose); **Availability:** *Inject:* 108 mg/vial (to deliver 90 mg/ml concentration); **Monitor:** Viral load, CD4 count, RR, temp, CBC, LFTs, cough, inject site reactions (pain, discomfort, induration, erythema, nodules and cysts, pruritus, ecchymosis); **Notes:** Patients with ↓ CD4 count, high initial viral load, IV drug use, smoking, and prior history of lung disease are at ↑ risk of pneumonia. Administer in upper arm, abdomen, or anterior thigh. Rotate sites; do not inject into sites with previous inject site reactions, moles, scars, bruises, or within 2 in. of the navel.

enoxaparin (Lovenox) **Uses:** Prevention of DVT and PE in surgical and medical patients; Treatment of DVT (with warfarin); Treatment of ACS (UA/NSTEMI or STEMI); **Class:** antithrombotics, heparins (low molecular weight); **Preg:** B; **CIs:** Hypersensitivity to enoxaparin, heparin, pork products, or benzyl alcohol; Active bleeding; Thrombocytopenia related to previous enoxaparin or heparin therapy; Spinal or epidural anesthesia; Peds (safety not established); **ADRs:** ↑ LFTs, BLEEDING, thrombocytopenia, pain at inject site; **Interactions:** ↑ risk of bleeding with antiplatelets, thrombolytics, or other anticoagulants; **Dose:** *Subcut: Adults: Knee replacement surgery*—30 mg q 12 hr × 7–10 days (start 12–24 hr after surgery). *Hip replacement*—30 mg q 12 hr (start 12–24 hr after surgery) *or* 40 mg/day (start 12 hr before surgery) (continue for up to 3 wk after hospital discharge). *Abdominal surgery*—40 mg/day × 7–10 days (start 2 hr before surgery). *Medical patients with acute illness*—40 mg/day × 6–11 days. *Treatment of DVT (with or without PE)*—Inpatient: 1 mg/kg q 12 hr or 1.5 mg/kg q 24 hr; Outpatient: 1 mg/kg q 12 hr. *Treatment of UA/NSTEMI*—1 mg/kg q 12 hr × 2–8 days. *Treatment of STEMI*—30 mg IV × 1 dose, then 1 mg/kg q 12 hr (max for 1st 2 doses = 100 mg/dose) × 8 days or hospital discharge (whichever occurs first). *Subcut (Geriatric Patients ≥75 yr) Treatment of STEMI*—0.75 mg/kg q 12 hr (max for 1st 2 doses = 75 mg/dose) (no initial IV bolus). *Renal Impairment Subcut: Adults:* ↓ dose if CrCl <30 ml/min; **Availability:** *Inject:* 30 mg/0.3 ml, 40 mg/0.4 ml, 60 mg/0.6 ml, 80 mg/0.8 ml, 100 mg/ml, 120 mg/0.8 ml, 150 mg/ml; **Monitor:** BUN/SCr, CBC, LFTs, anti-Xa (if renal dysfunction or obese), bleeding; **Notes:** Anti-Xa levels can be monitored after 3–4 doses; obtain 4 hr after a dose. For treatment of DVT/PE, warfarin should be started within 72 hr; enoxaparin should be continued for ≥5 days or until therapeutic INR achieved (INR >2 for two consecutive days).

entacapone (Comtan) Uses: Parkinson's disease (with levodopa/carbidopa) when signs/symptoms of end-of-dose "wearing-off" occur; **Class:** catechol-*O*-methyltransferase inhibitors; **Preg:** C; **CIs:** Hypersensitivity; Concurrent nonselective MAOI therapy; **ADRs:** NMS, dizziness, hallucinations, syncope, pulmonary infiltrates, pleural effusion, orthostatic hypotension, N/V/D, abdominal pain, constipation, urine discoloration (brownish-orange), RHABDOMYOLYSIS, dyskinesia; **Interactions:** Concurrent use with selective MAOIs is not recommended; both agents inhibit the metabolic pathways of catecholamines; ↑ risk of ↑ HR, ↑ BP and arrhythmias with drugs that are metabolized by COMT (e.g., isoproterenol, epinephrine, norepinephrine, dopamine, dobutamine, and methyldopa); Probenecid, cholestyramine, erythromycin, rifampin, ampicillin, and chloramphenicol may ↓ biliary elimination of entacapone; **Dose:** *PO: Adults:* 200 mg with each dose of levodopa/carbidopa up to a maximum of 8 ×/day; **Availability:** *Tabs:* 200 mg; **Monitor:** S/S Parkinson's, EPS, diarrhea; **Notes:** Always administer with levodopa/carbidopa (has no antiparkinsonism effects of its own). Taper gradually to discontinue.

entecavir (Baraclude) Uses: Chronic active HBV; **Class:** nucleoside analogues; **Preg:** C; **CIs:** Hypersensitivity; Lactation; Peds <16 yr (safety not established); Pregnancy (use only if clearly needed, considering benefits and risks); **ADRs:** dizziness, fatigue, HA, ↑ LFTs, nausea, LACTIC ACIDOSIS; **Interactions:** Nephrotoxic drugs may ↑ levels/toxicity; **Dose:** *PO: Adults and Peds: >16 yr:* 0.5 mg/day. *Refractory to lamivudine*—1 mg/day. *Renal Impairment PO: Adults and Peds: >16 yr:* ↓ dose if CrCl <50 ml/min; **Availability:** *Tabs:* 0.5, 1 mg. *Oral soln:* 0.05 mg/ml; **Monitor:** S/S hepatitis, BUN/SCr, LFTs, HBV DNA, HIV status (prior to starting therapy); **Notes:** Give on empty stomach ≥2 hr before or after a meal. Give soln undiluted. May ↑ risk of HIV resistance.

epinephrine (Adrenalin, EpiPen, Primatene) Uses: *Subcut, IV, Inhaln:* Reversible airway disease due to asthma or COPD. *Subcut, IV:* Severe allergic reactions; *IV, Endotracheal, Intraosseous (part of ACLS and*

PALS guidelines): Cardiac arrest; **Inhaln:** Upper airway obstruction and croup (racemic epinephrine); *Local/Spinal:* Adjunct in the localization/ prolongation of anesthesia; **Class:** adrenergics; **Preg:** C; **CIs:** Hypersensitivity to adrenergic amines; Arrhythmias; Narrow-angle glaucoma; **ADRs:** nervousness, restlessness, tremor, HA, insomnia, paradoxical bronchospasm (excessive use of inhalers), ARRHYTHMIAS, angina, ↑ BP, ↑ HR, N/V, ↑ BG; **Interactions:** ↑ risk of adrenergic side effects with other adrenergic agents; Use with MAOIs may lead to hypertensive crisis; Beta blockers may negate therapeutic effect; **Dose:** *IV: Adults: Anaphylactic reactions*—0.1 mg (of 1:10,000 soln). *Cardiac arrest (asystole, PEA, pulseless VT/VF)*—1 mg q 3–5 min; may also be given by intraosseous route. *Bradycardia*—1 mg q 3–5 min; may also be given as infusion of 2–10 mcg/ min. *ET: Adults: Cardiac arrest*—2–2.5 mg (diluted in 10 ml of NS or distilled water) administered down ET tube q 3–5 min. *Subcut: Adults: Bronchodilator*—0.3–0.5 mg of 1:1000 soln q 20 min × 3 doses. *IM: Adults: Anaphylactic reactions*—0.3 mg (EpiPen). *Subcut, IM: Adults: Anaphylactic reactions*—0.3–0.5 mg of 1:1000 soln q 15–20 min if needed. *Inhaln: Adults: MDI*—1 inhaln, may be repeated after 1–2 min; additional doses may be repeated q 3 hr. *Inhaln soln*—1–3 inhaln of 1% soln; additional doses may be given q 3 hr. *Racepinephrine*—Via hand nebulizer, 2–3 inhaln of 2.25% soln; may repeat in 5 min with 2–3 more inhaln, may repeat q 3–4 hr. *Topical: Adults and Peds: ≥6 yr Nasal decongestant*—Apply 0.1% solution as gtt, spray, or with a swab. *Intraspinal: Adults and Peds:* 0.2–0.4 ml of 1:1000 soln. *With Local Anesthetics: Adults and Peds:* Use 1:200,000 soln with local anesthetic. *IV: Peds: Cardiac arrest*—0.01 mg/kg (max: 1 mg) q 3–5 min; may also be given by intraosseous route. *ET: Peds Cardiac arrest*—0.1 mg/kg (max: 10 mg) (diluted in 3–5 ml NS) administered down ET tube q 3–5 min. *Subcut: Peds: >1 month Bronchodilator*—0.01 mg/kg of 1:1000 soln (max: 0.5 mg/dose) q 20 min for 3 doses. *Subcut, IV: Peds: Anaphylactic reactions*—0.01 mg/kg q 20 min. *IM: Peds: >1 month Anaphylactic reactions*—<30 kg: 0.15 mg (EpiPen Jr); >30 kg: 0.3 mg (EpiPen). *Inhaln: Peds: >1 month Inhaln soln*—1–3 inhaln of 1% soln; additional doses may be given q 3 hr. *Racepinephrine*—0.05 ml/kg (max: 0.5 ml/dose) of 2.25% racemic epinephrine solution diluted in 3 ml NS; may repeat q 2 hr; **Availability (G):** *Inhaln aerosol:* 0.22 mg/inhaln^{OTC}. *Inhaln soln:* 1% (1:100)^{OTC}. *Inhaln soln (racepinephrine):* 2.25%^{OTC}. *Inject:* 0.1 mg/ml (1:10,000) 1 mg/ml (1:1000). *Autoinjector (EpiPen):* 0.15 mg/0.3 ml (1:2000), 0.3 mg/0.3 ml (1:1000). *Top soln:* 0.1%; **Monitor:** BP, HR, RR, ECG, lung sounds; **Notes: High Alert:** Patient harm or fatalities have occurred from medication errors with epinephrine. Epinephrine is available in various concentrations, strengths, and percentages and is used for different purposes. Packaging labels may be easily confused or the products incorrectly diluted. Dilutions should be prepared by a pharmacist. IV doses should be expressed in milligrams, not ampules, concentration, or volume. Prior to administration, have second practitioner independently check original order, dose calculations, concentration, route of administration, and infusion pump settings. Avoid IM administration in gluteal muscle. For cardiac arrest, give via intraosseous or ET route if cannot obtain IV access.

epirubicin (Ellence) Uses: Component of adjuvant therapy for evidence of axillary tumor involvement following resection of primary breast CA; **Class:** anthracyclines; **Preg:** D; **CIs:** Hypersensitivity to epirubicin or other anthracyclines; Baseline neutrophil count <1500; Severe myocardial insufficiency or recent MI; Severe arrhythmias; Previous anthracycline therapy; Severe hepatic dysfunction; Pregnancy/lactation; Concurrent cimetidine therapy; **ADRs:** lethargy, CARDIOTOXICITY (dose-related), mucositis, N/V/D, anorexia, alopecia, flushing, photosensitivity, rash, skin/nail hyperpigmentation, gonadal suppression, LEUKOPENIA, anemia, thrombocytopenia, treatment-related leukemia/myelodysplastic syndromes, inject site reactions, phlebitis at IV site, hot flashes, ↑ uric acid, ANAPHYLAXIS, INFECTION; **Interactions:** ↑ bone marrow suppression with other antineoplastics or radiation therapy; Cardiotoxicity may be additive with other cardiotoxic agents (e.g., cyclophosphamide, doxorubicin, daunorubicin); Cimetidine ↑ levels (contraindicated); **Dose:** *IV: Adults:* 100–120 mg/m² repeated in 3–4 wk cycles (total dose may be given on Day 1 or split and given in equally divided doses on Day 1 and Day 8 of each cycle) (combination regimens may also include 5-fluorouracil and cyclophosphamide). *Hepatic/Renal Impairment IV: Adults:* ↓ dose if serum bilirubin ≥1.2 mg/dl, AST ≥2 × ULN or SCr >5 mg/dl; **Availability (G):** *Powder for inject:* 50 mg, 200 mg. *Soln for inject:* 2 mg/ml; **Monitor:** BP, HR, temp, BUN/SCr, CBC (with diff), uric acid, LFTs, S/S infection, S/S HF, bleeding, echo (LVEF), ECG, infusion site; **Notes: High Alert:** Fatalities have occurred with incorrect administration of chemotherapeutic agents. Before administering, clarify all ambiguous orders; double-check single, daily, and course-of-therapy dose limits; have second practitioner independently double-check original order, calculations, and infusion pump settings. ↑ risk of cardiotoxicity with cumulative dose regimen >900 mg/m² and mediastinal radiation. Leukocyte count nadir = 10–14 days (recovery in 21 days after administration). Potent vesicant. Patients receiving 120 mg/m² regimen should receive prophylactic anti-infective therapy with trimethoprim/sulfamethoxazole or a FQ.

eplerenone (Inspra) Uses: HTN; HF post-MI; **Class:** aldosterone antagonists; **Preg:** B; **CIs:** Serum K >5.5 mEq/L; CrCl ≤30 ml/min; Concurrent use of strong CYP3A4 inhibitors (ketoconazole, itraconazole, nefazodone, clarithromycin, ritonavir, nelfinavir); Type 2 DM with microalbuminuria (for HTN only); SCr >2.0 mg/dl (males) or >1.8 mg/dl (females) (for HTN only); CrCl <50 ml/min (for HTN only); Concurrent use of K+ supplements or K+ sparing diuretics (for HTN only); Lactation; Pregnancy (use only if clearly needed); **ADRs:** dizziness, ↑ LFTs, diarrhea, ↑ K+, ↑ TGs; **Interactions:** Strong

CYP3A4 inhibitors (e.g., ketoconazole, itraconazole, nefazodone, clarithromycin, nelfinavir, and ritonavir) ↑ levels (contraindicated); Moderate CYP3A4 inhibitors (erythromycin, saquinavir, verapamil, and fluconazole) may ↑ levels; ↑ risk of hyperkalemia with ACEIs, ARBs, K+ supplements, K+ salt substitutes, K+ sparing diuretics, or NSAIDs; NSAIDs may ↓ effectiveness; **Dose:** *PO: Adults: HTN*—50 mg/day initially; may ↑ to 50 mg bid. *Patients with HTN receiving concurrent moderate CYP3A4 inhibitors (erythromycin, saquinavir, verapamil, fluconazole)*—25 mg/day initially. *HF post-MI*—25 mg/day; titrate to 50 mg/day within 4 wk; **Availability (G):** *Tabs:* 25, 50 mg; **Monitor:** BP, HR, wt, edema, BUN/SCr, K+, LFTs, S/S HF; **Notes:** Monitor K+ within 1 wk after starting, then at 1 mo, then monthly thereafter.

epoetin alfa (Epogen, Procrit) **Uses:** Anemia in chronic renal failure; Anemia secondary to zidovudine therapy in patients with HIV; Chemotherapy-induced anemia in non-myeloid malignancies; Reduction of need for transfusions after surgery; **Class:** colony-stimulating factors; **Preg:** C; **CIs:** Hypersensitivity to albumin or mammalian cell-derived products; Uncontrolled HTN; **ADRs:** SEIZURES, HA, cough, dyspnea, ARRHYTHMIAS, HF, MI, STROKE, THROMBOTIC EVENTS (esp. with Hgb >12 g/dl), edema, ↑ BP, CP, abdominal pain, N/V/D, constipation, rash, pruritus, arthralgia, allergic reactions, fever, ↑ MORTALITY (esp. with Hgb ≥12 g/dl), TUMOR GROWTH (esp. with Hgb ≥12 g/dl), fever; **Interactions:** None reported; **Dose:** *IV, Subcut: Adults: Chronic renal failure*—50–100 units/kg 3 ×/wk; adjust dose to attain target Hgb of 10–12 g/dl; if Hgb ↑ by >1.0 g/dl in 2 wk or if the Hgb is ↑ and nearing 12 g/dl, ↓ dose by 25%; if Hgb <10 g/dl and ↑ by <1.0 g/dl after 4 wk of therapy (with adequate iron stores), ↑ dose by 25%. Do not ↑ dose more frequently than q 4 wk. *Zidovudine-treated HIV patients*—100 units/kg 3 ×/wk × 8 wk; if inadequate response, may ↑ by 50–100 units/kg q 4–8 wk, up to 300 units/kg 3 ×/wk. *Subcut: Adults: CA patients on chemotherapy*—150 units/kg 3 ×/week *or* 40,000 units once weekly; target Hgb should not exceed 12 g/dl. If Hgb ↑ by >1.0 g/dl in 2 wk, if Hgb >12 g/dl, or if Hgb reaches level to avoid transfusion, ↓ dose by 25%. If Hgb ↑ by <1.0 g/dl after 4–8 wk of therapy, ↑ dose to 300 units/kg *or* 60,000 units once weekly. Discontinue after chemotherapy completed. *Surgery patients*—300 units/kg daily × 10 days before surgery, on the day of surgery, and for 4 days after surgery *or* 600 units/kg 21, 14, and 7 days before surgery and on day of surgery. *Subcut, IV: Peds: Chronic renal failure*—50 units/kg 3 ×/week; adjust dose to attain target Hgb of 10–12 g/dl. If Hgb ↑ by >1.0 g/dl in 2 wk or if the Hgb is ↑ and nearing 12 g/dl, ↓ dose by 25%. If Hgb <10 g/dl and ↑ by <1.0 g/dl after 4 wk of therapy (with adequate iron stores), ↑ dose by 25%. Do not ↑ dose more frequently than q 4 wk. *Zidovudine-treated HIV patients*—50–400 units/kg 2–3 ×/week. *IV: Peds: CA patients on chemotherapy*—600 units/kg weekly (max: 40,000 units/wk); target Hgb should not exceed 12 g/dl. If Hgb ↑ by >1.0 g/dl in 2 wk, if Hgb >12 g/dl, or if Hgb reaches level to avoid transfusion, ↓ dose by 25%. If Hgb ↑ by <1.0 g/dl after 4 wk of therapy, ↑ dose to 900 units/kg (max: 60,000 units/wk). Discontinue after chemotherapy completed; **Availability:** *Inject:* 2000 units/ml, 3000 units/ml, 4000 units/ml, 10,000 units/ml, 20,000 units/ml, 40,000 units/ml; **Monitor:** BP, S/S thrombosis, Hgb/Hct, serum ferritin, transferrin, iron levels; **Notes:** IV route recommended for HD patients. Most patients require supplemental iron during therapy. Correct folate and vitamin B_{12} deficiencies before therapy. ↑ risk of VTE in surgery patients (use DVT prophylaxis in these patients). Patients receiving zidovudine with endogenous serum erythropoietin levels >500 mUnits/ml may not respond to epoetin therapy.

E

eprosartan (Teveten) **Uses:** HTN; **Class:** angiotensin II receptor antagonists; **Preg:** C (1st tri), **D** (2nd and 3rd tri); **CIs:** Hypersensitivity; Pregnancy/lactation; Peds <18 yr (safety not established); **ADRs:** dizziness, ↓ BP, ↑ SCr, ↑ K+, ANGIOEDEMA; **Interactions:** ↑ effects with other antihypertensives; ↑ risk of hyperkalemia with ACEIs, K+ supplements, K+ salt substitutes, K+ sparing diuretics, and NSAIDs; NSAIDs may ↓ effectiveness; ↑ lithium levels; **Dose:** *PO: Adults:* 600 mg/day; may be ↑ to 800 mg/day if needed (in 1–2 divided doses). *Renal Impairment PO: Adults: CrCl <60 ml/min*—Do not exceed 600 mg/day; **Availability:** *Tabs:* 400, 600 mg; **Monitor:** BP, HR, BUN/SCr, K+; **Notes:** Can be used in patients intolerant to ACEI (due to cough); just as likely as ACEI to cause ↑ K+ and ↑ SCr. Avoid K+ salt substitutes.

eptifibatide (Integrilin) **Uses:** ACS (UA/NSTEMI), including patients who will be managed medically and those who will undergo PCI; Treatment of patients undergoing PCI; **Class:** glycoprotein IIb/IIIa inhibitors; **Preg:** B; **CIs:** Hypersensitivity; Active bleeding or history of bleeding in last 30 days; Severe uncontrolled HTN (SBP >200 mmHg and/or DBP >110 mmHg); Major surgery in previous 6 wk; History of any stroke in previous 30 days or any history of hemorrhagic stroke; Concurrent use of another GP IIb/IIIa receptor inhibitor; Receiving HD; Platelet count <100,000; **ADRs:** ↓ BP, BLEEDING, thrombocytopenia; **Interactions:** ↑ risk of bleeding with anticoagulants, thrombolytics, or other antiplatelet agents; **Dose:** *IV: Adults: ACS*—180 mcg/kg bolus dose, followed by 2 mcg/kg/min infusion until hospital discharge or CABG surgery (up to 72 hr); if patient undergoes PCI, continue infusion for up to 18–24 hr after procedure or until discharge, whichever comes first. *PCI*—180 mcg/kg as bolus dose immediately before PCI, followed by 2 mcg/kg/min infusion; a second bolus of 180 mcg/kg is given 10 min after first bolus; continue infusion for up to 18–24 hr after procedure or until discharge, whichever comes first (minimum of 12 hr recommended). *Renal Impairment IV: Adults:* ↓ dose if CrCl <50 ml/min; **Availability:** *Inject:* 0.75 mg/ml, 2 mg/ml; **Monitor:** BP, HR, CBC,

BUN/SCr, ACT, aPTT, bleeding; **Notes: High Alert:** Accidental overdose of antiplatelet medications has resulted in patient harm or death from internal hemorrhage or intracranial bleeding. Have second practitioner independently check original order, dose calculations, and infusion pump settings. Usually used concurrently with aspirin and heparin; heparin usually discontinued after PCI. If platelets ↓ to <100,000 or ↓ by >50% from baseline, discontinue eptifibatide and heparin.

ergocalciferol (Drisdol, vitamin D^2) **Uses:** Familial hypophosphatemia; Hypoparathyroidism; Vitamin D-resistant rickets; **Class:** fat-soluble vitamins; **Preg:** C; **CIs:** Hypersensitivity; Hypercalcemia; Vitamin D toxicity; Malabsorption problems; Lactation; **ADRs:** weakness, anorexia, constipation, nausea, polydipsia, ↓ wt, polyuria, ↑ Ca++, bone pain, metastatic calcification; **Interactions:** Cholestyramine, colestipol, or mineral oil ↓ absorption; ↑ risk of hypercalcemia with thiazide diuretics; Ca++ containing drugs may ↑ risk of hypercalcemia; Ingestion of foods high in Ca++ content may lead to hypercalcemia; **Dose:** *PO: Adults and Peds: Familial hypophosphatemia*—10,000–80,000 units/day (with phosphorus 1–2 g/day). *Hypoparathyroidism*—50,000–200,000 units/day (with Ca++ supplements). *Vitamin-resistant rickets*—12,000–500,000 units/day (with PO_4 supplements); **Availability (G):** *Liquid:* 8000 units/ml. *Caps:* 50,000 units. *Tabs:* 400 units; **Monitor:** Bone pain, Ca++, PO_4, S/S hypocalcemia, ht/wt (in peds); **Notes:** Toxicity appears as hypercalcemia, hypercalciuria, and hyperphosphatemia.

ergotamine (Ergomar) **Uses:** Migraine or cluster HAs; **Class:** ergot alkaloids; **Preg:** X; **CIs:** PAD; Ischemic heart disease; Uncontrolled HTN; Severe renal or liver disease; Pregnancy/lactation; Concurrent use of potent CYP3A4 enzyme inhibitors (macrolides, azole antifungals, and protease inhibitors); Concurrent use with other vasoconstrictors (including 5-HT_3 agonists); Peds (safety not established); **ADRs:** dizziness, PULMONARY FIBROSIS, rhinitis, MI, ↑ BP, angina pectoris, intermittent claudication, VALVULAR HEART DISEASE, nausea, altered taste, diarrhea, vomiting, muscle pain, leg weakness, numbness or tingling in fingers or toes; **Interactions:** ↑ risk of life-threatening ischemia with potent CYP3A4 inhibitors, including macrolides, azole antifungals, and protease inhibitors (contraindicated); ↑ risk of peripheral vasoconstriction with beta blockers, oral contraceptives, or nicotine; ↑ risk of HTN with vasoconstrictors (contraindicated); ↑ risk of prolonged vasoconstriction with 5-HT_3 agonists (allow 24 hr between use); **Dose:** *SL: Adults:* 2 mg initially; then 2 mg q 30 min until attack subsides or total of 6 mg has been given (max: 6 mg/day or 10 mg/wk); **Availability:** *SL tabs:* 2 mg; **Monitor:** BP, peripheral pulses, pain, signs of ergotism (cold/numb fingers/toes; N/V; HA; muscle pain; weakness); **Notes:** May give metoclopramide to minimize N/V. Administer as soon as patient reports prodromal symptoms or HA. Not to be used chronically. Do not allow patient to eat, drink, or smoke while tablet is dissolving.

erlotinib (Tarceva) **Uses:** Locally advanced/metastatic non–small-cell lung CA which has not responded to previous chemotherapy; Locally advanced/unresectable/metastatic pancreatic CA (with gemcitabine); **Class:** enzyme inhibitors; **Preg:** D; **CIs:** Pregnancy/lactation; **ADRs:** CVA, fatigue, conjunctivitis, INTERSTITIAL LUNG DISEASE, cough, dyspnea, MYOCARDIAL ISCHEMIA, abdominal pain, N/V/D, stomatitis, ↑ LFTs, pruritus, rash, dry skin; **Interactions:** CYP3A4 inhibitors may ↑ levels/toxicity; CYP3A4 inducers may ↓ levels/effects; May ↑ risk of bleeding with warfarin; **Dose:** *PO: Adults: Non–small-cell lung CA*—150 mg/day. *Pancreatic CA*—100 mg/day; **Availability:** *Tabs:* 25, 100, 150 mg; **Monitor:** RR, temp, cough, LFTs; **Notes:** Give ≥1 hr ac or 2 hrs pc. ↑ risk of hepatotoxicity in patients with hepatic impairment.

E

ertapenem (Invanz) **Uses:** CAP, skin/skin structure infections, UTIs, gynecological infections, or intra-abdominal infections due to susceptible organisms (e.g., *S. pneumo*, *S. aureus*, *S. pyogenes*, *E. coli*, *H. flu*, *Klebsiella*, *P. mirabilis*, *M. catarrhalis*, *B. fragilis*); Surgical prophylaxis after elective colorectal surgery; **Class:** carbapenems; **Preg:** B; **CIs:** Hypersensitivity (cross-sensitivity to other beta-lactam antibiotics may exist); Hypersensitivity to lidocaine (may be used as diluent for IM administration); **ADRs:** SEIZURES, HA, PSEUDOMEMBRANOUS COLITIS, N/V/D, rash, pruritis, vaginitis, phlebitis, pain at IM site, ANAPHYLAXIS; **Interactions:** Probenecid ↓ excretion and ↑ levels; May ↓ valproic acid levels; **Dose:** *IV, IM: Adults and Peds: ≥13 yr:* 1 g/day. *Surgical prophylaxis*—1 g given 1 hr before surgical incision. *IV, IM: Peds: 3 mo–12 yr:* 15 mg/kg q 12 hr (max: 1 g/day). *Renal Impairment IM, IV: Adults:* ↓ dose if CrCl ≤30 ml/min; **Availability:** *Inject:* 1 g; **Monitor:** BP, HR, temp, sputum, U/A, BUN/SCr, CBC; **Notes:** Does not cover *Pseudomonas*. Use with caution in patients with seizure disorders. Use with caution in patients with beta-lactam allergy (do not use if history of anaphylaxis or hives).

erythromycin (Akne-Mycin, E.E.S, Eryderm, Erygel, EryPed, Erythrocin, PCE, Romycin) **Uses:** **PO, IV:** Respiratory tract infections, skin/skin structure infections, urethritis, syphilis, or PID due to susceptible organisms (e.g., *S. pneumo*, *S. pyogenes*, *H. flu*, *Chlamydia*, *Legionella*, *Mycoplasma*, *N. gonorrhoeae*, *Treponema*); *Topical:* Acne; *Ophth:* Conjunctivitis; **Class:** macrolides; **Preg:** B; **CIs:** Hypersensitivity; Concurrent use of pimozide (for PO or IV); **ADRs:** VENTRICULAR ARRHYTHMIAS, QT interval prolongation, PSEUDOMEMBRANOUS COLITIS, N/V, abdominal pain, cramping, diarrhea, hepatitis, rash, pruritis, phlebitis at IV site, allergic reactions; **Interactions:** CYP3A4 inhibitors may ↑ levels/toxicity; CYP3A4 inducers may ↓ levels/effects; May ↑ levels/toxicity of CYP3A4 substrates; ↑ risk of arrhythmias with pimozide (contraindicated); May

↑ digoxin levels; May ↑ risk of bleeding with warfarin; **Dose:** *PO: Adults: Base or stearate*—250 mg q 6 hr *or* 500 mg q 12 hr. *Ethylsuccinate*— 400 mg q 6 hr *or* 800 mg q 12 hr. *IV: Adults:* 500–1000 mg q 6 hr. *PO: Peds: >1 mo:* 30–50 mg/kg/day in 2–4 divided doses (max: 2 g/day as base or stearate or estolate; 3.2 g/day as ethylsuccinate). *IV: Peds: >1 mo:* 15–50 mg/kg/day divided q 6 hr (max: 4 g/day). *Ophth: Adults and Peds:* 1/2 in. in affected eye 2–6 times/day. *Topical: Adults and Peds: >12 yr:* Apply bid; **Availability (G):** *DR, EC tabs (base):* 250 mg, 333 mg, 500 mg. *Tabs with polymer-coated particles (base):* 333 mg, 500 mg. *Film-coated tabs (base):* 250 mg, 500 mg. *DR, EC caps (base):* 250 mg. *Tabs (ethylsuccinate):* 400 mg. *Oral susp (ethylsuccinate):* 200 mg/5 ml, 400 mg/5 ml. *Gtt (ethylsuccinate):* 100 mg/2.5 ml. *Oral susp (estolate):* 125 mg/5 ml, 250 mg/5 ml. *Film-coated tabs (stearate):* 250 mg, 500 mg. *Inject:* 500 mg, 1 g. *Gel:* 2%. *Top oint:* 2%. *Top soln:* 2%. *Ophth oint:* 0.5%; **Monitor:** BP, HR, temp, sputum, U/A, CBC, LFTs, ECG (QT interval), inject site, acne lesions; **Notes:** 250 mg of erythromycin base, estolate or stearate = 400 mg of erythromycin ethylsuccinate. Film-coated tabs (base and stearate) are absorbed better on empty stomach (≥1 hr ac or 2 hr pc); may be taken with food if GI irritation occurs. Ethylsuccinate should be taken with meals. Do not crush or chew DR caps or tabs (DR caps may be opened and sprinkled on applesauce, jelly, or ice cream immediately before taking). For top oint, cleanse area before applying.

E

escitalopram (Lexapro) **Uses:** Depression; GAD; **Class:** SSRIs; **Preg:** C; **CIs:** Hypersensitivity; Concurrent MAOI or pimozide therapy; May ↑ risk of suicidal thoughts/behaviors, esp. during early treatment or dose adjustment; risk may be ↑ in peds and adolescents; **ADRs:** SUICIDAL THOUGHTS, HA, insomnia, dizziness, drowsiness, fatigue, dry mouth, nausea, diarrhea, ↑ appetite, ejaculatory delay, ED, ↓ libido, ↑ sweating; **Interactions:** ↑ risk of toxicity with MAOIs (discontinue for ≥2 wk); ↑ risk of QT_C prolongation with pimozide (contraindicated); Use cautiously with other centrally acting drugs (including alcohol, antihistamines, opioid analgesics, and sedative/hypnotics; use with alcohol not recommended); Cimetidine may ↑ levels; ↑ risk of serotonin syndrome with lithium, 5-HT_1 agonists, linezolid, tramadol, or St. John's wort; May ↑ levels of metoprolol; May ↑ risk of bleeding with antiplatelets, NSAIDs, or warfarin; **Dose:** *PO: Adults:* 10 mg/day; may be ↑ to 20 mg/day after 1 wk. *Hepatic Impairment PO: Adults:* 10 mg/day; **Availability:** *Tabs:* 5, 10, 20 mg. *Oral soln:* 1 mg/ml; **Monitor:** Mental status, suicidal thoughts/behaviors, sexual dysfunction; **Notes:** Do not confuse with citalopram (Celexa). Should not abruptly discontinue (should taper to ↓ withdrawal).

esmolol (Brevibloc) **Uses:** SVT (for ventricular rate control); Intra/postoperative tachycardia and/or HTN; **Class:** beta blockers; **Preg:** C; **CIs:** Hypersensitivity; Decompensated HF; Pulmonary edema;

Cardiogenic shock; Bradycardia or ≥2nd-degree heart block (in absence of pacemaker); **ADRs:** agitation, confusion, dizziness, drowsiness, HA, PULMONARY EDEMA, bronchospasm, HF, ↓ BP, ↓ HR, nausea, ↓ BG, inject site reactions; **Interactions:** ↑ risk of bradycardia with digoxin, diltiazem, verapamil, or clonidine; ↑ effects with other antihypertensives; ↑ risk of hypertensive crisis if concurrent clonidine discontinued; May alter the effectiveness of insulins or oral hypoglycemic agents; May ↓ the effects of $beta_1$ agonists (e.g., dopamine or dobutamine); **Dose:** *IV: Adults: SVT*—LD of 500 mcg/kg given over 1 min, then infusion of 50 mcg/kg/min × 4 min; if desired response not achieved, repeat 500 mcg/kg LD over 1 min, then ↑ infusion rate to 100 mcg/kg/min × 4 min; if desired response not achieved, repeat 500 mcg/kg LD over 1 min, then ↑ infusion rate to 150 mcg/kg/min; if further HR control needed, may ↑ infusion rate to max of 200 mcg/kg/min. *Intra/postoperative tachycardia/HTN*—For immediate control: give LD of 80 mg over 30 sec, then infusion of 150 mcg/kg/min; may gradually ↑ infusion rate, as needed, up to 300 mcg/kg/min. For gradual control: follow dosage regimen for SVTs (max infusion rate: 300 mcg/kg/min); **Availability (G):** *Inject:* 10 mg/ml, 20 mg/ml; **Monitor:** HR, BP, ECG, S/S HF, edema, wt, BG (if DM); **Notes:** Do not abruptly discontinue. To convert to oral rate-control agents, administer the 1st dose of the oral agent and ↓ esmolol dose by 50% after 30 min; if adequate response is maintained for 1 hr following the 2nd dose of oral agent, discontinue esmolol.

esomeprazole (Nexium) **Uses:** GERD/erosive esophagitis; Hypersecretory conditions (Zollinger-Ellison Syndrome); *H. pylori* eradication in patients with duodenal ulcer disease (with amoxicillin and clarithromycin); Prevention of NSAID-induced gastric ulcers; **Class:** proton pump inhibitors; **Preg:** B; **CIs:** Hypersensitivity; **ADRs:** HA, abdominal pain, constipation, diarrhea, dry mouth, flatulence, nausea; **Interactions:** May ↓ absorption of digoxin, ketoconazole, iron salts, and atazanavir (use with atazanavir not recommended); May ↑ risk of bleeding with warfarin; **Dose:** *PO: Adults: GERD (healing of erosive esophagitis)*—20–40 mg/day × 4–8 wk. *GERD (maintenance of healing of erosive esophagitis)*—20 mg/day. *Symptomatic GERD*—20 mg/day × 4 wk. *Prevention of NSAID-induced gastric ulcers*—20–40 mg/day for up to 6 mo. *H. pylori eradication*—40 mg/day × 10 days (with amoxicillin and clarithromycin). *Hypersecretory conditions, including Zollinger-Ellison syndrome*—40 mg bid. *PO: Peds: 12–17 yr Short-term treatment of GERD*—20–40 mg/day for up to 8 wk. *PO: Peds: 1–11 yr Short-term treatment of GERD*—10 mg/day for up to 8 wk. *Healing of erosive esophagitis*—<20 kg: 10 mg/day for up to 8 wk; ≥20 kg: 10–20 mg/day for up to 8 wk. *IV: Adults: GERD (with history of erosive esophagitis)*—20–40 mg/day. *Hepatic Impairment PO, IV: Adults: Severe hepatic impairment.* Should not exceed 20 mg/day; **Availability:** *DR caps:* 20, 40 mg. *DR oral susp packets:* 10, 20, 40 mg. *Inject:* 20, 40 mg; **Monitor:** S/S GERD/PUD, bleeding, CBC,

LFTs; **Notes:** Administer caps ≥1 hr ac. Caps may be opened; mix pellets with applesauce and swallow immediately (do not crush or chew pellets). Can be administered down NG tube (open caps, empty intact granules into 60-ml syringe and mix with 60 ml water; suspension can also be given down NG tube).

estradiol (Alora, Climara, Delestrogen, Depo-Estradiol, Divigel, Elestrin, Estrace, Estraderm, Estrasorb, Estring, EstroGel, EvaMist, Femring, Femtrace, Gynodiol, Menostar, Vagifem, Vivelle-DOT) Uses: *PO, IM, Topical, Transdermal, Vag:* Replacement of estrogen to diminish moderate-to-severe vasomotor symptoms of menopause and of various estrogen deficiency states (female hypogonadism, primary ovarian failure). *PO: Transdermal:* Prevention of postmenopausal osteoporosis; *PO:* Inoperable metastatic postmenopausal breast or prostate CA; *Topical Transdermal: Vag:* Vulvar or vaginal atrophy; **Class:** estrogens; **Preg:** X; **CIs:** Thromboembolic disease (e.g., DVT, PE, MI, Stroke); Undiagnosed vaginal bleeding; Liver disease; History of estrogen-dependent CA; Pregnancy/lactation; **ADRs:** HA, dizziness, MI, THROMBOEMBOLISM, edema, HTN, nausea, wt changes, anorexia, jaundice, vomiting, women—amenorrhea, breast tenderness, dysmenorrhea, breakthrough bleeding, ↓ libido, men—ED, testicular atrophy, oily skin, acne, gynecomastia, ↑ BG, ↑ TGs; **Interactions:** CYP3A4 inhibitors may ↑ levels/toxicity; CYP3A4 inducers may ↓ levels/effects; May alter requirement for warfarin, oral hypoglycemic agents, or insulins; **Dose:** *PO: Adults: Hypogonadism, symptoms of menopause*—1–2 mg/day × 3 wk, then off × 1 wk. *Osteoporosis prevention*—0.5 mg/day × 3 wk, then off × 1 wk. *Postmenopausal breast CA or prostate CA*—10 mg tid. *IM: Adults: Symptoms of menopause, hypogonadism*—1–5 mg monthly (estradiol cypionate) *or* 10–20 mg (estradiol valerate) monthly. *Prostate CA*—30 mg q 1–2 wk (estradiol valerate). *Topical Emulsion (Estrasorb): Adults: Menopausal symptoms*—Apply two 1.74 g pouches/day. *Topical Gel: Adults: Menopausal symptoms*—Divigel: 0.25–1 g/day; Elestrin: 0.87 g/day; EstroGel: 1.25 g/day. *Atrophic vaginitis*—Estrogel: 1.25 g/day; *Topical Spray (EvaMist): Adults: Menopausal symptoms*—1 spray/day, may be ↑ to 2–3 sprays/day. *Transdermal: Adults: Symptoms of menopause, atrophic vaginitis, female hypogonadism, ovarian failure, osteoporosis prevention*—Alora, Estraderm: 0.05 mg/day patch (0.025 mg/day for Alora for osteoporosis prevention) applied twice weekly; may adjust dose based on response. Climara: 0.025 mg/day patch applied weekly; may adjust dose based on response. Vivelle-DOT: 0.0375 mg/day (0.025 mg/day for osteoporosis prevention) patch applied twice weekly; may adjust dose based on response. *Osteoporosis prevention*—Menostar: 14 mcg/day patch applied q 7 days. Progestin may be administered for 14 days q 6–12 mo in women with a uterus. *Vag: Adults: Atrophic vaginitis*—Cream: 2–4 g/day (0.2–0.4 mg estradiol) × 1–2 wk, then ↓ to 1–2 g/day × 1–2 wk; then MD of 1 g 1–3 times weekly × 3 wk, then off × 1 wk; then repeat cycle once vaginal mucosa has been restored. Estring (ring): 2 mg (releases 7.5 mcg estradiol/24 hr) inserted q 3 mo. Femring (ring): 0.05 mg (releases 50 mcg estradiol/24 hr) inserted q 3 mo; may ↑ to 0.1 mg (releases 100 mcg estradiol/24 hr) inserted q 3 mo based on symptoms (may also be used to treat vasomotor symptoms of menopause). Vagifem (tabs): 1 tab/day × 2 wk, then twice weekly; **Availability (G):** *Tabs:* 0.45 mg, 0.5 mg, 0.9 mg, 1 mg, 1.8 mg, 2 mg. *Inject (valerate):* 10 mg/ml, 20 mg/ml, 40 mg/ml. *Inject (cypionate):* 5 mg/ml. *Top emulsion:* 4.35 mg/1.74 g pouch. *Top gel packet (0.1%) (Divigel):* 0.25 g, 0.5 g, 1 g. *Top gel pump (0.06%) (Elestrin, EstroGel):* 0.87 g/actuation, 1.25 g/actuation. *Top spray:* 1.53 mg/spray. *Transdermal system:* 14 mcg/24-hr release rate, 25 mcg/24-hr release rate, 37.5 mcg/24-hr release rate, 50 mcg/24-hr release rate, 60 mcg/24-hr release rate, 75 mcg/24-hr release rate, 100 mcg/24-hr release rate. *Vag cream:* 0.1 mg/g. *Vag ring (Estring):* 2 mg (releases 7.5 mcg/day over 90 days). *Vag ring (Femring):* 0.05 mg (releases 0.05 mg/day over 90 days), 0.1 mg (releases 0.1 mg/day over 90 days). *Vag tabs:* 25 mcg; **Monitor:** BP, edema, wt, vasomotor symptoms, lipid panel, S/S thromboembolism; **Notes:** Concurrent use of progestin is recommended during cyclical therapy to ↓ risk of endometrial CA in women with an intact uterus. Should be used in lowest doses for shortest period of time. Follow manufacturer's directions regarding site of application for top emulsion, gel, or spray.

estrogens, conjugated (Cenestin, Enjuvia, Premarin)
Uses: PO: Moderate-to-severe vasomotor symptoms of menopause; Estrogen deficiency states, including: Female hypogonadism, Ovariectomy, Primary ovarian failure; Prevention of postmenopausal osteoporosis; Atrophic vaginitis; Advanced inoperable metastatic breast and prostatic CA; **IM, IV:** Abnormal uterine bleeding; **Vag:** Atrophic vaginitis; **Class:** estrogens; **Preg:** X; **CIs:** Hypersensitivity; Thromboembolic disease (e.g., DVT, PE, MI, stroke); Undiagnosed vaginal bleeding; History of breast CA; History of estrogen-dependent CA; Liver disease; Pregnancy/lactation; **ADRs:** HA, insomnia, MI, THROMBOEMBOLISM, edema, ↑ BP, nausea, wt changes, ↑ appetite, jaundice, vomiting, amenorrhea, breakthrough bleeding, dysmenorrhea, ↓ libido, vag candidiasis, ED, testicular atrophy, acne, oily skin, gynecomastia, breast tenderness, ↑ TGs; **Interactions:** CYP1A2 inhibitors and CYP3A4 inhibitors may ↑ levels/toxicity; CYP1A2 inducers and CYP3A4 inducers may ↓ levels/effects; Smoking ↑ risk of adverse CV reactions; **Dose:** *PO: Adults: Ovariectomy/Primary ovarian failure*—1.25 mg/day administered cyclically (3 wk on, 1 wk off). *Osteoporosis prevention/Menopausal symptoms/Atrophic vaginitis* 0.3–1.25 mg/day or in a cycle. *Female hypogonadism*—0.3–0.625 mg/day administered cyclically (3 wk on, 1 wk off). *Inoperable breast CA (men and postmenopausal women)*—10 mg tid. *Inoperable prostate CA*—1.25–2.5 mg tid. *IM, IV: Adults: Uterine bleeding*—25 mg, may repeat in 6–12 hr if needed. *Vag: Adults: Atrophic vaginitis*—1.25–2.5 mg/day (2–4 g cream) for 3 wk, off for 1 wk, then repeat; **Availability:** *Tabs:* 0.3, 0.45, 0.625, 0.9,

1.25 mg. *Inject:* 25 mg. *Vag cream:* 0.625 mg/g; **Monitor:** BP, edema, wt, vasomotor symptoms, lipid panel, LFTs, S/S thromboembolism; **Notes:** Concurrent use of progestin is recommended during cyclical therapy to ↓ risk of endometrial carcinoma in women with an intact uterus. Should be used in lowest doses for shortest period of time. IV is preferred parenteral route because of rapid response.

eszopiclone (Lunesta) Uses: Insomnia; **Class:** cyclopyrrolones; **Preg:** C; **CIs:** Peds <18 yr (safety not established); **ADRs:** HA, abnormal thinking, behavior changes, dizziness, hallucinations, sleep-driving, unpleasant taste, dry mouth, rash; **Interactions:** ↑ CNS depression with alcohol, antidepressants, sedative hypnotics, antihistamines, and opioids; CYP3A4 inhibitors may ↑ levels/effects; CYP3A4 inducers may ↓ levels/effects; **Dose:** *PO: Adults:* 2 mg immediately before bedtime; may ↑ to 3 mg if needed (more effective for sleep maintenance). *Concurrent therapy with potent CYP3A4 inhibitors*—1 mg immediately before bedtime, may ↑ to 2 mg if needed. *PO: (Geriatric Patients):* 1 mg immediately before bedtime for patients with difficulty falling asleep, 2 mg for patients who have difficulty staying asleep. *Hepatic Impairment PO: Adults: Severe hepatic impairment*—1 mg immediately before bedtime; **Availability:** *Tabs:* 1, 2, 3 mg; **Monitor:** Mental status, sleep patterns; **Notes:** Schedule IV controlled substance. Potential for dependence/abuse with long-term use (use with caution in patients at risk for addiction). Should be given only on nights when patient is able to get ≥8 hr of sleep. Do not break, crush, or chew tabs.

etanercept (Enbrel) Uses: RA (as monotherapy or with methotrexate); Juvenile idiopathic arthritis; Psoriatic arthritis (with methotrexate); Ankylosing spondylitis; Plaque psoriasis; **Class:** DMARDs, anti-TNF agents; **Preg:** B; **CIs:** Hypersensitivity; Sepsis; Active infection; Lactation; Concurrent use of cyclophosphamide or anakinra; **ADRs:** CNS DEMYELINATING DISORDERS, SEIZURES, HA, dizziness, weakness, rhinitis, optic neuritis, pharyngitis, sinusitis, cough, abdominal pain, dyspepsia, rash, PANCYTOPENIA, inject site reactions, INFECTIONS (including reactivation of tuberculosis and hepatitis), MALIGNANCY, allergic reactions, ANAPHYLAXIS; **Interactions:** ↑ risk of infection with anakinra (not recommended); ↑ risk of malignancy with cyclophosphamide (not recommended); May ↓ antibody response to live-virus vaccines and ↑ risk of ADRs (do not administer concurrently); **Dose:** *Subcut: Adults: RA, ankylosing spondylitis, psoriatic arthritis*—50 mg once weekly. *Plaque psoriasis*—50 mg twice weekly × 3 mo, then 50 mg once weekly; may also be given as 25–50 mg once weekly as an initial dose. *Subcut: Peds: 4–17 yr Juvenile idiopathic arthritis*—0.8 mg/kg once weekly (max: 50 mg/wk); **Availability:** *Prefilled syringes:* 50 mg/ml. *Powder for inject:* 25 mg; **Monitor:** Pain scale, ROM, S/S infection, S/S anaphylaxis, CBC; **Notes:** Place PPD prior to initiation (may reactivate latent TB).

Discontinue if serious infection develops. Use with caution in LV dysfunction (may cause or worsen HF). Needle cap of prefilled syringe contains latex. Methotrexate, analgesics, NSAIDs, corticosteroids, and/or salicylates may be continued during therapy.

ethambutol (Myambutol) **Uses:** Active TB or other mycobacterial diseases (with ≥1 other drug); **Class:** antituberculars; **Preg:** C; **CIs:** Hypersensitivity; Optic neuritis; Peds <13 yr (safety not established); **ADRs:** confusion, hallucinations, HA, optic neuritis, pulmonary infiltrates, HEPATITIS, abdominal pain, N/V, hyperuricemia, leukopenia, thrombocytopenia, joint pain, peripheral neuritis, anaphylactoid reactions, fever; **Interactions:** Aluminum hydroxide may ↓ absorption; **Dose:** *PO: Adults and Peds: ≥13 yr* 15–25 mg/kg/day (max: 2.5 g/day) *or* 50 mg/kg (up to 4 g) twice weekly *or* 25–30 mg/kg (up to 2.5 g) 3 ×/week. *Renal Impairment Adults:* ↓ dose if CrCl ≤50 ml/min; **Availability (G):** *Tabs:* 100, 400 mg; **Monitor:** Ophth exam, BUN/SCr, CBC, LFTs, uric acid; **Notes:** Should be administered with other antitubercular meds.

etoposide (Toposar, VePesid) **Uses:** Refractory testicular CA (IV only) (with other chemotherapy agents); Small-cell lung CA (PO and IV) (with other chemotherapy agents); **Class:** antineoplastics; **Preg:** D; **CIs:** Hypersensitivity; Pregnancy/lactation; **ADRs:** ↓ BP (IV), anorexia, N/V/D, abdominal pain, stomatitis, alopecia, pruritis, rash, urticaria, sterility, anemia, leukopenia, thrombocytopenia, phlebitis at IV site, peripheral neuropathy, ANAPHYLAXIS, fever; **Interactions:** ↑ bone marrow depression with other antineoplastics or radiation therapy; **Dose:** *IV: Adults: Testicular CA*—Dosage ranges from 50–100 mg/m^2 daily × 5 days up to 100 mg/m^2 daily on days 1, 3, and 5; repeat at 3–4 wk intervals. *Small-cell lung CA*—Dosage ranges from 35 mg/m^2 daily × 4 days up to 50 mg/m^2 daily × 5 days; repeat at 3–4 wk intervals. *IV: Peds:* 60–150 mg/m^2 × 2–5 days q 3–6 weeks (refer to individual protocols). *PO: Adults: Small-cell lung CA*—Dosage ranges from 70 mg/m^2 daily × 4 days up to 100 mg/m^2 daily × 5 days (round dose to nearest 50 mg); repeat at 3–4 wk intervals. *Renal Impairment IV, PO: Adults and Peds:* ↓ dose if CrCl ≤50 ml/min; **Availability (G):** *Caps:* 50 mg. *Inject:* 20 mg/ml; **Monitor:** BP, HR, RR, temp, BUN/SCr, CBC (with diff), LFTs, S/S infection, bleeding, S/S hypersensitivity reaction (fever, chills, dyspnea, pruritus, urticaria, bronchospasm, ↑ HR, ↓ BP); **Notes:** **High Alert:** Fatalities have occurred with incorrect administration of chemotherapeutic agents. Before administering, clarify all ambiguous orders; double-check single, daily, and course-of-therapy dose limits; have second practitioner independently double-check original order, calculations, and infusion pump settings. Do not confuse etoposide (Toposar) with etoposide phosphate (Etopophos). Leukocyte nadir = 7–14 days; platelet nadir = 9–16 days (bone marrow recovery occurs ~20 days after administration). Avoid rapid IV infusion. Refrigerate caps.

exenatide (Byetta) **Uses:** Type 2 DM uncontrolled by metformin, sulfonylurea, and/or thiazolidinedione; **Class:** incretrin mimetic agents; **Preg:** C; **CIs:** Hypersensitivity; Type 1 diabetes or DKA; Severe renal disease (CrCl <30 ml/min); Severe GI disease; Peds (safety not established); **ADRs:** dizziness, HA, jitteriness, weakness, PANCREATITIS, N/V/D, dyspepsia, GI reflux, hyperhidrosis, ↓ wt, ↓ BG (esp. with sulfonylurea); **Interactions:** Use with sulfonlyureas may ↑ risk of hypoglycemia; Due to slowed gastric emptying, may ↓ absorption of orally administered meds, esp. those requiring rapid GI absorption or specific level for efficacy (e.g., antibiotics, oral contraceptives); May ↑ warfarin levels; **Dose:** *Subcut: Adults:* 5 mcg within 60 min before morning and evening meal; after 1 mo, may ↑ to 10 mcg bid based on response; **Availability:** *Inject:* 250 mcg/ml; **Monitor:** BG, A1C, S/S hypoglycemia; **Notes:** Give oral meds ≥1 hr before exenatide. May cause hypoglycemia, esp. when used with sulfonylurea (consider ↓ dose of sulfonylurea). Do not give pc. Administer in thigh, abdomen, or upper arm. Available in prefilled pen.

F

ezetimibe (Zetia) **Uses:** Dyslipidemia; **Class:** cholesterol absorption inhibitors; **Preg:** C; **CIs:** Hypersensitivity; Acute liver disease (when used with HMG-CoA reductase inhibitor); Pregnancy, lactation, or peds <10 yr (safety not established); **ADRs:** diarrhea, ↑ LFTs (esp. with HMG-CoA reductase inhibitors), myalgia (esp. with HMG-CoA reductase inhibitors), arthralgia; **Interactions:** Cholestyramine or colestipol may ↓ absorption (give ezetimibe ≥2 hr before or ≥4 hr after these drugs); ↑ risk of cholelithiasis with fibrates (should only use fenofibrate); Cyclosporine may ↑ levels; May ↑ cyclosporine levels; May ↑ effects of warfarin; **Dose:** *PO: Adults and Peds: ≥10 yr:* 10 mg/day; **Availability:** *Tabs:* 10 mg; **Monitor:** Lipid panel, LFTs, CK (if symptoms); **Notes:** Used primarily for ↓ LDL-C. Can be used with or without HMG-CoA reductase inhibitor.

famciclovir (Famvir) **Uses:** Herpes zoster (shingles); Treatment/suppression of recurrent genital herpes in immunocompetent patients; Treatment of recurrent herpes labialis (cold sores) in immunocompetent patients; Treatment of recurrent mucocutaneous herpes simplex infections in HIV-infected patients; **Class:** antivirals; **Preg:** B; **CIs:** Hypersensitivity to famciclovir or penciclovir; Peds <18 yr (safety not established); **ADRs:** HA, fatigue, N/V/D; **Interactions:** None significant; **Dose:** *PO: Adults: Herpes zoster*—500 mg q 8 hr × 7 days. *Genital herpes treatment (immunocompetent)*—1000 mg bid × 1 day. *Genital herpes treatment (HIV)*—500 mg bid × 7 days. *Genital herpes suppression*—250 mg bid for up to 1 yr. *Cold sores*—1500 mg as single dose. *Renal Impairment PO: Adults: Single-dose regimens and treatment of herpes zoster*—↓ dose if CrCl <60 ml/min. *Multiple-day dosing regimens (other than for herpes zoster)*—↓ dose if CrCl < 40 ml/min; **Availability:** *Tabs:* 125, 250, 500 mg; **Monitor:** Lesions, postherpetic neuralgia; **Notes:** Initiate treatment as soon as herpes diagnosed (within 72 hr for herpes zoster; within 6 hr for recurrent genital herpes). Avoid sexual contact when lesions present. Prodrug of penciclovir.

famotidine (Pepcid, Pepcid AC, Pepcid AC Maximum Strength) **Uses:** Short-term treatment of duodenal and gastric ulcers; Maintenance therapy for duodenal ulcers; GERD; Heartburn (OTC use); Gastric hypersecretory states (Zollinger-Ellison syndrome); **Class:** histamine H_2 antagonists; **Preg:** B; **CIs:** Hypersensitivity; **ADRs:** dizziness, HA, constipation, diarrhea; **Interactions:** ↓ absorption of ketoconazole and itraconazole; **Dose:** *PO: Adults: Short-term treatment of active ulcers*—40 mg at bedtime *or* 20 mg bid for up to 8 wk. *Duodenal ulcer prophylaxis*—20 mg at bedtime. *GERD*—20 mg bid for up to 6 wk; 40 mg bid for up to 12 wk can be used for esophagitis with erosions or ulcerations. *Gastric hypersecretory conditions*—20 mg q 6 hr (max: 160 mg q 6 hr). *OTC use*—10–20 mg q 12 hr (15–60 min before eating foods that cause heartburn). *IV: Adults:* 20 mg q 12 hr. *PO, IV: Peds: 1–16 yr Peptic ulcer*—0.5 mg/kg/day as single bedtime dose or in 2 divided doses (max: 40 mg/day). *GERD*—1 mg/kg/day in 2 divided doses (max: 80 mg/day). *PO: Infants: ≥3 mo–1 yr GERD*—0.5 mg/kg bid. *PO: Infants and Neonates: <3 mo GERD*—0.5 mg/kg/day. *Renal Impairment PO: Adults:* ↓ dose if CrCl <50 ml/min; **Availability (G):** *Tabs:* 10, 20, 40 mg. *Gelcaps:* 10 mg[OTC]. *Oral susp:* 40 mg/5 ml. *Inject:* 10 mg/ml; **Monitor:** S/S GERD/PUD, bleeding, BUN/SCr; **Notes:** Should not take OTC for >2 wk. Administer once daily dose at bedtime.

felodipine (Plendil) **Uses:** HTN; **Class:** Calcium channel blockers; **Preg:** C; **CIs:** Hypersensitivity; Pregnancy, lactation, and peds (safety not established); **ADRs:** <u>HA</u>, dizziness, <u>peripheral edema</u>, ↓ BP, ↑ HR, gingival hyperplasia, flushing; **Interactions:** NSAIDs may ↓ effectiveness; ↑ effects with other antihypertensives; CYP3A4 inhibitors may ↑ levels; CYP3A4 inducers may ↓ levels; **Dose:** *PO: Adults:* 5 mg/day (2.5 mg/day in geriatric patients); may increase q 2 wk (max: 10 mg/day); **Availability: (G):** *Tabs:* 2.5, 5, 10 mg; **Monitor:** BP, HR, peripheral edema; **Notes:** Do not crush, break, or chew. Avoid grapefruit juice (may ↑ effects).

fenofibrate (Antara, Fenoglide, Lipofen, Lofibra, Tricor, Triglide) **Uses:** Hypercholesterolemia or mixed dyslipidemia; Hypertriglyceridemia; **Class:** fibric acid derivatives; **Preg:** C; **CIs:** Hypersensitivity; Hepatic impairment (including primary biliary cirrhosis); Gallbladder disease; Severe renal impairment; Pregnancy, lactation, and peds (safety not established); **ADRs:** constipation, ↑ LFTs, nausea, PANCREATITIS, rash, RHABDOMYOLYSIS; **Interactions:** May ↑ effects of warfarin; Use with HMG-CoA reductase inhibitors may ↑ risk of rhabdomyolysis; ↓ absorption with bile acid sequestrants; ↑ risk of nephrotoxicity with cyclosporine; **Dose:** *Primary hypercholesterolemia/mixed dyslipidemia PO: Adults: Antara*—130 mg/day. *Fenoglide*—120 mg/day.

Lipofen—150 mg/day. *Lofibra*—160–200 mg/day. *Tricor*—145 mg/day. *Triglide*—160 mg/day. *Hypertriglyceridemia PO: Adults: Antara*—43–130 mg/day. *Fenoglide*—40–120 mg/day. *Lipofen*—50–150 mg/day. *Lofibra*—54–200 mg/day. *Tricor*—48–145 mg/day. *Triglide*—50–160 mg/day. *Renal Impairment PO: Adults:* ↓ dose in renal impairment for most formulations; **Availability (G):** *Caps (Lipofen):* 50, 150 mg. *Micronized caps (Antara):* 43, 130 mg. *Micronized caps (Lofibra):* 67, 134, 200 mg. *Micronized tabs (Lofibra):* 54, 160 mg. *Tabs (Fenoglide):* 40, 120 mg. *Tabs (Tricor):* 48, 145 mg. *Tabs (Triglide):* 50, 160 mg; **Monitor:** Lipid panel, BUN/SCr, LFTs, CK (if symptoms); **Notes:** Primarily used to ↓ TGs. Brands are not interchangeable. Give *Fenoglide, Lipofen,* and *Lofibra* products with meals. Take ≥1 hr before or ≥4–6 hr after bile acid resins.

F

fenoldopam (Corlopam) **Uses:** Hypertensive emergency; **Class:** vasodilators; **Preg:** B; **CIs:** Hypersensitivity to fenoldopam or sulfites; Concurrent beta blocker therapy; **ADRs:** HA, ↓ BP, ↑ HR, nausea, flushing, ↓ K+, inject site reactions; **Interactions:** Concurrent use with beta blockers may ↑ risk of hypotension and prevent reflex tachycardia (contraindicated); **Dose:** *IV: Adults:* 0.1–0.3 mcg/kg/min; may titrate by 0.05–0.1 mcg/kg/min q 15 min (max: 1.6 mcg/kg/min). *IV: Peds:* 0.2 mcg/kg/min; may titrate by 0.05–0.1 mcg/kg/min q 20–30 min up to 0.3–0.5 mcg/kg/min (max: 0.8 mcg/kg/min); **Availability (G):** *Inject:* 10 mg/ml; **Monitor:** BP, HR, ECG, K+; **Notes:** Administer via continuous infusion; do not use bolus doses. Should be used for <48 hr. Use with caution in patients with glaucoma or intraocular HTN (may ↑ IOP). Can be abruptly discontinued (no need to taper).

fentanyl (Actiq, Duragesic, Fentora, Ionsys, Sublimaze) **Uses: PO:** Breakthrough CA pain in opioid-tolerant patients (for buccal and transmucosal dosage forms); **Transdermal:** Acute postoperative pain in hospitalized patients (iontophoretic transdermal system); Moderate-to-severe chronic pain (transdermal patch); **IM, IV:** Adjunct to general or regional anesthesia; pre-/postoperative analgesia; sedation and analgesia; **Class:** opioid agonists; **Preg:** C; **CIs:** Hypersensitivity; *PO: Transdermal:* Acute/postoperative pain, Opioid non-tolerant patients, Lactation; *Transdermal:* Significant respiratory depression, Paralytic ileus, Patients requiring short-term therapy, Intermittent therapy; **ADRs:** dizziness, drowsiness, HA, confusion, depression, fatigue, insomnia, weakness, RESPIRATORY DEPRESSION, cough, dyspnea, ↓ HR, ↓ BP, constipation, N/V, abdominal pain, anorexia, ileus, application site reactions, itching, physical/psychological dependence; **Interactions:** CYP3A4 inhibitors may ↑ levels/toxicity; CYP3A4 inducers may ↓ levels/effects; CNS depressants, opioids, sedative/hypnotics, general anesthetics, phenothiazines, skeletal muscle relaxants, antihistamines, and alcohol may ↑ CNS depression, hypoventilation, and hypotension; **Dose:** *Buccal: Adults:* 100 mcg; additional 100 mcg dose may be started 30 min after 1st dose if needed;

dose can be titrated if needed (max: 2 doses/breakthrough pain episode q 4 hr). *Transmucosal: Adults:* 200-mcg unit dissolved in mouth; additional unit may be used 15 min after 1st unit is completed. Use should be limited to ≤4 units/day. *Transdermal: Adults: (iontophoretic system):* Assure adequate analgesia before initiating iontophoretic system. System delivers 40 mcg q 10 min prn; system can deliver max of 6 doses/hr and total of 80 doses/24 hr. Max duration of therapy = 72 hr. *Transdermal: Adults and Peds: ≥2 yr:* To calculate the dosage of transdermal fentanyl required in patients already receiving opioid analgesics, assess 24-hr requirement of currently used opioid. Using an equianalgesic table, convert this to an equivalent amount of morphine/24 hr. Conversion to fentanyl transdermal may be accomplished by using a fentanyl conversion table. During dosage titration, additional short-acting opioids should be available for any breakthrough pain that may occur. Transdermal patch lasts 72 hr in most patients; some patients may require new patch q 48 hr. *IM, IV: Adults and Peds: >12 yr Preop use*—50–100 mcg 30–60 min before surgery. *Postoperative use*—50–100 mcg; may repeat in 1–2 hr. *Adjunct to general anesthesia*—Low dose (minor surgery): 2 mcg/kg; Moderate dose (major surgery): 2–20 mcg/kg; High dose (major surgery): 20–50 mcg/kg. *Adjunct to regional anesthesia*—50–100 mcg. *Sedation/analgesia*—0.5–1 mcg/kg/dose, may repeat after 30–60 min. *IV: Peds: 1–12 yr Sedation/analgesia*—Bolus of 1–2 mcg/kg/dose, may repeat at 30–60 min intervals, then continuous infusion of 1–5 mcg/kg/hr; **Availability (G):** *Buccal tabs:* 100, 200, 300, 400, 600, 800 mcg. *Iontophoretic system:* 40 mcg/dose. *Loz.:* 200, 400, 600, 800, 1200, 1600 mcg. *Transdermal patch:* 12.5 mcg/hr, 25 mcg/hr, 50 mcg/hr, 75 mcg/hr, 100 mcg/hr. *Inject:* 0.05 mg/ml; **Monitor:** BP, HR, RR, pain, bowel function; **Notes: High Alert:** Accidental overdosage of opioid analgesics has resulted in fatalities. Before administering, clarify all ambiguous orders; have second practitioner independently check original order and dose calculations. Schedule II controlled substance. Patients considered opioid-tolerant are those taking ≥60 mg of PO morphine/day, ≥25 mcg transdermal fentanyl/hr, ≥30 mg of oxycodone/day, ≥8 mg of hydromorphone/day or an equianalgesic dose of another opioid for ≥1 wk. Do not substitute fentanyl buccal for fentanyl oral transmucosal; doses are not equivalent. For patients not previously using transmucosal fentanyl, initial dose of buccal should be 100 mcg. For patients switching from oral transmucosal fentanyl to fentanyl buccal, if transmucosal dose is 200–400 mcg, switch to 100 mcg buccal; if transmucosal dose is 600–800 mcg, switch to 200 mcg buccal; if transmucosal dose is 1200–1600 mcg, switch to 400 mcg buccal fentanyl. Do not suck, chew, or swallow buccal tabs; they should be placed between cheek and gum above a molar and allowed to dissolve. Do not chew or swallow loz. Patients must have access to supplemental analgesics during treatment with iontophoretic system; each system may be used for 24 hr from completion of 1st dose or until 80 doses have been delivered. (System then deactivates and cannot deliver more doses; do not apply >1 system at the same time.) If >100 mcg/hr is required, may use multiple transdermal patches at one time; do not cut patches. Naloxone is antidote.

ferrous gluconate (12% elemental iron) (Fergon) **Uses: PO:** Iron deficiency anemia; **Class:** iron supplements; **Preg:** A; **CIs:** Hypersensitivity to iron products; Anemia not due to iron deficiency; Hemochromatosis; Hemosiderosis; **ADRs:** N/V, constipation, dark stools, epigastric pain, GI bleeding, temporary staining of teeth (liquid preparations); **Interactions:** ↓ absorption of tetracyclines, fluoroquinolones, bisphosphonates, levothyroxine, levodopa, and mycofenolate mofetil; Use of PPIs, H_2 antagonists, and cholestyramine may ↓ absorption; **Dose:** *PO: Adults: Treatment of iron deficiency anemia*—60 mg elemental iron bid (max: 240 mg/day). *Prophylaxis of iron deficiency anemia*—60 mg elemental iron/day. *PO: (Infants and Children) Treatment of severe iron deficiency*—4–6 mg/kg/day of elemental iron in 3 divided doses. *Treatment of mild-to-moderate iron deficiency*—3 mg/kg/day elemental iron in 1–2 divided doses. *Prophylaxis of iron deficiency anemia*—1–2 mg/kg/day elemental iron in 1–2 divided doses; **Availability (G):** *Tabs:* 240, 246, 300, 325 mg; **Monitor:** CBC, reticulocyte count, serum ferritin, iron levels, TIBC, bowel function; **Notes:** Take with water or juice on empty stomach (may be given with food to ↓ GI upset). Separate interacting meds by >2–4 hr. Stool may turn black. Keep out of reach of peds.

ferrous sulfate (20% elemental iron) (Feosol, Feratab, Fer-Gen-Sol, Fer-In-Sol, Fer-Iron, Slow FE) **Uses: PO:** Iron deficiency anemia; **Class:** iron supplements; **Preg:** A; **CIs:** Hypersensitivity to iron products; Anemia not due to iron deficiency; Hemochromatosis; Hemosiderosis; **ADRs:** N/V, constipation, dark stools, epigastric pain, GI bleeding, temporary staining of teeth (liquid preparations); **Interactions:** ↓ absorption of tetracyclines, FQs, bisphosphonates, levothyroxine, levodopa, and mycofenolate mofetil; Use of PPIs, H_2 antagonists, and cholestyramine may ↓ absorption; **Dose:** *PO: Adults: Treatment of iron deficiency anemia*—60 mg elemental iron bid (max: 240 mg/day). *Prophylaxis of iron deficiency anemia*—60 mg elemental iron/day. *PO: (Infants and Peds) Treatment of severe iron deficiency*—4–6 mg/kg/day of elemental iron divided tid. *Treatment of mild-to-moderate iron deficiency*—3 mg/kg/day elemental iron in 1–2 divided doses. *Prophylaxis of iron deficiency anemia*—1–2 mg/kg/day elemental iron in 1–2 divided doses; **Availability (G):** *Tabs:* 200, 300, 325 mg. *Timed-release tabs:* 160 mg. *Elixir:* 220 mg/5 ml (44 mg elemental iron/5 ml). *Gtt:* 75 mg/0.6 ml (15 mg elemental iron/0.6 ml); **Monitor:** CBC, reticulocyte count, serum ferritin, iron levels, TIBC, bowel function; **Notes:** Take with water or juice on empty stomach (may be given with food to ↓ GI upset). Separate interacting meds by >2–4 hr. Stool may turn black. Keep out of reach of peds. Do not crush or chew EC or timed-release tabs.

F

fexofenadine (Allegra, Allegra ODT) Uses: Seasonal allergic rhinitis; Chronic idiopathic urticaria; **Class:** antihistamines; **Preg:** C; **CIs:** Hypersensitivity; **ADRs:** dizziness, HA, drowsiness, diarrhea, vomiting; **Interactions:** Mg++ and aluminum-containing antacids ↓ absorption; Erythromycin and ketoconazole may ↑ levels; Apple, orange, and grapefruit juice ↓ absorption; **Dose:** *PO: Adults and Peds: ≥12 yr:* 60 mg bid or 180 mg/day. *PO: Peds: 2–11 yr:* 30 mg bid. *PO: Peds: 6 mo–2 yr:* 15 mg bid. *Renal Impairment Adults and Peds:* ↓ dose if CrCl <80 ml/min; **Availability (G):** *Tabs:* 30, 60, 180 mg. *ODT:* 30 mg. *Susp:* 30 mg/5 ml; **Monitor:** Allergy symptoms; **Notes:** Give tabs with water. ODTs can be taken with or without water and on empty stomach.

filgrastim (Neupogen, G-CSF) Uses: Stimulation of granulocyte production in the following conditions: CA patients (with non-myeloid malignancies) receiving myelosuppressive chemotherapy, Patients with acute myeloid leukemia receiving induction or consolidation chemotherapy, CA patients (with non-myeloid malignancies) receiving BMT, Patients undergoing PBPC collection and therapy, Patients with severe chronic neutropenia; **Class:** colony-stimulating factors; **Preg:** C; **CIs:** Hypersensitivity to filgrastim or *E. coli*–derived proteins; **ADRs:** HA, splenomegaly, N/V, petechiae, pain, redness at subcut site, ↑ alk phos, bone pain; **Interactions:** None significant; **Dose:** *IV: Subcut: Adults: Chemotherapy-induced neutropenia*—5 mcg/kg daily for up to 2 wk or until ANC >10,000; may ↑ by 5 mcg/kg during each chemotherapy cycle, based on duration and severity of ANC nadir. Avoid use for 24 hr before and 24 hr after chemotherapy. *BMT*—10 mcg/kg daily; initiate ≥24 hr after chemotherapy and ≥24 hr after BMT; adjust dosage based on neutrophil response. *Subcut: Adults: PBPC collection*—10 mcg/kg daily; give for ≥4 days before first leukopheresis and continue until last leukopheresis; dosage modification suggested if WBC >100,000. *Congenital neutropenia*—6 mcg/kg bid; adjust dosage based on clinical response and ANC. *Idiopathic/cyclic neutropenia*—5 mcg/kg daily; adjust dosage based on clinical response and ANC; **Availability:** *Inject:* 300 mcg/ml, 600 mcg/ml; **Monitor:** BP, HR, RR, temp, CBC (with diff), ANC, bone pain; **Notes:** Bone pain can usually be controlled with nonopioid analgesics (may require treatment with opioid analgesics). If subcut dose requires >1 ml of solution, may be divided into 2 inject sites.

finasteride (Propecia, Proscar) Uses: BPH (can be used with doxazosin); Male pattern baldness (in men only); **Class:** androgen inhibitors; **Preg:** X; **CIs:** Hypersensitivity; Women; Peds; **ADRs:** impotence, ↓ libido; **Interactions:** None noted; **Dose:** *PO: Adults: BPH*—5 mg/day (Proscar). *Male pattern baldness*—1 mg/day (Propecia); **Availability (G):** *Tabs:* 1 mg (Propecia), 5 mg (Proscar); **Monitor:** S/S BPH, DRE, PSA; **Notes:** May take ≥6–12 mo to see response. Women who are pregnant or may become pregnant should avoid exposure to semen of a partner taking finasteride and should not handle crushed finasteride because of the potential for absorption (may adversely affect male fetus).

flecainide (Tambocor) **Uses:** Life-threatening ventricular arrhythmias, including VT; PSVT; Paroxysmal AF/AFl; **Class:** antiarrhythmics (Class Ic); **Preg:** C; **CIs:** Hypersensitivity; Cardiogenic shock; HF; ≥2nd-degree heart block (in absence of pacemaker); CAD; Pregnancy, lactation, or peds (safety not established); **ADRs:** dizziness, fatigue, HA, blurred vision, dyspnea, ARRHYTHMIAS, CP, HF, heart block, constipation, nausea, stomach pain, tremor; **Interactions:** CYP2D6 inhibitors may ↑ levels/toxicity; ↑ risk of arrhythmias with other antiarrhythmics; May ↑ digoxin levels; Concurrent beta blocker therapy may ↑ levels of beta blocker and flecainide; **Dose:** *PO: Adults: PSVT or AF/AFl (maintenance of sinus rhythm)*—50 mg q 12 hr initially; may ↑ by 50 mg q 12 hr q 4 days until efficacy achieved (max: 300 mg/day). *Conversion of AF ("pill-in-the-pocket")*—200 mg (<70 kg) or 300 mg (≥70 kg) single dose. *VT*—100 mg q 12 hr initially; may ↑ by 50 mg q 12 hr q 4 days until efficacy achieved (max: 400 mg/day). *PO: Peds:* 3–6 mg/kg/day divided tid (range 1–8 mg/kg/day). *Renal Impairment PO: Adults:* ↓ dose if CrCl ≤35 ml/min; **Availability (G):** *Tabs:* 50, 100, 150 mg; **Monitor:** BP, HR, ECG, S/S HF, electrolytes; **Notes:** Usually initiated in hospital. Not recommended for patients with structural heart disease.

fluconazole (Diflucan) **Uses: PO, IV:** Fungal infections, including: Oropharyngeal, esophageal, or vag candidiasis, Systemic candidal infections, UTIs, Peritonitis, Cryptococcal meningitis; Prevention of candidiasis in patients who have undergone BMT; **Class:** antifungals; **Preg:** C; **CIs:** Hypersensitivity to fluconazole or other azole antifungals; Lactation; **ADRs:** HA, QT interval prolongation, HEPATOTOXICITY, abdominal discomfort, N/V/D, rash, exfoliative skin disorders including SJS, allergic reactions, including ANAPHYLAXIS; **Interactions:** May ↑ levels of CYP2C9 substrates, CYP2C19 substrates, and CYP3A4 substrates; Rifampin may ↓ levels; May ↑ hypoglycemic effects of glyburide or glipizide; May ↑ risk of bleeding with warfarin; **Dose:** *PO, IV: Adults: Vag candidiasis*—150 mg × 1. *Oropharyngeal candidiasis*—200 mg on 1st day, then 100 mg/day for ≥2 wk. *Esophageal candidiasis*—200 mg on 1st day, then 100 mg/day for ≥3 wk (may use up to 400 mg/day). *UTIs/ peritonitis*—50–200 mg/day. *Candidemia*—400–800 mg/day × 14 days after last positive blood culture and resolution of S/S. *Cryptococcal meningitis (treatment)*—400 mg on 1st day, then 200–400 mg/day × 10–12 wk after CSF becomes negative. *Cryptococcal meningitis (suppressive therapy)*—200 mg/day. *Prophylaxis in BMT*—400 mg/day; begin several days before procedure if severe neutropenia is expected, and continue × 7 days after ANC >1000. *PO, IV: Peds: Oropharyngeal candidiasis*—6 mg/kg on 1st day, then 3 mg/kg/day for ≥2 wk. *Esophageal candidiasis*—6 mg/kg on 1st day, then 3 mg/kg/day for ≥3 wk (max: 12 mg/kg/day). *Candidemia*—6 mg/kg q 12 hr × 28 days. *Cryptococcal meningitis (treatment)*—12 mg/kg on 1st day, then 6 mg/kg/day × 10–12 wk after CSF becomes negative. *Cryptococcal meningitis (suppressive therapy)*—6 mg/kg/day. *Renal Impairment PO, IV: Adults:* ↓ dose if CrCl ≤50 ml/min; **Availability (G):** *Tabs:* 50, 100, 150, 200 mg. *Oral susp:* 10, 40 mg/ml. *Inject:* 2 mg/ml; **Monitor:** BP, HR, temp, sputum, U/A, CBC, BUN/SCr, LFTs; **Notes:** When converting between IV and PO, use same dose.

F

fludrocortisone (Florinef) Uses: Partial replacement therapy for adrenocortical insufficiency associated with Addison's disease (given with hydrocortisone or cortisone); Management of Na^+ loss due to congenital adrenogenital syndrome (congenital adrenal hyperplasia); **Class:** corticosteroids; **Preg:** C; **CIs:** Hypersensitivity; Systemic fungal infection; **ADRs:** dizziness, HA, cataracts, HF, edema, ↑ BP, anorexia, nausea, adrenal suppression, ↑ BG, ↑ wt, ↓ K+, acne, muscle weakness, tendon rupture; **Interactions:** ↑ risk of hypokalemia with thiazide or loop diuretics or amphotericin B; ↑ risk of tendon rupture with FQs; May produce prolonged neuromuscular blockade following the use of nondepolarizing neuromuscular blocking agents; Phenobarbital or rifampin may ↓ levels; **Dose:** *PO: Adults: Adrenocortical insufficiency*—0.1 mg/day (range: 0.1 mg 3 ×/wk–0.2 mg/day). Use with 10–37.5 mg cortisone daily *or* 10–30 mg hydrocortisone daily. *Adrenogenital syndrome*—0.1–0.2 mg/day. *PO: Peds:* 0.05–0.1 mg/day; **Availability (G):** *Tabs:* 0.1 mg; **Monitor:** BP, HR, edema, wt, electrolytes; **Notes:** Do not abruptly discontinue (may result in Addisonian crisis).

flumazenil (Romazicon) Uses: Complete/partial reversal of sedative effects of BZs; Management of BZ overdose; **Class:** benzodiazepines; **Preg:** C; **CIs:** Hypersensitivity to flumazenil or BZs; Receiving BZ for life-threatening medical problems (e.g., status epilepticus, ↑ ICP); Serious cyclic antidepressant overdose; Mixed CNS depressant overdose; **ADRs:** SEIZURES, dizziness, agitation, drowsiness, HA, blurred vision, N/V, flushing, ↑ sweating, pain/inject-site reactions, phlebitis; **Interactions:** None significant; *Dose: IV: Adults: Conscious sedation or general anesthesia reversal*—0.2 mg; additional doses may be given q 1 min until desired results obtained (max total dose: 1 mg). If resedation occurs, regimen may be repeated at 20-min intervals (max: 3 mg/hr). *IV: Peds: ≥1 yr Conscious sedation reversal*—0.01 mg/kg (max: 0.2 mg); additional doses may be given q 1 min until desired results obtained (max total dose = 0.05 mg/kg or 1 mg, whichever is lower). *IV: Adults: BZ overdose*—0.2 mg; if desired results not obtained after 30 sec, give additional 0.3 mg; if needed, further doses of 0.5 mg may be given q 1 min (max total dose: 3 mg). If resedation occurs, additional doses of 1 mg may be given q 20 min (max: 3 mg/hr); **Availability (G):** *Inject:* 0.1 mg/ml; **Monitor:** RR, level of consciousness, seizure activity; **Notes:** Ensure patient has patent airway before administration. Observe patient for ≥2 hr after administration for appearance of resedation. Seizures may be treated with BZs, barbiturates, or phenytoin. Does not consistently reverse the amnestic effects of BZs.

flunisolide (AeroBid, AeroBid-M, Nasarel) Uses: Inhaln: Maintenance treatment of asthma (prophylactic therapy); **Intranasal:** Seasonal or perennial allergic rhinitis; **Class:** corticosteroids; **Preg:** C; **CIs:** Hypersensitivity; Acute asthma attack/status asthmaticus; **ADRs:** HA, dizziness, irritability, hoarseness, nasal burning sensation, nasal congestion, pharyngitis, dysphonia, epistaxis, nasal irritation, oropharyngeal fungal infections, rhinorrhea, sinusitis, sneezing, tearing eyes, bronchospasm, cough, wheezing, N/V/D, taste disturbances, adrenal suppression (increased dose, long-term therapy only), ↓ growth (peds); **Interactions:** CYP3A4 inhibitors may ↑ levels; CYP3A4 inducers may ↓ levels; **Dose:** *Inhaln: Adults and Peds: >15 yr:* 2 inhaln bid (max: 4 inhaln bid). *Intranasal: Adults and Peds: >14 yr:* 2 sprays in each nostril bid; may ↑ to 2 sprays in each nostril tid after 4–7 days, if needed (max: 8 sprays in each nostril/day). *Inhaln: Peds: 6–15 yr:* 2 inhaln bid (max: 2 inhaln bid). *Intranasal: Peds: 6–14 yr:* 1 spray in each nostril tid *or* 2 sprays in each nostril bid (max: 4 sprays in each nostril/day); **Availability (G):** *Inhaln aerosol (Aerobid):* 250 mcg/metered inhaln. *Inhaln aerosol-menthol (Aerobid-M):* 250 mcg/metered inhaln. *Nasal spray (Nasarel):* 25 mcg/metered spray, 29 mcg/metered spray; **Monitor:** RR, lung sounds, PFTs, growth rate (in peds), S/S asthma/allergies; **Notes:** After desired effect achieved, ↓ dose to lowest amount required to control symptoms (if possible). For asthma, use bronchodilator first and allow 5 min to elapse before using flunisolide. Allow ≥1 min between oral inhaln of aerosol. Inhaler should not be used to treat acute asthma attack. When using inhaler, rinse mouth with water or mouthwash after each use to minimize fungal infections, dry mouth, and hoarseness.

fluocinolone (Capex, Derma-Smoothe/FS, FS Shampoo) Uses: Management of inflammation and pruritis associated with various dermatoses; **Class:** corticosteroids; **Preg:** C; **CIs:** Hypersensitivity; **ADRs:** burning sensation, dryness, folliculitis, hypersensitivity reactions, hirsutism, hypopigmentation, irritation, secondary infection, striae, adrenal suppression (with use of occlusive dressings or long-term therapy); **Interactions:** None significant; **Dose:** *Topical: Adults:* Apply 2–4 ×/day (depends on product, preparation, and condition being treated). *Topical: Peds: ≥3 mo:* Apply bid (depends on product, preparation, and condition being treated); **Availability (G):** *Cream:* 0.01%, 0.025%. *Oint:* 0.025%. *Soln/Shampoo/Oil:* 0.01%; **Monitor:** Skin condition (inflammation, erythema, pruritis); **Notes:** Oints are more occlusive and preferred for dry, scaly lesions. Creams should be used on oozing or intertriginous areas (may cause more skin drying than oint). Soln and shampoo are useful in hairy areas. Apply oil and shampoo to scalp.

fluocinonide (Vanos) Uses: Management of inflammation and pruritis associated with various dermatoses; **Class:** corticosteroids; **Preg:** C; **CIs:** Hypersensitivity; **ADRs:** burning sensation, dryness, folliculitis, hypersensitivity reactions, hirsutism, hypopigmentation, irritation, secondary infection, striae, adrenal suppression (with use of occlusive dressings or long-term therapy); **Interactions:** None significant; **Dose:** *Topical: Adults:* Apply 2–4 ×/day (depends on product, preparation, and condition being treated). *Topical: Peds:* Apply once daily; **Availability (G):** *Cream:* 0.05%, 0.1%. *Gel/Oint/Soln:* 0.05%; **Monitor:** Skin condition (inflammation, erythema, pruritis); **Notes:** Oints are more occlusive and preferred for dry, scaly lesions. Creams should be used on oozing or intertriginous areas (may cause more skin drying than oint). Gels and soln are useful in hairy areas.

fluorouracil (Adrucil, Carac, Efudex, Fluoroplex) Uses: IV: Used alone and/or in combination in the treatment of Colon CA, Breast CA, Rectal CA, Gastric CA, Pancreatic CA; **Topical:** Management of multiple actinic (solar) keratoses and superficial basal cell carcinomas; **Class:** antimetabolites; **Preg:** D (inject), **X** (top); **CIs:** Hypersensitivity; Pregnancy/lactation; Infections; Bone marrow depression; **ADRs:** N/V/D, stomatitis, alopecia, maculopapular rash, hand-foot syndrome, local inflammatory reactions (top only), photosensitivity, sterility, anemia, leukopenia, thrombocytopenia, thrombophlebitis; **Interactions:** Combination chemotherapy with irinotecan may produce unacceptable toxicity (dehydration, neutropenia, sepsis); ↑ bone marrow suppression with other antineoplastics or radiation therapy; **Dose:** *IV: Adults: Initial dose*—12 mg/kg/day × 4 days (max: 800 mg/day), then 1 day of rest, then 6 mg/kg every other day × 5 doses. *Maintenance*—Repeat initial course of therapy q 30 days *or* 10–15 mg/kg q wk (max: 1000 mg/wk). *Topical: Adults: Actinic/solar keratoses*—Efudex or Fluoroplex: Apply bid × 2–4 wk (Efudex) or 2–6 wk (Fluoroplex); Carac: Apply once daily for up to 4 wk. *Superficial basal cell carcinomas*—Efudex (5% solution or cream): Apply bid × 3–6 wk (up to 12 wk); **Availability (G):** *Inject:* 50 mg/ml. *Cream:* 0.5%, 1%, 5%. *Soln:* 2%, 5%; **Monitor:** BP, HR, temp, CBC (with diff), S/S infection, bleeding, mucous membranes, infusion site, skin lesions, I/Os; **Notes: High Alert:** Fatalities have occurred with chemotherapeutic agents. Before administering, clarify all ambiguous orders; double-check single, daily, and course-of-therapy dose limits; have second practitioner independently double-check original order, calculations, and infusion pump settings. Leukocyte count nadir = 9–14 days (recovery in 30 days after administration). Apply top formulation with gloves. For top, erythema, scaling, blistering with pruritus, and burning sensation are expected. Therapy is discontinued when erosion, ulceration, and necrosis occur.

fluoxetine (Prozac, Prozac Weekly, Sarafem) Uses: Depression; OCD; Bulimia nervosa; Panic disorder; **Sarafem:** PMDD;

Class: SSRIs; **Preg:** C; **CIs:** Hypersensitivity to fluoxetine or other SSRIs; Concurrent use of pimozide or thioridazine; Concurrent or recent (within 14 days) use of MAOIs (fluoxetine should be discontinued 5 wk before MAOI therapy is initiated); May ↑ risk of suicidal thoughts/behaviors. esp. during early treatment or dose adjustment; risk may be ↑ in peds and adolescents; Pregnancy (esp. in 3rd tri, as neonates are at ↑ risk for drug discontinuation syndrome [including respiratory distress, feeding difficulty, and irritability] and pulmonary HTN); Lactation; **ADRs:** SEIZURES, SUICIDAL THOUGHTS, anxiety, drowsiness, HA, insomnia, nervousness, abnormal dreams, weakness, anorexia, diarrhea, nausea, abdominal pain, constipation, dyspepsia, ↓ wt, sexual dysfunction, pruritus, rash, ↑ sweating, tremor, allergic reactions, fever, flu-like syndrome; **Interactions:** CYP2C9 inhibitors and CYP2D6 inhibitors may ↑ levels/toxicity; CYP2C9 inducers may ↓ levels/effects; May ↑ levels/toxicity of CYP1A2 substrates, CYP2C9 substrates, and CYP2D6 substrates; Serious, potentially fatal reactions (serotonin syndrome) may occur with MAOIs (discontinue MAOIs for ≥14 days before starting fluoxetine; discontinue fluoxetine for ≥5 wk before starting MAOI); ↑ levels of pimozide and thioridazine (contraindicated); ↑ risk of serotonin syndrome with 5-HT_1 agonists, linezolid, lithium, or trazodone; ↑ levels of alprazolam, diazepam, and lithium; ↑ CNS depression with alcohol, antihistamines, other antidepressants, opioid analgesics, or sedative/hypnotics; **Dose:** *PO: Adults: Depression*—20 mg in AM; may ↑ by 20 mg/day q 2–3 wk (max: 80 mg/day); doses >20 mg/day may be given daily or bid (in AM and at noon). Patients stabilized on the 20 mg/day dose may be switched over to DR caps (Prozac Weekly) at dose of 90 mg weekly (initiated 7 days after the last 20 mg/day dose). *Panic disorder*—10 mg/day; after 1 wk, may ↑ to 20 mg/day; additional dosage ↑ may be made if necessary after several wk (max: 60 mg/day). *Bulimia nervosa*—60 mg/day (may ↑ dosage over several days). *PMDD*—20 mg/day *or* 20 mg/day starting 14 days prior to expected onset of menses, continued through 1st full day of menstruation, repeated with each cycle. *PO: Peds: 8–17 yr Depression*—10 mg/day; after 1 wk, may ↑ to 20 mg/day. *PO: Peds: 7–17 yr OCD*—10 mg/day; after 2 wk, may ↑ to 20 mg/day; additional dosage ↑ may be made if necessary after several wk (max: 60 mg/day); **Availability (G):** *Tabs:* 10, 20 mg. *Caps:* 10, 20, 40 mg. *DR caps (Prozac Weekly):* 90 mg. *Oral soln:* 20 mg/5 ml; **Monitor:** Mental status, OCD behaviors, binge eating/vomiting, suicidal thoughts/behaviors; **Notes:** Should not abruptly discontinue (should taper to ↓ withdrawal). May take 4–6 wk to see effect.

fluphenazine (Prolixin, Prolixin Decanoate) **Uses:** Acute and chronic psychoses; **Class:** phenothiazines; **Preg:** C; **CIs:** Hypersensitivity (cross-sensitivity with other phenothiazines may exist); Subcortical brain damage; Severe depression; Coma; Bone marrow depression; Liver disease; Hypersensitivity to sesame oil (decanoate salt);

F

Concurrent use of drugs that prolong the QT interval; Lactation; Peds <12 yr (safety not established); **ADRs:** NMS, EPS, sedation, tardive dyskinesia, blurred vision, ↑↓ BP, QT interval prolongation, ↑ HR, anorexia, constipation, ↑ LFTs, dry mouth, ileus, nausea, ↑ wt, urinary retention, photosensitivity, rash, galactorrhea, AGRANULOCYTOSIS, leukopenia, thrombocytopenia, allergic reactions; **Interactions:** ↑ risk of QT prolongation with other QT-prolonging drugs; CYP2D6 inhibitors may ↑ levels; Additive hypotension with antihypertensives; ↑ CNS depression with other CNS depressants including alcohol, antidepressants, antihistamines, opioids, and sedative/hypnotics; May ↑ risk of lithium toxicity; May ↓ effects of levodopa and bromocriptine; ↑ risk of anticholinergic effects with other anticholinergic agents; Metoclopramide may ↑ the risk of EPS; **Dose:** *IM (as decanoate): Adults:* 12.5–25 mg initially; may be repeated q 3 wk. Dosage may be slowly ↑ as needed (max: 100 mg/dose). *IM (as hydrochloride): Adults:* 1.25–2.5 mg q 6–8 hr. *PO: Adults:* 0.5–10 mg/day divided q 6–8 hr (max: 40 mg/day); **Availability (G):** *Decanoate inject:* 25 mg/ml. *Hydrochloride tabs:* 1, 2.5, 5, 10 mg. *Hydrochloride elixir:* 2.5 mg/5 ml. *Hydrochloride oral concentrate:* 5 mg/ml. *Hydrochloride inject:* 2.5 mg/ml; **Monitor:** BP, HR, RR, ECG, mental status, EPS, tardive dyskinesia, S/S NMS, CBC, LFTs; **Notes:** IM dose (of hydrochloride) is 30–50% of PO dose. 12.5 mg q 3 wk of decanoate = 10 mg/day of hydrochloride. Decanoate is used for long-term therapy. Benztropine or diphenhydramine can be used to treat EPS.

flurazepam (Dalmane) Uses: Short-term management of insomnia (<4 wk); **Class:** benzodiazepines; **Preg:** X; **CIs:** Hypersensitivity (cross-sensitivity with other BZs may exist); Acute narrow-angle glaucoma; Severe hepatic disease; Severe pulmonary impairment; Sleep apnea; Pregnancy/lactation; Peds <15 yr (safety not established); **ADRs:** ataxia, confusion, depression, dizziness, drowsiness, hallucinations, sleep-driving, blurred vision, respiratory depression, constipation, N/V/D, ↑ wt, physical/psychological dependence, tolerance; **Interactions:** ↑ CNS depression with alcohol, antidepressants, other BZs, antihistamines, and opioids; CYP3A4 inhibitors may ↑ levels; CYP3A4 inducers may ↓ levels; **Dose:** *PO: Adults and Peds: ≥15 yr:* 15–30 mg at bedtime. *PO: Geriatric Patients or Debilitated Patients:* 15 mg initially, may be ↑; **Availability (G):** *Caps:* 15, 30 mg; **Monitor:** Mental status, sleep patterns; **Notes:** Schedule IV controlled substance. Potential for dependence/abuse with long-term use (use with caution in patients at risk for addiction). Flumazenil is antidote. Do not discontinue abruptly; taper to ↓ risk of withdrawal.

fluticasone (Cutivate, Flonase, Flovent Diskus, Flovent HFA, Veramyst) Uses: Inhaln: Maintenance treatment of asthma (prophylactic therapy); **Intranasal:** Seasonal or perennial allergic or nonallergic rhinitis; **Topical:** Inflammation and pruritis associated with various allergic/immunologic skin problems; **Class:** corticosteroids;

Preg: C; **CIs:** Hypersensitivity; Acute asthma attack/status asthmaticus (inhaln); Active untreated infections (top); **ADRs:** HA, dizziness, dysphonia, epistaxis, nasal irritation, nasal stuffiness, oropharyngeal fungal infections, pharyngitis, rhinorrhea, sinusitis, sneezing, tearing eyes, bronchospasm, cough, wheezing, N/V/D, allergic contact dermatitis, atrophy, burning sensation, dryness, folliculitis, hirsutism, irritation, ↓ wound healing, adrenal suppression (increased dose, long-term therapy only), ↓ growth (peds); **Interactions:** CYP3A4 inhibitors may ↑ levels; CYP3A4 inducers may ↓ levels; **Dose:** *Inhaln: Adults and Peds: ≥12 yr (Flovent HFA) Previously on bronchodilators alone*—88 mcg bid (max: 440 mcg bid). *Previously on inhaled corticosteroids*—88–220 mcg bid (max: 440 mcg bid). *Previously on PO corticosteroids*—440 mcg bid (max: 880 mcg bid). *Inhaln: Adults and Peds: ≥12 yr (Flovent Diskus) Previously on bronchodilators alone*—100 mcg bid (max: 500 mcg bid); *Previously on inhaled corticosteroids*—100–250 mcg bid (max: 500 mcg bid); *Previously on PO corticosteroids*—500–1000 mcg bid. *Intranasal: Adults:* 2 sprays in each nostril daily *or* 1 spray in each nostril bid (max: 2 sprays in each nostril/day); after several days, ↓ to 1 spray in each nostril daily. *Topical: Adults:* Apply bid. *Inhaln: Peds 4–11 yr (Flovent HFA)*—88 mcg bid. *Inhaln: Peds 4–11 yr (Flovent Diskus)*—50 mcg bid (max: 100 mcg bid). *Intranasal: Peds ≥4 yr:* 1 spray in each nostril daily (max: 2 sprays in each nostril/day); **Availability (G):** *Inhaln aerosol (Flovent HFA):* 44 mcg/metered inhaln, 110 mcg/metered inhaln, 220 mcg/metered inhaln. *Powder for inhaln (Flovent Diskus):* 50 mcg. *Nasal spray:* 27.5 mcg/metered spray (Veramyst), 50 mcg/metered spray (Flonase). *Cream/Lotion:* 0.05%. *Oint:* 0.005%; **Monitor:** RR, lung sounds, PFTs, growth rate (in peds), S/S asthma/allergies, skin condition (inflammation, erythema, pruritis); **Notes:** After desired effect achieved, ↓ dose to lowest amount required to control symptoms (if possible). For asthma, use bronchodilator first and allow 5 min to elapse before using fluticasone. Allow ≥1 min between oral inhaln of aerosol. Inhaler should not be used to treat acute asthma attack. When using inhaler, rinse mouth with water or mouthwash after each use to minimize fungal infections, dry mouth, and hoarseness. Oints are more occlusive and preferred for dry, scaly lesions. Creams should be used on oozing or intertriginous areas (may cause more skin drying than oint). Lotions are useful in hairy areas.

fluvastatin (Lescol, Lescol XL) **Uses:** Hypercholesterolemia; Secondary prevention of coronary revascularization procedures; Slows progression of coronary atherosclerosis in patients with CAD; **Class:** hmg CoA reductase inhibitors; **Preg:** X; **CIs:** Hypersensitivity; Liver disease; Pregnancy/lactation; Peds <9 yr (safety not established); **ADRs:** HA, abdominal cramps, diarrhea, dyspepsia, flatulence, ↑ LFTs, nausea, rash, RHABDOMYOLYSIS, myalgia; **Interactions:** CYP2C9 inhibitors may ↑ levels/toxicity; May ↑ levels/toxicity of CYP2C9 substrates; ↑ risk of myopathy with cyclosporine, gemfibrozil, erythromycin, niacin (≥1 g/day), or fluconazole; May ↑ digoxin levels; May ↑ effects of warfarin; Cholestyramine or colestipol may ↓ absorption (separate by ≥2 hr); *Dose: PO: Adults: IR*—20–40 mg at bedtime; may ↑ to 40 mg bid, if needed. *ER*—80 mg at bedtime. *PO: Peds: ≥9 yr:* 20 mg at bedtime; may ↑ to 40 mg bid (IR) *or* 80 mg at bedtime (ER), if needed; **Availability (G):** *Caps:* 20, 40 mg. *ER tabs:* 80 mg; **Monitor:** Lipid panel, LFTs, CK (if symptoms); **Notes:** Do not crush, break, or chew ER tabs.

F

fluvoxamine (Luvox, Luvox CR) **Uses:** OCD (IR and CR); SAD (CR only); **Class:** SSRIs; **Preg:** C; **CIs:** Hypersensitivity to fluvoxamine or other SSRIs; Concurrent use of alosetron, pimozide, ramelteon, thioridazine, or tizanidine; Concurrent or recent (within 14 days) use of MAOIs; May ↑ risk of suicidal thoughts/behaviors, esp. during early treatment or dose adjustment; risk may be ↑ in peds and adolescents; Pregnancy (esp. in 3rd tri, as neonates are at ↑ risk for drug discontinuation syndrome [including respiratory distress, feeding difficulty, and irritability] and pulmonary HTN); Lactation; **ADRs:** SUICIDAL THOUGHTS, dizziness, HA, insomnia, nervousness, sedation, weakness, agitation, anxiety, emotional lability, manic reactions, palpitations, anorexia, diarrhea, dry mouth, dyspepsia, nausea, constipation, vomiting, ↓ libido/sexual dysfunction, ↑ sweating, tremor, ↑ yawning; **Interactions:** CYP1A2 inhibitors and CYP2D6 inhibitors may ↑ levels/toxicity; CYP1A2 inducers may ↓ levels/effects; May ↑ levels/toxicity of CYP1A2 substrates, CYP2C19 substrates, and CYP3A4 substrates; Serious, potentially fatal reactions (serotonin syndrome) may occur with MAOIs (contraindicated); ↑ levels of alosetron, pimozide, ramelteon, thioridazine, and tizanidine (contraindicated); ↑ risk of serotonin syndrome with 5-HT_1 agonists, linezolid, lithium, or trazodone; ↑ clozapine levels/toxicity (dosage adjustments may be necessary); **Dose:** *PO: Adults: IR*—50 mg at bedtime; may ↑ by 50 mg/day q 4–7 days until desired effect (max: 300 mg/day); if dose >50 mg/day, give in 2 divided doses. *CR*—100 mg/day; may ↑ by 50 mg/day on weekly basis until desired effect (max: 300 mg/day). *PO: Peds: 8–17 yr OCD*—25 mg at bedtime, may ↑ by 25 mg/day q 4–7 days (max: 200 mg/day); if dose >50 mg/day, give in 2 divided doses; **Availability: (G):** *Tabs:* 25, 50, 100 mg. *CR caps:* 100, 150 mg; **Monitor:** Mental status, suicidal thoughts/behaviors; **Notes:** Should not abruptly discontinue (should taper to ↓ withdrawal symptoms). Do not crush or chew CR caps. May take 4–6 wk to see effect.

folic acid (folate, Folvite, vitamin B) **Uses:** Megaloblastic and macrocytic anemias due to folate deficiency; Prevents neural tube defects during pregnancy; **Class:** water soluble vitamins; **Preg:** A; **CIs:** Anemia due to vitamin B_{12} deficiency; **ADRs:** rash; **Interactions:** Sulfonamides (including sulfasalazine) and cholestyramine ↓ absorption; Folic acid requirements ↑ by phenytoin, phenobarbital, primidone, or carbamazepine; May ↓ phenytoin levels; **Dose:** *PO: IM IV: Subcut: Adults:*

Anemia—0.4 mg/day (0.8 mg/day in pregnancy/lactation). *Prevention of neural tube defects*—0.4 mg/day. *PO: IM IV: Subcut: Peds: Anemia*—>4 yr: 0.4 mg/day; <4 yr: up to 0.3 mg/day; **Availability: (G):** *Tabs:* 0.4, 0.8, 1 mg. *Inject:* 5 mg/ml; **Monitor:** CBC, folate levels, reticulocyte count; **Notes:** Do not confuse with folinic acid (leucovorin calcium). Foods high in folic acid include vegetables, fruits, and organ meats.

fondaparinux (Arixtra) **Uses:** Prevention of DVT/PE in surgical patients (hip fracture, hip/knee replacement, abdominal); Treatment of DVT/PE; **Class:** active factor X inhibitors; **Preg:** B; **CIs:** Hypersensitivity; Severe renal impairment (CrCl <30 ml/min; ↑ risk of bleeding); Wt <50 kg (for prophylaxis; ↑ risk of bleeding); Active major bleeding; IE; Thrombocytopenia due to fonaparinux antibodies; **ADRs:** ↑ LFTs, hematoma, purpura, rash, BLEEDING, thrombocytopenia, fever; **Interactions:** ↑ risk of bleeding with antiplatelets, thrombolytics, or other anticoagulants; **Dose:** *Subcut: Adults: DVT/PE prophylaxis*—2.5 mg/day, starting 6–8 hr after surgery, continuing for 5–9 days (up to 10 days for abdominal surgery; up to 11 days for hip/knee replacement surgery); extended prophylaxis recommended for hip fracture surgery (total duration of peri-operative and extended prophylaxis may be up to 32 days). *DVT/PE treatment*—<50 kg: 5 mg/day; 50–100 kg: 7.5 mg/day; >100 kg: 10 mg/day; continue treatment for ≥5 days until therapeutic anticoagulation with warfarin achieved (INR >2 for 2 consecutive days); warfarin may be started within 72 hr of fondaparinux; **Availability:** *Inject:* 2.5 mg/0.5 ml, 5 mg/0.4 ml, 7.5 mg/0.6 ml, 10 mg/0.8 ml; **Monitor:** BUN/SCr, CBC, LFTs, S/S bleeding; **Notes:** Use with caution in elderly (at ↑ risk for bleeding). Do not administer within 6 hr after surgery (↑ risk of bleeding). If platelets <100,000, discontinue. PT and aPTT cannot be used to monitor efficacy/safety.

formoterol (Foradil, Perforomist) **Uses:** Asthma (aerolizer only); COPD (aerolizer and nebulizer); Acute prevention of exercise-induced bronchospasm (aerolizer only); **Class:** adrenergics; **Preg:** C; **CIs:** Hypersensitivity; Acute attack of asthma or COPD (onset of action is delayed); Peds <5 yr (safety not established); **ADRs:** dizziness, insomnia, nervousness, PARADOXICAL BRONCHOSPASM, angina, ARRHYTHMIAS, ↑ BP, palpitations, ↑ HR, dry mouth, muscle cramps, tremor, ANAPHYLAXIS; **Interactions:** ↑ risk of arrhythmias with MAOIs, TCAs, or other agents that may prolong the QT interval; ↑ risk of hypokalemia with theophylline, corticosteroids, or diuretics; Beta blockers may ↓ therapeutic effects; ↑ adrenergic effects may occur with concurrent use of adrenergics; **Dose:** *Inhaln: Adults and Peds: ≥5 yr Asthma or COPD*—1 cap q 12 hr using Aerolizer Inhaler. *Prevention of exercise-induced bronchospasm*—1 cap using Aerolizer Inhaler ≥15 min before exercise on a prn basis. *Inhaln: Adults: COPD*—20 mcg bid via nebulization; **Availability:** *Caps for Aerolizer:* 12 mcg. *Nebulization* *soln:* 20 mcg/2 ml; **Monitor:** Lung sounds, HR, BP, RR, PFTs, ECG (QT interval); **Notes:** Not for acute asthma symptoms; should use short-acting beta$_2$ agonist for acute relief of symptoms. Do not exceed recommended dose (may ↑ risk of asthma-related death). Caps are only to be used with Aerolizer Inhaler and should not be taken orally. Do not use spacer with Aerolizer Inhaler.

F

fosamprenavir calcium (Lexiva) **Uses:** HIV (with other antiretrovirals); **Class:** protease inhibitors; **Preg:** C; **CIs:** Hypersensitivity to fosamprenavir or sulfonamides; Severe hepatic impairment; Concurrent use with flecainide, propafenone, rifampin, ergot derivatives, St. John's wort, lovastatin, simvastatin, pimozide, delavirdine, midazolam, or triazolam; Peds <2 yr (safety not established); **ADRs:** HA, N/V/D, abdominal pain, ↑ LFTs, rash, ↑ BG, fat redistribution, ↑ TGs, neutropenia, SJS; **Interactions:** CYP3A4 inhibitors may ↑ levels/toxicity; CYP3A4 inducers may ↓ levels/effects; May ↑ levels/toxicity of CYP3A4 substrates; ↑ levels of flecainide, propafenone, ergot derivatives, lovastatin, simvastatin, pimozide, midazolam, and triazolam (contraindicated); Rifampin and St. John's wort ↓ levels (contraindicated); ↓ levels of delavirdine (contraindicated); Efavirenz ↓ levels (if added to fosamprenavir/ritonavir once daily regimen, an additional 100 mg of ritonavir (total of 300 mg) should be given); Lopinavir/ritonavir, saquinavir, and H$_2$ antagonists ↓ levels; Nevirapine ↓ levels (need to use fosamprenavir with ritonavir when used together); Indinavir and nelfinavir ↑ levels; May ↓ levels of methadone and paroxetine; ↑ rifabutin levels (↓ rifabutin dose by 50% when used with fosamprenavir, or by 75% when used with fosamprenavir and ritonavir); ↑ risk of myopathy with atorvastatin or rosuvastatin (consider using fluvastatin or pravastatin); ↑ levels of sildenafil, vardenafil, and tadalafil (↓ dose of these agents); May alter the effects of warfarin or hormonal contraceptives (use alternative method of contraception); **Dose:** *PO: Adults: Treatment-naive without ritonavir*—1400 mg bid. *Treatment-naive with ritonavir*—1400 mg/day with ritonavir 100 or 200 mg/day *or* 700 mg bid with ritonavir 100 mg bid. *Protease inhibitor–experienced*—700 mg bid with ritonavir 100 mg bid. *PO: Peds: 2–5 yr Treatment-naive*—30 mg/kg (max: 1400 mg/dose) of oral suspension bid. *PO: Peds: 6–18 yr Treatment-naive*—30 mg/kg (max: 1400 mg/dose) of oral susp bid *or* 18 mg/kg (max: 700 mg/dose) of oral susp bid with ritonavir 3 mg/kg (max: 100 mg/dose) bid. *PO: Peds: 6–18 yr Treatment-experienced*—18 mg/kg (max: 700 mg/dose) of oral susp bid with ritonavir 3 mg/kg (max: 100 mg/dose) bid. *Hepatic Impairment: Adults:* ↓ dose in mild, moderate, and severe hepatic impairment; **Availability:** *Tabs:* 700 mg. *Oral susp:* 50 mg/ml; **Monitor:** Viral load, CD4 count, BG, LFTs, lipid panel; **Notes:** Sulfa drug. Rash can occur within 1st 2 wk and usually resolves within 2 wk (must discontinue if severe skin reaction). Adults should take susp on empty stomach; peds should take susp with food.

foscarnet (Foscavir) Uses: Treatment of CMV retinitis in patients with AIDS; Treatment of acyclovir-resistant mucocutaneous HSV infections in immunocompromised patients; **Class:** antivirals; **Preg:** C; **CIs:** Hypersensitivity; **ADRs:** SEIZURES, HA, anxiety, confusion, depression, dizziness, fatigue, vision abnormalities, cough, dyspnea, N/V/D, abdominal pain, anorexia, renal impairment, genital irritation/ ulceration, ↑ sweating, rash, ↓ Ca++, ↓ K+, ↓ Mg++, ↓ ↑PO_4, anemia, leukopenia, pain/inflammation at inject site, involuntary muscle contraction, neuropathy, paresthesia, tremor, fever, chills, flu-like syndrome; **Interactions:** ↑ risk of hypocalcemia with IV pentamidine; ↑ risk of nephrotoxicity with other nephrotoxic drugs (e.g., amphotericin, aminoglycosides, vancomycin, cisplatin, cyclosporine); ↑ risk of electrolyte abnormalities with diuretics; ↑ risk of renal impairment with ritonavir or saquinavir; **Dose:** *IV: Adults: CMV retinitis*—60 mg/kg q 8 hr or 90 mg/ kg q 12 hr × 2–3 wk, then 90–120 mg/kg/day as a single daily infusion. *HSV*—40 mg/kg q 8–12 hr × 2–3 wk or until healing occurs. *IV: Adults:* ↓ dose if CrCl ≤1.4 ml/min/kg; **Availability (G):** *Inject:* 24 mg/ml; **Monitor:** BUN/SCr, CBC, electrolytes (also ionized Ca++), ophth exam, HSV lesions; **Notes:** Give 750–1000 ml of NS or D5W prior to 1st infusion, and then 750–1000 ml with 120 mg/kg of foscarnet or 500 ml with 40–60 mg/kg of foscarnet with each subsequent infusion to ↓ risk of renal impairment. Not a cure for CMV retinitis or HSV infections (progression or relapse may still occur). Risk factors for seizures include renal impairment, electrolyte abnormalities, history of seizures, and ↓ Ca++. Avoid rapid (bolus) administration (↑ risk of nephrotoxicity). Must be diluted if administering through peripheral line (can be given undiluted through central line). CrCl should be calculated even if SCr is in normal range.

fosinopril (Monopril) Uses: HTN; HF; **Class:** ACEIs; **Preg:** C (1st tri), **D** (2nd and 3rd tri); **CIs:** Previous sensitivity/intolerance to ACEIs; Peds <6 yr (safety not established); Pregnancy/lactation; **ADRs:** dizziness, cough, ↓ BP, ↑ SCr, ↑ K+, rash, ANGIOEDEMA; **Interactions:** ↑ effects with other antihypertensives; ↑ risk of hyperkalemia with ARBs, K+ supplements, K+ salt substitutes, K+–sparing diuretics, or NSAIDs; NSAIDs may ↓ effectiveness; ↑ lithium levels; **Dose:** *PO: Adults: HTN*—10 mg/day, may be ↑ up to 80 mg/day. *HF*—10 mg/day (5 mg/day if recently diuresed); titrate up to target dose of 40 mg/day. *PO: Peds: ≥6 yr and >50 kg HTN*—5–10 mg/day; **Availability (G):** *Tabs:* 10, 20, 40 mg; **Monitor:** BP, HR, wt, edema, BUN/SCr, K+; **Notes:** Correct volume depletion. Advise on S/S angioedema. Avoid K+ salt substitutes.

fosphenytoin (Cerebyx) Uses: Short-term (<5 day) management of generalized, convulsive status epilepticus or treatment/prevention of seizures during neurosurgery when phenytoin use is not feasible; **Class:** anticonvulsants; **Preg:** D; **CIs:** Hypersensitivity; Sinus bradycardia, ≥2nd-degree heart block or Adams-Stokes syndrome (in absence of pacemaker); Lactation; **ADRs:** dizziness, drowsiness, nystagmus, agitation,

F

HA, stupor, vertigo, amblyopia, diplopia, tinnitus, ↓ BP (with rapid IV administration), ↑ HR, dry mouth, N/V, taste perversion, tongue disorder, pruritus, rash, SJS, ataxia, dysarthria, EPS, incoordination, paresthesia, tremor; **Interactions:** CYP2C9 inhibitors or CYP2C19 inhibitors may ↑ levels/toxicity; CYP2C9 inducers or CYP2C19 inducers may ↓ levels/effects; May ↓ levels/effects of CYP2C9 substrates; CYP2C19 substrates, and CYP3A4 substrates; Additive CNS depression with other CNS depressants, alcohol, antihistamines, antidepressants, opioids, and sedative/hypnotics; **Dose:** *Dosage is expressed in phenytoin sodium equivalents (PE) IV: Adults: Status epilepticus*—15–20 mg PE/kg. *IV, IM: Adults and Peds: >16 yr: LD*—10–20 mg PE/kg. *MD*—4–6 mg PE/kg/day. *IV, IM: Peds: 10–16 yr:* 6–7 mg PE/kg/day. *IV, IM: Peds: 7–9 yr:* 7–8 mg PE/kg/day. *IV, IM: Peds: 4–6 yr:* 7.5–9 mg PE/kg/day. *IV, IM: Peds: 0.5–3 yr:* 8–10 mg PE kg/day. *IV, IM: Infants:* 5 mg PE kg/day. *IV, IM: Neonates:* 5–8 mg PE/kg/day; **Availability (G):** *Inject:* 50 mg PE/ml; **Monitor:** BP, HR, RR, seizure activity, mental status, ECG, phenytoin levels; **Notes:** Should always be prescribed in PE. IM should not be used for status epilepticus. Contains 0.0037 mmol PO_4 per mg PE; may cause ↑ serum PO_4 in patients with renal dysfunction; therapeutic phenytoin concentrations = 10–20 mcg/ml (unbound = 1–2 mcg/ml). When converting from oral phenytoin to fosphenytoin, give same total daily dose as single dose. Do not administer faster than 150 mg PE/min (to ↓ risk of hypotension). Advise females to use additional non-hormonal method of contraception during therapy. Do not confuse with Celexa (citalopram), Celebrex (celecoxib), or Zyprexa (olanzapine).

frovatriptan (Frova) **Uses:** Acute treatment of migraines; **Class:** 5-HT_1 agonists; **Preg:** C; **CIs:** Hypersensitivity; CAD or significant CV disease; Uncontrolled HTN; Use of other 5-HT_1 agonists or ergot derivatives within 24 hr; Basilar or hemiplegic migraine; CV risk factors (use only if CV status has been determined to be safe and 1st dose is administered under supervision); Peds <18 yr (safety not established); **ADRs:** dizziness, fatigue, CORONARY ARTERY VASOSPASM, MI/ISCHEMIA, VT/VF, dry mouth, nausea, paresthesia; **Interactions:** Use with other 5-HT_1 agonists or ergot derivatives may ↑ risk of vasospasm (avoid use within 24 hr of each other); Use with SSRIs or SNRIs may ↑ risk of serotonin syndrome; **Dose:** *PO: Adults:* 2.5 mg; if HA recurs, may repeat after ≥2 hr if first dose provided some relief (max: 7.5 mg/24 hr or treatment of 4 HAs/mo); **Availability:** *Tabs:* 2.5 mg; **Monitor:** Pain/associated symptoms; **Notes:** Only aborts migraines (should not be used for prophylaxis). Administer as soon as migraine symptoms occur.

furosemide (Lasix) **Uses:** Edema due to HF, hepatic disease, or renal impairment; HTN; **Class:** loop diuretics; **Preg:** C; **CIs:** Hypersensitivity (cross-sensitivity with thiazides and sulfonamides may occur); Hepatic coma; Anuria; Severe electrolyte depletion; **ADRs:** dizziness,

HA, hearing loss, tinnitus, ↓ BP, photosensitivity, rash, ↑ BG, ↑ uric acid, dehydration, ↓ Ca++, ↓ K+, ↓ Mg++, ↓ Na+, hypovolemia, metabolic alkalosis, muscle cramps, azotemia; **Interactions:** ↑ effects with other antihypertensives; May ↑ lithium levels; ↑ risk of ototoxicity with aminoglycosides; NSAIDs may ↓ effectiveness; **Dose:** *PO: Adults: Edema*—20–80 mg/day as single dose initially, may repeat in 6–8 hr; may ↑ dose by 20–40 mg q 6–8 hr until desired response (may be titrated up to 600 mg/day for severe edema); MD may be given daily or bid. *HTN*—10–40 mg bid. *PO: Peds: >1 month Edema*—2 mg/kg as single dose; may ↑ by 1–2 mg/kg q 6–8 hr (max: 6 mg/kg). *IM, IV: Adults:* 20–40 mg, may repeat in 1–2 hr and ↑ by 20 mg q 1–2 hr until desired response; MD usually given q 6–12 hr. *Continuous infusion*—Bolus of 0.1 mg/kg followed by 0.1 mg/kg/hr; may double q 2 hr until desired response (max: 0.4 mg/kg/hr). *IM, IV: Peds:* 1–2 mg/kg q 6–12 hr; may ↑ by 1 mg/kg q 6–12 hr until desired response (max: 6 mg/kg/dose). *Continuous infusion*—0.05 mg/kg/hr; titrate to clinical effect; **Availability (G):** *Tabs:* 20, 40, 80 mg. *Oral soln:* 8 mg/ml, 10 mg/ml. *Inject:* 10 mg/ml; **Monitor:** BP, HR, electrolytes, BUN/SCr, BG, uric acid, wt, I/Os, edema; **Notes:** If giving bid, give last dose no later than 5 PM. IV dose = 0.5 × (PO dose). IV route preferred over IM route. Advise patient to wear sunscreen.

gabapentin (Neurontin) **Uses:** Partial seizures (adjunct treatment); Post-herpetic neuralgia; **Class:** anticonvulsants; **Preg:** C; **CIs:** Hypersensitivity; **ADRs:** dizziness, drowsiness, concentration difficulties (peds), emotional lability (peds), HA, hostility (peds), hyperkinesia (peds), blurred vision, nystagmus, edema, anorexia, constipation, flatulence, N/V/D, ataxia, tremor, ↑ wt; **Interactions:** Antacids may ↓ absorption; ↑ risk of CNS depression with other CNS depressants, alcohol, antihistamines, opioids, and sedative/hypnotics; **Dose:** *PO: Adults: Post-herpetic neuralgia*—300 mg on Day 1, then 300 mg bid on Day 2, then 300 mg tid on Day 3; may ↑ prn for pain relief up to 600 mg tid. *PO: Adults and Peds: >12 yr Partial seizures*—300 mg tid initially; may ↑ prn up to 1800 mg/day in divided doses (doses up to 2400–3600 mg/day have also been well tolerated). *PO: Peds: 3–12 yr Partial seizures*—10–15 mg/kg/day in 3 divided doses initially; ↑ over a period of 3 days to 25–35 mg/kg day in 3 divided doses (in peds ≥5 yr) or 40 mg/kg day in 3 divided doses (in peds 3–4 yr). *Renal Impairment PO: Adults and Peds: >12 yr:* ↓ dose if CrCl <60 ml/min; **Availability (G):** *Caps:* 100, 300, 400 mg. *Tabs:* 100, 300, 400, 600, 800 mg. *Oral soln:* 250 mg/5 ml; **Monitor:** Seizure activity, pain, mental status; **Notes:** Do not abruptly discontinue (taper over 1 wk). 600-mg and 800-mg tabs are scored and can be broken in half. If half-tab is used, administer other half at next dose; discard half-tabs not used within several days. Do not exceed 12 hr between doses. Separate from antacids by ≥2 hr.

galantamine (Razadyne, Razadyne ER) **Uses:** Mild-to-moderate dementia of the Alzheimer's type; **Class:** cholinergics; **Preg:** B; **CIs:** Hypersensitivity; Severe hepatic or renal impairment; Peds or lactation; **ADRs:** depression, dizziness, fatigue, HA, syncope, ↓ HR, heart block, N/V, anorexia, diarrhea, dyspepsia, tremor, ↓ wt; **Interactions:** ↑ neuromuscular blockade from succinylcholine-type neuromuscular blocking agents; ↑ effects of other cholinesterase inhibitors or other cholinergic agonists, including bethanechol; ↓ effectiveness of anticholinergic medications; CYP2D6 inhibitors and CYP3A4 inhibitors may ↑ levels/toxicity; CYP3A4 inducers may ↓ levels/effects; **Dose:** *PO: Adults: IR*—4 mg bid; may ↑ to 8 mg bid after 4 wk, then ↑ to 12 mg bid after another 4 wk. *ER*—8 mg/day; may ↑ to 16 mg/day after 4 wk, then ↑ to 24 mg/day after another 4 wk. *Renal Impairment PO: Adults: Moderate renal impairment*—Do not exceed dose of 16 mg/day. *Hepatic Impairment PO: Adults: Moderate hepatic impairment*—Do not exceed dose of 16 mg/day; **Availability:** *IR tabs:* 4, 8, 12 mg. *ER caps:* 8, 16, 24 mg. *Oral soln:* 4 mg/ml; **Monitor:** HR, cognitive function; **Notes:** To convert from IR to ER, use same total daily dose. ER caps should be taken in AM with food. IR tabs and soln should be taken in AM and PM with meals. Maintain on stable dose for ≥4 wk before ↑ dose. If therapy is interrupted for ≥3 days, restart at lowest dose and ↑ to current dose. Mix soln with 3–4 oz of beverage.

ganciclovir (Cytovene, Vitrasert) **Uses: IV:** Treatment of CMV retinitis in immunocompromised patients; **PO:** Maintenance treatment of CMV retinitis in immunocompromised patients; Prevention of CMV infection in transplant patients and patients with advanced HIV infection; **Ophth** Treatment of CMV retinitis; **Class:** antivirals; **Preg:** C; **CIs:** Hypersensitivity to ganciclovir or acyclovir; ANC <500/mm³ or platelets <25,000/mm³; Pregnancy/lactation; **ADRs:** SEIZURES, confusion, HA, retinal detachment, anorexia, N/V/D, ↑ LFTs, gonadal suppression, nephrotoxicity, pruritus, rash, anemia, neutropenia, thrombocytopenia, pain/phlebitis at IV site, neuropathy, fever; **Interactions:** May ↑ didanosine levels; ↑ risk of bone marrow depression with antineoplastics, radiation therapy, or zidovudine; Probenecid may ↑ levels/toxicity; ↑ risk of seizures with imipenem/cilastatin; ↑ risk of nephrotoxicity with other nephrotoxic drugs (e.g., amphotericin, aminoglycosides, vancomycin, cisplatin, cyclosporine); **Dose:** *IV: Adults and Peds: CMV treatment (induction)*—5 mg/kg q 12 hr × 14–21 days. *CMV treatment (maintenance)*—5 mg/kg/day *or* 6 mg/kg/day × 5 days/wk. If progression occurs, retreat with induction regimen. *CMV prevention*—5 mg/kg q 12 hr × 7–14 days, then 5 mg/kg/day *or* 6 mg/kg/day × 5 days/wk. *PO: Adults: CMV treatment (maintenance)*—1000 mg tid *or* 500 mg 6 ×/day. *CMV prevention*—1000 mg tid. *PO: Peds: CMV prevention:* 30 mg/kg q 8 hr. *Intravitreal: Adults:* 4.5-mg implant × 5–8 mo, then may be removed and replaced if infection progressing. *Renal Impairment IV, PO:*

Adults: ↓ dose if CrCl <70 ml/min; **Availability (G):** *Caps:* 250, 500 mg. *Inject:* 500 mg/vial. *Intravitreal insert:* 4.5 mg; **Monitor:** BUN/SCr, CBC (with diff), LFTs, ophth exam, S/S infection; **Notes:** Non-hormonal method of contraception should be used during and for ≥90 days after therapy. Give caps with food (to ↑ absorption). Recovery of neutrophils and platelets begins within 3–7 days of discontinued therapy. Maintain adequate hydration. Avoid rapid administration. Not a cure for CMV retinitis (progression may still occur).

gefitinib (Iressa) **Uses:** Locally advanced/metastatic non–small-cell lung CA (after failure of platinum-based and docetaxel chemotherapies) in patients who experienced benefit from gefitinib; **Class:** enzyme inhibitors; **Preg:** D; **CIs:** Hypersensitivity; Pregnancy/lactation; **ADRs:** weakness, aberrant eyelash growth, corneal erosion/ulcer, eye pain, PULMONARY TOXICITY, cough, dyspnea, HEPATOTOXICITY, N/V/D, anorexia, ↑ LFTs, acne, dry skin, rash, pruritus, ↓ wt, ANGIOEDEMA; **Interactions:** CYP3A4 inhibitors may ↑ levels/toxicity; CYP3A4 inducers may ↓ levels/effects (consider ↑ dose of gefitinib to 500 mg/day with strong inducers); Drugs that ↑ gastric pH (e.g., H_2 antagonists, Na bicarbonate) may ↓ absorption; May ↑ risk of bleeding with warfarin; **Dose:** *PO: Adults:* 250 mg/day; **Availability:** *Tabs:* 250 mg; **Monitor:** LFTs, CXR, ophth exam; **Notes:** Discontinue if interstitial lung disease develops. If difficulty swallowing, may place tab in half-glass of water (do not crush, let tab dissolve while stirring). May interrupt therapy for 14 days for patients with poorly tolerated diarrhea or skin ADRs. Distribution limited to patients enrolled in Iressa Access Program.

gemcitabine (Gemzar) **Uses:** Locally advanced/metastatic pancreatic CA; Inoperable locally advanced/metastatic non–small-cell lung CA (with cisplatin); Metastatic breast CA that has failed anthracycline-based therapy (with paclitaxel); Advanced ovarian CA that has relapsed ≥6 mo after completion of platinum-based therapy (with carboplatin); **Class:** antimetabolites, nucleoside analogues; **Preg:** D; **CIs:** Hypersensitivity; Pregnancy/lactation; **ADRs:** PULMONARY TOXICITY, dyspnea, bronchospasm, edema, HEPATOTOXICITY, constipation, ↑ LFTs, N/V/D, stomatitis, HEMOLYTIC UREMIC SYNDROME, hematuria, proteinuria, alopecia, rash, anemia, neutropenia, thrombocytopenia, inject site reactions, paresthesias, fever, flu-like symptoms, anaphylactoid reactions; **Interactions:** ↑ bone marrow depression with other antineoplastics or radiation therapy; **Dose:** *IV: Adults: Pancreatic CA*—1000 mg/m²/wk for up to 7 wk, followed by 1 wk of rest; may be followed by cycles of once-weekly administration × 3 wk followed by 1 wk of rest; *Non–small-cell lung CA*—1000 mg/m² on Days 1, 8, and 15 of each 28-day cycle (cisplatin is also given on Day 1) *or* 1250 mg/m² on Days 1 and 8 of each 21-day cycle (cisplatin is also given on Day 1). *Breast CA*—1250 mg/m² on Days 1 and 8 of each

21-day cycle (paclitaxel is also given on Day 1). *Ovarian CA*—1000 mg/m^2 on Days 1 and 8 of each 21-day cycle (carboplatin is also given on Day 1); **Availability:** *Inject:* 200 mg, 1 g; **Monitor:** BP, HR, RR, temp, BUN/SCr, CBC (with diff), LFTs, U/A, S/S infection, bleeding, CXR, infusion site; **Notes: High Alert:** Fatalities have occurred with incorrect administration of chemotherapeutic agents. Before administering, clarify all ambiguous orders; double-check single, daily, and course-of-therapy dose limits; have second practitioner independently double-check original order, calculations, and infusion pump settings. Need to adjust dose if ↓ ANC or platelets.

G

gemfibrozil (Lopid) Uses: Hypertriglyceridemia; **Class:** fibric acid derivatives; **Preg:** C; **CIs:** Hypersensitivity; Concurrent use of HMG-CoA reductase inhibitors; Gallbladder disease; Liver disease (including primary biliary cirrhosis); Severe renal impairment; Pregnancy, lactation, or peds (safety not established); **ADRs:** abdominal pain, dyspepsia, diarrhea, gallstones, ↑ LFTs, N/V, RHABDOMYOLYSIS, myalgia; **Interactions:** May ↑ levels/toxicity of CYP2C9 substrates and CYP2C19 substrates; May ↑ effects of warfarin, sulfonylureas, or repaglinide; ↑ risk of rhabdomyolysis with HMG-CoA reductase inhibitors (avoid concurrent use); May ↓ cyclosporine levels; **Dose:** *PO: Adults:* 600 mg bid; **Availability (G):** *Tabs:* 600 mg; **Monitor:** Lipid panel, LFTs, CK (if symptoms); **Notes:** If fibrate needed in patient on statin, use fenofibrate. Give 30 min before breakfast and dinner.

gemifloxacin (Factive) Uses: Acute bacterial exacerbations of chronic bronchitis or CAP due to susceptible organisms (e.g., *S. pneumo, Mycoplasma, Chlamydia pneumoniae, Klebsiella, H. flu, M. catarrhalis*; **Class:** FQs; **Preg:** C; **CIs:** Hypersensitivity (cross-sensitivity within class may exist); QT interval prolongation; Pregnancy, lactation, or peds <18 yr (safety not established); **ADRs:** dizziness, HA, QT interval prolongation, PSEUDOMEMBRANOUS COLITIS, abdominal pain, ↑ LFTs, N/V/D, photosensitivity, rash, SJS, ↑↓ BG, tendonitis, tendon rupture, peripheral neuropathy, ANAPHYLAXIS; **Interactions:** ↑ risk of QT prolongation with other QT-prolonging drugs; Use with antacids, Ca++ supplements, iron salts, zinc, didanosine, or sucralfate may ↓ absorption; May ↑ effects of warfarin; Probenecid may ↑ levels; May ↑ risk of hypoglycemia with sulfonylureas; ↑ risk of tendon rupture with corticosteroids; Absorption ↓ by dairy products; **Dose:** *PO: Adults:* 320 mg/day × 5–7 days. *Renal Impairment PO: Adults:* ↓ dose if CrCl ≤ 40 ml/min; **Availability:** *Tabs:* 320 mg; **Monitor:** HR, BP, temp, sputum, U/A, CBC, BG (in patients with DM), LFTs; **Notes:** Give ≥2 hr before or ≥3 hr after products/foods containing Ca++, Mg++, aluminum, iron, or zinc. Advise patients to use sunscreen.

gentamicin (Gentak) Uses: Treatment of serious infections due to Gram (–) organisms (e.g., *P. aeruginosa, E. coli, Proteus, Klebsiella,*

Enterobacter, *Serratia*, *Citrobacter*) and Gram (+) organisms (*Staphylococci*, *Enterococci*); **Topical, Ophth:** Treatment of localized infections due to susceptible organisms; **Class:** aminoglycosides; **Preg:** C (topical, ophth), D (inject); **CIs:** Hypersensitivity to aminoglycosides; **ADRs:** vertigo, ototoxicity (vestibular and cochlear), nephrotoxicity; **Interactions:** May ↑ effects of neuromuscular blockers; ↑ risk of ototoxicity with loop diuretics; ↑ risk of nephrotoxicity with other nephrotoxic drugs (e.g., amphotericin, vancomycin, acyclovir, cisplatin); **Dose:** *IM, IV: Adults:* 1–2 mg/kg q 8 hr. *Once-daily dosing*—4–7 mg/kg q 24 hr. *IM, IV: Peds: ≥5 yr* 2–2.5 mg/kg q 8 hr. *Once daily dosing*—5–7.5 mg/kg q 24 hr. *IM, IV: Peds: <5 yr:* 2.5 mg/kg q 8 hr. *Once daily dosing*—5–7.5 mg/kg q 24 hr. *IT: Adults:* 4–8 mg/day. *IT: Infants >3 months and Peds:* 1–2 mg/day. *Topical: Adults and Peds: > 1 month:* Apply cream or oint 3–4 times daily. *Ophth: Adults and Peds: Ointment*—Instill 1/2 in. q 3–4 hr; *Soln*—Instill 1–2 gtt q 2–4 hr. *Renal Impairment IM, IV: Adults: CrCl <60 ml/min*— ↓ frequency of administration or dose by levels; **Availability (G):** *Inject:* 10 mg/ml, 40 mg/ml. *Ophth oint/soln:* 0.3%. *Top cream/oint:* 0.1%; **Monitor:** HR, BP, temp, sputum, U/A, CBC, BUN/SCr, I/Os, hearing; **Notes:** Use cautiously in renal dysfunction. Monitor blood levels (traditional dosing: peak 6–10 mcg/ml (synergy for Gram (+) organisms 3–5 mcg/ml); trough <1 mcg/ml; q 24 h dosing: trough <1 mcg/ml). Used with another antibiotic (e.g., penicillin, vancomycin) for synergy against Gram (+) organisms.

G

glimepiride (Amaryl) **Uses: PO:** Type 2 DM; **Class:** sulfonylureas; **Preg:** C; **CIs:** Hypersensitivity to sulfonamides (cross-sensitivity may occur); Type 1 DM; Diabetic coma or DKA; Pregnancy or lactation (safety not established; insulin recommended during pregnancy); Peds (safety not established); **ADRs:** dizziness, HA, diarrhea, dyspepsia, ↑ LFTs, ↑ appetite, nausea, photosensitivity, rash, ↓ BG, ↓ Na+, ↑ wt, AGRANULOCYTOSIS, APLASTIC ANEMIA, leukopenia, thrombocytopenia; **Interactions:** CYP2C9 inhibitors may ↑ levels/effects; CYP2C9 inducers may ↓ levels/effects; Diuretics, corticosteroids, phenothiazines, oral contraceptives, estrogens, thyroid preparations, phenytoin, niacin, sympathomimetics, and isoniazid may ↓ effects; ↑ risk of hypoglycemia with alcohol, chloramphenicol, FQs, MAOIs, NSAIDs, probenecids, salicylates, sulfonamides, and warfarin; Beta blockers may mask S/S of hypoglycemia; **Dose:** *PO: Adults:* 1–2 mg/day initially; may ↑ q 1–2 wk (max: 8 mg/day) (usual range 1–4 mg/day); **Availability (G):** *Tabs:* 1, 2, 4 mg; **Monitor:** BG, A1C, LFTs, CBC, S/S hypoglycemia; **Notes:** Give before breakfast. Advise patients to wear sunscreen.

glipiZIDE (Glucotrol, Glucotrol XL) **Uses: PO:** Type 2 DM; **Class:** sulfonylureas; **Preg:** C; **CIs:** Hypersensitivity to sulfonamides (cross-sensitivity may occur); Type 1 DM; Diabetic coma or DKA; Pregnancy or lactation (safety not established; insulin recommended during pregnancy); Peds (safety not established); **ADRs:** diarrhea, dyspepsia, ↑ LFTs, ↑ appetite, nausea, photosensitivity, rash, ↓ BG, ↓ Na+, ↑ wt,

AGRANULOCYTOSIS, APLASTIC ANEMIA, leukopenia, thrombocytopenia; **Interactions:** CYP2C9 inhibitors may ↑ levels/effects; CYP2C9 inducers may ↓ levels/effects; Diuretics, corticosteroids, phenothiazines, oral contraceptives, estrogens, thyroid preparations, phenytoin, niacin, sympathomimetics, and isoniazid may ↓ effects; ↑ risk of hypoglycemia with alcohol, chloramphenicol, FQs, MAOIs, NSAIDs, probenecid, salicylates, sulfonamides, and warfarin; May ↑ effects of warfarin; Beta blockers may mask S/S of hypoglycemia; **Dose:** *PO: Adults:* 5 mg/day initially; may ↑ by 2.5–5 mg/day increments (max: 40 mg/day of IR, 20 mg/day XL) (doses >15 mg/day of IR should be divided bid); XL is given once daily; **Availability (G):** *Tabs:* 5, 10 mg. *ER tabs (XL):* 2.5, 5, 10 mg; **Monitor:** BG, A1C, LFTs, CBC, S/S hypoglycemia; **Notes:** Preferred over glyburide in elderly (less risk of hypoglycemia). Give IR tabs 30 min before a meal. Give ER tabs before breakfast. Advise patients to wear sunscreen. Do not crush, chew, or break ER tabs.

G

glucagon (GlucaGen) Uses: Severe hypoglycemia; Facilitation of radiographic examination of the GI tract (↓ motility); Beta blocker or CCB overdose; **Class:** pancreatics; **Preg:** B; **CIs:** Hypersensitivity; Pheochromocytoma; **ADRs:** ↓ BP, N/V, ANAPHYLAXIS; **Interactions:** May ↑ risk of bleeding with warfarin (with glucagon doses ≥50 mg); Negates the response to insulin and oral hypoglycemic agents; **Dose:** *IV, IM, Subcut: Adults and Peds: ≥20 kg Hypoglycemia*—1 mg; may be repeated in 15 min if needed. *IV, IM, Subcut: Peds: <20 kg Hypoglycemia*—0.5 mg or 0.02–0.03 mg/kg; may be repeated in 15 min if needed. *IM, IV: Adults: Diagnostic aid*—0.25–2 mg; depending on location and duration of examination (0.5 mg IV or 2 mg IM for relaxation of stomach, 2 mg IM for examination of the colon). *IV: Adults: Beta blocker or CCB overdose*—5–10 mg initially, followed by 1–10 mg/hr infusion; **Availability:** *Inject:* 1 mg (equivalent to 1 unit); **Monitor:** BP, HR, BG, S/S hypoglycemia, mental status; **Notes:** Severe hypoglycemia should be treated with IV glucose, if possible. For doses ≤2 mg, use diluent provided by manufacturer. For doses >2 mg, use sterile water for inject instead of diluent supplied by manufacturer to ↓ risk of thrombophlebitis, CNS toxicity, and myocardial depression from phenol preservative in manufacturer's diluent. Once patient is alert after hypoglycemia, administer oral glucose.

glyBURIDE (DiaBeta, Glynase PresTab, Micronase) Uses: PO: Type 2 DM; **Class:** sulfonylureas; **Preg:** B (Glynase PresTab only), C; **CIs:** Hypersensitivity to sulfonamides (cross-sensitivity may occur); Type 1 DM; Diabetic coma or DKA; Pregnancy or lactation (safety not established; insulin recommended during pregnancy); Peds (safety not established); **ADRs:** diarrhea, dyspepsia, ↑ LFTs, ↑ appetite, nausea, photosensitivity, rash, ↓ BG, ↓ Na+, ↑ wt, AGRANULOCYTOSIS, APLASTIC ANEMIA, leukopenia, thrombocytopenia; **Interactions:** Diuretics, corticosteroids, phenothiazines, oral contraceptives, estrogens, thyroid preparations, phenytoin, niacin, sympathomimetics, and isoniazid may ↓ effects; ↑ risk of hypoglycemia with alcohol, chloramphenicol, FQs, MAOIs, NSAIDs, probenecids, salicylates, sulfonamides, and warfarin; May ↑ effects of warfarin; Beta blockers may mask S/S of hypoglycemia; **Dose:** *PO: Adults: DiaBeta/Micronase*—2.5–5 mg/day initially; may ↑ by 2.5 mg/day q wk (range: 1.25–20 mg/day). *Glynase PresTab*—1.5–3 mg/day initially; may ↑ by 1.5 mg/day q wk (range: 0.75–12 mg/day; doses >6 mg/day should be divided); **Availability (G):** *Tabs:* 1.25, 2.5, 5 mg. *Micronized tabs (Glynase PresTab):* 1.5, 3, 6 mg; **Monitor:** BG, A1C, LFTs, CBC, S/S hypoglycemia; **Notes:** DiaBeta/Micronase are not interchangeable with Glynase PresTabs. Give with meals. Advise patients to wear sunscreen.

G

glycopyrrolate (Robinul, Robinul-Forte) **Uses:** Inhibits salivation and excessive respiratory secretions preop; Reverses some of the secretory and vagal actions of cholinesterase inhibitors used to treat nondepolarizing neuromuscular blockade (cholinergic adjunct); Adjunctive management of PUD; **Class:** anticholinergics; **Preg:** B; **CIs:** Hypersensitivity; Narrow-angle glaucoma; Obstructive disease of GI tract; Ulcerative colitis; Acute hemorrhage; Myasthenia gravis; Obstructive uropathy; Paralytic ileus; Infants <1 mo (injection contains benzyl alcohol); **ADRs:** confusion, drowsiness, blurred vision, cycloplegia, dry eyes, mydriasis, photophobia, ↑ HR, orthostatic hypotension, palpitations, dry mouth, constipation, N/V, urinary hesitancy/retention, ↓ sweating; **Interactions:** ↑ risk of anticholinergic effects with other anticholinergic agents; May alter the absorption of other orally administered drugs by ↓ motility of GI tract; May ↑ GI mucosal lesions from oral KCl tabs; **Dose:** *IM: Adults and Peds: Preop use*—0.004 mg/kg 30–60 min prior to induction of anesthesia (infants 1 mo–2 yr may require up to 0.009 mg/kg). *IV: Adults and Peds: Neuromuscular blockade reversal*—0.2 mg for each 1 mg of neostigmine or 5 mg of pyridostigmine (give at same time). *IV: Adults: Intraoperative use*—0.1 mg q 2–3 min prn. *IV: Peds: Control of secretions*—0.004–0.01 mg/kg/dose q 3–4 hrs. *Intraoperative use*—0.004 mg/kg (max: 0.1 mg) q 2–3 min prn. *PO: Adults: PUD*—1–2 mg bid–tid. *IM, IV: Adults: PUD*—0.1–0.2 mg tid–qid up to 0.4 mg qid. *PO: Peds: Control of secretions*—0.04–0.1 mg/kg/dose tid–qid; **Availability (G):** *Tabs:* 1, 2 mg. *Inject:* 0.2 mg/ml; **Monitor:** HR, BP, RR, I/Os, bowel function, secretions; **Notes:** Paradoxical hyperexcitability may occur in peds. Neostigmine is antidote. Use with caution in elderly (↑ risk of sedation and anticholinergic effects).

granisetron (Granisol, Kytril, Sancuso) **Uses:** Prevention of N/V associated with emetogenic chemotherapy or radiation therapy; Prevention and treatment of PONV (IV only); **Class:** 5-HT_3 antagonists; **Preg:** B; **CIs:** Hypersensitivity; Peds <2 yr (safety not established for IV); <18 yr (safety not established for PO); **ADRs:** HA, agitation, anxiety, dizziness, drowsiness, insomnia, weakness, constipation, diarrhea, ↑ LFTs, taste disorder, fever; **Interactions:** None significant; **Dose:** *PO:*

Adults: Prevention of chemotherapy-induced N/V—1 mg bid with 1st dose taken up to 60 min prior to chemotherapy and 2nd dose 12 hr later only on days when chemotherapy is administered; may also be taken as 2 mg/day up to 60 min prior to chemotherapy. *Prevention of radiation-induced N/V*—2 mg/day taken within 1 hr of radiation therapy. *IV: Adults and Peds: 2–16 yr Prevention of chemotherapy-induced N/V*—10 mcg/kg within 30 min prior to chemotherapy (give only on days of chemotherapy). *IV: Adults: Prevention of PONV*—1 mg prior to induction of anesthesia or just prior to reversal of anesthesia. *Treatment of PONV*—1 mg. *IV: Peds: ≥4 yr Prevention and treatment of PONV*—20–40 mcg/kg single dose (max: 1 mg); *Transdermal: Adults:* Apply 1 patch ≥24 hr prior to chemotherapy. Remove a minimum of 24 hr after chemotherapy (max duration of wearing patch = 7 days); **Availability (G):** *Tabs:* 1 mg. *Oral soln:* 2 mg/10 ml. *Inject:* 0.1 mg/ml, 1 mg/ml; Transdermal patch: 3.1 mg/24 hr; **Monitor:** N/V, I/Os, LFTs; **Notes:** Administer PO and IV only on days of chemotherapy or radiation. Not effective for treatment of breakthrough N/V.

halcinonide (Halog) **Uses:** Management of inflammation and pruritis associated with various dermatoses; **Class:** corticosteroids; **Preg:** C; **CIs:** Hypersensitivity; **ADRs:** burning sensation, dryness, folliculitis, hypersensitivity reactions, hypertrichosis, hypopigmentation, irritation, secondary infection, striae, adrenal suppression (with use of occlusive dressings or long-term therapy); **Interactions:** None significant; **Dose:** *Topical: Adults:* Apply 1–3 ×/day (depends on product, preparation, and condition being treated). *Topical: Peds:* Apply once daily; **Availability:** *Cream/Oint/Soln:* 0.1%; **Monitor:** Skin condition (inflammation, erythema, pruritis); **Notes:** Oints are more occlusive and preferred for dry, scaly lesions. Creams should be used on oozing or intertriginous areas (may cause more skin drying than oint). Solution is useful in hairy areas.

halobetasol (Ultravate) **Uses:** Management of inflammation and pruritis associated with various dermatoses; **Class:** corticosteroids; **Preg:** C; **CIs:** Hypersensitivity; **ADRs:** burning sensation, dryness, folliculitis, hypersensitivity reactions, hirsutism, hypopigmentation, irritation, secondary infection, striae, adrenal suppression (with use of occlusive dressings or long-term therapy); **Interactions:** None significant; **Dose:** *Topical: Adults and Peds: ≥12 yr:* Apply 1–2 ×/day; **Availability (G):** *Cream/Oint:* 0.05%; **Monitor:** Skin condition (inflammation, erythema, pruritis); **Notes:** Oints are more occlusive and preferred for dry, scaly lesions. Creams should be used on oozing or intertriginous areas (may cause more skin drying than oint).

haloperidol (Haldol, Haldol Decanoate) **Uses:** Schizophrenia; Agitation; Tourette's syndrome; Severe behavioral problems in children; **Class:** butyrophenones; **Preg:** C; **CIs:** Hypersensitivity; Parkinson's disease; Bone marrow depression; CNS depression; Severe liver or CV disease (QT interval–prolonging conditions); QT interval prolongation; Lactation; **ADRs:** NMS, SEIZURES, EPS, confusion, drowsiness, restlessness, tardive dyskinesia, blurred vision, dry eyes, TORSADE DE POINTES, ↓ BP, QT interval prolongation, ↑ HR, constipation, dry mouth, anorexia, ↑ LFTs, ↑ wt, urinary retention, galactorrhea; **Interactions:** CYP2D6 inhibitors and CYP3A4 inhibitors may ↑ levels/toxicity; May ↑ levels/toxicity of CYP2D6 substrates and CYP3A4 substrates; CYP3A4 inducers may ↓ levels/effects; ↑ risk of QT prolongation with other QT-prolonging drugs; ↑ risk of hypotension with other antihypertensives; ↑ risk of anticholinergic effects with other anticholinergic agents; ↑ CNS depression with other CNS depressants, alcohol, antihistamines, opioid analgesics, and sedative/hypnotics; May ↓ therapeutic effects of levodopa; ↑ risk of acute encephalopathic syndrome with lithium; **Dose:** *PO: Adults: Psychosis*—0.5–5 mg 2–3 ×/day. Patients with severe symptoms may require up to 100 mg/day. *PO: (Geriatric Patients or Debilitated Patients):* 0.5–2 mg bid initially; may be gradually ↑ prn. *PO: Peds: 3–12 yr or 15–40 kg:* 0.05 mg/kg/day in 2–3 divided doses; may ↑ by 0.25–0.5 mg/day q 5–7 days prn (max: 0.075 mg/kg/day for nonpsychotic disorders or Tourette's syndrome; max: 0.15 mg/kg/day for psychoses). *IM: Adults: (as lactate) Psychosis*—2–5 mg q 1–8 hr prn. *IM: Peds (as lactate):* 1–3 mg q 4–8 hr; may ↑ as needed up to 0.15 mg/kg/day. *IV: Adults: Agitation*—0.5–5 mg, may be repeated q 30 min until calmness achieved, then give 25% of this dose q 6 hr. *IM: Adults: (as decanoate):* 10–15 times the previous daily PO dose, not to exceed 100 mg/day initially; given monthly, not to exceed 450 mg/month; **Availability (G):** *Tabs:* 0.5, 1, 2, 5, 10, 20 mg. *Oral concentrate:* 2 mg/ml. *Inject (lactate):* 5 mg/ml. *Inject (decanoate):* 50 mg/ml, 100 mg/ml; **Monitor:** BP, HR, ECG (QT interval), mental status, EPS, tardive dyskinesia, NMS, LFTs; **Notes:** Lactate is short-acting formulation. Decanoate is long-acting depot formulation (should never be administered IV). Benztropine used to treat EPS.

heparin (Hep-Lock, Hep-Lock U/P) **Uses:** Prophylaxis and treatment of thromboembolic disorders; **Class:** antithrombotics; **Preg:** C; **CIs:** Hypersensitivity; Active bleeding; Severe thrombocytopenia; Intracranial hemorrhage; History of HIT; **ADRs:** rash, urticaria, BLEEDING, anemia, thrombocytopenia (can occur up to several wk after discontinuation of therapy), pain at inject site, osteoporosis (long-term use), fever, hypersensitivity; **Interactions:** ↑ risk of bleeding with antiplatelets, thrombolytics, or other anticoagulants; **Dose:** *IV: Adults: ACS*—60–70 units/kg bolus (max: 5000 units, 4000 units with thrombolytic), then continuous infusion of 12–15 units/kg/hr (max: 1000 units/hr) (titrate to aPTT). *DVT/PE treatment*—80 units/kg bolus, then continuous infusion of 18 units/kg/hr (titrate to aPTT). *PCI*—Maintain ACT of 300–350 sec (without GPIIb/IIIa inhibitor) or ACT of 200–250 sec (with a GPIIb/IIIa inhibitor). *IV: Peds: >1 yr:* 75 units/kg over 10 min, then 20 units/kg/hr (titrate to aPTT). *IV: Peds: <1 yr:* 75 units/kg over 10 min, then 28 units/kg/hr (titrate to aPTT). *Subcut: Adults: VTE* *prophylaxis*—5000 units q 8–12 hr. *DVT treatment*—17,500 units q 12 hr; **Availability (G):** *Inject:* 10 units/ml, 100 units/ml, 1000 units/ml, 5000 units/ml, 10,000 units/ml, 20,000 units/ml. *Premixed soln:* 1000 units/ 500 ml, 2000 units/1000 ml, 10,000 units/100 ml, 12,500 units/250 ml, 20,000 units/500 ml, 25,000 units/250 ml, 25,000 units/500 ml; **Monitor:** BP, HR, CBC, ACT, aPTT, bleeding; **Notes:** Discontinue and send off HIT panel if platelets ↓ to <100,000 or ↓ by 50% of baseline. Protamine is antidote.

quadravalent human papillomavirus (types 6, 11, 16, 18) recombinant vaccine (Gardasil) **Uses:** Prevention of cervical CA, other cervical and vaginal neoplasias, and genital warts in females 9–26 yr; **Class:** vaccines/immunizing agents; **Preg:** B; **CIs:** Hypersensitivity; Peds <9 yr (safety not established); **ADRs:** inject site reactions, ANAPHYLAXIS (RARE), fever; **Interactions:** Immunosuppressants or antineoplastics may ↓ antibody response; **Dose:** *IM: Adults and Peds:* 0.5-ml doses at 0, 2, and 6 months; **Availability:** *Inject:* 20 mcg of HPV 6 L1 protein, 40 mcg of HPV 11 L1 protein, 40 mcg of HPV 16 L1 protein, and 20 mcg of HPV 18 L1 protein/ 0.5-mL dose; **Monitor:** Temp, inject site reactions; **Notes:** Not intended for treatment of active genital warts or cervical CA; administer IM in the deltoid or in the high anterolateral area of the thigh.

H

hydrALAZINE (Apresoline) **Uses:** HTN; HF (must be used with isosorbide dinitrate); **Class:** vasodilators; **Preg:** C; **CIs:** Hypersensitivity; CAD; Mitral valve rheumatic heart disease; **ADRs:** dizziness, HA, edema, ↑ HR, angina, orthostatic hypotension, palpitations, anorexia, N/V/D, rash, arthralgias, lupus-like syndrome; **Interactions:** ↑ effects with other antihypertensives; ↑ risk of hypotension with MAOIs; NSAIDs may ↓ effectiveness; **Dose:** *PO: Adults: HTN*—10 mg 4 ×/day initially; may ↑ by 25–50 mg/dose q 2–5 days (max: 300 mg/ day). *HF*—10–25 mg 3–4 ×/day (target dose = 225–300 mg/day in divided doses; must be used with isosorbide dinitrate). *PO: Peds: >1 month HTN*—0.75–1 mg/kg/day in 2–4 divided doses; may ↑ over 3–4 wk up to 7.5 mg/kg/day in 2–4 divided doses (max: 200 mg/day). *IM, IV: Adults: HTN*—10–40 mg q 4–6 hr prn. *Eclampsia*—5–10 mg q 20–30 min prn; if no response after a total of 20 mg, consider an alternative agent. *IM, IV: Peds: >1 month HTN*—0.1–0.2 mg/kg (max: 20 mg/ dose) q 4–6 hr prn; may ↑ up to 1.7–3.5 mg/kg/day in 4–6 divided doses; **Availability (G):** *Tabs:* 10, 25, 50, 100 mg. *Inject:* 20 mg/ml; **Monitor:** BP, HR, S/S SLE (joint pain, pleuritic chest pain, rash), S/S HF, ANA titer; **Notes:** Often given with diuretics and beta blockers (to minimize edema and tachycardia, respectively).

hydrochlorothiazide (HCTZ, HydroDIURIL, Microzide) **Uses:** HTN; Edema due to HF, hepatic disease, or renal impairment;

Class: thiazide diuretics; **Preg:** B; **CIs:** Hypersensitivity (cross-sensitivity with other sulfonamides may occur); Anuria; Lactation; **ADRs:** dizziness, ↓ BP, N/V/D, photosensitivity, rash, ↑ BG, ↑ uric acid, dehydration, ↑ Ca++, ↓ K+, ↓ Mg++, ↓ Na+, hypovolemia, metabolic alkalosis, muscle cramps, azotemia; **Interactions:** ↑ effects with other antihypertensives; May ↑ requirement for insulin or oral hypoglycemic agents; May ↑ lithium levels; Cholestyramine or colestipol may ↓ absorption; NSAIDs may ↓ effectiveness; **Dose:** *PO: Adults:* 12.5–100 mg/day in 1–2 doses (max: 200 mg/day for edema; 50 mg/day for HTN). *PO: Peds: >1 mo HTN*—1–3 mg/kg/day (max: 50 mg/day). *PO: Peds: >6 mo Edema*—2 mg/kg/day divided bid (max: 200 mg/day). *PO: Peds: <6 mo* 2–3.3 mg/kg/day divided bid (max: 37.5 mg/day); **Availability (G):** *Tabs:* 25, 50 mg. *Caps:* 12.5 mg; **Monitor:** BP, HR, electrolytes, BUN/SCr, BG, uric acid, weight, I/Os, edema; **Notes:** Administer in AM. Advise patient to use sunscreen. Ineffective if CrCl <30 ml/min. If giving bid, give last dose no later than 5 PM.

H

hydrocodone/acetaminophen (Anexsia, Co-Gesic, Lorcet, Lortab, Norco, Vicodin, Xodol, Zydone) **Uses:** Moderate-to-severe pain; **Class:** opioid agonists, nonopioid analgesic combinations; **Preg:** C; **CIs:** Hypersensitivity (cross-sensitivity may exist to other opioids); Severe respiratory depression; **ADRs:** confusion, dizziness, sedation, euphoria, hallucinations, HA, blurred vision, miosis, respiratory depression, ↓ BP, ↓ HR, HEPATOTOXICITY (overdose), constipation, N/V, renal failure (high doses/chronic use), urinary retention, physical/psychological dependence, tolerance; **Interactions:** Use with extreme caution in patients receiving MAOIs (do not use within 14 days of each other); Additive CNS depression with alcohol, antihistamines, and sedative/hypnotics; Administration of partial antagonist opioids (buprenorphine, butorphanol, nalbuphine, or pentazocine) may ↓ analgesia or precipitate opioid withdrawal in physically dependent patients; Chronic high-dose acetaminophen (>2 g/day) may ↑ risk of bleeding with warfarin; ↑ risk of hepatotoxicity with alcohol, isoniazid, rifampin, rifabutin, phenytoin, barbiturates, or carbamazepine (for acetaminophen); ↑ risk of nephrotoxicity with NSAIDs (for acetaminophen); **Dose:** *PO: Adults:* 2.5–10 mg q 3–6 hr prn; acetaminophen dosage should not exceed 4 g/day (2 g/day in patients with hepatic/renal impairment). *PO: Peds: 2–13 yr:* 0.14 mg/kg q 4–6 hr prn; acetaminophen dosage should not exceed 2.6 g/day; **Availability (G):** *Tabs:* 2.5 mg hydrocodone/500 mg acetaminophen, 5 mg hydrocodone/300 mg acetaminophen, 5 mg hydrocodone/325 mg acetaminophen, 5 mg hydrocodone/400 mg acetaminophen, 5 mg hydrocodone/500 mg acetaminophen, 7 mg hydrocodone/300 mg acetaminophen, 7.5 mg hydrocodone/325 mg acetaminophen, 7.5 mg hydrocodone/400 mg acetaminophen, 7.5 mg hydrocodone/500 mg acetaminophen, 7.5 mg hydrocodone/650 mg acetaminophen, 7.5 mg hydrocodone/750 mg acetaminophen, 10 mg hydrocodone/300 mg acetaminophen, 10 mg hydrocodone/325 mg acetaminophen, 10 mg hydrocodone/400 mg acetaminophen, 10 mg hydrocodone/500 mg acetaminophen, 10 mg hydrocodone/650 mg acetaminophen, 10 mg hydrocodone/660 mg acetaminophen, 10 mg hydrocodone/750 mg acetaminophen. *Caps:* 5 mg hydrocodone/500 mg acetaminophen. *Elixir:* 7.5 mg hydrocodone plus 500 mg acetaminophen/15 ml. *Oral soln:* 7.5 mg hydrocodone plus 325 mg acetaminophen/15 ml; **Monitor:** BP, HR, RR, BUN/SCr, LFTs, pain, bowel function; **Notes:** Schedule III controlled substance. Prolonged use may lead to physical and psychological dependence and tolerance. Naloxone is the antidote for hydrocodone, acetylcysteine for acetaminophen.

H

hydrocortisone (Anucort-HC, Anusol HC, Beta-HC, Caldecort, Cetacort, Colocort, Cortaid, Cortef, Cortenema, Cortifoam, Cortizone, Dermacort, Dermtex HC, Hemril-HC, Hytone, Locoid, Nutracort, Pandel, Proctocort, Proctosert, Solu-Cortef, Texacort, Westcort) **Uses: PO, IM, IV:** Wide variety of chronic diseases including: Inflammatory, Allergic, Hematologic, Neoplastic, Autoimmune disorders, Adrenocortical insufficiency; **Topical:** Inflammation and pruritis associated with various allergic/immunologic skin problems; **Class:** corticosteroids; **Preg:** C; **CIs:** Hypersensitivity; Active untreated infections; **ADRs:** depression, euphoria, personality changes, restlessness, cataracts, ↑ BP, PUD, anorexia, N/V, acne, hirsutism, petechiae, allergic contact dermatitis, atrophy, burning, dryness, folliculitis irritation, ↓ wound healing, adrenal suppression, ↑ BG, fluid retention (long-term high doses), ↓ K+, THROMBOEMBOLISM, ↑ wt, muscle wasting, osteoporosis, muscle pain, cushingoid appearance, infection; **Interactions:** Additive hypokalemia with thiazide and loop diuretics, or amphotericin B; May ↑ requirement for insulins or oral hypoglycemic agents; Phenytoin, phenobarbital, and rifampin may ↓ levels; ↑ risk of adverse GI effects with NSAIDs; **Dose:** *PO: Adults:* 20–240 mg/day in 1–4 divided doses. *IM, IV: Adults:* 100–500 mg q 2–6 hr (range: 100–8000 mg/day). *Rect: Adults:* 10–100 mg 1–2 ×/day × 2–3 wk. *Topical: Adults and Peds:* Apply 1–4 ×/day (depends on product, preparation, and condition being treated). *PO: Peds: Anti-inflammatory*—2.5–10 mg/kg/day divided q 6–8 hr. *Physiologic replacement*—0.5–0.75 mg/kg/day divided q 8 hr. *IM, IV: Peds: Acute adrenal insufficiency*—1–2 mg/kg bolus then 25–250 mg/day divided q 6–8 hr. *Other uses*—1–8 mg/kg/day; **Availability (G):** *Tabs:* 5, 10, 20 mg. *Rect enema:* 100 mg/60 ml. *Rect aerosol:* 90 mg/applicator. *Rect supp:* 25 mg, 30 mg. *Inject:* 100 mg, 250 mg, 500 mg, 1 g. *Cream:* 0.1%, 0.2%, 0.5%^{OTC}, 1%^{OTC}, 2.5%. *Gel:* 1%^{OTC}. *Oint:* 0.1%, 0.2%, 0.5%^{OTC}, 1%^{OTC}, 2.5%. *Lotion:* 1%^{OTC}, 2.5%. *Soln:* 0.1%, 1%, 2.5%. *Spray:* 0.5%^{OTC}, 1%^{OTC}; **Monitor:** Systemic therapy: S/S adrenal insufficiency, wt/ht (peds), edema, electrolytes, BG, pain; Topical: skin condition (inflammation, erythema, pruritis); **Notes:** IM doses should not be administered when rapid effect is desirable. Oints are more occlusive and preferred for dry, scaly lesions. Creams should be used on oozing or intertriginous areas (may cause more skin drying than oint). Gels, solns, and lotions are useful in hairy areas.

hydromorphone (Dilaudid, Dilaudid-HP) Uses: Moderate-to-severe pain (alone and in combination with nonopioid analgesics); **Class:** opioid agonists; **Preg:** C; **CIs:** Hypersensitivity (cross-sensitivity may exist with other opioids); Status asthmaticus; Severe respiratory depression (in absence of ventilator); Pregnancy/lactation; **ADRs:** confusion, dizziness, sedation, euphoria, hallucinations, HA, unusual dreams, blurred vision, diplopia, miosis, respiratory depression, ↓ BP, ↓ HR, constipation, dry mouth, N/V, urinary retention, flushing, pruritis, sweating, physical/psychological dependence, tolerance; **Interactions:** Exercise extreme caution with MAOIs (may produce severe, unpredictable reactions—↓ initial dose of hydromorphone by 25%; discontinue MAOIs 2 wk prior to hydromorphone); ↑ risk of CNS depression with alcohol, antidepressants, antihistamines, and sedative/hypnotics; Use of partial antagonists (buprenorphine, butorphanol, nalbuphine, or pentazocine) may precipitate opioid withdrawal in physically dependent patients; **Dose:** *PO: Adults and Peds: ≥50 kg:* 2–8 mg q 3–4 prn. *IV: Adults and Peds: ≥50 kg:* 0.2–0.6 mg q 2–3 prn; may be ↑. *IV: Adults: Continuous infusion (unlabeled)*—0.5–1 mg/hr depending on previous opioid use. *IM, Subcut: Adults:* 0.8–2 mg q 3–6 hr prn. *Rect: Adults:* 3 mg q 4–8 hr prn. *PO: Peds: ≥6 mo and <50 kg:* 0.03–0.08 mg/kg q 3–4 hr prn. *IV: Peds: ≥6 mo and <50 kg:* 0.015 mg/kg q 3–6 hr prn; **Availability (G):** *Tabs:* 2, 4, 8 mg. *Oral soln:* 1 mg/ml. *Inject:* 1 mg/ml, 2 mg/ml, 4 mg/ml, 10 mg/ml. *Supp:* 3 mg; **Monitor:** BP, HR, RR, pain, bowel function; **Notes: High Alert:** Accidental overdosage of opioid analgesics has resulted in fatalities. Before administering, clarify all ambiguous orders; have second practitioner independently check original order, dose calculations, and infusion pump settings. Do not confuse high-potency (HP) dose forms with regular dose forms. Schedule II controlled substance. Give stimulant laxatives to minimize constipation if used >2–3 days. When titrating opioid doses, ↑ of 25–50% should be administered until there is either a 50% ↓ in patient's pain rating or patient reports satisfactory pain relief. Patients on continuous infusion should have additional bolus doses provided q 15–30 min prn for breakthrough pain. Use equianalgesic dose chart when converting between opioids or changing routes of administration. May lead to physical/psychological dependence and tolerance. Naloxone is the antidote. When discontinued, should taper to prevent withdrawal.

hydroxychloroquine (Plaquenil) Uses: Suppression and treatment of acute attacks of malaria; SLE; RA; **Class:** dmards; **Preg:** C; **CIs:** Hypersensitivity to hydroxychloroquine or chloroquine; Previous visual damage from hydroxychloroquine or chloroquine; Pregnancy or lactation (avoid use unless treating/preventing malaria or treating amebic abscess); Peds (long-term use); **ADRs:** SEIZURES, anxiety, dizziness, HA, irritability, personality changes, psychoses, keratopathy, retinopathy, tinnitus, visual disturbances, ECG changes, HEPATOTOXICITY, abdominal cramps, anorexia, N/V/D, alopecia, bleaching of hair, hyperpigmentation, photosensitivity, pruritis, SJS, AGRANULOCYTOSIS, APLASTIC ANEMIA, anemia, leukopenia, thrombocytopenia, myopathy, neuromyopathy; **Interactions:** ↑ risk of hepatotoxicity with other hepatotoxic drugs; **Dose:** *All doses expressed as hydroxychloroquine base. PO: Adults: Malaria suppression*—310 mg once weekly; start 2 wk prior to entering malarious area; continue for 8 wk after leaving area. *Malaria treatment*—620 mg initially, then 310 mg at 6 hr, 24 hr, and 48 hr after initial dose. *SLE*—400 mg 1–2 ×/day initially, then MD of 200–400 mg/day. *RA*—400–600 mg/day initially, then MD of 200–400 mg/day. *PO: Peds: Malaria suppression*—5 mg/kg once weekly (max: 310 mg/wk); start 2 wk prior to entering malarious area; continue for 8 wk after leaving area. *Malaria treatment*—10 mg/kg (max: 620 mg) initially, then 5 mg/kg (max: 310 mg) at 6 hr, 24 hr, and 48 hr after initial dose; **Availability (G):** *Tabs:* 200 mg (155 mg base); **Monitor:** Pain scale, ROM, CBC, LFTs, ophth exam; **Notes:** 200 mg hydroxychloroquine sulfate = 155 mg hydroxychloroquine base. If visual abnormalities develop, discontinue. Give with food or milk. Instruct patient to use sunscreen. May require up to 6 mo to see benefit in RA.

hydrOXYzine (Vistaril) **Uses:** Anxiety; Preop sedation; N/V; Pruritis; **Class:** antihistamines; **Preg:** C; **CIs:** Hypersensitivity; Pregnancy (1st tri)/lactation; **ADRs:** drowsiness, agitation, ataxia, dizziness, dry mouth, constipation, urinary retention, pain at IM site; **Interactions:** Additive CNS depression with other CNS depressants, alcohol, antidepressants, antihistamines, opioid analgesics, and sedative/hypnotics; ↑ risk of anticholinergic effects with other anticholinergic agents; **Dose:** *PO: Adults: Antianxiety*—50–100 mg qid. *Preop sedation*—50–100 mg single dose. *Antipruritic*—25 mg tid-qid. *PO: Peds: <6 yr Antianxiety or antipruritic*—50 mg/day in divided doses. *PO: Peds: ≥6 yr Antianxiety or antipruritic*—50–100 mg/day in divided doses. *PO: Peds: Preop sedation*—0.6 mg/kg single dose. *IM: Adults: Antianxiety*—50–100 mg qid. *Preop sedation*—25–100 mg single dose. *Antiemetic*—25–100 mg q 4–6 hr prn. *IM: Peds: Preop sedation*—0.5–1 mg/kg single dose; **Availability (G):** *Tabs:* 10, 25, 50 mg. *Caps:* 25, 50, 100 mg. *Syrup:* 10 mg/5 ml. *Oral susp:* 25 mg/5 ml. *Inject:* 25 mg/ml, 50 mg/ml; **Monitor:** Mental status, N/V, itching; **Notes:** Should NOT be given IV. Inject can be very painful.

hyoscyamine (Anaspaz, Cystospaz, Levbid, Levsin, Levsinex, NuLev) **Uses:** Infant colic or GI disorders caused by spasm; Adjunctive therapy in PUD, irritable bowel, neurogenic bladder/bowel disturbances; ↓ rigidity, tremors, sialorrhea, and hyperhidrosis associated with parkinsonism; *IM, IV: Subcut:* Facilitation of diagnostic hypotonic duodenography; may also ↑ radiologic visibility of the kidneys; Preop administration ↓ secretions and blocks bradycardia associated with some forms of anesthesia; Management of some forms of heart block due to vagal activity; ↓ pain and hypersecretion associated with pancreatitis; **Class:** anticholinergics; **Preg:** C; **CIs:** Hypersensitivity, Angle-closure glaucoma; Tachycardia or unstable CV status; GI obstructive disease, paralytic ileus, intestinal atony, severe ulcerative colitis; Obstructive uropathy; Myasthenia gravis; **ADRs:** confusion/excitement (esp in geriatric patients), dizziness, HA, insomnia, nervousness, blurred vision, ↑ IOP, mydriasis, palpitations, ↑ HR, nausea, bloating, constipation, dry mouth, paralytic ileus, vomiting, impotence, urinary retention, ↓ sweating, local irritation (IM, IV, subcut), ANAPHYLAXIS, suppression of lactation; **Interactions:** ↑ risk of anticholinergic effects with other anticholinergic agents; **Dose:** *PO, SL: Adults:* 0.125–0.25 mg q 4 hr prn (max 1.5 mg/day). *Cystospaz*—0.15–0.3 mg up to 4 ×/day. *Levsinex*—0.375–0.75 mg q 12 hr. *PO: Peds: 2–<12 yr: ODT (NuLev)*—0.0625–0.125 mg (1/2–1 tablet) q 4 hr, up to 6 ×/day. *PO: Peds: 34–36 kg:* 125–187 mcg q 4 hr prn. *PO: Peds: 22.7–33 kg:* 94–125 mcg q 4 hr prn. *PO: Peds: 13.6–22.6 kg:* 63 mcg q 4 hr prn. *PO: Peds: 9.1–13.5 kg:* 31.3 mcg q 4 hr prn. *PO: Peds: 6.8–9 kg:* 25 mcg q 4 hr prn. *PO: Peds: 4.5–6.7 kg:* 18.8 mcg q 4 hr prn. *PO: Peds: 3.4–4.4 kg:* 15.6 mcg q 4 hr prn. *PO: Peds: 2.3–3.3 kg:* 12.5 mcg q 4 hr prn. *IM, IV, Subcut: Adults: GI anticholinergic*—0.25–0.5 mg 3–4 ×/day prn. *Preop prophylaxis of secretions*—0.005 mg/kg 30–60 min before anesthesia. *Reduce bradycardia during surgery*—0.125 mg IV repeated prn. *IM, IV, Subcut: Peds: ≥2 yr Preop prophylaxis of secretions*—0.005 mg/kg 30–60 min before anesthesia; **Availability (G):** *Tabs:* 0.125, 0.15 mg. *SL tabs:* 0.125 mg. *ODT:* 0.125 mg. *ER tabs:* 0.375 mg. *Timed-release caps:* 0.375 mg. *Oral soln (gtt):* 0.125 mg/ml. *Elixir:* 0.125 mg/5 ml. *Inject:* 0.5 mg/ml; **Monitor:** BP, HR, I/Os, bowel sounds/function; **Notes:** Physostigmine is antidote. Give PO ac.

ibandronate (Boniva) Uses: Treatment/prevention of postmenopausal osteoporosis (IV is used for treatment only); **Class:** biphosphonates; **Preg:** C; **CIs:** Esophageal disease (that may delay emptying); Unable to stand or sit upright for ≥60 min; Hypocalcemia; Severe renal insufficiency (CrCl <30 ml/min); Peds <18 yr (safety not established); **ADRs:** HA, dyspepsia, dysphagia, esophagitis, gastritis, N/V/D, musculoskeletal pain, osteonecrosis (of jaw), inject site reactions; **Interactions:** Antacids, Ca++, iron, and Mg++ ↓ absorption; ↑ risk of GI effects with NSAIDs or aspirin; Food, coffee, and orange juice ↓ absorption; **Dose:** *PO: Adults:* 2.5 mg/day *or* 150 mg/mo. *IV: Adults:* 3 mg q 3 mo; **Availability:** *Tabs:* 2.5, 150 mg. *Inject:* 1 mg/ml; **Monitor:** BMD, Ca++; **Notes:** Take first thing in AM with 6–8 oz plain water ≥60 min before other meds, beverages, or food. Remain upright for ≥60 min after dose and after eating. Ca++ and vitamin D supplements recommended. Avoid dental procedures during therapy. Administer once-monthly tabs on same date each month.

ibuprofen, oral (Advil, Genpril, Midol Maximum Strength Cramp Formula, Motrin) Uses: Mild-to-moderate pain; Dysmenorrhea; RA (including juvenile); OA; Fever; **Class:** NSAIDs; **Preg:** C (1st and 2nd tri), D (3rd tri); **CIs:** Hypersensitivity (cross-sensitivity may exist with other NSAIDs or ASA); Active GI bleeding or ulcer disease; Peri-operative pain from CABG surgery; Infants <6 mo (safety not established); **ADRs:** dizziness, HA, tinnitus, edema, GI BLEEDING, dyspepsia, N/V, abdominal discomfort, constipation, diarrhea, ↑ LFTs, hematuria, renal failure, EXFOLIATIVE DERMATITIS, SJS, TEN, rash, anemia, ANAPHYLAXIS; **Interactions:** May ↓ cardioprotective effects of low-dose aspirin; ↑ risk of GI side effects with aspirin, oral K^+ supplements, other NSAIDs, corticosteroids, or alcohol; May ↓ effectiveness of antihypertensives; May ↑ levels/toxicity of lithium and methotrexate; ↑ risk of bleeding with antiplatelet agents or anticoagulants; ↑ risk of nephrotoxicity with cyclosporine; **Dose:** *PO: Adults: Anti-inflammatory*—400–800 mg tid–qid (max: 3200 mg/day). *Analgesic/antidysmenorrheal/antipyretic*—200–400 mg q 4–6 hr (max: 1200 mg/day). *PO: Peds: 6 mo–12 yr Anti-inflammatory*—30–50 mg/kg/day in 3 divided doses (max: 2.4 g/day). *Antipyretic*—5 mg/kg for temp <102.5°F or 10 mg/kg for higher temp (max: 40 mg/kg/day); may be repeated q 6–8 hr. *Analgesic*—4–10 mg/kg q 6–8 hr; **Availability (G):** *Tabs:* 100, 200, 400, 600, 800 mg. *Caps (liqui-gels):* 200 mg. *Chew tabs:* 50, 100 mg. *Oral susp:* 100 mg/5 ml. *Pediatric drops:* 40 mg/ml; **Monitor:** BP, temp, BUN/SCr, LFTs, CBC, bleeding, S/S PUD, pain scale, S/S anaphylaxis; **Notes:** For rapid initial effect, administer 30 min ac or 2 hr pc. Caution on use of other OTC cough/cold/pain products (may also contain ibuprofen).

I

ibutilide (Corvert) Uses: Rapid conversion of recent-onset AF/AFl to sinus rhythm; **Class:** antiarrhythmics (class III); **Preg:** C; **CIs:** Hypersensitivity; QT interval prolongation (>440 msec); Hypokalemia; Hypomagnesemia; Pregnancy, lactation, or peds <18 yr (safety not established); **ADRs:** HA, ARRHYTHMIAS, nausea; **Interactions:** Amiodarone, disopyramide, procainamide, quinidine, and sotalol should not be given concurrently or within 4 hr because of additive effects on refractoriness; ↑ risk of QT prolongation with other QT-prolonging drugs; **Dose:** *IV: Adults: ≥60 kg:* 1-mg infusion over 10 min; may be repeated 10 min after end of first infusion. *IV: Adults: <60 kg:* 0.01-mg/kg infusion; may be repeated 10 min after end of first infusion; **Availability:** *Inject:* 0.1 mg/ml; **Monitor:** BP, HR, ECG (QT interval); **Notes:** Correct hypokalemia and/or hypomagnesemia before administering. Discontinue if proarrhythmia occurs. May start oral antiarrhythmic therapy ≥4 hr after ibutilide infusion.

idarubicin (Idamycin) Uses: AML in adults (with other agents); **Class:** anthracyclines; **Preg:** D; **CIs:** Bone marrow suppression; Serum bilirubin >5 mg/dl; Pregnancy/lactation; Peds (safety not established); **ADRs:** HA, mental status changes, pulmonary toxicity, ARRHYTHMIAS, CARDIOTOXICITY, HF, abdominal cramps, mucositis, N/V/D, ↑ LFTs, alopecia, rash, gonadal suppression, BLEEDING, anemia, NEUTROPENIA, thrombocytopenia, phlebitis at IV site, ↑ uric acid, peripheral neuropathy, fever; **Interactions:** ↑ myelosuppression with other antineoplastics or radiation therapy; **Dose:** *IV: Adults:* 12 mg/m²/day × 3 days in combination with cytarabine. *IV: Peds: Leukemia*—10–12 mg/m²/day × 3 days q 3 wk; *Solid tumors*—5 mg/m²/day × 3 days q 3 wk; **Availability (G):** *Inject:* 1 mg/ml; **Monitor:** BP, HR, RR, temp, BUN/SCr, CBC (with diff), uric acid, LFTs, S/S infection, S/S HF, bleeding, echo (LVEF), ECG, CXR, infusion site; **Notes:** **High Alert:** Fatalities have occurred with incorrect administration of chemotherapeutic agents. Before administering, clarify all ambiguous orders; double-check single, daily, and course-of-therapy dose limits; have second practitioner independently double-check original order, calculations, and infusion pump settings. Do not confuse with doxorubicin or daunorubicin. Leukocyte count nadir = 10–14 days (recovery in 21 days after administration). Withhold therapy if mucositis develops; after recovery, ↓ subsequent doses by 25%. Potent vesicant.

ifosfamide (Ifex) **Uses:** Germ cell testicular carcinoma (with other agents); **Class:** alkylating agents; **Preg:** D; **CIs:** Hypersensitivity; Pregnancy/lactation; Bone marrow suppression; **ADRs:** confusion, hallucinations, sedation, disorientation, dizziness, N/V, HEPATOTOXICITY, hemorrhagic cystitis, dysuria, sterility, renal impairment, alopecia, anemia, NEUTROPENIA, thrombocytopenia, phlebitis, allergic reactions; **Interactions:** ↑ myelosuppression with other antineoplastics or radiation therapy; **Dose:** *IV: Adults:* 1.2 g/m²/day × 5 days; give with mesna. May repeat cycle q 3 wk. *IV: Peds:* 1200–1800 mg/m²/day × 3–5 days q 3–4 wk *or* 5 g/m² once q 3–4 wk *or* 3 g/m²/day × 2 days q 3–4 wk; **Availability (G):** *Inject:* 1 g, 3 g; **Monitor:** BP, HR, RR, temp, I/Os, U/A, neuro exam, CBC (with diff), BUN/SCr, LFTs; **Notes:** To prevent hemorrhagic cystitis, give hydration (≥3000 ml/day for adults and 1000–2000 ml/day for peds) and mesna. Patient should also void frequently to ↓ bladder irritation. Withhold dose if WBC <2000 or platelets <50,000. Leukocyte and platelet count nadir = 7–14 days (recovery in 21 days after administration).

imatinib (Gleevec) **Uses:** Newly diagnosed Ph+ CML; CML in blast crisis, accelerated phase, or in chronic phase after failure of interferon-alpha treatment; Kit (CD117) positive metastatic/unresectable malignant GIST; Pediatric patients with Ph+ CML in chronic phase; Adult patients with relapsed or refractory Ph+ ALL; MDS/MPD; ASM; HES/CEL; DFSP; **Class:** enzyme inhibitors; **Preg:** D; **CIs:** Hypersensitivity;

I

Pregnancy/lactation; Concurrent use of strong CYP3A4 inducers (e.g., dexamethasone, phenytoin, carbamazepine, rifampin, rifabutin, phenobarbital); Peds <2 yr (safety not established); **ADRs:** depression, dizziness, fatigue, HA, insomnia, cough, dyspnea, nasopharyngitis, pneumonia, HEPATOTOXICITY, abdominal pain, anorexia, constipation, N/V/D, petechiae, pruritus, rash, HF, edema, ↓ K+, BLEEDING, NEUTROPENIA, THROMBOCYTOPENIA, ↑ wt, arthralgia, muscle cramps, myalgia, fever, night sweats; **Interactions:** CYP3A4 inhibitors may ↑ levels/toxicity; CYP3A4 inducers may ↓ levels/effects; May ↑ levels/toxicity of CYP3A4 substrates or CYP2D6 substrates; May ↑ risk of bleeding with warfarin; May ↑ acetaminophen levels/toxicity; **Dose:** *PO: Adults: Newly diagnosed Ph+ CML (chronic phase)*—400 mg/day, may ↑ to 600 mg/day based on response and circumstances. *Ph+ CML (accelerated phase or blast crisis)*—600 mg/day; may ↑ to 400 mg bid based on response and circumstances. *Ph+ ALL*—600 mg/day. *MDS/MPD*—400 mg/day. *ASM or HES/CEL*—100–400 mg/day. *DFSP*—400 mg bid. *GIST*—400–600 mg/day. *PO: Peds: Newly diagnosed Ph+ CML*—340 mg/m^2/day (max: 600 mg/day); *Ph+ chronic phase CML recurrent after failure of stem cell transplant or resistant to interferon-alpha*—260 mg/m^2/day. *Hepatic Impairment PO: Adults and Peds:* ↓ dose if severe hepatic impairment; **Availability:** *Tabs:* 100, 400 mg; **Monitor:** BP, HR, RR, temp, edema, electrolytes, CBC (with diff), LFTs, bilirubin; **Notes: High Alert:** Fatalities have occurred with incorrect administration of chemotherapeutic agents. Before administering, clarify all ambiguous orders; double-check single, daily, and course-of-therapy dose limits; have second practitioner independently double-check original order and dose calculations. Therapy should be initiated by physician experienced in the treatment of patients with chronic myeloid leukemia. If serum bilirubin ↑ to >3 × ULN or LFTs ↑ to >5 × ULN, hold therapy until bilirubin <1.5 × ULN and LFTs <2.5 × ULN, and then ↓ dose. Also need to adjust dose if neutropenia and/or thrombocytopenia develop. Patients requiring anticoagulation while receiving imatinib should receive LMWH or UFH (not warfarin). Give with food and water to ↓ GI irritation. If unable to take tab, can dissolve in water or apple juice.

imipenem/cilastatin (Primaxin) **Uses:** Respiratory tract infections, skin/skin structure infections, UTIs, gynecological infections, septicemia, bone/joint infections, IE, polymicrobic infections, or intra-abdominal infections due to susceptible organisms (e.g., *S. pneumo, S. aureus, S. epidermidis, S. pyogenes, Enterococcus faecalis, E. coli, H. flu, Klebsiella, P. mirabilis, M. catarrhalis, Enterobacter, Serratia, Acinetobacter, Pseudomonas, B. fragilis*); **Class:** carbapenems; **Preg:** C; **CIs:** Hypersensitivity (cross-sensitivity to other beta-lactam antibiotics may exist); **ADRs:** SEIZURES, PSEUDOMEMBRANOUS COLITIS, N/V/D, rash, pruritis, phlebitis, pain at IM site, ANAPHYLAXIS; **Interactions:** Probenecid ↓ excretion and ↑ levels; May ↓ valproic acid levels;

↑ risk of seizures with ganciclovir (avoid concurrent use); **Dose:** *IV: Adults: Mild infections*—250–500 mg q 6 hr. *Moderate infections*—500 mg q 6–8 hr *or* 1 g q 8 hr. *Serious infections*—500 mg q 6 hr *or* 1 g q 6–8 hr. *IV: Peds:* ≥*3 mo:* 15–25 mg/kg q 6 hr; higher doses have been used in older peds with cystic fibrosis. *IV: Peds: 4 wk–3 mo* 25 mg/kg q 6 hr. *IV: Peds: 1–4 wk:* 25 mg/kg q 8 hr. *IV: Peds: <1 wk:* 25 mg/kg q 12 hr. *IM: Adults:* 500–750 mg q 12 hr. *Renal Impairment IV: Adults:* ↓ dose if CrCl ≤ 70 ml/min; **Availability:** *Inject:* 250 mg imipenem/250 mg cilastatin, 500 mg imipenem/500 mg cilastatin; **Monitor:** BP, HR, temp, sputum, U/A, BUN/SCr, CBC; **Notes:** IM should not be used for severe infections. IM formulation/vial is different than IV formulation/vial. Use with caution in patients with seizure disorders. Use with caution in patients with beta-lactam allergy (do not use if history of anaphylaxis or hives).

imipramine (Tofranil, Tofranil PM) **Uses:** Depression; Enuresis in peds; **Class:** tricyclic antidepressants; **Preg:** D; **CIs:** Hypersensitivity; Concurrent use with MAOIs; Post-MI; May ↑ risk of suicidal thoughts/behaviors, esp. during early treatment or dose adjustment; risk may be ↑ in peds and adolescents; Pregnancy/lactation; Peds <6 yr (safety not established); **ADRs:** confusion, lethargy, sedation, blurred vision, dry mouth, ARRHYTHMIAS, ↓ BP, constipation, hepatitis, ↑ appetite, ↑ wt, urinary retention, ↓ libido, gynecomastia, blood dyscrasias, SUICIDAL THOUGHTS; **Interactions:** CYP2D6 inhibitors (e.g., phenothiazines, quinidine, cimetidine, class Ic antiarrhythmics) may ↑ levels; ↑ risk of hypertensive crises, seizures, or death with MAOIs (discontinue for ≥2 wk); ↑ risk of toxicity with SSRIs (discontinue fluoxetine for ≥5 wk); ↑ risk of arrhythmias with other drugs that prolong QT_C interval; ↑ CNS depression with other CNS depressants including alcohol, antihistamines, opioids, and sedative/hypnotics; ↑ risk of anticholinergic effects with other anticholinergic agents; **Dose:** *PO: Adults:* 25–50 mg 3–4/day (max: 300 mg/day); total daily dose may be given at bedtime. *PO: (Geriatric Patients):* 25 mg at bedtime initially, up to 100 mg/day in divided doses. *PO: Peds: >12 yr Depression*—30–40 mg/day in divided doses (max: 100 mg/day). *PO: Peds* ≥*6 yr Enuresis*—25 mg 1 hr before bedtime; ↑ if necessary by 25 mg q wk to 50 mg/day in children <12 yr, or 75 mg/day in children >12 yr; **Availability (G):** *Tabs:* 10, 25, 50 mg. *Caps:* 75, 100, 125, 150 mg; **Monitor:** BP, HR, ECG, mental status, suicidal thoughts/behaviors, wt, frequency of bedwetting, serum concentrations (if treatment refractory); **Notes:** May take 4–6 wk to see effect. May give entire dose at bedtime. Taper to avoid withdrawal. Use with caution in elderly (↑ risk of sedation and anticholinergic effects).

indapamide (No Trade) **Uses:** HTN; Edema due to HF or nephrotic syndrome; **Class:** thiazide-like diuretics; **Preg:** B; **CIs:** Hypersensitivity (cross-sensitivity with sulfonamides may occur); Hypersensitivity; Anuria; **ADRs:** dizziness, drowsiness, lethargy, arrhythmias,

↓ BP, anorexia, cramping, N/V, photosensitivity, rash, ↑ BG, ↓ K+, dehydration, metabolic alkalosis, ↓ Na+, hypovolemia, ↑ uric acid, muscle cramps; **Interactions:** ↑ effects with other antihypertensives; Additive hypokalemia with corticosteroids or amphotericin B; May ↑ requirement for insulin or oral hypoglycemic agents; May ↑ lithium levels; ↑ risk of ototoxicity with aminoglycosides; NSAIDs may ↓ effectiveness; **Dose:** *PO: Adults: HTN*—1.25–5 mg/day. *Edema*—2.5–5 mg/day; **Availability (G):** *Tabs:* 1.25, 2.5 mg; **Monitor:** BP, HR, electrolytes, BUN/SCr, BG, uric acid, wt, I/Os, edema; **Notes:** Administer in AM.

indomethacin (Indocin) Uses: Arthritis, Ankylosing spondylitis; **IV:** PDA closure in neonates; **Class:** NSAIDs; **Preg:** B (1st tri), C (3rd tri); **CIs:** Hypersensitivity to aspirin or NSAIDs; Active bleeding, Perioperative pain in setting of CABG surgery; NEC in neonates; Thrombocytopenia; Severe renal disease; **ADRs:** dizziness, HA, tinnitus, GI bleeding, N/V/D, ↑ SCr, rash; **Interactions:** ↑ GI effects with aspirin and corticosteroids; ↓ effects of aspirin, diuretics, or antihypertensives; ↑ risk of bleeding with warfarin and drugs affecting platelet function; ↑ nephrotoxicity with cyclosporine; ↑ levels of methotrexate, lithium, aminoglycosides, and vancomycin; **Dose:** *PO: Adults: Arthritis*—25–50 mg bid–qid *or* 75-mg SR cap daily or bid (max: 200 mg/day or 150 mg SR/day). *PO: Peds:* 1–2 mg/kg/day divided bid–qid (max: 4 mg/kg/day). *IV: (Neonates):* 0.2 mg/kg followed by 2 PNA-dependent doses (PNA <48 hr: 0.1 mg/kg q 12 hr; PNA 2–7 days: 0.2 mg/kg q 12 hr; PNA >7 days: 0.25 mg/kg q 12 h); **Availability (G):** *Caps:* 25 mg, 50 mg. *SR caps:* 75 mg. *Susp:* 25 mg/5 ml. *Inject:* 1 mg; **Monitor:** Pain, bleeding, BUN/SCr, CBC. In PDA: BP, HR, RR, ECG; **Notes:** Avoid use in oliguria/anuria. Do not give IV, intra-arterially, or via umbilical catheter. Give PO with food.

infliximab (Remicade) Uses: RA; Crohn's disease; Psoriatic arthritis; Ankylosing spondylitis; Ulcerative colitis; Plaque psoriasis; **Class:** dmards, monoclonal antibodies; **Preg:** B; **CIs:** Hypersensitivity to murine proteins; HF (NYHA Class III/IV); Concurrent use of anakinra; Active infection; **ADRs:** fatigue, HA, laryngitis, HTN, abdominal pain, nausea, diarrhea, dyspepsia, ↑ LFTs, rash, anemia, INFECTIONS (including reactivation TB), MALIGNANCY; **Interactions:** ↑ infection risk with anakinra; Do not give with live vaccines; **Dose:** *IV: Adults: RA*—3 mg/kg at 0, 2, and 6 wk then q 8 wk; may ↑ dose up to 10 mg/kg or give q 4 wk if incomplete response. *Crohn's disease, ulcerative colitis, plaque psoriasis, psoriatic arthritis*—5 mg/kg IV at 0, 2, and 6 wk, then q 8 wk (q 6 wk for ankylosing spondylitis). *IV: Peds: Crohn's disease*—5 mg/kg IV at 0, 2, and 6 wk, then q 8 wk; **Availability:** *Inject:* 100 mg; **Monitor:** Vital signs, LFTs, CBC, S/S of infection/malignancy, pain scale, ROM; **Notes:** Premedicate with antihistamines, acetaminophen, and/or corticosteroids to ↓ infusion-related reactions; place PPD prior to initiation (may reactivate latent TB).

insulin aspart (NovoLog) **Uses:** Control of hyperglycemia in DM; **Class:** pancreatics; **Preg:** B; **CIs:** Hypoglycemia; Allergy or hypersensitivity to insulin aspart; **ADRs:** ↓ BG, lipodystrophy, pruritis, erythema, swelling, ALLERGIC REACTIONS; **Interactions:** Beta blockers and clonidine may mask S/S of hypoglycemia; Corticosteroids, thyroid supplements, oral contraceptives, niacin, and diuretics may ↑ insulin requirements; Alcohol, MAOIs, pentamidine, oral hypoglycemics, and salicylates may ↓ insulin requirements; **Dose:** *Subcut: Adults and Peds:* Varies; usually 0.5–1 unit/kg/day total. 50–70% may be given as insulin aspart, and the remainder as intermediate- or long-acting insulin; **Availability:** *Inject:* 100 units/ml vials and pens; **Monitor:** BG, urine sugar/ketones, A1C, electrolytes, S/S hypo/hyperglycemia; **Notes:** Rapid-acting insulin. Give within 5–10 min ac. Use with long-acting insulin. Renal impairment may require ↓ dose.

insulin detemir (Levemir) **Uses:** Control of hyperglycemia in DM; **Class:** pancreatics; **Preg:** C; **CIs:** Hypoglycemia; Allergy or hypersensitivity to insulin detemir; **ADRs:** ↓ BG, lipodystrophy, pruritis, erythema, swelling, ALLERGIC REACTIONS; **Interactions:** Beta blockers and clonidine may mask S/S of hypoglycemia; Corticosteroids, thyroid supplements, oral contraceptives, niacin, and diuretics may ↑ insulin requirements; Alcohol, MAOIs, pentamidine, oral hypoglycemics, and salicylates may ↓ insulin requirements; **Dose:** *Subcut: Adults and Peds: ≥6 yr Insulin-naive*—0.1–0.2 units/kg/day in the evening or 10 units/day in 1 or 2 doses. *Basal insulin or basal bolus*—may substitute on an equal unit-per-unit basis; **Availability:** *Inject:* 100 units/ml vials and pens; **Monitor:** BG, urine sugar/ketones, A1C, electrolytes, S/S hypo/hyperglycemia; **Notes:** Long-acting. Do not give IV. Give with evening meal or at bedtime. Renal impairment may require ↓ dose.

insulin glargine (Lantus) **Uses:** Control of hyperglycemia in DM; **Class:** pancreatics; **Preg:** C; **CIs:** Hypoglycemia; Allergy, or hypersensitivity to insulin glargine; **ADRs:** ↓ BG, lipodystrophy, pruritus, erythema, swelling, ALLERGIC REACTIONS; **Interactions:** Beta blockers and clonidine may mask S/S of hypoglycemia; Corticosteroids, thyroid supplements, oral contraceptives, niacin, and diuretics may ↑ insulin requirements; Alcohol, MAOIs, pentamidine, oral hypoglycemics, and salicylates may ↓ insulin requirements; **Dose:** *Subcut: Adults and Peds: ≥6 yr Concurrent treatment with oral antidiabetic agents*—10 units/day; adjust based on response (range: 2–100 units/day). *Conversion from NPH insulin*—Once daily NPH: give same dose. NPH bid: Use 80% of the total daily NPH dose and give once daily; adjust based on response; **Availability:** *Inject:* 100 units/ml vials and pens; **Monitor:** BG, urine sugar/ketones, A1C, electrolytes, S/S hypo/hyperglycemia; **Notes:** Long-acting insulin. Do not give IV. Renal impairment may require ↓ dose.

insulin glulisine (Apidra) **Uses:** Control of hyperglycemia in DM; **Class:** pancreatics; **Preg:** C; **CIs:** Hypoglycemia; Allergy or hypersensitivity to insulin glulisine; **ADRs:** ↓ BG, lipodystrophy, pruritis, erythema, swelling, ALLERGIC REACTIONS; **Interactions:** Beta blockers and clonidine may mask S/S of hypoglycemia; Corticosteroids, thyroid supplements, oral contraceptives, niacin, and diuretics may ↑ insulin requirements; Alcohol, MAOIs, pentamidine, oral hypoglycemics, and salicylates may ↓ insulin requirements; **Dose:** *Subcut: IV: Adults:* Varies; range: 0.2–1.2 units/kg/day; **Availability:** *Inject:* 100 units/ml in vials and pens; **Monitor:** BG, urine sugar/ketones, A1C, electrolytes, S/S hypo/hyperglycemia; **Notes:** Rapid-acting insulin. Give 15 min prior to or 20 min after starting meal. Use with long-acting insulin. Renal impairment may require ↓ dose.

I

insulin lispro (Humalog) **Uses:** Control of hyperglycemia in DM; **Class:** pancreatics; **Preg:** B; **CIs:** Hypoglycemia; Allergy or hypersensitivity to insulin lispro; **ADRs:** ↓ BG, lipodystrophy, pruritus, erythema, swelling, ALLERGIC REACTIONS; **Interactions:** Beta blockers and clonidine may mask S/S of hypoglycemia; corticosteroids, thyroid supplements, oral contraceptives, niacin, and diuretics may ↑ insulin requirements; Alcohol, MAOIs, pentamidine, oral hypoglycemics, and salicylates may ↓ insulin requirements; **Dose:** *Subcut: Adults and Peds: Initial*—0.2–0.6 units/kg/day. *MD*—0.5–1.2 units/kg/day. *Adolescents*—≤1.5 units/kg/day; **Availability:** *Inject:* 100 units/ml vials and pens; **Monitor:** BG, urine sugar/ketones, A1C, electrolytes, S/S hypo/hyperglycemia; **Notes:** Rapid-acting insulin. Give within 15 min before or immediately after meal. Use with long-acting insulin. Renal impairment may require ↓ dose.

NPH insulin (Humulin N, Novolin N) **Uses:** Control of hyperglycemia in DM; **Class:** pancreatics; **Preg:** B; **CIs:** Hypoglycemia; Allergy or hypersensitivity to NPH insulin; **ADRs:** ↓ BG, lipodystrophy, pruritus, erythema, swelling, ALLERGIC REACTIONS; **Interactions:** Beta blockers and clonidine may mask S/S of hypoglycemia; Corticosteroids, thyroid supplements, oral contraceptives, niacin, and diuretics may ↑ insulin requirements; Alcohol, MAOIs, pentamidine, oral hypoglycemics, and salicylates may ↓ insulin requirements; **Dose:** *Subcut: Adults and Peds: Initial*—0.2–0.6 units/kg/day in 1 or 2 doses. *MD*—0.5–1.2 units/kg/day. *Adolescents*—≤1.5 units/kg/day; **Availability:** *Inject:* 100 units/ml vials and pens; **Monitor:** BG, urine sugar/ketones, A1C, electrolytes, S/S hypo/hyperglycemia; **Notes:** Do not give IV. Give 30–60 min ac. Renal impairment may require ↓ dose.

insulin, regular (Humulin R, Novolin R, Humulin R U-500 (Concentrated)) **Uses:** Control of hyperglycemia in DM; Hyperkalemia; **Class:** pancreatics; **Preg:** B; **CIs:** Hypoglycemia;

Allergy or hypersensitivity to insulin; **ADRs:** ↓ BG, lipodystrophy, pruritus, erythema, swelling, ALLERGIC REACTIONS; **Interactions:** Beta blockers and clonidine may mask S/S of hypoglycemia; corticosteroids, thyroid supplements, oral contraceptives, niacin, and diuretics may ↑ insulin requirements; Alcohol, MAOIs, pentamidine, oral hypoglycemics, and salicylates may ↓ insulin requirements; **Dose:** *IV: Adults and Peds:* 0.1 unit/kg/hr as continuous infusion. *Subcut: Adults and Peds: Initial*—0.2–0.6 units/kg/day. *MD*—0.5–1.2 units/kg/day. *Adolescents*—≤1.5 units/kg/day. *Subcut: IV: Adults and Peds: Hyperkalemia*—Dextrose 0.5–1 g/kg with 1 unit of insulin for every 4–5 g dextrose given; **Availability:** *Inject:* 100 units/ml vials and pens. *Concentrated inject:* 500 units/ml; **Monitor:** BG, urine sugar/ketones, A1C, electrolytes, S/S hypo/hyperglycemia; **Notes:** Give 15–30 min ac. Do not give U-500 concentrate IV. Renal impairment may require ↓ dose.

interferon alfa-2b (Intron A) Uses: Treatment of: Hairy cell leukemia, Malignant melanoma, AIDS-related KS, Condylomata acuminata (intralesional), Chronic HBV, Chronic HCV, Follicular non-Hodgkin's lymphoma; **Class:** interferons; **Preg:** C; **CIs:** Hypersensitivity to alfa interferons or human serum albumin; Autoimmune hepatitis; Hepatic decompensation (Child-Pugh class B and C) before or during therapy; Severe CV, pulmonary, or renal disease; Active infections; Underlying CNS pathology or psychiatric history; Decreased bone marrow reserve or underlying immunosuppression; Childbearing potential, pregnancy, lactation, and peds <3 yr (safety not established); **ADRs:** NEUROPSYCHIATRIC DISORDERS, <u>confusion</u>, <u>depression</u>, <u>dizziness</u>, <u>fatigue</u>, <u>HA</u>, <u>insomnia</u>, <u>irritability</u>, anxiety, blurred vision, <u>nosebleeds</u>, <u>rhinitis</u>, ISCHEMIC DISORDERS, arrhythmias, CP, <u>edema</u>, COLITIS, PANCREATITIS, <u>anorexia</u>, <u>abdominal pain</u>, <u>N/V/D</u>, <u>dry mouth</u>, <u>taste disorder</u>, ↓ <u>wt</u>, hepatitis, flatulence, <u>alopecia</u>, <u>dry skin</u>, <u>pruritus</u>, <u>rash</u>, <u>sweating</u>, thyroid disorders, LEUKOPENIA, THROMBOCYTOPENIA, <u>anemia</u>, <u>hemolytic anemia (with ribavirin)</u>, <u>arthralgia</u>, <u>myalgia</u>, leg cramps, paresthesia, <u>cough</u>, <u>dyspnea</u>, inject site reactions, AUTOIMMUNE DISORDERS, INFECTION, allergic reactions including ANAPHYLAXIS, <u>chills</u>, <u>fever</u>, <u>flu-like syndrome</u>; **Interactions:** Additive myelosuppression with other antineoplastic agents or radiation therapy; ↑ CNS depression with other CNS depressants, including alcohol, antihistamines, sedative/hypnotics, and opioids; May ↓ metabolism and ↑ levels and toxicity of theophylline and methadone; ↑ risk of adverse reactions with zidovudine; May ↓ effects of immunosuppressant agents; **Dose:** *IV: Adults: Malignant melanoma (induction)*—20 million units/m² × 5 days of each wk × 4 wk initially, followed by subcut maintenance dosing. *IM, Subcut: Adults: Hairy cell leukemia*—2 million units/m² 3 ×/wk for 2–6 mo. *Malignant melanoma (maintenance)*—10 million units/m² subcut 3 ×/wk × 48 wk, following initial IV dosing. *AIDS-related KS*—30 million units/m² 3 ×/wk. *Chronic HCV*—3 million units 3 ×/wk. If normalization of ALT occurs after 16 wk of therapy, continue treatment for total of 18–24 mo. If normalization of ALT does not occur after 16 wk of therapy, consider treatment discontinuation. *Chronic HBV*—5 million units/day *or* 10 million units 3 ×/wk × 16 wk. *Follicular non-Hodgkin's lymphoma*—5 million units subcut 3 ×/wk for up to 18 mo (to be used following completion of anthracycline-containing chemotherapy). *Subcut: Peds: >3 yr Chronic HBV*—3 million units/m^2 3 ×/wk for the 1st wk of therapy then ↑ to 6 million units/m^2 3 ×/wk (max: 10 million units/dose) × 16–24 wk. *Intralesional Adults: Condylomata acuminata*—1 million units/lesion 3 ×/wk × 3 wk; treat only 5 lesions per course. An additional course of treatment may be initiated at 12–16 wk; **Availability:** *Powder for inject:* 10 million units, 18 million units, 50 million units. *Soln for inject:* 6 million units/ml, 10 million units/ml. *Prefilled pens for inject:* 18 million units (3 million units/0.2 ml), 30 million units (5 million units/0.2 ml), 60 million units (10 million units/0.2 ml); **Monitor:** CXR, ECG, CBC, LFTs, TFTs, electrolytes, wt; **Notes:** Should be discontinued if ANC <500 or platelets <25,000 and then may be restarted at a lower dose if the ANC >1000. Discontinue drug therapy in cases of severe infection, pancreatitis, colitis, or if AST/ALT >5 × ULN.

interferon beta-1a (Avonex, Rebif) **Uses:** MS; **Class:** interferons; **Preg:** C; **CIs:** Hypersensitivity to recombinant interferons or albumin; Severe depression/psychosis; seizures; Hepatic/renal impairment; **ADRs:** SEIZURES, dizziness, fatigue, HA, abdominal pain, nausea, ↑ LFTs, UTI, rash, leukopenia, fever, flu-like symptoms, pain; **Interactions:** ↑ risk of granulocytopenia with ACEIs, Hepatotoxic agents ↑ hepatotoxicity risk; ↑ effects of warfarin and zidovudine; **Dose:** *IM: Adults:* 30 mcg once weekly. *Subcut: Adults: Target dose of 22 mcg 3 ×/wk*—4.4 mcg 3 ×/wk × 2 wk, then 11 mcg 3 ×/wk × 2 wk, then 22 mcg 3 ×/wk. *Target dose of 44 mcg 3 ×/wk*—8.8 mcg 3 ×/wk × 2 wk, then 22 mcg 3 ×/wk × 2 wk, then 44 mcg 3 ×/wk; **Availability:** **Avonex** *Inject:* 30 mcg. **Rebif** *Inject:* 8.8 mcg, 22 mcg, 44 mcg; **Monitor:** S/S depression, LFTs, CBC, TFTs; **Notes:** Give inject ≥48 hr apart at different sites; may premedicate with antipyretics for fever/flu-like S/S.

interferon beta-1b (Betaseron) **Uses:** MS; **Class:** interferons; **Preg:** C; **CIs:** Hypersensitivity to *E. coli*–derived products, recombinant interferons, or albumin; Severe depression/psychosis; Seizures; Hepatic/renal impairment; **ADRs:** HA, edema, CP, abdominal pain, constipation, N/V/D, ↑ LFTs, rash, neutropenia, fever, flu-like symptoms, pain; **Interactions:** ↓ metabolism of theophylline; **Dose:** *Subcut: Adults:* 0.0625 mg (2 million units) every other day then ↑ by 0.0625 mg q 2 wk to 0.25mg (8 million units) every other day; **Availability:** *Inject:* 0.3 mg (9.6 million units); **Monitor:** S/S depression, LFTs, CBC, TFTs; **Notes:** Hydrate well prior to treatment; may premedicate with antipyretics for fever/flu-like S/S.

ipratropium (Atrovent, Atrovent HFA) **Uses:** **Inhaln:** Bronchospasm associated with COPD; **Intranasal:** Rhinorrhea associated with common cold or allergic/nonallergic rhinitis; **Class:** anticholinergics; **Preg:** B; **CIs:** Hypersensitivity to ipratropium, atropine, belladonna alkaloids, or bromide; Bladder neck obstruction, BPH, or glaucoma; **ADRs:** dizziness, HA, dyspnea, nasal dryness/irritation, bronchospasm, cough, palpitations, GI irritation, nausea, rash, allergic reactions; **Interactions:** ↑ toxicity with anticholinergics or drugs with anticholinergic properties; **Dose:** *Inhaln: Adults and Peds: >12 yr MDI*—2 inhaln qid (max 12 inhaln/24 hr). *Neb*—500 mcg tid–qid. *Inhaln: Peds: <12 yr MDI*—1–2 inhaln tid (max 6 inhaln/24 hr). *Neb*—125–250 mcg tid. *Inhaln: (Neonates) Neb*—25 mcg/kg/dose tid. *Intranasal: Adults and Peds: >6yr 0.03% soln*—Allergic/nonallergic rhinitis: 2 sprays in each nostril bid–tid. *Intranasal: Adults and Peds: ≥5 yr 0.06% soln*—Cold: 2 sprays in each nostril tid–qid; **Availability (G):** *MDI (CFC-free):* 17 mcg/spray. *Neb soln:* 0.02% (500 mcg/2.5 ml). *Nasal spray:* 0.03% soln (21 mcg/spray), 0.06% soln (42 mcg/spray); **Monitor:** RR, PFTs, relief of bronchospasm/rhinorrhea; **Notes:** Do not use for acute episodes of bronchospasm. MDI does not contain soy and may be used safely in soy allergy.

I

irbesartan (Avapro) **Uses:** HTN; Diabetic nephropathy in patients with type 2 DM; **Class:** angiotensin II receptor antagonists; **Preg:** C (1st tri), D (2nd/3rd tri); **CIs:** Hypersensitivity; Pregnancy/lactation; **ADRs:** dizziness, fatigue, ↓ BP, ↑ HR, dyspepsia, N/V/D, ↑ SCr, ↑ K+, ANGIOEDEMA; **Interactions:** ↑ effects with other antihypertensives; ↑ risk of hyperkalemia with ACEIs, K+ supplements, K+ salt substitutes, K+ sparing diuretics, or NSAIDs; NSAIDs may ↓ effectiveness; ↑ levels/effects of amiodarone, fluoxetine, glimepiride, glipizide, phenytoin, rosiglitazone, or warfarin; **Dose:** *PO: Adults and Peds: >12 yr HTN*—150–300 mg/day; 75 mg/day in volume-depleted patients. *Nephropathy*—300 mg/day. *PO: Peds: 6–12 yr:* 75–150 mg/day; **Availability:** *Tabs:* 75 mg, 150 mg, 300 mg; **Monitor:** BP, HR, wt, edema, BUN/SCr, K+; **Notes:** Can be use in patients intolerant to ACEI (due to cough); just as likely as ACEI to cause ↑ K+ and ↑ SCr.

irinotecan (Camptosar) **Uses:** Metastatic colorectal CA; **Class:** enzyme inhibitors; **Preg:** D; **CIs:** Hypersensitivity; Pregnancy; **ADRs:** dizziness, HA, insomnia, cough, dyspnea, edema, vasodilation, DIARRHEA, ↑ LFTS, abdominal pain/cramping, anorexia, constipation, dyspepsia, flatulence, N/V, stomatitis, alopecia, rash, dehydration, anemia, leukopenia, neutropenia, thrombocytopenia, ↓ wt, back pain, chills, fever; **Interactions:** ↑ toxicity/effects with fluorouracil, atazanavir, azole antifungals, erythromycin, isoniazid, or verapamil; Laxatives ↑ diarrhea; ↓ effects with St. John's wort, carbamazepine, phenobarbital, phenytoin, or rifampin; **Dose:** *IV: Adults: Single-agent treatment*—125 mg/m^2 once weekly × 4 wk. *Once-every-3-wk schedule*—350 mg/m^2 q 3 wk. *IV: Adults: Combination treatment with fluorouracil: Regimen 1*—125 mg/m^2 once weekly × 4 wk; *Regimen 2*—180 mg/m^2 q 2 wk × 3 doses; *Hepatic Impairment IV: Adults: Bilirubin 1–2 mg/dl—100 mg/m^2*; **Availability:** *Inject:* 20 mg/ml; **Monitor:** HR, BP, RR, CBC (with diff), BUN/SCr, LFTs, electrolytes, hydration status, S/S bleeding, diarrhea; **Notes:** Diarrhea may be life-threatening. Causes severe myelosuppression.

iron dextran (DexFerrum, InFeD) **Uses:** Iron deficiency anemia; **Class:** iron supplements; **Preg:** C; **CIs:** Anemia not due to iron deficiency; Hemolytic anemia; Hemochromatosis; Hypersensitivity; **ADRs:** HA, dizziness, ↓ BP, N/V, metallic taste, flushing, ANAPHYLAXIS, pain at IM site, fever; **Interactions:** Chloramphenicol may ↓ response; **Dose:** *IM, IV: Adults and Peds:* Test dose 25 mg. *IM, IV: Infants:* Test dose 12.5 mg. *IM, IV: Adults and Peds: >15 kg Iron deficiency anemia*—Total dose (ml) = 0.0442 (14.8–actual Hgb) × IBW in kg + (0.26 × IBW in kg). *IM, IV: Peds: 5–15 kg Iron deficiency anemia*—Total dose (ml) = 0.0442 (12–actual Hgb) × ABW in kg + (0.26 × ABW in kg) (max: 25 mg/day if <5 kg; 50 mg/day if 5–15 kg; and 100 mg/day if >15 kg or adult). *IM, IV: Adults: Blood loss*—Dose (mg) = (Blood loss [ml] × Hct). *IV: Neonates:* 0.2–1 mg/kg/day or 20 mg/kg/wk with epoetin alfa therapy; **Availability:** *Inject:* 50 mg/ml; **Monitor:** BP, HR, Hgb/Hct, retic count, serum ferritin, serum iron, TIBC, S/S anaphylaxis; **Notes:** May stain skin at inject site; use Z track technique for IM inject.

iron sucrose (Venofer) **Uses:** Iron deficiency anemia; **Class:** iron supplements; **Preg:** B; **CIs:** Anemia not due to iron deficiency; Hemochromatosis, hemosiderosis, or evidence of iron overload; Hypersensitivity; **ADRs:** HA, dizziness, ↓ BP, N/V/D, metallic taste, flushing, ANAPHYLAXIS, fever; **Interactions:** Chloramphenicol may ↓ response; **Dose:** *IV: Adults: HD patients*—100 mg during dialysis session for total cumulative dose of 1000 mg. *Non-dialysis patients*—200 mg on 5 different days within a 2 wk period to a total dose of 1000 mg *or* 500 mg on Day 1 and Day 14. *Peritoneal dialysis patients*—Total cumulative dose of 1000 mg in 3 divided doses, 14 days apart; **Availability:** *Inject:* 20 mg/ml; **Monitor:** BP, HR, Hgb/Hct, retic count, serum ferritin, serum iron, TIBC, S/S anaphylaxis; **Notes:** Give 100 mg by slow IV infusion over 2–5 minutes.

isoniazid (INH) **Uses:** TB prevention/treatment; **Class:** none assigned; **Preg:** C; **CIs:** Hypersensitivity; Acute liver disease; Previous hepatitis from INH; **ADRs:** psychosis, seizures, visual disturbances; HEPATITIS, N/V, rash, ↑ BG, blood dyscrasias, peripheral neuropathy, fever; **Interactions:** ↓ metabolism of phenytoin; Aluminum-containing antacids may ↓ absorption; ↑ hepatotoxicity/levels of carbamazepine and rifampin; ↓ levels/effects of ketoconazole; **Dose:** *PO: Adults:* 300 mg once or twice daily *or* 15 mg/kg (up to 900 mg) 2–3 ×/wk. *PO: Peds:* 10–20 mg/kg/day (max: 300 mg/day) *or* 20–40 mg/kg (up to 900 mg) 2–3 ×/wk. *Renal Impairment PO: Adults:* ↓ dose by 50% if CrCl <10 ml/min; **Availability**

(G): *Tabs:* 100 mg, 300 mg. *Syrup:* 50 mg/5 ml; **Monitor:** LFTs, sputum cultures, S/S neuropathy; **Notes:** Pyridoxine 10–50 mg/day recommended for patients prone to neuropathy.

isosorbide dinitrate/mononitrate (Dilatrate-SR, Isordil, Imdur, Ismo, Isochron, Monoket) **Uses:** Acute treatment of anginal attacks (SL only); Prophylactic management of angina pectoris; Chronic HF (to be used with hydralazine); **Class:** nitrates; **Preg:** C; **CIs:** Hypersensitivity; Concurrent use of sildenafil, vardenafil, or tadalafil; Volume-depleted patients; Right ventricular infarction; Hypertrophic cardiomyopathy; Pregnancy (may compromise maternal/fetal circulation) or lactation; Peds (safety not established); **ADRs:** dizziness, HA, ↓ BP, ↑ HR, syncope, N/V, flushing, tolerance; **Interactions:** ↑ risk of hypotension with sildenafil, tadalafil, or vardenafil (do not use these drugs within 24 hr of isosorbide dinitrate or mononitrate); Additive hypotension with antihypertensives, acute ingestion of alcohol, and phenothiazines; **Dose:** *SL Adults: Acute attack of angina pectoris*—2.5–5 mg; may be repeated q 5–10 min for 3 doses in 15–30 min. *Prophylaxis of angina pectoris*—2.5–5 mg given 15 min prior to activities known to provoke angina. *PO: Adults: Prophylaxis of angina pectoris*—Dinitrate: 5–20 mg bid–tid; usual MD is 10–40 mg qid (IR) or 40 mg q 8–12 hr (SR). Mononitrate (ISMO, Monoket): 5–20 mg bid given 7 hr apart. Mononitrate (Imdur): 30–60 mg/day; may ↑ to 120 mg/day (max: 240 mg/day). *HF*—Dinitrate: 20 mg tid–qid (with hydralazine); ↑ to target dose of 120–160 mg/day in 3–4 divided doses; **Availability (G):** *SL tabs (dinitrate):* 2.5, 5 mg. *Tabs (dinitrate):* 5, 10, 20, 30, 40 mg. *Tabs (Ismo, Monoket):* 10, 20 mg. *ER tabs (dinitrate):* 40 mg. *ER tabs (Imdur):* 30, 60, 120 mg. *SR caps (dinitrate):* 40 mg; **Monitor:** BP, HR, anginal pain; **Notes:** Do not crush, break, or chew ER/SR caps/tabs. SL tabs should be held under tongue until dissolved. Take last dose of day no later than 7 PM to prevent development of tolerance.

isradipine (DynaCirc, DynaCirc CR) **Uses:** HTN; Angina; **Class:** calcium channel blockers; **Preg:** C; **CIs:** Hypersensitivity; SBP <90; Severe hepatic/renal impairment; **ADRs:** dizziness, HA, edema, CP, ↓ BP, palpitations, ↑ HR, ↑ LFTs, N/V/D, rash; **Interactions:** CYP3A4 inhibitors may ↑ levels/toxicity, CYP3A4 inducers may ↓ levels/effects; ↓ antihypertensive effects with NSAIDs; Grapefruit juice ↑ serum levels and effect; **Dose:** *PO: Adults: IR*—2.5 mg bid; may ↑ q 2–4 wk (max: 10 mg/day). *CR* —5 mg/day; may ↑ q 2–4 wk (max: 10 mg/day); **Availability:** *Caps:* 2.5 mg, 5 mg. *CR tabs:* 5 mg, 10 mg; **Monitor:** BP, HR, BUN/SCr, LFTs; **Notes:** Taper off gradually. Do not crush, break, or chew CR tabs.

itraconazole (Sporanox) **Uses:** Histoplasmosis; Blastomycosis; Aspergillosis; Onychomycosis of the fingernail or toenail; Oral/esophageal candidiasis; **Class:** antifungals (azole); **Preg:** C; **CIs:** Previous sensitivity to other azole antifungals; Concurrent use of quinidine, dofetilide, pimozide, midazolam, triazolam, ergot alkaloids, simvastatin, or lovastatin; Severe renal/hepatic impairment; HF; **ADRs:** dizziness, fatigue, HA, HF, edema, HTN, N/V/D, ↑ LFTs, albuminuria, ED, photosensitivity, pruritus, rash, ↓ K+, fever; **Interactions:** ↑ risk of potentially fatal arrhythmias with quinidine, dofetilide, or pimozide (contraindicated); ↑ sedation with midazolam or triazolam (contraindicated); ↑ risk of myopathy with simvastatin or lovastatin (contraindicated); ↑ risk of vasoconstriction with ergot alkaloids (contraindicated); May ↑ levels of CYP3A4 substrates; CYP3A4 inhibitors may ↑ levels/toxicity; CYP3A4 inducers may ↓ levels/effects; Absorption ↓ by antacids, H_2 blockers, sucralfate, PPIs, and buffered didanosine (take 2 hr after itraconazole); **Dose:** *PO: Adults:* 100–400 mg/day. *PO: Peds:* 5 mg/kg/day; **Availability (G):** *Caps:* 100 mg. *Oral soln:* 10 mg/ml; **Monitor:** CBC, LFTs, K+, S/S infection, and HF; **Notes:** Do not give with antacids. Give caps with food and solution without food. Instruct patient to use sunscreen.

K

ketoconazole (Nizoral) **Uses:** Candidiasis; Chromomycosis; Coccidioidomycosis; Histoplasmosis; Paracoccidioidomycosis; **Class:** antifungals (azole); **Preg:** C; **CIs:** Previous sensitivity to azole antifungals; Concurrent use with ergot derivatives or triazolam; **ADRs:** dizziness, photophobia, ↑ LFTs, N/V/D, abdominal pain, thrombocytopenia, rash, gynecomastia; **Interactions:** CYP3A4 inhibitors may ↑ levels/toxicity, CYP3A4 inducers may ↓ levels/effects; May ↑ levels/toxicity of CYP1A2 substrates, CYP2C9 substrates, CYP2C19 substrates, CYP2D6 substrates, and CYP3A4 substrates; Absorption ↓ by antacids, histamine H_2 blockers, sucralfate, PPIs, and buffered didanosine; Sucralfate and INH ↓ bioavailability; ↑ hepatotoxicity with other hepatotoxic agents; **Dose:** *PO: Adults:* 200–400 mg/day. *PO: Peds:* 3.3–6.6 mg/kg/day; **Availability (G):** *Tabs:* 200 mg; **Monitor:** CBC, LFTs, S/S of infection; **Notes:** Do not give with antacids; give with food. Concurrent alcohol use can cause disulfiram-like reaction.

ketoprofen (Orudis) **Uses:** RA; OA; Pain/fever; **Class:** NSAIDs; **Preg:** B (1st tri); **CIs:** Hypersensitivity to aspirin or NSAIDs; Active bleeding; Perioperative pain from CABG surgery; CV disease; Severe renal disease; **ADRs:** HA, dizziness, tinnitus, edema, ↑ BP, GI BLEEDING, N/V/D, ↑ SCr, rash; **Interactions:** ↑ GI effects with aspirin and corticosteroids; ↓ effects of aspirin or antihypertensives; ↑ risk of bleeding with antiplatelet agents or anticoagulants; ↑ risk of nephrotoxicity with cyclosporine; ↑ levels of methotrexate and lithium; **Dose:** *PO: Adults: Anti-inflammatory*—IR: 50–75 mg tid–qid (max: 300 mg/day); ER: 200 mg/day. *Analgesic*—25–50 mg q 6–8 hr. *Renal Impairment PO: Adults:* Max dose of 100 mg/day if CrCl <25 ml/min; **Availability (G):** *Caps:* 50 mg, 75 mg. *ER caps:* 200 mg; **Monitor:** BP, Pain, temp, S/S GI upset/bleeding, BUN/SCr, LFTs, CBC; **Notes:** Avoid use in oliguria/anuria. Give with food. Do not crush, break, or chew ER caps.

ketorolac (Toradol) Uses: Pain; **Class:** NSAIDs; **Preg:** C; **CIs:** Hypersensitivity to aspirin or NSAIDs; Active bleeding; Perioperative pain from CABG surgery; CV disease; Severe renal disease; **ADRs:** HA, dizziness, tinnitus, edema, ↑ BP, GI BLEEDING, N/V/D, ↑SCr, rash; **Interactions:** ↑ adverse GI effects with aspirin and corticosteroids; ↓ effects of aspirin, or antihypertensives; ↑ risk of bleeding with antiplatelet agents or anticoagulants; ↑ nephrotoxicity with cyclosporine; ↑ levels of methotrexate and lithium; **Dose:** *PO: Adults: <65 yr* 20 mg, then 10 mg q 4–6 hr prn (max: 40 mg/day). *PO: Adults: ≥65 yr, <50 kg, or with renal impairment* 10 mg q 4–6 hr prn (max: 40 mg/day). *IV: IM Adults: <65 yr* 60 mg × 1 *or* 30 mg q 6 hr (max: 120 mg/day). *IV: IM Adults: ≥65 yr, <50 kg, or with renal impairment* 30 mg × 1 *or* 15 mg q 6 hr (max: 60 mg/day). *Renal Impairment IV, IM, PO: Adults:* ↓ dose by 50% in moderate renal impairment; **Availability (G):** *Tabs:* 10 mg. *Inject:* 15 mg/ml, 30 mg/ml; **Monitor:** Pain, S/S GI upset/bleeding, BUN/SCr, LFTs, CBC; **Notes:** Duration of therapy should not exceed 5 days.

labetalol (Trandate) Uses: HTN; **Class:** beta blockers; **Preg:** C; **CIs:** Hypersensitivity; Decompensated HF; Pulmonary edema, Cardiogenic shock; Bradycardia or ≥2nd-degree heart block (in absence of pacemaker); **ADRs:** fatigue, weakness, depression, dizziness, drowsiness, nightmares, blurred vision, bronchospasm, BRADYCARDIA, HF, PULMONARY EDEMA, ↓ BP, diarrhea, nausea, vomiting, ED, ↓ libido, ↑↓ BG; **Interactions:** ↑ risk of bradycardia with digoxin, diltiazem, verapamil, or clonidine; ↑ effects with other antihypertensives; ↑ risk of hypertensive crisis if concurrent clonidine discontinued; May alter the effectiveness of insulins or oral hypoglycemic agents, May ↓ the effects of $beta_1$ agonists (e.g., dopamine or dobutamine); **Dose:** *PO: Adults:* 100–400 mg bid (max: 2.4 g/day). *IV: Adults:* 20 mg (0.25 mg/kg), then 40–80 mg q 10 min prn (max: 300 mg total cumulative dose) *or* 2 mg/min infusion (range: 50–300 mg total cumulative dose). *PO: Peds:* 3–20 mg/kg/day in 2 divided doses. *IV: Peds:* 0.3–1 mg/kg/dose *or* 0.4–1 mg/kg/hr infusion (max: 3 mg/kg/hr); **Availability (G):** *Tabs:* 100, 200, 300 mg. *Inject:* 5 mg/ml; **Monitor:** HR, BP, ECG, S/S HF, edema, wt, BG (in DM); **Notes:** Abrupt withdrawal may cause life-threatening arrhythmias, hypertensive crises, or myocardial ischemia. May mask S/S of hypoglycemia (esp. tachycardia) in DM.

lactulose (Chronulac, Enulose, Kristalose) Uses: Constipation; PSE; **Class:** osmotic diuretics; **Preg:** B; **CIs:** Galactosemia; **ADRs:** abdominal discomfort, flatulence, N/V/D, ↑ BG; **Interactions:** ↓ effects with PO neomycin, laxatives, and antacids; **Dose:** *PO: Adults: Diarrhea*—15-60 ml/day in 1–2 divided doses. *PSE*—30–45 ml tid–qid; may be given q 1–2 hr initially to induce laxation, titrate dose to 2–3 soft stools. *PO: Peds: Diarrhea*—7.5 ml/day. *PSE*—40–90 ml/day divided tid–qid. *PO: Infants: PSE*—2.5–10 ml/day divided tid-qid. *Rect: Adults: PSE*—300 ml diluted with 700 ml water or NS administered as a retention enema q 4–6 hr; **Availability (G):** *Syrup:* 10 g/15 ml. *Packets (Kristalose):* 10 g, 20 g (equal to 30 ml liquid lactulose); **Monitor:** BP, K+, BG (in DM), stools, fluid status, mental status, serum ammonia; **Notes:** May mix syrup with juice, water, milk, carbonated beverages. Diarrhea may indicate overdosage.

lamivudine (Epivir, Epivir HBV, 3TC) **Uses:** HIV (with other antiretrovirals); HBV; **Class:** nucleoside reverse transcriptase inhibitors; **Preg:** C; **CIs:** Hypersensitivity; Impaired renal/hepatic function; Peds with a history of pancreatitis; **ADRs:** SEIZURES, fatigue, HA, insomnia, cough, PANCREATITIS, N/V/D, ↑ LFTs, rash, neutropenia, musculoskeletal pain, neuropathy; **Interactions:** Trimethoprim/sulfamethoxazole ↑ levels; ↑ risk of pancreatitis with other drugs causing pancreatitis; ↑ risk of neuropathy with other drugs causing neuropathy; Concurrent use with tenofovir and abacavir may lead to virologic nonresponse; **Dose:** *PO: Adults: HIV*—150 mg bid (or 4 mg/kg bid if <50 kg) or 300 mg/day. *HBV*—100 mg/day. *PO: Peds: HIV*—4 mg/kg bid (max: 300 mg/day). *HBV*—≥2yr: 3 mg/kg/day (max: 100 mg/day). *Renal Impairment PO: Adults:* ↓ dose if CrCl <50 ml/min; **Availability:** *Tabs:* 100 mg (HBV), 150 mg, 300 mg. *Oral soln:* 5 mg/ml (HBV), 10 mg/ml; **Monitor:** CD4 count, viral load, LFTs, amylase, lipase, CBC, bilirubin, S/S pancreatitis and neuropathy; **Notes:** Do not substitute Epivir for Epivir HBV. Not to be used as monotherapy for HIV.

L

lamotrigine (Lamictal) **Uses:** Seizures; Lennox-Gastaut syndrome; Bipolar disorder; **Class:** anticonvulsants; **Preg:** C; **CIs:** Previous sensitivity or rash to lamotrigine; **ADRs:** ataxia, dizziness, HA, insomnia, blurred vision, nystagmus, rhinitis, N/V, dysmenorrhea, rash, back pain; **Interactions:** Carbamazepine, phenobarbital, phenytoin, oral contraceptives, and primidone ↓ levels; Concurrent use with valproic acid ↑ lamotrigine levels and ↓ valproic acid levels; **Dose:** *PO: Adults and Peds: >12 yr (Seizures) Patients taking enzyme-inducing anticonvulsants (without valproic acid)*—50 mg/day × 2 wk, then 50 mg bid × 2 wk; then ↑ by 100 mg/day weekly to 150–250 mg bid (max: 500 mg/day). *Patients taking regimen containing valproic acid*—25 mg every other day × 2 wk, then 25 mg/day × 2 wk; then ↑ by 25–50 mg/day q 1–2 wk to 50–200 mg bid (max: 400 mg/day). *Patients taking other anti-epileptic drugs*—25 mg/day × 2 wk, then 50 mg/day × 2 wk, then ↑ by 50 mg/day weekly to 225–375 mg/day. *PO: Peds: 2–12 yr (Seizures) Patients taking enzyme-inducing anticonvulsants without valproic acid*—0.6 mg/kg/day in 2 divided doses × 2 wk, then 1.2 mg/kg/day × 2 wk, then ↑ by 1.2 mg/kg/day q 1–2 wk to 5–15 mg/kg/day (400 mg/day). *Patients taking regimen containing valproic acid*—0.15 mg/kg/day in 1–2 divided doses × 2 wk, then 0.3 mg/kg/day × 2 wk, then ↑ by 0.3 mg/kg/day q 1–2 wk to 1–5 mg/kg/day (max: 200 mg/day). *Patients taking other anti-epileptic drugs*—0.3 mg/kg/day in 1–2 divided doses × 2 wk, then 0.6 mg/kg/day × 2 wk, then ↑ by 0.6 mg/kg/day q 1–2 wk to 9–15 mg/kg day (max: 300 mg/day). *PO: Adults: ≥16 yr (Seizures) Conversion to lamotrigine monotherapy*—50 mg/day × 2 wk, then 100 mg/day × 2 wk, then ↑ by 100 mg/day q 1–2 wk to 300–500 mg/day; when target level reached, wean other antiepileptics over 4 wk. *PO: Adults: (Bipolar Disorder) Patients not taking valproic acid or enzyme-inducing anticonvulsants*—25 mg/day × 2 wk, then 50 mg/day × 2 wk, then 100 mg/day × 1 wk, then 200 mg/day. *Patients taking valproic acid*—25 mg every other day × 2 wk, then 25 mg/day × 2 wk, then 50 mg/day × 1 wk, then 100 mg/day. *Patients taking enzyme inducers without valproic acid*—50 mg/day × 2 wk, then 100 mg/day × 2 wk, then 200 mg/day × 1 wk, then 300 mg/day × 1 wk, then 400 mg/day; **Availability (G):** *Tabs:* 25, 100, 150, 200 mg. *Chew tabs:* 2, 5, 25 mg; **Monitor:** Seizure frequency, mood, LFTs, lamotrigine levels (range: 1–5 mcg/ml), rash; **Notes:** Discontinue therapy at first sign of rash. Round doses down to nearest whole tab. Do not discontinue abruptly.

lansoprazole (Prevacid) **Uses:** Esophagitis, PUD *H. pylori* eradication, GERD; Hypersecretory conditions; **Class:** proton pump inhibitors; **Preg:** B; **CIs:** Hypersensitivity; Severe hepatic impairment; **ADRs:** dizziness, HA, N/V/D, abdominal pain, rash; **Interactions:** Sucralfate ↓ absorption; ↓ absorption of ketoconazole, itraconazole, ampicillin, iron, and digoxin; ↑ risk of bleeding with warfarin; **Dose:** *PO: Adults and Peds: ≥12 yr PUD*—15–30 mg/day; *H. pylori eradication*—30 mg bid–tid. *GERD*—15 mg/day. *Esophagitis*—15 mg/day. *Hypersecretory conditions*—60–180 mg/day. *PO: Peds:* 0.5–1.6 mg/kg/day or 7.5–30 mg/day; **Availability:** *Caps:* 15, 30 mg. *SoluTabs:* 15, 30 mg. *Packets:* 15, 30 mg; **Monitor:** Hgb/Hct, LFTs, BUN/SCr, S/S abdominal pain/GI bleeding; **Notes:** Capsule contents may be mixed in juice for NG use. Mix in Na bicarbonate for NG use.

L

lanthanum carbonate (Fosrenol) **Uses:** Hyperphosphatemia in ESRD; **Class:** phosphate binders; **Preg:** C; **CIs:** None; **ADRs:** N/V/D; **Interactions:** None noted; **Dose:** *PO: Adults:* 750–1500 mg/day in divided doses with meals; titrate up q 2–3 wk up to 3750 mg/day to an acceptable serum PO_4 level; **Availability:** *Chew tabs:* 500, 750, 1000 mg; **Monitor:** Serum PO_4; **Notes:** Give with meals. Chew tabs, do not swallow whole.

lapatinib (Tykerb) **Uses:** HER2+ metastatic breast CA; **Class:** enzyme inhibitors, kinase inhibitors; **Preg:** D; **CIs:** Pregnancy; **ADRs:** fatigue, QT interval prolongation, INTERSTITIAL LUNG DISEASE, pneumonitis, ↓ LVEF, N/V/D, ↑ LFTs, palmar-plantar erythrodysesthesia, rash, extremity pain; **Interactions:** ↑ levels/effects with CYP3A4 inhibitors; ↓ levels/effects with CYP3A4 inducers; **Dose:** *PO: Adults:* 1250 mg daily × 21 days. *Hepatic Impairment PO: Adults: Severe hepatic impairment*—750 mg/day; **Availability:** *Tabs:* 250 mg; **Monitor:** CXR, RR, LFTs, ECG, LVEF, electrolytes; **Notes:** Manage diarrhea promptly. Give 1 hr ac or pc. Consider dose ↓ with strong CYP3A4 inhibitors or gradual dose ↑ with CYP3A4 inducers.

leflunomide (Arava) **Uses:** RA; **Class:** dmards; **Preg:** X; **CIs:** Hypersensitivity; Pregnancy; **ADRs:** HA, dizziness, respiratory tract infection, HTN, N/V/D, HEPATOTOXICITY, stomatitis, UTI, alopecia, rash, ↓ wt, tenosynovitis; **Interactions:** Cholestyramine ↓ levels of active metabolite; ↑ risk of hepatotoxicity and bone marrow suppression with methotrexate; Rifampin ↑ levels of the active metabolite; ↑ effects of warfarin; Live-virus vaccines ↑ infection risk; **Dose:** *PO: Adults: RA*—100 mg/day × 3 days, then 20 mg/day; **Availability:** *Tabs:* 10 mg, 20 mg, 100 mg; **Monitor:** CBC, LFTs, albumin, wt, S/S infection; **Notes:** ↓ dose to 10 mg/day if intolerant or if LFTs >2 × but <3 × ULN. If LFTs >3× ULN, discontinue therapy.

lepirudin (Refludan) **Uses:** Anticoagulation in patients with HIT; **Class:** thrombin inhibitors; **Preg:** B; **CIs:** Hypersensitivity; Patients at ↑ risk for bleeding; **ADRs:** BLEEDING, bronchospasm, ALLERGIC REACTIONS; **Interactions:** ↑ risk of bleeding with antiplatelets, thrombolytics, or other anticoagulants; **Dose:** *IV: Adults:* 0.4 mg/kg bolus (max: 44 mg) over 15–20 sec, then 0.15 mg/kg/hr infusion (max: 16.5 mg/hr); adjust according to aPTT (do not exceed max infusion rate of 0.21 mg/kg/hr without checking for coagulation abnormalities). *Renal Impairment IV: Adults:* ↓ dose if CrCl <60 ml or SCr >1.5 mg/dl; **Availability:** *Inject:* 50 mg; **Monitor:** BP, HR, aPTT, CBC, BUN/SCr, LFTs, S/S of bleeding; **Notes:** Do not use if CrCl <15 ml/min (ARF or dialysis patients).

letrozole (Femara) **Uses:** Metastatic breast CA; **Class:** aromatase inhibitors; **Preg:** D; **CIs:** Hypersensitivity; Pregnancy; Severe hepatic impairment; **ADRs:** fatigue, HA, cough, dyspnea, CP, edema, HTN, N/V/D, anorexia, alopecia, hot flashes, rash, ↑ Ca++, ↑ cholesterol, ↓ wt, musculoskeletal pain, ↓ BMD, fractures; **Interactions:** ↑ levels/effects of dexmedetomidine and ifosfamide; **Dose:** *PO: Adults*—2.5 mg/day. *Hepatic Impairment PO: Adults: Severe hepatic impairment*—2.5 mg every other day; **Availability:** *Tabs:* 2.5 mg; **Monitor:** CBC, cholesterol, electrolytes, LFTs, BUN/SCr, BMD; **Notes:** Do not use in premenopausal women; Ca++ and vitamin D supplementation recommended.

leucovorin calcium (folinic acid) **Uses:** Colorectal CA (with 5-FU); Prevent toxicity from folic acid antagonists; Folic acid deficiency (when PO therapy not possible or working); **Class:** folic acid analogues; **Preg:** C; **CIs:** Pernicious anemia; **ADRs:** thrombocytosis, allergic reactions (rash, urticaria, wheezing); **Interactions:** ↓ effects of barbiturates, phenytoin, or primidone; ↓ effects of trimethoprim/sulfamethoxazole; ↑ effects/toxicity of fluorouracil; **Dose:** *PO: Adults and*

Peds: Folic acid antagonist overdosage—2–15 mg/day × 3 days *or* 5 mg q 3 days until blood counts are normal. *IM: Adults and Peds: Folate-deficient megaloblastic anemia*—1 mg/day. *Dihydrofolate reductase-deficient megaloblastic anemia*—3–6 mg/day. *PO, IM, IV: Adults and Peds: Rescue dose*—10 mg/m^2 × 1 dose, then 10–15 mg/m^2 q 6 hr until MTX level <0.05 micromole/L; may need to ↑ to 20–100 mg/m^2 q 6 hr if MTX level still elevated after 48–72 hrs; **Availability (G):** *Tabs:* 5, 10, 15, 25 mg. *Inject:* 10 mg/ml; **Monitor:** MTX levels, urine pH, BUN/SCr, Hgb/Hct, S/S allergic reactions; **Notes:** Give within 24 hr of MTX therapy.

leuprolide (Eligard, Lupron, Viadur) Uses: Advanced prostate CA; Central precocious puberty; Endometriosis; Uterine fibroids; **Class:** hormones, gonadotropin-releasing hormones; **Preg:** X; **CIs:** Hypersensitivity to LHRH (GnRH); Pregnancy/lactation; Undiagnosed vag bleeding; **ADRs:** dizziness, HA, insomnia, PE, MI, angina, weakness/paresthesia, edema, N/V/D, GI BLEEDING, ↑ LFTs, ↓ testicular size, testicular/prostate pain, rash, breast tenderness, urinary obstruction, anemia, ↓ BMD, ↑ PO_4, ↓ K+, body odor, epistaxis; **Interactions:** ↑ antineoplastic effects with megestrol or flutamide; **Dose:** *Subcut: Adults: Prostate CA*—Lupron: 1 mg/day; Eligard: 7.5 mg q mo *or* 22.5 mg q 3 mo *or* 30 mg q 4 mo *or* 45 mg q 6 mo. *IM: Adults: Prostate CA*—Lupron Depot: 7.5 mg q mo *or* 22.5 mg q 3 mo *or* 30 mg q 4 mo. *Endometriosis*—Lupron Depot: 3.75 mg/mo × 6 mo *or* 11.25 mg q 3 mo × 2 doses. *Fibroids*—Lupron Depot: 3.75 mg/month × 3 mo *or* 11.25 mg × 1 dose. *Implant: Adults: Prostate CA*—One implant (65 mg) q 12 mo. *Subcut: Peds: Central precocious puberty*—Lupron: 50 mcg/kg/day; may ↑ by 10 mcg/kg/day prn based on response. *IM: Peds: Central precocious puberty*—Lupron Depot Ped: 0.3 mg/kg/dose q 28 days as depot inject (min dose: 7.5 mg); **Availability (G):** *Soln for inject (Lupron):* 5 mg/ml. *Depot inject (Lupron Depot):* 3.75 mg, 7.5 mg. *Depot inject (Lupron Depot-Ped):* 7.5 mg, 11.25 mg, 15 mg. *Depot inject (Lupron Depot–3 mo):* 11.25 mg, 22.5 mg. *Depot inject (Lupron Depot–4 mo):* 30 mg. *Depot inject (Eligard):* 7.5 mg, 22.5 mg, 30 mg, 45 mg. *Implant (Viadur):* 65 mg; **Monitor:** LH/FSH, serum testosterone/estradiol, PSA, BMD, LFTs, BUN/SCr, electrolytes, S/S of urinary obstruction and weakness/paresthesias; **Notes:** Weakness/paresthesias can be a sign of spinal cord compression in prostate CA patients.

levalbuterol (Xopenex) Uses: Bronchospasm due to reversible airway disease; **Class:** adrenergics; **Preg:** C; **CIs:** Hypersensitivity to levalbuterol or albuterol; **ADRs:** anxiety, dizziness, HA, nervousness, cough, paradoxical bronchospasm, nasal edema, ↑ HR, dyspepsia, ↑ BG, ↓ K+, tremor; **Interactions:** TCAs, sympathomimetics, inhaled anesthetics, or MAOIs may ↑ risk of CV reactions; Beta blockers ↓ effects; ↑ risk of hypokalemia from medications that deplete K+; ↓ digoxin levels; **Dose:** *Inhaln: Adults and Peds: >12 yr:* 0.63–1.25 mg via nebulization tid *or*

2 puffs via MDI q 4–6 hr. *Inhaln: Peds 6–11 yr:* 0.31 mg via nebulization tid (max: 0.63 mg tid); **Availability:** *Inhaln soln:* 0.31 mg/3 ml, 0.63 mg/3 ml, 1.25 mg/3 ml. *MDI:* 45 mcg/actuation; **Monitor:** BP, HR, K+, BG, PFTs, relief of bronchospasm; **Notes:** Does not require dilution prior to nebulization; shake MDI well before use.

levetiracetam (Keppra) Uses: Seizures; **Class:** anticonvulsants; **Preg:** C; **CIs:** Hypersensitivity; **ADRs:** <u>dizziness</u>, <u>weakness</u>, behavioral abnormalities (peds > adults), somnolence, leukopenia, coordination difficulties; **Interactions:** CNS depressants may ↑ toxicity; **Dose:** *PO: IV: Adults and Peds: ≥12 yr Myoclonic seizures*—500 mg bid, then ↑ by 1000 mg/day q 2 wk to 3000 mg/day. *PO, IV: Adults and Peds: ≥16 yr Partial-onset or tonic-clonic seizures*—500 mg bid, then ↑ by 1000 mg/day q 2 wk to 3000 mg/day. *PO: Peds: 4–15 yr Partial-onset seizures*—10 mg/kg bid; may ↑ by 20 mg/kg/day q 2 wk (max: 60 mg/kg/day). *PO: Peds: 6–15 yrs Tonic-clonic seizures*—10 mg/kg bid; may ↑ by 20 mg/kg/day q 2 wk (max: 60 mg/kg/day). *Renal Impairment PO: Adults:* ↓ dose if CrCl <80 ml/min; **Availability:** *Tabs:* 250, 500, 750, 1000 mg. *Oral soln:* 100 mg/ml. *Inject:* 100 mg/ml; **Monitor:** Seizure activity, S/S behavioral abnormalities, LFTs, CBC; **Notes:** Infuse IV over 15 min. Discontinue gradually to minimize seizure risk.

levofloxacin (Iquix, Levaquin, Quixin) Uses: Treatment of respiratory tract infections, UTIs, and skin/skin structure infections due to *S. aureus*, *S. pneumoniae*, *E. faecalis*, *H. flu*, and enteric GNRs; Post-exposure treatment of inhalational anthrax; **Ophth:** Conjunctivitis, corneal ulceration; **Class:** fluoroquinolones; **Preg:** C; **CIs:** Prior sensitivity to levofloxacin or other FQs; Peds <18 yr; **ADRs:** SEIZURES, confusion, dizziness, HA, insomnia, ARRHYTHMIAS, QT interval prolongation, PSEUDOMEMBRANOUS COLITIS, abdominal pain, hepatotoxicity, N/V/D, vaginitis, photosensitivity, rash, ↑↓ BG, phlebitis at IV site, peripheral neuropathy, tendon rupture, ANAPHYLAXIS; **Interactions:** ↑ risk of QT interval prolongation with other QT_C-prolonging drugs; Use with antacids, Ca++ supplements, iron salts, zinc, didanosine, or sucralfate may ↓ absorption; May ↑ the effects of warfarin; May ↑ risk of hypoglycemia with sulfonylureas; May ↑ risk of seizures when used with NSAIDs; ↑ risk of tendon rupture with corticosteroids; Absorption ↓ by dairy products; **Dose:** *PO, IV: Adults:* 250–750 mg/day. *Anthrax*—500 mg/day × 60 days. *Ophth: Adults and Peds: Conjunctivitis*—1–2 gtt q 2 hr up to 8 ×/day × 2 days then q 4 hr up to qid × 5 days. *Corneal ulcer*—1–2 gtt q 30 min–2 hr while awake and at bedtime × 3 days. *Renal Impairment PO, IV: Adults:* ↓ dose if CrCl <50 ml/min; **Availability:** *Tabs:* 250, 500, 750 mg. *Oral soln:* 25 mg/ml. *Inject:* 25 mg/ml. *Ophth soln:* 0.5%, 1.5%; **Monitor:** BP, HR, temp, sputum, U/A, CBC, BG (in patients with DM), tendon pain; **Notes:** Space doses 2 hr apart from products/foods containing Ca++, Mg++, aluminum, iron, or zinc. Give IV over 60–90 min. Advise patient to use sunscreen.

levothyroxine (Levothroid, Levoxyl, Synthroid, Tirosint, Unithroid) **Uses:** Thyroid supplementation; **Class:** thyroid preparations; **Preg:** A; **CIs:** Recent MI; Hyperthyroidism; Uncorrected adrenal disorders; **ADRs:** HA, insomnia, irritability, ARRHYTHMIAS, angina, ↑ HR, abdominal cramps, diarrhea, vomiting, hyperhidrosis, hyperthyroidism, menstrual irregularities, ↓ wt, heat intolerance; **Interactions:** ↓ absorption with bile acid sequestrants; ↑ effects of warfarin; ↓ effects of oral hypoglycemics; Estrogen may ↑ levothyroxine requirements; ↑ BP and HR with ketamine; **Dose:** *PO: Adults: Hypothyroidism*—50 mcg/day; may ↑ q 2–3 wk by 25 mcg/day up to 1.7 mcg/kg/day. *PO: Geriatric Patients:* 12.5–25 mcg/day; may ↑ q 6–8 wk up to 75 mcg/day. *PO: Peds: >12 yr:* 2–3 mcg/kg/day. *PO: Peds: 6–12 yr:* 4–5 mcg/kg/day. *PO: Peds: 1–5 yr:* 5–6 mcg/kg/day. *PO: Peds: 6–12 mo:* 6–8 mcg/kg/day. *PO: Infants: 3–6 mo:* 8–10 mcg/kg/day. *PO: Infants: 0–3 mo:* 10–15 mcg/kg/day. *IM, IV: Adults and Peds: Hypothyroidism*—Give 50% of oral dose. *Myxedema coma/stupor*—200–500 mcg IV; then 100–300 mcg on the next day if needed; **Availability (G):** *Tabs:* 13, 25, 50, 75, 88, 100, 112, 125, 137, 150, 175, 200, 300 mcg; *Inject:* 200, 500 mcg; **Monitor:** BP, HR, wt, TFTs; **Notes:** Dilute IV to 100 mcg/ml and give at a rate of 100 mcg/min.

lidocaine (Anestacon, Lidoderm, LidoPen, L-M-X 4, L-M-X 5, Solarcaine Aloe Extra Burn Relief, Xylocaine, Xylocaine Viscous, Zilactin-L) **Uses:** **IV:** Ventricular arrhythmias, **IM:** Self-injected or when IV unavailable (during transport to hospital facilities); **Local:** Infiltration/mucosal/top anesthetic; **Patch:** Pain due to post-herpetic neuralgia; **Class:** antiarrhythmics (class Ib); **Preg:** B; **CIs:** Hypersensitivity to lidocaine or other amide type anesthetics; ≥2nd-degree heart block (in absence of pacemaker); Peds (safety not established for transdermal patch); **ADRs:** SEIZURES, confusion, drowsiness, blurred vision, dizziness, nervousness, slurred speech, tremor, ARRHYTHMIAS, ↓ HR, heart block, N/V, bronchospasm, stinging, burning sensation, contact dermatitis, erythema, ANAPHYLAXIS; **Interactions:** Applies to systemic use; CYP2D6 inhibitors and CYP3A4 inhibitors may ↑ levels/toxicity; CYP3A4 inducers may ↓ levels/effects; May ↑ levels of CYP1A2 substrates, CYP2D6 substrates, and CYP3A4 substrates; **Dose:** *IV: Adults: Antiarrhythmic*—1–1.5 mg/kg bolus; may repeat doses of 0.5–0.75 mg/kg q 5–10 min up to a total dose of 3 mg/kg; may then start continuous infusion of 1–4 mg/min. *ET: Adults: Antiarrhythmic*—Give 2–2.5 × the IV LD down the ET tube, followed by a 10-ml NS flush. *IM: Adults and Peds: ≥50 kg Antiarrhythmic*—300 mg (4.5 mg/kg); may be repeated in 60–90 min. *Local Infiltration: Adults and Peds:* Infiltrate affected area as needed. *Topical: Adults:* Apply 2–3 ×/day. *Mucosal: Adults: For anesthetizing oral surfaces*—20 mg as 2 sprays/quadrant (max: 30 mg/quadrant) may be used. 15 ml of the viscous soln may be used q 3 hr for oral or pharyngeal pain. *For anesthetizing the female urethra*—3–5 ml of the jelly or 20 mg as 2% soln may be used. *For* *anesthetizing the male urethra*—5–10 ml of the jelly or 5–15 ml of 2% soln may be used before catheterization or 30 ml of jelly before cystoscopy or similar procedures. *Patch: Adults:* Up to 3 patches may be applied once for up to 12 hr in any 24-hr period; consider smaller areas of application in geriatric or debilitated patients. *IV: Peds: Antiarrhythmic*—1 mg/kg bolus (max: 100 mg), followed by 20–50 mcg/kg/min continuous infusion (range: 20–50 mcg/kg/min); may administer second bolus of 0.5–1 mg/kg if delay between bolus and continuous infusion. *ET: Peds: Antiarrhythmic*—Give 2–3 mg/kg down the ET tube followed by a 5 ml NS flush; **Availability (G):** *Autoinjector for IM inject:* 300 mg/3 ml. *Direct IV inject:* 10 mg/ml (1%), 20 mg/ml (2%). *For IV admixture:* 100 mg/ml (10%). *Premixed solution for IV infusion:* 4 mg/ml (0.4%), 8 mg/ml (0.8%). *Inject for local infiltration/nerve block:* 0.5%, 1%, 2%, 4%. *Cream:* 4% OTC. *Gel:* 0.5%OTC, 2.5%OTC. *Jelly:* 2%. *Liquid:* 5%. *Oint:* 5%. *Transdermal system:* 5% patch. *Soln:* 4%. *Spray:* 10%. *Viscous soln:* 2%; **Monitor:** BP, HR, RR, ECG, serum lidocaine levels (IV use >24 hr); degree of numbness (anesthetic use); **Notes:** Topical solns may also be used to anesthetize mucous membranes of the larynx, trachea, or esophagus. Ensure that gag reflex is intact before allowing patient to drink or eat after using in the mouth or throat. Therapeutic serum lidocaine levels: 1.5–5 mcg/ml. **High Alert:** Lidocaine is readily absorbed through mucous membranes. Inadvertent overdosage of lidocaine jelly and spray has resulted in patient harm or death from neurologic and/or cardiac toxicity. Do not exceed recommended dosages. Apply patch to intact skin to cover the most painful area. Patch may be cut to smaller sizes with scissors before removing release liner. Clothing may be worn over patch. If irritation or burning sensation occurs during application, remove patch until irritation subsides. Wash hands after application; avoid contact with eyes. Dispose of used patch to avoid access by children or pets.

linezolid (Zyvox) Uses: Treatment of: Infections caused by VRE, Skin/skin structure infections, nosocomial pneumonia, or CAP caused by *S. aureus* (MSSA and MRSA) or *S. pneumoniae* (including MDRSP); **Class:** oxazolidinones; **Preg:** C; **CIs:** Hypersensitivity, Phenylketonuria (susp only); Concurrent or recent use (< 2 wk) of MAOIs; Concurrent use of MAOIs, SSRIs, TCAs, 5-HT_1 agonists, meperidine, sympathomimetics, or buspirone; **ADRs:** HA, insomnia, PSEUDOMEMBRANOUS COLITIS, N/V/D, ↑ LFTs, taste alteration, lactic acidosis, anemia, leukopenia, thrombocytopenia, optic neuropathy, peripheral neuropathy; **Interactions:** Linezolid has MAOI properties; may cause ↑ response to indirect-acting sympathomimetics, vasopressors, or dopaminergic agents; ↑ risk of serotonin syndrome with MAOIs, SSRIs, TCAs, 5-HT agonists, meperidine, or buspirone (should discontinue for 2 wk before initiating therapy); Because of MAOI properties, consumption of large amounts of foods or beverages containing tyramine should be avoided (↑ risk of pressor response); **Dose:** *PO, IV: Adults and Peds: ≥12 yr:* 600 mg q 12 hrs × 10-14 days. *PO, IV: Peds: <12 yr:* 10 mg/kg q 8–12 hr × 10–14 days; **Availability:** *Oral susp:* 20 mg/ml. *Tabs:* 400, 600 mg. *Inject:* 2 mg/ml; **Monitor:** BP, temp, CBC, cultures, vision (if therapy ≥3 mo); **Notes:** CBC should be performed weekly if therapy >2 wk or if receiving other myelosuppressive agents. IV = PO dose. Protect infusion from light.

lisinopril (Prinivil, Zestril) Uses: HTN; HF; Post-MI; **Class:** ACE inhibitors; **Preg:** C (1st tri), D (2nd and 3rd tri); **CIs:** Previous sensitivity/intolerance to ACEIs; **ADRs:** dizziness, cough, ↓ BP, ↑ SCr, ↑ K+, ANGIOEDEMA; **Interactions:** ↑ effects with other antihypertensives; ↑ risk of hyperkalemia with ARBs, K+ supplements, K+ salt substitutes, K+ sparing diuretics, or NSAIDs; NSAIDs may ↓ effectiveness; ↑ lithium levels; **Dose:** *PO: Adults: HTN*—5–40 mg/day. *CHF*—2.5–40 mg/day. *Post-MI*—5 mg/day × 2 days, then 10 mg/day. *PO: Peds: ≥6 yr HTN*—0.07 mg/kg/day (max: 5 mg/day) up to 0.6 mg/kg/day (max: 40 mg/day). *Renal Impairment PO: Adults:* ↓ dose if CrCl <30 ml/min; **Availability (G):** *Tabs:* 2.5, 5, 10, 20, 30, 40 mg; **Monitor:** BP, HR, wt, edema, BUN/SCr, K+; **Notes:** Correct volume depletion. Advise patients on S/S angioedema and instruct them to avoid K+ salt substitutes.

L

lithium (Lithobid) Uses: Bipolar disorders and mania; **Class:** none assigned; **Preg:** D; **CIs:** Pregnancy; Severe CV or renal disease; Sodium depletion or dehydration; **ADRs:** SEIZURES, fatigue, HA, ataxia, confusion, dizziness, psychomotor retardation, restlessness, stupor, aphasia, blurred vision, ARRHYTHMIAS, ECG changes, edema, ↓ BP, abdominal pain, anorexia, N/V/D, dry mouth, metallic taste, polyuria, glycosuria, DI, ↑ BUN/SCr, folliculitis, alopecia, rash, hypo/hyperthyroidism, goiter, ↑ BG, ↓ Na+, leukocytosis, ↑ wt, muscle weakness, tremor; **Interactions:** ↑ effects of neuromuscular blocking agents; ↑ toxicity with haloperidol and SSRIs; Diuretics, ACEIs, COX-2 inhibitors, losartan, TCAs, carbamazepine, phenytoin MAOIs, and NSAIDs may ↑ lithium levels/toxicity; **Dose:** *PO: Adults:* 900–2400 mg/day in 3–4 divided doses (IR) or bid (ER). *PO: Renal Impairment Adults:* ↓ dose if CrCl <50 ml/min; **Availability (G):** *Caps:* 150, 300, 600 mg. *Tabs:* 300 mg. *ER tabs:* 300, 450 mg. *Syrup:* 300 mg/5 ml; **Monitor:** BP, HR, lithium levels, mental status, BUN/SCr, Na+, BG, CBC, TFTs, I/Os; **Notes:** Therapeutic level 0.6–1.2 mEq/L. Low Na+ levels may ↑ toxicity. Do not crush or chew ER tabs.

loperamide (Imodium A-D) Uses: Acute/chronic diarrhea; **Class:** none assigned; **Preg:** B; **CIs:** Hypersensitivity; Acute dysentery, bacterial enterocolitis, acute ulcerative colitis; Abdominal pain without diarrhea; Peds <2 yr; **ADRs:** drowsiness, dizziness, constipation, abdominal pain/distention/discomfort, dry mouth, N/V, allergic reactions; **Interactions:** ↑ CNS depression with CNS depressants, alcohol, antihistamines, opioid analgesics, and sedative/hypnotics; **Dose:** *PO: Adults:* 4 mg × 1, then 2 mg after each loose stool (max: 16 mg/day). *PO: Peds: ≥2 yr:* For the 1st 24 hours: 1–2 mg bid–tid then 0.1 mg/kg/dose after each loose stool; **Availability (G):** *Tabs:* 2 mg[OTC]. *Caps:* 2 mg. *Liquid:* 1 mg/5 ml[OTC]; **Monitor:** Frequency of stools, fluid status, electrolytes; **Notes:** Do not use with diarrhea accompanied by fever or blood in stool.

lopinavir/ritonavir (Kaletra) **Uses:** HIV infection (with other antiretrovirals); **Class:** protease inhibitors; **Preg:** C; **CIs:** Prior sensitivity to lopinavir or ritonavir; Concurrent use of ergot derivatives, midazolam, pimozide, triazolam, rifampin, lovastatin, simvastatin, or St. John's wort; **ADRs:** HA, insomnia, weakness, PANCREATITIS, N/V/D, abdominal pain, taste aversion, rash; **Interactions:** Lopinavir is a substrate of CYP3A4. Ritonavir is a substrate of CYP2D6 and CYP3A4. Ritonavir is also an inhibitor of CYP2D6 and CYP3A4; CYP3A4 inhibitors and CYP2D6 inhibitors may ↑ levels; CYP3A4 inducers may ↓ levels; May ↑ levels of CYP2D6 substrates and CYP3A4 substrates; ↑ levels of ergotamine, ergonovine, dihydroergotamine, methylergonovine, midazolam, triazolam, pimozide, lovastatin, and simvastatin (contraindicated); Rifampin and St. John's wort ↓ levels (contraindicated); Nevirapine and efavirenz ↓ levels (when used together, use lopinavir/ritonavir BID); ↑ risk of bleeding with warfarin; ↑ tenofovir and indinavir levels (↓ indinavir dose); ↓ abacavir and zidovudine levels; ↑ levels of clarithromycin (↓ clarithromycin dose by 50–75%); ↑ levels of rifabutin (↓ rifabutin dose by 75%); ↑ risk of myopathy with atorvastatin or rosuvastatin; ↑ levels of fluticasone; consider alternative therapy; May ↓ levels of hormonal contraceptives; use alternative non-hormonal contraceptive; **Dose:** *PO: Adults and Peds: >40 kg Therapy-naive*—400/100 mg bid *or* 800/200 mg once daily. *Therapy-experienced*—400/100 mg bid. *Dosage with concomitant use of efavirenz, fosamprenavir, nelfinavir, or nevirapine*—Therapy-naive: 400/100 mg bid; Therapy-experienced: 600/150 mg (tab) *or* 533/133 mg (soln) bid. *Dosage with concomitant use of maraviroc or saquinavir*—400/100 mg bid. *PO: Peds: 15–40 kg:* 10 mg/kg lopinavir content bid. *PO: Peds: 7–15 kg:* 12 mg/kg lopinavir content bid; **Availability:** *Tabs:* 100 mg lopinavir/25 mg ritonavir, 200 mg lopinavir/50 mg ritonavir; *Soln:* 80 mg lopinavir/20 mg ritonavir per ml; **Monitor:** Viral load, CD4 count, BG, LFTs, bilirubin, amylase/lipase, lipids; **Notes:** Not to be used as monotherapy. Give solution with food. Tabs may be taken without regard to meals. Do not crush tabs.

loratadine (Alavert, Claritin, Tavist ND) **Uses:** Seasonal allergic rhinitis, Chronic idiopathic urticaria; **Class:** antihistamines; **Preg:** B; **CIs:** Hypersensitivity, Children <2 yr (safety not established); **ADRs:** confusion, drowsiness (rare), paradoxical excitation, blurred vision, dry mouth, GI upset, rash, ↑ wt; **Interactions:** MAOIs may ↑ effects; ↑ CNS depression may occur with other CNS depressants, including alcohol, antidepressants, opioid analgesics, and sedative/

hypnotics; **Dose:** *PO: Adults and Peds: ≥6 yr:* 10 mg/day. *PO: Peds: 2–5 yr:* 5 mg/day. *Renal Impairment PO: Adults:* ↓ dose if CrCl <30 ml/min. *Hepatic Impairment PO: Adults:* 10 mg every other day; **Availability (G):** *Rapidly disintegrating tabs:* 5, 10 mg. *Tabs:* 10 mg. *Chew tabs:* 5 mg. *Syrup:* 5 mg/5 ml; **Monitor:** Allergy symptoms, secretions; **Notes:** Disintegrating tabs may be taken with or without water.

lorazepam (Ativan) Uses: PO: Anxiety, N/V; **IV:** Status epilepticus, sedation, N/V; **Class:** benzodiazepines; **Preg:** D; **CIs:** Hypersensitivity (cross-sensitivity with other BZs may exist); Acute narrow-angle glaucoma; Severe hepatic/renal/pulmonary disease; Sleep apnea; Pregnancy/lactation; **ADRs:** sedation, amnesia, ataxia, confusion, HA, mental depression, slurred speech, blurred vision, APNEA, resp depression, CARDIAC ARREST, ↓ HR, ↓ BP, constipation, N/V/D, rash, physical/psychological dependence, tolerance; **Interactions:** ↑ CNS depression with alcohol, antidepressants, other BZs, antihistamines, and opioids; **Dose:** *PO: Adults: Anxiety/sedation*—1–10 mg in 2–3 divided doses. *Insomnia*—2–4 mg/day at bedtime. *N/V*—0.5–2 mg 30 min prior to chemotherapy; may repeat q 4 hr prn. *IV, IM: Adults: Preop sedation*—0.05 mg/kg. *N/V*—0.5–2 mg 30 min prior to chemotherapy; may repeat q 4 hr prn. *Status epilepticus*—4 mg × 1; may repeat after 10–15 min (max dose: 8 mg). *PO, IM, IV: Infants and Peds Anxiety/sedation*—0.02–0.1 mg/kg/dose (max: 2 mg/dose) q 4–8 hr. *Preop sedation*—0.02–0.09 mg/kg/dose. *N/V*—0.05 mg/kg/dose prior to chemotherapy (max dose: 2 mg), then q 6 hr prn. *Status epilepticus*—0.1 mg/kg (0.05 mg/kg in neonates); may repeat with 0.05 mg/kg (max dose: 4 mg); **Availability (G):** *Tabs:* 0.5, 1, 2 mg. *Oral soln:* 2 mg/ml. *Inject:* 2 mg/ml, 4 mg/ml; **Monitor:** BP, HR, RR, S/S CNS depression, seizure frequency, LFTs; **Notes:** Schedule IV controlled substance. Flumazenil is antidote. Elderly may require ↓ doses. Inject contains propylene glycol and benzyl alcohol. Max IV rate 2 mg/min.

losartan (Cozaar) Uses: HTN; Diabetic nephropathy in patients with type 2 DM; Stroke prevention in patients with HTN and LVH; **Class:** angiotensin II receptor antagonists; **Preg:** C (1st tri), D (2nd and 3rd tri); **CIs:** Hypersensitivity; Pregnancy/lactation; **ADRs:** fatigue, weakness, CP, edema, ↓ BP, cough, hypoglycemia, ↑ wt, diarrhea, anemia, nausea, ↑ SCr, ↑ K+, back pain, myalgia, ANGIOEDEMA; **Interactions:** ↑ effects with other antihypertensives; ↑ risk of hyperkalemia with ACEIs, K+ supplements, K+ salt substitutes, K+ sparing diuretics, or NSAIDs; NSAIDs may ↓ effectiveness; CYP2C9 inhibitors may ↑ levels/effects; CYP2C9 inducers may ↓ levels/effects; May ↑ levels/effects of CYP2C9 substrates; **Dose:** *PO: Adults: HTN*—25–100 mg/day. *Stroke prevention*—50 mg/day in combination with a thiazide diuretic (max: 100 mg/day). *Nephropathy*—50–100 mg/day. *PO: Peds: 6–16 yr:* 0.7 mg/kg/day (max: 50 mg/day). *Renal Impairment PO: Peds: 6–16 yr:*

L

Do not use if CrCl <30 ml/min; **Availability:** *Tabs:* 25, 50, 100 mg; **Monitor:** BP, HR, wt, edema, BUN/SCr, K+; **Notes:** Can be used in patients intolerant to ACEIs (due to cough); just as likely as ACEIs to cause ↑ K+ and ↑ SCr.

lovastatin (Altoprev, Mevacor) **Uses:** Hyperlipidemia; Primary prevention of CV disease; Slows progressions of coronary atherosclerosis in patients with CAD; **Class:** hmg coa reductase inhibitors; **Preg:** X; **CIs:** Hypersensitivity; Liver disease; Pregnancy/lactation; Concurrent use with itraconazole, ketoconazole, erythromycin, clarithromycin, protease inhibitors, or nefazodone; **ADRs:** HA, abdominal cramps, constipation, diarrhea, dyspepsia, flatulence, ↑ LFTs, nausea, rash, RHABDOMYOLYSIS, myalgia; **Interactions:** CYP3A4 inhibitors may ↑ levels/toxicity, CYP3A4 inducers may ↓ levels/effects, ↑ risk of myopathy with amiodarone, cyclosporine, gemfibrozil, erythromycin, clarithromycin, protease inhibitors, nefazodone, niacin (≥1 g/day), verapamil, and azole antifungals; May ↑ effects of warfarin; **Dose:** *PO: Adults:* 20–80 mg/day in 1–2 divided doses (max: 80 mg/day of IR; 60 mg/day of ER). *Dosing with concomitant meds*—Max dose of 20 mg/day with fibrates, niacin (>1 g/day), cyclosporine, or danazol; max dose of 40 mg/day (IR) or 20 mg/day (ER) with amiodarone or verapamil. *PO: Peds: >10 yr:* 10–40 mg/day (IR). *Renal Impairment PO: Adults:* ↓ dose if CrCl <30 ml/min; **Availability (G):** *Tabs:* 10, 20, 40 mg. *ER tabs:* 20, 40, 60 mg; **Monitor:** Lipid panel, LFTs, CK (if symptoms); **Notes:** Discontinue if LFTs persistently >3 × ULN. Give IR tabs with meals; give ER tabs at bedtime. Instruct patient to avoid grapefruit juice. Do not crush or chew ER tabs.

magnesium hydroxide/aluminum hydroxide (Alamag, Rulox) **Uses:** Indigestion/heartburn; **Class:** antacids; **Preg:** C; **CIs:** Severe abdominal pain of unknown cause; Renal failure (CrCl <30 ml/min); **ADRs:** constipation, diarrhea, ↑ Mg++, ↓ PO_4; **Interactions:** ↓ absorption of tetracyclines, ketoconazole, itraconazole, iron salts, FQs, bisphosphonates, and isoniazid (separate by ≥2 hr); **Dose:** *PO: Adults and Peds: ≥12 yr:* 5–30 ml or 1–2 tabs 1–3 hr pc and at bedtime; **Availability (G):** *Chew Tabs:* 300 mg aluminum hydroxide/150 mg Mg hydroxide[OTC]. *Susp:* 225 mg aluminum hydroxide/200 mg Mg hydroxide per 5 ml, 500 mg aluminum hydroxide/500 mg Mg hydroxide per 5 ml; **Monitor:** Heartburn, indigestion, PO_4, Mg, BUN/SCr; **Notes:** Do not take within 2 hr of taking other meds.

magnesium oxide (Mag-Ox 400, Uro-Mag) **Uses:** Treatment/prevention of hypomagnesemia; **Class:** minerals electrolytes; **Preg:** B; **CIs:** Hypermagnesemia; Anuria; Active labor or within 2 hr of delivery (unless used for preterm labor); **ADRs:** diarrhea, flushing, sweating; **Interactions:** Potentiates neuromuscular blocking agents;

May ↓ absorption of FQs, bisphosphonates, and tetracyclines; **Dose:** *PO: Adults:* 400–800 mg/day (Mag-Ox 400) *or* 140–280 mg tid (Uro-Mag). *PO: Peds:* 10–20 mg/kg elemental Mg per dose qid; **Availability (G):** *Tabs:* 400 mg (242 mg Mg)OTC. *Caps:* 140 mg (84.5 mg Mg)OTC; **Monitor:** S/S hypo/hypermagnesemia, Mg, BUN/SCr; **Notes:** Do not take within 2 hr of taking other meds.

magnesium sulfate (IV) (NO TRADE) **Uses:** Treatment/prevention of hypomagnesemia; Anticonvulsant associated with severe eclampsia, pre-eclampsia, or acute nephritis; Torsades de pointes; **Class:** minerals electrolytes; **Preg:** A; **CIs:** Hypermagnesemia; Hypocalcemia; Anuria; Heart block; Active labor or within 2 hr of delivery (unless used for preterm labor); Renal insufficiency; **ADRs:** drowsiness, ↓ RR, ARRHYTHMIAS, ↓ HR, ↓ BP, diarrhea, muscle weakness, flushing, sweating, hypothermia; **Interactions:** Potentiates CCBs and neuromuscular blocking agents; **Dose:** *IM, IV: Adults: Severe deficiency*—250 mg/kg IM *or* 5 g over 3 hr IV. *Mild deficiency*—1 g q 6 hr × 4 doses. *Seizures*—1 g IV q 6 hr × 4 doses as needed. *Eclampsia/Pre-eclampsia*—4–5 g by IV infusion, concurrently with up to 5 g IM in each buttock; then 4–5 g IM q 4 hr *or* 4 g by IV infusion followed by 1–2 g/hr continuous infusion (max: 40 g/day or 20 g/48 hr if severe renal insufficiency). *Torsades de pointes*—1–2 g IV over 5–20 min. *IM, IV: Peds: >1 mo Hypomagnesemia*—25–50 mg/kg/dose q 4–6 hr × 3–4 doses (max dose: 2 g); **Availability (G):** *Inject:* 125 mg/ml, 500 mg/ml; **Monitor:** BP, HR, RR, ECG, Mg, BUN/SCr, deep tendon reflexes; **Notes:** Dilute to 60 mg/ml and give IV at a rate not to exceed 150 mg/min.

M

mannitol (Osmitrol, Resectisol) **Uses: IV:** Acute oliguric renal failure; ↑ ICP or IOP; Toxic overdose; GU irrigant: During transurethral procedures; **Class:** osmotic diuretics; **Preg:** C; CIs: Hypersensitivity; Anuria; Dehydration; Active intracranial bleeding; ADRs: confusion, HA, blurred vision, rhinitis, transient volume expansion, CP, HF, pulmonary edema, ↑ HR, N/V, thirst, ↑ BUN/SCr, urinary retention, dehydration, ↑↓ K+, ↑↓ Na+, phlebitis at IV site; **Interactions:** Hypokalemia ↑ risk of digoxin toxicity; **Dose:** *IV: Adults: Edema, oliguric renal failure*—50–100 g. *Reduction of ICP/IOP*—0.25–2 g/kg over 30–60 min. *Diuresis in drug intoxications*—50–200 g titrated to maintain UO of 100–500 ml/hr. *IV: Peds: Edema, oliguric renal failure*—0.25–2 g/kg over 2–6 hr. *Reduction of ICP/IOP*—1–2 g/kg over 30–60 min. *Diuresis in drug intoxications*—up to 2 g/kg; **Availability (G):** Inject: 5, 10, 15, 20%; GU irrigant: 5%; **Monitor:** Electrolytes, UO, BUN/SCr, CVP, ICP; **Notes:** Administer undiluted with in-line filter; soln may contain crystals and will dissolve upon warming; cool to body temp before administration.

maraviroc (Selzentry) **Uses:** HIV infection (with only CCR5-tropic HIV-1 detectable); **Class:** CCR5 co-receptor antagonists;

Preg: B; **CIs:** Hypersensitivity; **ADRs:** dizziness, cough, respiratory tract infection, abdominal pain, appetite disorder, HEPATOTOXICITY, RASH, musculoskeletal pain, ALLERGIC REACTIONS, fever, immune reconstitution syndrome, ↑ risk of infection; **Interactions:** CYP3A4 inhibitors may ↑ levels, CYP3A4 inducers may ↓ levels; **Dose:** *PO: Adults: Concurrent CYP3A4 inhibitors (except tipranavir/ritonavir) or delavirdine*—150 mg bid. *Concurrent NRTIs, tipranavir/ritonavir, nevirapine, and other drugs that are not strong inhibitors/inducers of CYP3A4*—300 mg bid. *Concurrent CYP3A4 inducers including efavirenz (with no strong CYP3A4 inhibitor)*—600 mg bid; **Availability:** *Tabs:* 150, 300 mg; **Monitor:** CD4 count, viral load, LFTs, CBC, S/S rash/hepatitis; **Notes:** Patients with CrCl <50 ml/min and on a CYP3A4 inhibitor have ↑ risk for toxicity. Do not crush, break, or chew tabs.

meclizine (Antivert, Bonine) **Uses:** Management/prevention of: Motion sickness, Vertigo; **Class:** antihistamines; **Preg:** B; **CIs:** Hypersensitivity, BPH, Angle-closure glaucoma; **ADRs:** drowsiness, fatigue, blurred vision, dry mouth; **Interactions:** ↑ CNS depression with CNS depressants, including alcohol, antihistamines, opioid analgesics, and sedative/hypnotics; ↑ risk of anticholinergic effects with other anticholinergic agents; **Dose:** *PO: Adults: Motion sickness*—25–50 mg 1 hr before exposure; may repeat in 24 hr. *Vertigo*—25–100 mg/day in divided doses; **Availability (G):** *Tabs:* 12.5, 25, 50 mg; *Chew tabs:* 25 mg; *Caps:* 15, 25, 30 mg; **Monitor:** N/V, sedation; **Notes:** Give with food, water, or milk to ↓ GI irritation. Chewable tab may be chewed or swallowed whole.

M

medroxyPROGESTERone (Depo-Provera, Depo-Sub Q Provera 104, Provera) **Uses:** Endometrial hyperplasia in postmenopausal women receiving estrogen; Secondary amenorrhea and abnormal uterine bleeding; **IM:** Endometrial or renal carcinoma; Endometriosis-associated pain (Depo-Sub Q Provera 104 only); Prevention of pregnancy; **Class:** hormones, progestins; **Preg:** X; **CIs:** Hypersensitivity; Pregnancy; Missed abortion; Thromboembolic disease; Cerebrovascular disease; Severe liver disease; Breast or genital CA; **ADRs:** depression, THROMBOEMBOLIC EVENTS (E.G., STROKE/TIA, MI, VTE), edema, ↑ LFTs, gingival bleeding, cervical erosions, melasma, rash, amenorrhea, breakthrough bleeding, breast tenderness, changes in menstrual flow, galactorrhea, ↑ BG, spotting, bone loss, ANAPHYLAXIS/ANGIOEDEMA, wt changes; **Interactions:** ↓ effects of bromocriptine when used for galactorrhea/amenorrhea; CYP3A4 inhibitors may ↑ levels/toxicity; CYP3A4 inducers may ↓ levels/effects; **Dose:** *PO: Adults: Postmenopausal women receiving concurrent estrogen*—2.5–5 mg/day with 0.625 mg conjugated estrogens (monophasic regimen) *or* 5 mg/day on Days 15–28 of the cycle with 0.625 mg conjugated estrogens taken daily throughout cycle (biphasic regimen). *Amenorrhea*—5–10 mg/day

× 5–10 days. *Abnormal uterine bleeding*—5–10 mg/day × 5–10 days, starting on Day 16 or Day 21 of menstrual cycle. *IM: Adults: Endometrial or renal carcinoma*—400–1000 mg/wk; if improvement occurs, attempt to ↓ dosage to 400 mg/mo. *Contraception*—Depo-Provera: 150 mg q 3 mo. *Subcut: Adults: Endometriosis*—104 mg q 3 mo, beginning on Day 5 of normal menses. *Contraception*—104 mg q 3 mo. *Hepatic Impairment Adults:* ↓ dose in mild-to-moderate liver impairment; **Availability (G):** *Tabs:* 2.5, 5, 10 mg; *Depot inject (IM):* 150 mg/ml, 400 mg/ml; *Subcut inject (Depo-Sub Q Provera 104):* 104 mg/0.65 ml; **Monitor:** BP, LFTs, menstrual cycle, visual changes, wt, S/S bleeding, thromboembolic events, depression; **Notes:** Rule out pregnancy prior to use. Maintain adequate amounts of dietary Ca and vitamin D to prevent bone loss with injectable use.

megestrol (Megace, Megace ES) **Uses:** Palliative treatment of endometrial and breast CA; AIDS-related anorexia, wt loss, and cachexia; **Class:** progestins; **Preg:** D (tabs), X (susp); **CIs:** Hypersensitivity, Pregnancy, missed abortion, or lactation; **ADRs:** THROMBOEMBOLISM, edema, GI irritation, alopecia, adrenal suppression (chronic therapy), thrombophlebitis, vag bleeding; **Interactions:** None significant; **Dose:** *PO: Adults: Breast CA*—40 mg 4 ×/day. *Endometrial CA*—40–320 mg/day in divided doses. *AIDS-related anorexia*—400–800 mg/day (Megace); 625 mg/day (Megace ES). **Availability (G):** *Tabs:* 20, 40 mg; *Oral susp:* 40 mg/ml, 125 mg/ml (Megace ES); **Monitor:** S/S thromboembolism/vag bleeding, wt, appetite; **Notes:** May give with food. Teratogenic—instruct patients to use contraception.

M

meloxicam (Mobic) **Uses:** OA; RA; Juvenile RA; **Class:** NSAIDs; **Preg:** C, D (3rd tri); **CIs:** Hypersensitivity to aspirin or NSAIDs, Active bleeding; Perioperative pain from CABG surgery; **ADRs:** HA, dizziness, tinnitus, edema, GI BLEEDING, N/V/D, ↑ SCr, rash; **Interactions:** ↑ adverse GI effects with aspirin and corticosteroids; ↓ effects of aspirin and antihypertensives; ↑ risk of bleeding with antiplatelet agents and anticoagulants; ↑ risk of nephrotoxicity with cyclosporine; ↑ levels of methotrexate and lithium; **Dose:** *PO: Adults:* 7.5–15 mg/day. *PO: Peds: ≥2 yr:* 0.125 mg/kg once daily (max: 7.5 mg/day); **Availability (G):** *Tabs:* 7.5 mg, 15 mg; *Oral susp:* 7.5 mg/5 ml; **Monitor:** Pain, temp, S/S of GI upset/bleeding, BUN/SCr, LFTs, CBC; **Notes:** Avoid use in oliguria/anuria. Give with food.

memantine (Namenda) **Uses:** Moderate-to-severe Alzheimer's dementia; **Class:** N-Methyl-D-Aspartate antagonist; **Preg:** B; **CIs:** Hypersensitivity; **ADRs:** dizziness, fatigue, HA, sedation, HTN, rash, ↑ wt, urinary frequency, anemia; **Interactions:** Medications that ↑ urine pH lead to ↓ excretion/↑ blood levels (carbonic anhydrase inhibitors, Na bicarbonate); **Dose:** *PO: Adults:* 5 mg/day × 1 wk, then ↑ to 10 mg/day × 1 wk, then ↑ to 15 mg/day × 1 wk, then ↑ to 20 mg/day (as 10 mg bid).

Renal Impairment Adults: ↓ dose if CrCl <30 ml/min; **Availability:** *Tabs:* 5, 10 mg. *Oral soln:* 2 mg/ml; **Monitor:** Cognitive function, wt, CBC; **Notes:** May give without regard to meals.

meperidine (Demerol, Meperitab) **Uses:** Moderate-to-severe pain; Anesthesia adjunct; Analgesic during labor; Preop sedation; **Class:** opioid agonists; **Preg:** C; **CIs:** Hypersensitivity; Pregnancy/lactation (chronic use); Current or recent use (14 days) of MAOIs; **ADRs:** SEIZURES, confusion, sedation, dysphoria, euphoria, hallucinations, HA, blurred vision, diplopia, miosis, respiratory depression, ↓ BP, ↓ HR, constipation, N/V, urinary retention, flushing, sweating, physical/psychological dependence, tolerance; **Interactions:** Do not use in patients receiving MAOIs or procarbazine (may cause fatal reaction—contraindicated within 14 days of MAOI therapy); ↑ CNS depression with alcohol, antihistamines, and sedative/hypnotics; Administration of agonist/antagonist opioid analgesics may precipitate withdrawal in physically dependent patients; Nalbuphine or pentazocine may ↓ analgesia; Protease inhibitors may ↑ effects and ADRs (avoid use); Phenytoin ↓ levels; Acyclovir may ↑ plasma concentrations of meperidine and normeperidine; **Dose:** *PO, IM, Subcut, IV: Adults: Analgesia*—50–150 mg q 3–4 hr. *Analgesia during labor*—50–100 mg IM or subcut when contractions become regular; may repeat q 1–3 hr. *Preop sedation*—50–100 mg IM or subcut 30–90 min before anesthesia. *IV: Adults: PCA*—10 mg initially; with a range of 1–5 mg/incremental dose, recommended lockout interval is 6–10 min (min: 5 min). *PO, IM, Subcut, IV: Peds: Analgesia*—1–1.5 mg/kg q 3–4 hr (max: 100 mg/dose). *Preop sedation*—1–2 mg/kg 30–90 min before anesthesia (not to exceed adult dose). *Renal Impairment Adults and Peds:* ↓ dose if CrCl <50 ml/min; **Availability (G):** *Tabs:* 50, 100 mg. *Syrup:* 50 mg/5 ml. *Inject:* 25 mg/ml, 50 mg/ml, 75 mg/ml, 100 mg/ml; **Monitor:** BP, HR, RR, pain, mental status, BUN/SCr; **Notes:** Schedule II controlled substance. ↑ intake of fluids and bulk and use laxatives to minimize constipating effects. Taper gradually to avoid withdrawal. Avoid repeated administration in renal dysfunction to prevent accumulation of active metabolite, normeperidine. Naloxone is antidote.

M

meropenem (Merrem) **Uses:** Skin/skin structure infections, meningitis, or intra-abdominal infections due to susceptible organisms (e.g., *S. pneumo*, *S. aureus*, S. *epidermidis*, *S. pyogenes*, *Enterococcus faecalis*, *E. coli*, *H. flu*, *Klebsiella*, *P. mirabilis*, *N. meningitidis*, *Pseudomonas*, *B. fragilis*); **Class:** carbapenems; **Preg:** B; **CIs:** Hypersensitivity (cross-sensitivity to other beta-lactam antibiotics may exist); **ADRs:** SEIZURES, PSEUDOMEMBRANOUS COLITIS, N/V/D, rash, pruritis, phlebitis, ANAPHYLAXIS; **Interactions:** Probenecid ↓ excretion and ↑ levels; May ↓ valproic acid levels; **Dose:** *IV: Adults:* 0.5–1 g q 8 hr. *Meningitis*—2 g q 8 hr; *IV: Peds: ≥3 mo–12 yr Intra-abdominal infections*—20 mg/kg q 8 hr. *Meningitis*—40 mg/kg q 8 hr (max: 2 g q 8 hr). *IV: Neonates*

<7 *days:* 20 mg/kg/dose q 12 hr. *Neonates >7 days, 1200–2000 g*—20 mg/kg/dose q 12 hr. *Neonates >7 days, >2000 g*—20 mg/kg/dose q 8 hr. *Renal Impairment IV: Adults:* ↓ dose if CrCl <50 ml/min; **Availability:** *Inject:* 500 mg, 1 g; **Monitor:** BP, HR, temp, sputum, U/A, BUN/SCr, CBC; **Notes:** Use with caution in patients with seizure disorders. Use with caution in patients with beta-lactam allergy (do not use if history of anaphylaxis or hives).

mesalamine (Asacol, Canasa, Lialda, Pentasa, Rowasa) Uses: IBD; **Class:** 5–aminosalicylic acid derivative; **Preg:** B; **CIs:** Hypersensitivity reactions to sulfonamides, salicylates, mesalamine, or sulfasalazine; **ADRs:** HA, dizziness, malaise, weakness, pharyngitis, rhinitis, pericarditis, N/V/D, eructation (PO), flatulence, interstitial nephritis, PANCREATITIS, ↑ BUN/SCr, hair loss, rash, anal irritation (enema, suppository), back pain, ANAPHYLAXIS, acute intolerance syndrome, fever; **Interactions:** May ↓ metabolism and ↑ effects/toxicity of mercaptopurine or thioguanine; **Dose:** *PO: Adults:* 800 mg tid × 6 wk (DR tabs) *or* 1 g qid (CR caps) *or* 2.4–4.8 g once daily with a meal (Lialda). *Rect: Adults:* 4-g enema at bedtime, retained for 8 hr *or* 1 g at bedtime; **Availability (G):** *DR tabs:* 400 mg, 1.2 g (Lialda). *CR caps:* 250, 500 mg. *Supp:* 1 g. *Rect susp:* 4 g/60 ml; **Monitor:** I/Os, stool frequency, S/S IBD, BUN/SCr, LFTs, amylase/lipase; **Notes:** Give with a full glass of water. Do not chew, crush, or break tabs or caps. Use rectal suspension at bedtime and retain all night.

M

mesna (Mesnex) Uses: Prevention of ifosfamide-induced hemorrhagic cystitis; **Class:** ifosfamide detoxifying agents; **Preg:** B; **CIs:** Hypersensitivity to mesna or other thiol compounds; **ADRs:** dizziness, drowsiness, HA, anorexia, N/V/D, unpleasant taste, flushing, inject site reactions, flu-like symptoms; **Interactions:** None significant; **Dose:** *IV: Adults and Peds:* Mesna dose equal to 60% of the ifosfamide dose given at the same time as ifosfamide and 4 and 8 hr after. *PO, IV: Adults and Peds:* Mesna dose equal to 20% of the ifosfamide dose given IV at the same time as ifosfamide; then give PO mesna equal to 40% of the ifosfamide dose 2 and 6 hr after ifosfamide (total mesna dose is 100% of ifosfamide dose); **Availability (G):** *Tabs:* 400 mg. *Inject:* 100 mg/ml; **Monitor:** UA; **Notes:** If PO mesna is vomited within 2 hr, repeat dose or use IV mesna.

metaxalone (Skelaxin) Uses: Muscle spasm; **Class:** skeletal muscle relaxants; **Preg:** C; **CIs:** Hypersensitivity; Significant hepatic/renal impairment; History of drug-induced hemolytic anemia; **ADRs:** drowsiness, dizziness, HA, rash, hemolytic anemia, N/V, rash; **Interactions:** ↑ CNS depression with other CNS depressants; **Dose:** *PO: Adults:* 800 mg tid–qid; **Availability:** *Tabs:* 800 mg; **Monitor:** CBC, LFTs, pain, S/S CNS depression; **Notes:** Causes drowsiness/dizziness; advise patient to avoid driving and alcohol.

metformin (Fortamet, Glucophage, Glucophage XR, Glumetza, Riomet) Uses: Type 2 DM; **Class:** biguanides; **Preg:** B; **CIs:** Hypersensitivity; Metabolic acidosis; Renal dysfunction (SCr >1.5 mg/dl in men or >1.4 mg/dl in women); Radiographic studies requiring IV iodinated contrast media (withhold metformin); HF; **ADRs:** abdominal bloating, N/V/D, unpleasant metallic taste, ↓ BG, LACTIC ACIDOSIS, ↓ vitamin B_{12} levels; **Interactions:** Alcohol or iodinated contrast media ↑ risk of lactic acidosis; Amiloride, cimetidine, digoxin, furosemide, morphine, quinidine, ranitidine, triamterene, trimethoprim, CCBs, and vancomycin may ↑ levels/toxicity; **Dose:** *PO: Adults and Peds: ≥17 yr:* 500–1000 mg bid (max: 2550 mg/day) *or* 850 mg tid. *ER tabs*—500–1000 mg/day with evening meal (max: 2500 mg/day). *PO: Peds: 10–16 yr:* 500–1000 mg bid (max: 2000 mg/day); **Availability (G):** *Tabs:* 500, 850, 1000 mg. *ER tabs (Fortamet, Glucophage XR, Glumetza):* 500, 750, 1000 mg. *Oral soln (Riomet):* 100 mg/ml; **Monitor:** BUN/SCr, acid/base status, electrolytes, glucose, A1C, urine ketones, S/S hypoglycemia; **Notes:** Give with meals to minimize GI effects. Do not crush, break, or chew ER tabs. Discontinue for 48 hr before and after procedure requiring contrast.

M

methadone (Methadose) Uses: Severe pain; Suppresses withdrawal symptoms in opioid detoxification; **Class:** opioid agonists; **Preg:** C; **CIs:** Hypersensitivity; Concurrent MAOI therapy; Head trauma; ↑ ICP; Respiratory depression; **ADRs:** confusion, sedation, dizziness, dysphoria, euphoria, hallucinations, HA, blurred vision, diplopia, miosis, resp depression, ↓ BP, QT prolongation, TORSADES DE POINTES, constipation, N/V, urinary retention, flushing, sweating, physical/psychological dependence, tolerance; **Interactions:** Concurrent MAOI use may result in severe, unpredictable reactions—reduce methadone to 25% of usual dose; CYP3A4 inhibitors may ↑ levels/toxicity; CYP3A4 inducers may ↓ levels/effects; ↑ risk of QT prolongation with other QT-prolonging drugs; ↑ CNS depression with alcohol, antihistamines, and sedative/hypnotics; Agonist/antagonist opioids may precipitate withdrawal in physically dependent patients; Nalbuphine or pentazocine may ↓ analgesia; ↑ levels/effects of zidovudine and desipramine; ↓ level/effects of didanosine and stavudine; **Dose:** *PO: Adults and Peds: ≥50 kg Analgesic*—20 mg q 6–8 hr. *Opioid detoxification*—15–40 mg/day; dose may ↓ q 1–2 days; MD varies; *PO: Adults and Peds: <50 kg Analgesic*—0.2 mg/kg q 6–8 hr. *IM, Subcut: Adults and Peds: ≥50 kg Analgesic*—10 mg q 6–8 hr. *Opioid detoxification*—15–40 mg/day; dose may ↓ q 1–2 days; MD varies; *IM, Subcut: Adults and Peds: <50 kg:* 0.1 mg/kg q 6–8 hr; **Availability (G):** *Tabs:* 5, 10 mg. *Dispersible tabs (diskettes):* 40 mg. *Oral soln (contains alcohol):* 5 mg/5 ml, 10 mg/5 ml. *Oral concentrate:* 10 mg/ml; **Monitor:** BP, RR, HR, ECG, pain, S/S withdrawal/sedation; **Notes:** Schedule II-controlled substance. Prevent constipation with ↑ intake of fluids, bulk, and laxatives. Discontinue gradually after long-term use to prevent withdrawal symptoms.

Naloxone is antidote. Dilute 10 mg/ml oral concentrate doses with at least 30 ml of water.

methimazole (Tapazole) **Uses:** Hyperthyroidism; **Class:** antihyroid agents; **Preg:** D; **CIs:** Hypersensitivity; Lactation; Agranulocytosis or myelosuppression; Patients >40 yr (↑ risk of agranulocytosis); Pregnancy; **ADRs:** drowsiness, HA, vertigo, ↑ wt, ↑ LFTs, loss of taste, N/V/D, parotitis, rash, skin discoloration, urticaria, AGRANULOCYTOSIS, anemia, leukopenia, thrombocytopenia, arthralgia, fever, lymphadenopathy; **Interactions:** ↑ bone marrow depression with antineoplastics or radiation therapy; Antithyroid effect ↓ by potassium iodide or amiodarone; ↑ agranulocytosis with phenothiazines; ↓ effects of warfarin; **Dose:** *PO: Adults: Thyrotoxic crisis*—15–20 mg q 4 hr × 24 hr. *Hyperthyroidism*—15–60 mg/day as a single dose or divided doses for 6–8 wk. *PO: Peds: Initial*—0.4 mg/kg/day in single dose or bid. *MD*—0.2 mg/kg/day in single dose or bid (max: 30 mg/day); **Availability (G):** *Tabs:* 5, 10 mg; **Monitor:** TFTs, CBC, LFTs, wt, S/S hyper/hypothyroidism; **Notes:** Give consistently with regard to meals.

methocarbamol (Robaxin) **Uses:** Muscle spasm associated with painful musculoskeletal conditions; **Class:** skeletal muscle relaxants; **Preg:** C; **CIs:** Hypersensitivity; Renal impairment (do not use IV form); Seizure disorders (parenteral form). **ADRs:** SEIZURES (IV, IM ONLY), dizziness, drowsiness, lightheadedness, blurred vision, nasal congestion, ↓ HR, ↓ BP, anorexia, nausea, flushing (IV only), pruritus, rash, urticaria, pain at IM site, phlebitis at IV site, ANAPHYLAXIS (IM, IV USE ONLY), fever; **Interactions:** ↑ CNS depression with CNS depressants, alcohol, antihistamines, opioid analgesics, and sedative/hypnotics; **Dose:** *PO: Adults:* 1.5 g qid (max: 8 g/day) × 2–3 days, then 4–4.5 g/day in 3–6 divided doses; then 750 mg q 4 hr or 1 g qid or 1.5 g tid. *IM, IV: Adults:* 1–3 g/day for not more than 3 days; course may be repeated after 48 hr; **Availability (G):** *Tabs:* 500, 750 mg. *Inject:* 100 mg/ml; **Monitor:** Pain, stiffness, HR, BP, BUN/SCr; **Notes:** Give with food to ↓ GI irritation. Max IV rate 300 mg/min.

methotrexate (Rheumatrex, Trexall) **Uses:** Treatment of: Trophoblastic neoplasms, Leukemias, Breast CA, Head/neck CA, Lung CA, Osteosarcoma; Severe psoriasis and RA unresponsive to conventional therapy; Mycosis fungoides (cutaneous T-cell lymphoma); **Class:** antimetabolites; **Preg:** X; **CIs:** Hypersensitivity; Pregnancy/lactation; Severe renal impairment (CrCl <10 ml/min); Severe hepatic impairment; Active infections; Decreased bone marrow reserve; **ADRs:** arachnoiditis (IT use only), dizziness, drowsiness, HA, malaise, blurred vision, dysarthria, transient blindness, PULMONARY FIBROSIS, interstitial pneumonitis, anorexia, ↑ LFTs, N/V, stomatitis, infertility, alopecia, painful plaque erosions (during psoriasis treatment), photosensitivity, rash, skin ulceration, urticaria, APLASTIC ANEMIA, anemia, leukopenia,

M

thrombocytopenia, ↑ uric acid, stress fracture, ↑ BUN/SCr, chills, fever; **Interactions:** ↑ hematologic toxicity with high-dose salicylates, NSAIDs, sulfonylureas, phenytoin, tetracyclines, probenecid, trimethoprim/sulfamethoxazole, pyrimethamine, and chloramphenicol, ↑ hepatotoxicity with other hepatotoxic drugs including azathioprine, sulfasalazine, and retinoids; ↑ nephrotoxicity with other nephrotoxic drugs; ↑ bone marrow depression with other antineoplastics or radiation therapy; May ↓ antibody response to live-virus vaccines and ↑ risk of ADRs; ↑ risk of neurologic reactions with acyclovir (IT only); Asparaginase may ↓ effects; **Dose:** *PO: Adults: Leukemia induction*—3.3 mg/m²/day, usually with prednisone. *RA*—7.5 mg once weekly *or* 2.5 mg q 12 hr × 3 doses/wk (max: 20 mg/wk); when response obtained, dosage should be ↓. *Psoriasis*—2.5–5 mg q 12 hr × 3 doses/wk; *PO, IM: Adults: Trophoblastic neoplasms*—15–30 mg/day × 5 days; repeat after ≥1 wk × 3–5 courses. *Cutaneous T-cell lymphoma*—5–50 mg once weekly *or* 15–37.5 mg twice weekly. *Leukemia maintenance*—20–30 mg/m² twice weekly. *Psoriasis*—10–25 mg once weekly. *IV: Adults: Trophoblastic neoplasms*—11 mg/m² on Days 1–5 q 3 wk. *Breast CA*—30–60 mg/m² on Days 1 and 8 q 3 wk. *Osteosarcoma*—8–12 g/m² once weekly × 2–4 wk. *Leukemia*—2.5 mg/kg q 2 wk; *PO, IM, IV: Adults: Head/neck CA*—25–50 mg/m² once weekly. *IT: Adults: Meningeal leukemia*—12 mg/m² or 15 mg. *PO, IM: Peds Juvenile RA*—10 mg/m² once weekly initially, then 5–15 mg/m² once weekly as single dose or in 3 divided doses given 12 hr apart. *IT: Peds Meningeal leukemia*—≥3 yr: 12 mg; 2 yr: 10 mg; 1 yr: 8 mg; 4–11 mo: 6 mg; ≤3 mo: 3 mg; **Availability (G):** *Tabs:* 2.5, 5, 7.5, 10, 15 mg. *Soln for Inject:* 25 mg/ml, Powder for inject: 20 mg, 1 g; **Monitor:** BP, HR, temp, BUN/SCr, CBC, uric acid, LFTs, methotrexate levels, S/S bleeding and pulmonary toxicity, CXR, I/Os, pain and ROM (for RA); **Notes: High Alert:** Fatalities have occurred with chemotherapeutic agents. Before administering, clarify all ambiguous orders; double-check single, daily, and course-of-therapy dose limits; have second practitioner independently double-check original order, calculations, and infusion pump settings. Methotrexate for non-oncologic use is given at a much lower dose and frequency. Do not confuse non-oncologic dosing regimens with dosing regimens for CA patients. Doses >500 mg/m² require leucovorin rescue (doses of 100–500 mg/² may require leucovorin rescue). Monitor serum methotrexate levels q 12–24 hr during high-dose therapy until levels are <5 × 10–8 M (micromolar).

methyldopa (Aldomet) **Uses:** HTN; **Class:** centrally acting antiadrenergics; **Preg:** B; **CIs:** Hypersensitivity; Active liver disease; **ADRs:** sedation, ↓ mental acuity, depression, nasal stuffiness, MYOCARDITIS, ↓ HR, edema, orthostatic hypotension, ↑ LFTs, diarrhea, dry mouth, ED, eosinophilia, hemolytic anemia, fever; **Interactions:** ↑ hypotension with antihypertensives, alcohol, anesthesia, and nitrates; Amphetamines, barbiturates, TCAs, NSAIDs, and phenothiazines ↓ antihypertensive effects; ↑ effects/psychoses with haloperidol;

↑ sympathetic stimulation with MAOIs or other adrenergics; ↑ lithium toxicity, ↑ hypotension and CNS toxicity with levodopa; ↑ CNS depression with alcohol, antihistamines, sedative/hypnotics, some antidepressants, and opioid analgesics; **Dose:** *PO: Adults:* 250–500 mg bid–tid; ↑ q 2 days prn (max: 3 g/day). *PO: Peds:* 10 mg/kg/day divided bid–qid; ↑ q 2 days up to 65 mg/kg/day in divided doses (max: 3 g/day). *IV: Adults:* 250–500 mg q 6 hr (max: 1 g q 6 hr). *IV: Peds:* 5–10 mg/kg q 6 hr; up to 65 mg/kg/day in divided doses (max: 3 g/day). *Renal Impairment: PO, IV: Adults and Peds:* ↓ dose if CrCl <50 ml/min; **Availability (G):** *Tabs:* 125, 250, 500 mg. *Inject:* 50 mg/ml; **Monitor:** BP, HR, LFTs, BUN/SCr, CBC, I/Os, wt, temp; **Notes:** Dose increases should be made with the evening dose to minimize effects of drowsiness.

methylphenidate (Concerta, Daytrana, Metadate CD, Metadate ER, Methylin, Methylin ER, Ritalin, Ritalin LA, Ritalin-SR) **Uses:** ADHD; Narcolepsy; **Class:** central nervous system stimulants; **Preg:** C; **CIs:** Hypersensitivity; Marked anxiety, agitation, or tension; Motor tics, family history or diagnosis of Tourette's; Current or recent (within 2 wk) use of MAOIs; Glaucoma; Serious CV disease or structural heart disease (may ↑ risk of sudden death); History of substance abuse; HTN; Peds <6 yr (safety not established); **ADRs:** <u>hyperactivity</u>, <u>insomnia</u>, <u>restlessness</u>, <u>tremor</u>, dizziness, HA, irritability, blurred vision, <u>HTN</u>, ↑ <u>HR</u>, <u>anorexia</u>, constipation, cramps, dry mouth, metallic taste, N/V/D, rash, akathisia, dyskinesia, fever, hypersensitivity reactions, physical/psychological dependence, tolerance; **Interactions:** Use with MAOIs can result in hypertensive crisis (contraindicated); May ↓ effects of antihypertensives; ↑ risk of serious ADRs with clonidine; May ↑ effects of warfarin, phenobarbital, phenytoin, TCAs, or SSRIs; **Dose:** *PO: Adults: ADHD*—5–20 mg 2–3 ×/day (IR). *Narcolepsy*—10 mg 2–3 ×/day (max: 60 mg/day). *PO: Peds: ≥6 yr IR tabs*—0.3 mg/kg/dose or 2.5–5 mg before breakfast and lunch; ↑ by 0.1 mg/kg/dose or by 5–10 mg/day at weekly intervals (max: 60 mg/day or 2 mg/kg/day). *Concerta (patients not on methylphenidate previously)*—18 mg/day in AM; may ↑ as needed up to 54 mg/day. *Concerta (patients currently on methylphenidate)*—18 mg/day in AM if previous methylphenidate dose was 5 mg 2–3 ×/day or 20 mg/day of SR product; 36 mg/day in AM if previous methylphenidate dose was 10 mg 2–3 ×/day or 40 mg/day of SR product; 54 mg daily in AM if previous methylphenidate dose was 15 mg 2–3 ×/day or 60 mg/day of SR product. *Metadate CD or Ritalin LA*—20 mg daily in AM; may ↑ by 10–20 mg/day at weekly intervals (max: 60 mg/day). *Transdermal: Peds: ≥6 yr:* 10 mg daily; remove up to 9 hr after application; may ↑ to next transdermal dose at weekly intervals; **Availability (G):** *IR tabs:* 5, 10, 20 mg. *ER tabs (Metadate ER, Methylin ER):* 10, 20 mg. *ER tabs (Concerta):* 18, 27, 36, 54 mg. *SR tabs (Ritalin SR):* 20 mg. *ER caps (Metadate CD):* 10, 20, 30, 40, 50, 60 mg. *ER caps (Ritalin LA):* 10, 20, 30, 40 mg. *Chew tabs (Methylin):* 2.5, 5, 10 mg. *Oral soln (Methylin):*

M

5 mg/5 ml, 10 mg/5 ml. *Transdermal system (Daytrana):* 10 mg/9 hr, 15 mg/9 hr, 20 mg/9 hr, 30 mg/9 hr; **Monitor:** BP, HR, ECG, mental status, ht/wt; **Notes:** Schedule II controlled substance. When MD is determined, may change to ER formulation. Do not give later than 6 PM to prevent insomnia. IR and SR tabs should be given on empty stomach (30–45 min ac). SR tabs should be swallowed whole; do not crush, break, or chew. Metadate CD and Ritalin LA caps may be sprinkled on applesauce; Concerta may be administered without regard to food, but must be taken with water, milk, or juice. Total wear time of patch should not exceed 9 hr. All children should have CV assessment prior to initiation. Potential for dependence/abuse with long-term use.

methylPREDNISolone (Depo-Medrol, Medrol, Solu-Medrol) **Uses:** Used systemically and locally for diseases including: Inflammatory, Allergic, Hematologic, Neoplastic, Autoimmune disorders, Immunosuppressant; Replacement therapy in adrenal insufficiency; **Class:** corticosteroids; **Preg:** C; **CIs:** Active untreated infections; Administration of live virus vaccines; **ADRs:** depression, euphoria, ↑ ICP (peds only), psychoses, ↑ IOP, HTN, PUD, anorexia, N/V, acne, ↓ wound healing, ecchymoses, fragility, hirsutism, petechiae, adrenal suppression, ↑ BG, fluid retention (long-term high doses), ↓ K+, THROMBOEMBOLISM, thrombophlebitis, ↑ wt, muscle wasting, osteoporosis, cushingoid appearance, ↑ susceptibility to infection; **Interactions:** ↑ hypokalemia with thiazide and loop diuretics, amphotericin B, piperacillin, or ticarcillin; ↑ requirement for insulins or oral hypoglycemic agents; CYP3A4 inihibitors may ↑ levels/toxicity; CYP3A4 inducers may ↓ levels/effects; ↑ risk of adverse GI effects with NSAIDs (including aspirin); At chronic doses that suppress adrenal function, may ↓ response to/↑ risk of ADRs from live-virus vaccines; May ↑ the risk of tendon rupture from FQs; **Dose:** *PO: Adults: MS*—160 mg/day × 7 days, then 64 mg every other day × 1 mo. *Other uses*—2–60 mg/day as a single dose or in 2–4 divided doses. *Asthma exacerbations*—120–180 mg/day in 3–4 divided doses × 48 hr, then 60–80 mg/day divided bid. *PO: Peds: Anti-inflammatory/ Immunosuppressive*—0.5–1.7 mg/kg/day or 5–25 mg/m²/day in divided doses q 6–12 hr. *Asthma exacerbations*—1 mg/kg q 6 hr × 48 hr, then 1–2 mg/kg/day (max: 60 mg/day) divided bid. *IM, IV: Adults: Most uses*—40–250 mg q 4–6 hr. *High-dose "pulse" therapy*—30 mg/kg IV q 4–6 hr for up to 72 hr. *MS*—160 mg/day × 7 days, then 64 mg every other day × 1 mo. *Adjunctive therapy of PCP in AIDS patients*—30 mg bid × 5 days, then 30 mg once daily × 5 days, then 15 mg once daily × 10 days. *Acute spinal cord injury*—30 mg/kg over 15 min initially, followed 45 min later with 5.4 mg/kg/hr for 23 hr (unlabeled). *IM, IV: Peds: Anti-inflammatory/Immunosuppressive*—0.5–1.7 mg/kg/day or 5–25 mg/m²/day in divided doses q 6–12 hr. *Acute spinal cord injury*—30 mg/kg over 15 min initially, then 45 min later initiate 5.4 mg/kg/hr for 23 hr (unlabeled).

Status asthmaticus—2 mg/kg/dose, then 0.5–1 mg/kg/dose q 6 hr. *Lupus nephritis*—30 mg/kg IV every other day × 6 doses. *IM: Adults: Acetate*—40–120 mg daily, weekly, or q 2 wk; **Availability (G):** *Tabs:* 2, 4, 8, 16, 24, 32 mg. *Soln for inject (succinate):* 40 mg, 125 mg, 500 mg, 1 g, 2 g. *Susp for inject (acetate):* 20 mg/ml, 40 mg/ml, 80 mg/ml; **Monitor:** CBC, electrolytes, BG, BP, wt, I/Os, growth (peds), S/S adrenal insufficiency; **Notes:** Do not give acetate form IV; succinate may be given IV or IM. Use lowest possible dose to treat condition. Give with food to minimize GI irritation; do not give with grapefruit juice. Therapy longer than 5 days may require tapering upon discontinuation.

metoclopramide (Reglan) Uses: Prevention of chemotherapy-induced N/V and PONV; Treatment of postsurgical and diabetic gastric stasis; Facilitation of small bowel intubation in radiographic procedures; GERD; **Class:** antiemetics; **Preg:** B; **CIs:** Hypersensitivity; GI obstruction, perforation, or hemorrhage; Seizure disorder; Pheochromocytoma; **ADRs:** drowsiness, EPS, restlessness, NMS, anxiety, depression, irritability, tardive dyskinesia, HTN, ↓ BP, constipation, N/V/D, dry mouth, gynecomastia, methemoglobinemia, neutropenia, leukopenia; **Interactions:** ↑ CNS depression with CNS depressants, alcohol, antidepressants, antihistamines, opioid analgesics, and sedative/hypnotics; May ↑ levels of cyclosporine and tacrolimus; ↑ risk of EPS with haloperidol or phenothiazines; Opioids and anticholinergics may antagonize the GI effects of metoclopramide; Use cautiously with MAOIs (causes release of catecholamines); ↑ neuromuscular blockade from succinylcholine; ↓ effects of levodopa; **Dose:** *PO, IV: Adults and Peds: Chemotherapy-induced N/V*—1–2 mg/kg 30 min before chemotherapy; may be given q 2–4 hr prn. *IV: Adults and Peds: >14 yr Facilitation of small bowel intubation*—10 mg over 1–2 min. *IV: Peds: 6–14 yr:* 2.5–5 mg (max 0.5 mg/kg) over 1–2 min. *IV: Peds: <6 yr:* 0.1 mg/kg over 1–2 min. *PO, IV: Adults: Diabetic gastroparesis*—10 mg 30 min ac and at bedtime. *PO, IM, IV: Adults: GERD*—10–15 mg 30 min ac and at bedtime (max: 0.5 mg/kg/day). *PO, IM, IV: Neonates, Infants, and Peds: GERD*—0.4–0.8 mg/kg/day in 4 divided doses. *IM, IV: Adults and Peds: >14 yr PONV*—10 mg at the end of surgical procedure, repeat in 6–8 hr if needed. *IM, IV: Peds: <14 yr Postoperative N/V*—0.1–0.2 mg/kg/dose, repeat in 6–8 hr if needed; **Availability (G):** *Tabs:* 5, 10 mg. *Syrup:* 5 mg/5 ml. *Inject:* 5 mg/ml; **Monitor:** BP, N/V, EPS; **Notes:** Diphenhydramine 1 mg/kg IV may be given prophylactically 15 min before high doses of metoclopramide (1–2 mg/kg IV) to ↓ risk of EPS.

metolazone (Zaroxolyn) Uses: HTN; Edema; **Class:** thiazide-like diuretics; **Preg:** B; **CIs:** Hypersensitivity to thiazides or sulfonamides; Anuria; Severe hepatic impairment; Pregnancy; **ADRs:** ↓ BP, palpitations, anorexia, hepatitis, N/V/D, photosensitivity, rash, ↑ BG, ↓ K+, dehydration, ↑ Ca++, metabolic alkalosis, ↓ Mg++, ↓ Na+, ↑ uric acid, muscle cramps; **Interactions:** ↑ effects with other antihypertensives; May ↑ lithium levels; NSAIDs may ↓ effectiveness; **Dose:** *PO: Adults: HTN*—2.5–5 mg/day. *Edema*—5–20 mg/day; **Availability (G):** *Tabs:* 2.5, 5, 10 mg; **Monitor:** BP, electrolytes, BUN/SCr, BG, uric acid, wt, I/Os, edema; **Notes:** Give daily in the AM with food. Advise patient to use sunscreen.

metoprolol (Lopressor, Toprol-XL) **Uses:** HTN; Angina/MI; Stable HF (XL only); **Class:** beta blockers; **Preg:** C; **CIs:** Hypersensitivity; Decompensated HF; Pulmonary edema; Cardiogenic shock; Bradycardia or ≥2nd-degree heart block (in absence of pacemaker); **ADRs:** fatigue, weakness, depression, dizziness, drowsiness, nightmares, blurred vision, bronchospasm, BRADYCARDIA, HF, PULMONARY EDEMA, ↓ BP, N/V/D, ED, ↓ libido, ↑↓ BG; **Interactions:** ↑ risk of bradycardia with digoxin, diltiazem, verapamil, or clonidine; ↑ effects with other antihypertensives; ↑ risk of hypertensive crisis if concurrent clonidine discontinued; May alter the effectiveness of insulins or oral hypoglycemic agents; May ↓ the effects of $beta_1$ agonists (e.g., dopamine or dobutamine); **Dose:** *PO: Adults: HTN/angina/post-MI*—25–100 mg/day in 2 divided doses (IR) or as a single daily dose (XL); may ↑ q 7 days up to 450 mg/day. *HF*—12.5–25 mg/day (XL), double dose q 2 wk up to target dose of 200 mg/day. *IV: Adults: MI*—5 mg q 2 min × 3 doses, followed by oral dosing; **Availability (G):** *Tabs (tartrate):* 25, 50, 100 mg. *ER tabs (succinate; XL):* 25, 50, 100, 200 mg. *Inject:* 1 mg/ml; **Monitor:** BP, HR, ECG, S/S HF, edema, wt, S/S angina, BG (in DM); **Notes:** Abrupt withdrawal may cause life-threatening arrhythmias, hypertensive crises, or myocardial ischemia. May mask S/S of hypoglycemia (esp. tachycardia) in DM. ER (succinate) tabs may be cut in half but should not be crushed.

metronidazole (Flagyl, Flagyl ER, MetroCream, MetroGel, MetroGel-Vaginal, MetroLotion, Noritate) **Uses: PO, IV:** Treatment of the following anaerobic infections: Intra-abdominal infections, Gynecologic infections, Skin and skin structure infections, Lower respiratory tract infections, Bone and joint infections, CNS infections, Septicemia, IE; **IV:** Perioperative prophylactic agent in colorectal surgery; **PO:** Amebicide in the management of amebic dysentery, amebic liver abscess, and trichomoniasis; PUD caused by *H. pylori*; **Topical:** Acne rosacea; **Vag:** Bacterial vaginosis; **Class:** antibodies; **Preg:** B; **CIs:** Hypersensitivity; Hypersensitivity to parabens (top only); Pregnancy (1st tri); **ADRs:** SEIZURES, dizziness, HA, abdominal pain, anorexia, N/V/D, dry mouth, furry tongue, glossitis, metallic taste, rash, urticaria, burning sensation, mild dryness, skin irritation, transient redness, leukopenia, phlebitis at IV site, peripheral neuropathy, superinfection; **Interactions:** May ↑ levels/toxicity of CYP3A4 substrates. Phenobarbital and rifampin ↑ metabolism/↓ effects; ↑ effects of phenytoin, lithium, and warfarin; Disulfiram-like reaction may occur with alcohol; **Dose:** *PO: Adults: Anaerobic infections*—500 mg q 6–8 hr (max: 4 g/day). *Trichomoniasis*—250 mg q 8 hr × 7 days *or* single 2-g dose *or* 1 g bid × 1 day. *Amebiasis*—500–750 mg q 8 hr × 5–10 days. *H. pylori*—250 mg qid *or* 500 mg bid × 1–2 wk. *Bacterial vaginosis*—750 mg once daily as ER tabs × 7 days. *Antibiotic-associated pseudomembranous colitis*—250–500 mg tid–qid × 10–14 days; *PO: Infants and Peds: Anaerobic infections*—30 mg/kg/day IV/PO divided q 6–8 hr (max: 4 g/day). *Trichomoniasis*—15–30 mg/kg/day divided q 8 hr × 7–10 days. *Amebiasis*—35–50 mg/kg/day divided q 8 hr × 5–10 days (max 750 mg/dose). *Antibiotic-associated pseudomembranous colitis*—30 mg/kg/day divided q 6 hr × 7–10 days. *H. pylori*—15–20 mg/kg/day divided bid × 4 wk. *IV, PO: Neonates: <7 days or <2000 g:* 7.5 mg/kg q 12–48 hr. *PNA >7 days*, >2000 g—15 mg/kg q 12 hr; *IV: Adults: Anaerobic infections*—500 mg q 6–8 hr (max: 4 g/day). *Perioperative prophylaxis*—15 mg/kg 1 hr before surgery, then 7.5 mg/kg q 6 h × 2 days. *Amebiasis*—500–750 mg q 8 hr × 5–10 days. *Hepatic Impairment IV, PO: Adults and Peds:* ↓ dose in severe liver disease. *Topical: Adults: Acne rosacea*—apply bid. *Vag: Adults: Bacterial vaginosis*—One applicatorful (37.5 mg) bid × 5 days; **Availability (G):** *Tabs:* 250, 500 mg. *ER tabs:* 750 mg. *Caps:* 375 mg. *Top gel/cream/lotion:* 0.75%; *Vag gel:* 0.75% (37.5 mg/5 g applicatorful); **Monitor:** CBC, WBC, temp, cultures/sensitivity, LFTs; **Notes:** Administer on an empty stomach, or with food or milk to minimize GI irritation. Do not crush or chew ER tabs.

mexiletine (Mexitil) **Uses:** Management of serious ventricular arrhythmias; **Class:** antiarrhythmics (class Ib); **Preg:** C; **CIs:** Hypersensitivity; Cardiogenic shock; ≥2nd-degree heart block (in absence of a pacemaker); Sinus node or intraventricular conduction abnormalities; Hypotension; Severe HF; **ADRs:** dizziness, nervousness, confusion, fatigue, HA, sleep disorder, blurred vision, tinnitus, dyspnea, ARRHYTHMIAS, CP, edema, ↑ HR, HEPATITIS, heartburn, N/V, rash, blood dyscrasias, tremor, paresthesia; **Interactions:** CYP1A2 and CYP2D6 inhibitors may ↑ levels/toxicity; CYP1A2 inducers may ↓ levels/effects; May ↑ levels/effects of CYP1A2 substrates; Drugs that alter urine pH may alter blood levels (alkalinization ↑ levels; acidification ↓ levels); **Dose:** *PO: Adults:* 200 mg q 8 hr; may ↑ q 2–3 days (max: 1200 mg/day); **Availability (G):** *Caps:* 150, 200, 250 mg; **Monitor:** BP, HR, ECG, LFTs, CBC; **Notes:** Give with food.

micafungin (Mycamine) **Uses:** Esophageal candidiasis; Prophylaxis of *Candida* infections during hematopoetic stem cell transplantation; **Class:** echinocandins; **Preg:** C; **CIs:** Hypersensitivity; Peds (safety not established); **ADRs:** ↑ LFTs, N/V/D, ↑ BUN/SCr, ↓ K+, ↓ Mg++, inject site reactions, allergic reactions including ANAPHYLAXIS; **Interactions:** None noted; **Dose:** *IV: Adults: Esophageal candidiasis*—150 mg daily × 15 days (range: 10–30 days). *Prevention of*

Candida infections in stem cell transplantation—50 mg/day × 19 days (range 6–51 days); **Availability:** *Inject:* 50, 100 mg; **Monitor:** BP, HR, temp, sputum, U/A, CBC, LFTs, S/S anaphylaxis, electrolytes; **Notes:** Infuse over 1 hr.

miconazole (Fungoid, Lotrimin AF, Micatin, Monistat, Zeasorb-AF) **Uses:** Cutaneous fungal infections, including tinea pedis, tinea cruris, tinea corporis, and vulvovaginal candidiasis; **Class:** antifungals (topical); **Preg:** C; **CIs:** Hypersensitivity; **ADRs:** burning sensation, itching, local hypersensitivity reactions, redness, stinging; **Interactions:** Concurrent use of warfarin with vag miconazole may ↑ risk of bleeding/bruising; **Dose:** *Topical: Adults and Peds: >2 yr:* Apply bid × 2 wk for tinea cruris, or 4 wk for tinea pedis or tinea corporis. *Vag: Adults and Peds: ≥12 yr Supp*—100 mg at bedtime × 7 days *or* 200 mg at bedtime × 3 days *or* 1200 mg × 1. *2% Cream*—1 applicatorful at bedtime × 7 days. *4% Cream*—1 applicatorful at bedtime × 3 days. *Combination packs*—bid × 7 days; **Availability (G):** *Top cream/oint/soln:* 2%. *Powder:* 2%. *Spray liquid/powder:* 2%. *Tincture:* 2%. *Vag cream:* 2%, 4%. *Vag supp:* 100, 200, 1200 mg; **Monitor:** Mucous membranes, resolution of skin infection; **Notes:** Vag therapy should be continued during menstrual period; patient should avoid tampon use during treatment.

M

midazolam (Versed) **Uses:** Conscious sedation; ICU sedation; Status epilepticus; Anesthesia induction aid; **Class:** benzodiazepines; **Preg:** D; **CIs:** Prior sensitivity to other BZs; Acute narrow-angle glaucoma; Sleep apnea; Concurrent use of potent CYP3A4 inhibitors; **ADRs:** agitation, drowsiness, HA, sedation, blurred vision, APNEA, RESPIRATORY DEPRESSION, bronchospasm, cough, ↓ BP, N/V, rash; **Interactions:** ↑ CNS depression with alcohol, antidepressants, other BZs, antihistamines, and opioids; CYP3A4 inhibitors may ↑ levels; CYP3A4 inducers may ↓ levels; **Dose:** *IM: Adults: Preop sedation*—0.07–0.08 mg/kg 30–60 min before surgery/procedure (↓ dose to 0.02–0.03 mg/kg [usual dose 1–3 mg] for patients with COPD, high-risk patients, or patients ≥60 yr). *IV: Adults: Preop sedation*—0.02–0.04 mg/kg; may repeat q 5 min until desired effect (max total dose: 0.1–0.2 mg/kg). *Conscious sedation*—0.5–2 mg initially (do not give more than 1.5 mg in elderly or debilitated); may ↑ as needed (↓ dose by 30% if other CNS depressants are used). MDs of 25% of the dose required for initial sedation may be given as necessary. *Anesthesia induction*—0.3–0.35 mg/kg initially (up to 0.6 mg/kg total). If patient is premedicated, initial dose should be 0.15–0.35 mg/kg. *Anesthesia maintenance*—0.05–0.3 mg/kg as needed *or* continuous infusion of 0.25–1.5 mcg/kg/min. *ICU sedation*—0.02–0.08 mg/kg (1–5 mg in most adults) initially; may repeat q 10–15 min until adequate sedations obtained; may be followed by continuous infusion at 0.02–0.1 mg/kg/hr (1–7 mg/hr in most adults). *PO: Peds: 6 mo–16 yr Preop or conscious sedation*—0.25–0.5 mg/kg 30–40 min before surgery/procedure (max: 20 mg), may require up to 1 mg/kg (max: 20 mg/dose). *IM: Peds Preop or* *conscious sedation*—0.1–0.15 mg/kg up to 0.5 mg/kg 30–60 min prior to surgery/procedure (max total dose: 10 mg). *IV: Peds: Preop or conscious sedation*—6 mo–5 yr: 0.05–0.1 mg/kg initially, may ↑ up to 0.6 mg/kg total (max total dose: 6 mg); 6–12 yr: 0.025–0.05 mg/kg initially, may ↑ up to 0.4 mg/kg total (max total dose: 10 mg). *Sedation in mechanical ventilation*—0.05–0.2 mg/kg initially; follow with continuous infusion at 0.06–0.12 mg/kg/min (1–2 mcg/kg/min), titrate to effect, range: 0.4–6 mcg/kg/min. *Status epilepticus*—>2 mo: 0.15 mg/kg load followed by a continuous infusion of 0.06 mg/kg/hr. Titrate q 5 min until seizure controlled, range: 0.06–1.1 mg/kg/hr; **Availability (G):** *Inject:* 1 mg/ml, 5 mg/ml. *Syrup:* 2 mg/ml; **Monitor:** BP, HR, RR, mental status, seizure activity, LFTs, BUN/SCr; **Notes:** Schedule IV controlled substance. Elderly may require ↓ doses. Flumazenil is antidote. Do not confuse Versed (midazolam) with VePesid (etoposide).

mifepristone (Mifeprex) Uses: Medical termination of pregnancy up to Day 49; **Class:** antiprogestational agents; **Preg:** X; **CIs:** Presence of an IUD; Ectopic pregnancy; Undiagnosed adnexal mass; Chronic adrenal failure; Concurrent long-term corticosteroid therapy; Bleeding disorders or concurrent anticoagulant therapy; Inherited porphyrias; **ADRs:** dizziness, fainting, HA, weakness, abdominal pain, N/V/D, uterine bleeding, uterine cramping, ruptured ectopic pregnancy, pelvic pain; **Interactions:** None noted; **Dose:** *PO: Adults:* 600 mg × 1 followed by misoprostol within 48 h; **Availability:** *Tabs:* 200 mg; **Monitor:** Hgb/Hct, CBC, ultrasound to confirm pregnancy termination, S/S infection; **Notes:** Do not use beyond day 49 of pregnancy. Remove IUD prior to therapy.

M

miglitol (Glyset) Uses: Type 2 DM; **Class:** alpha glucosidase inhibitors; **Preg:** B; **CIs:** Hypersensitivity; DKA; IBD or other obstructive GI conditions; **ADRs:** abdominal pain, diarrhea, flatulence; **Interactions:** ↓ absorption of ranitidine, digoxin, and propranolol; **Dose:** *PO: Adults:* 25–100 mg tid; **Availability:** *Tabs:* 25, 50, 100 mg; **Monitor:** BG, A1C, S/S hypoglycemia; **Notes:** Give with the first bite of each meal.

milrinone (Primacor) Uses: Short-term treatment of decompensated HF; **Class:** phosphodiesterase inhibitors; **Preg:** C; **CIs:** Hypersensitivity; Severe aortic or pulmonic valvular heart disease; Hypertrophic subaortic stenosis; Arrhythmias; Acute MI; **ADRs:** HA, tremor, ARRHYTHMIAS, angina, ↓ BP; **Interactions:** None significant; **Dose:** *IV: Adults and Peds:* LD of 50 mcg/kg followed by 0.375–0.75 mcg/kg/min infusion. *Renal Impairment IV: Adults and Peds:* ↓ dose if CrCl <50 ml/min; **Availability:** *Inject:* 1 mg/ml; **Monitor:** BP, HR, ECG, CI, PCWP, CVP, I/Os, peripheral pulses, BUN/SCr, electrolytes, S/S HF; **Notes:** Correct electrolyte abnormalities (↑ risk of arrhythmias with ↓ K+ or ↓ Mg++). LD does not need to be given (may just start infusion). May be used in HF patients on beta blocker therapy.

minocycline (Dynacin, Minocin, Myrac, Solodyn) Uses: Various infections caused by unusual organisms, including *Mycoplasma*, *Chlamydia*, and *Rickettsia*; Inhalational, gastrointestinal, or cutaneous anthrax (postexposure); Gonococcal and non-gonococcal urethritis; Acne; Acute intestinal amebiasis; **Class:** tetracyclines; **Preg:** D; **CIs:** Hypersensitivity; Pregnancy, lactation, or peds <8 yr—risk of permanent staining of teeth in infant/ped (for pregnancy, risk is ↑ during last half of pregnancy); Nephrogenic DI; **ADRs:** bulging fontanelles, dizziness, vestibular reactions, N/V/D, esophagitis, ↑ LFTs, photosensitivity, rash, pigmentation of skin and mucous membranes, blood dyscrasias, hypersensitivity reactions, superinfection; **Interactions:** Use with antacids, bismuth subsalicylate, or drugs containing Ca, aluminum, Mg++, iron, or zinc may ↓ absorption; May ↑ effects of warfarin; May ↓ effectiveness of estrogen-containing oral contraceptives; Ca in foods or dairy products may ↓ absorption; **Dose:** *PO: Adults:* 100–200 mg × 1, then 100 mg q 12 hr or 50 mg q 6 hr (max: 400 mg/day). *Acne*—50–100 mg/day (caps or IR tabs). *PO: Peds: ≥8 yr:* 4 mg/kg × 1, then 2 mg/kg q 12 hr. *PO: Adults and Peds: ≥12 yr and 91–136 kg Acne (Solodyn)*—135 mg/day × 12 wk. *PO: Adults and Peds: ≥12 yr and 60–90 kg Acne (Solodyn)*—90 mg/day × 12 wk. *PO: Adults and Peds: ≥12 yr and 45–59 kg Acne (Solodyn)*—45 mg/day × 12 wk. *Renal Impairment PO: Adults and Peds:* Max dose: 200 mg/day; **Availability:** *Caps:* 50, 75, 100 mg. *Tabs:* 50, 75, 100 mg. *ER tabs (Solodyn):* 45, 90, 135 mg; **Monitor:** BP, HR, temp, sputum, U/A, CBC, LFTs, acne lesions; **Notes:** Do not administer within 1–3 hr of other meds. Give with ≥8 oz of liquid ≥1 hr before bedtime, and have patient sit up for ≥30 min after dose to ↓ esophageal irritation. Give ≥1 hr ac or ≥2 hr pc (may be taken with food if GI irritation occurs). Advise patient to use sunscreen.

mirtazapine (Remeron, Remeron Soltabs) Uses: Depression; **Class:** tetracyclic antidepressants; **Preg:** C; **CIs:** Hypersensitivity; MAOI therapy within 14 days; **ADRs:** drowsiness, abnormal dreams, abnormal thinking, agitation, anxiety, apathy, confusion, dizziness, malaise, weakness, sinusitis, dyspnea, ↑ cough, edema, ↓ BP, constipation, dry mouth, ↑ appetite, abdominal pain, anorexia, ↑ LFTs, N/V, urinary frequency, pruritus, rash, ↑ thirst, AGRANULOCYTOSIS, ↑ wt, ↑ cholesterol, ↑ TGs, arthralgia, back pain, myalgia, hyperkinesia, hypesthesia, twitching, flu-like syndrome; **Interactions:** May cause HTN, seizures, and death when used with MAOIs (do not use within 14 days of MAOI therapy); ↑ CNS depression with other CNS depressants, alcohol, and BZs; CYP1A2, CYP2D6 and CYP3A4 inhibitors may ↑ levels/effects; CYP1A2 and CYP3A4 inducers may ↓ levels/effects; **Dose:** *PO: Adults:* 15 mg at bedtime; may ↑ q 1–2 wk up to 45 mg/day. *Hepatic/Renal Impairment PO: Adults:* ↓ dose if CrCl <40 ml/min; clearance ↓ by 30% in hepatic impairment; **Availability (G):** *Tabs:* 15, 30, 45 mg. *ODT:* 15, 30, 45 mg;

Monitor: Mental status, mood, BP, HR, wt, lipid panel, CBC, LFTs; **Notes:** ODTs can be taken without water.

misoprostol (Cytotec) **Uses:** Prevention of gastric mucosal injury from NSAIDs; Termination of pregnancy; **Class:** prostaglandins; **Preg:** X; **CIs:** Hypersensitivity to prostaglandins; Pregnancy or lactation; **ADRs:** HA, abdominal pain, N/V/D, constipation, dyspepsia, flatulence, miscarriage, menstrual disorders; **Interactions:** ↑ risk of diarrhea with Mg-containing antacids; **Dose:** *PO: Adults: Antiulcer*—100–200 mcg qid ac and at bedtime *or* 400 mcg bid. *Termination of Pregnancy*—400 mcg 24–48 h after mifepristone; **Availability (G):** *Tabs:* 100, 200 mcg; **Monitor:** Epigastric/abdominal pain, S/S GI bleeding; **Notes:** Causes spontaneous abortion; advise on use of contraception. Give with meals.

mitomycin (MitoExtra, Mutamycin) **Uses:** Disseminated adenocarcinoma of the stomach or pancreas; **Class:** antitumor antibiotics; **Preg:** D; **CIs:** Hypersensitivity; Pregnancy or lactation; Bleeding tendencies; Decreased bone marrow reserve; **ADRs:** PULMONARY TOXICITY, edema, N/V, anorexia, stomatitis, infertility, ↑ BUN/SCr, alopecia, desquamation, leukopenia, thrombocytopenia, anemia, phlebitis at IV site, HEMOLYTIC UREMIC SYNDROME, fever, prolonged malaise; **Interactions:** ↑ bone marrow depression with other antineoplastics or radiation therapy, ↓ antibody response to live-virus vaccines and ↑ risk of ADRs, Concurrent or sequential use with vinca alkaloids may ↑ respiratory toxicity; **Dose:** *IV: Adults:* 20 mg/m² q 6–8 wk. *Renal Impairment PO: Adults:* ↓ dose if CrCl <10 ml/min; do not give if SCr >1.7 mg/dl; **Availability (G):** *Inject:* 5, 20, 40 mg; **Monitor:** RR, BP, CBC (with diff), I/Os, BUN/SCr, S/S bleeding, or pulmonary toxicity; **Notes:** Nadirs of leukopenia and thrombocytopenia occur in 4–8 wk.

mitoxantrone (Novantrone) **Uses:** ANLL; Advanced hormone-refractory prostate CA; Relapsing MS; **Class:** antitumor antibiotics; **Preg:** D; **CIs:** Hypersensitivity; Pregnancy; LVEF <50%; Pre-existing myelosuppression; Previous mediastinal radiation; **ADRs:** SEIZURES, HA, blue-green sclera, conjunctivitis, cough, dyspnea, CARDIOTOXICITY, ARRHYTHMIAS, ECG changes, abdominal pain, HEPATOTOXICITY, N/V/D, stomatitis, blue-green urine, gonadal suppression, ↑ BUN/SCr, alopecia, rash, anemia, leukopenia, secondary leukemia, thrombocytopenia, ↑ uric acid, fever, hypersensitivity reactions; **Interactions:** ↑ bone marrow depression with other antineoplastics or radiation therapy; Risk of cardiomyopathy ↑ by previous anthracycline antineoplastics, or mediastinal radiation; ↓ antibody response to live-virus vaccines and ↑ risk of ADRs; **Dose:** *IV: Adults: Leukemia induction*—12 mg/m²/day × 3 days; if incomplete remission occurs, a 2nd induction course may be given. *Consolidation*—12 mg/m²/day × 2 days, given 6 wk after induction then again 4 wk later. *IV: Adults: Solid tumors*—12–14 mg/m² single dose. *IV: Adults: MS*—12 mg/m² q 3 mo; **Availability (G):** *Inject:* 2 mg/ml; **Monitor:** CBC, LFTs, BUN/SCr, uric acid, CXR, ECG, S/S HF/bleeding, LVEF; **Notes:** Give IV over 30 min. Nadir of leukopenia occurs within 10 days, and recovery by 21 days.

modafinil (Provigil) Uses: Narcolepsy, obstructive sleep apnea, or shift work sleep disorder; **Class:** central nervous system stimulants; **Preg:** C; **CIs:** Hypersensitivity; History of LVH, ischemia, angina, recent MI, or mitral valve prolapse; **ADRs:** <u>HA</u>, anxiety, depression, dizziness, insomnia, nervousness, <u>rhinitis</u>, abnormal vision, pharyngitis, dyspnea, ↑ HR, CP, HTN, <u>N/V/D</u>, anorexia, mouth ulcers, ↑ LFTs, eosinophilia, back pain, paresthesia, tremor; **Interactions:** CYP3A4 inhibitors may ↑ levels/effects; CYP3A4 inducers may ↓ levels/effects; May ↑ levels/effects of CYP2C19 substrates; **Dose:** *PO: Adults:* 200 mg/day. *Hepatic Impairment PO: Adults: Severe hepatic impairment*—100 mg/day; **Availability:** *Tabs:* 100, 200 mg; **Monitor:** LFTs, BP, frequency of narcoleptic episodes; **Notes:** Give dose daily in the AM.

moexipril (Univasc) Uses: HTN; **Class:** ACEIs; **Preg:** C (1st tri), D (2nd and 3rd tri); **CIs:** Previous sensitivity/intolerance to ACEIs; **ADRs:** <u>dizziness</u>, <u>cough</u>, ↓ <u>BP</u>, ↑ SCr, ↑ K+, ANGIOEDEMA; **Interactions:** ↑ effects with other antihypertensives; ↑ risk of hyperkalemia with ARBs, K+ supplements, K+ salt substitutes, K+ sparing diuretics, or NSAIDs; NSAIDs may ↓ effectiveness; ↑ lithium levels; **Dose:** *PO: Adults:* 3.75–30 mg/day as a single dose or 2 divided doses. *Renal Impairment PO: Adults:* ↓ dose if CrCl <40 ml/min; **Availability (G):** *Tabs:* 7.5, 15 mg; **Monitor:** BP, HR, wt, edema, BUN/SCr, K+; **Notes:** Correct volume depletion. Advise on S/S angioedema, avoidance of K+ salt substitutes, and taking on an empty stomach.

mometasone (Nasonex, Asmanex, Elocon) Uses: **Intranasal:** Treatment of nasal symptoms of seasonal and perennial allergic rhinitis; prophylaxis of seasonal allergic rhinitis; treatment of nasal polyps, **Topical:** Relief of dermatoses; **Inhaln:** Maintenance therapy of asthma; **Class:** corticosteroids; **Preg:** C; **CIs:** Hypersensitivity; Active untreated infections; Acute asthma attack (inhaln); **ADRs:** <u>HA</u>, <u>pharyngitis</u>, epistaxis, nasal burning/irritation, nasopharyngeal fungal infection, sinusitis, vomiting, allergic contact dermatitis, atrophy, dryness, edema, folliculitis, hypertrichosis, hypopigmentation, dysmenorrhea, adrenal suppression (high dose, long-term), ↓ growth (peds), pain, cough; **Interactions:** None known; **Dose:** *Intranasal: Adults and Peds: ≥12 yr Allergic rhinitis (treatment)*—2 sprays in each nostril daily (max: 2 sprays in each nostril daily). *Allergic rhinitis (prophylaxis)*—2 sprays in each nostril daily 2–4 wk prior to pollen season. *Intranasal: Peds: 2–11 yr Allergic rhinitis (treatment)*—1 spray in each nostril daily. *Intranasal: Adults: ≥18 yr Nasal polyps*—2 sprays in each nostril 1–2 ×/day (max: 2 sprays in each nostril bid). *Inhaln: Adults and Peds: >12 yr No oral steroid therapy*—1 inhaln 220 mcg daily (max: 440 mcg/day); *Oral steroid therapy*—440 mcg bid (max: 880 mcg/day). *Inhaln: Peds 4–11 yr:* 110 mcg daily in evening. *Topical: Adults:* Apply once daily; **Availability (G):** *Nasal spray:* 50 mcg/metered spray; *Powder for oral inhaln:* 110 mcg/inhaln, 220 mcg/inhaln; *Cream/Oint/Lotion:* 0.1%; **Monitor:** Nasal symptoms, RR, PFTs, frequency of asthma attacks, growth rate (peds); **Notes:** Oints are preferred for dry, scaly lesions. Creams should be used on oozing or intertriginous areas. Lotion is useful in hairy areas. Dose should be titrated to effect; use lowest possible dose.

montelukast (Singulair) **Uses:** Prevention/treatment of asthma; Allergic rhinitis; Exercise-induced bronchoconstriction; **Class:** leukotriene antagonists; **Preg:** B; **CIs:** Hypersensitivity; Acute attacks of asthma; Phenylketonuria (chew tabs contain aspartame); **ADRs:** fatigue, HA, weakness, otitis, sinusitis, cough, rhinorrhea, abdominal pain, diarrhea, dyspepsia, nausea, ↑ LFTs, rash; **Interactions:** CYP2C9 and CYP3A4 inhibitors may ↑ levels/effects; CYP2C9 and CYP3A4 inducers may ↓ levels/effects; **Dose:** *PO: Adults and Peds: ≥15 yr:* Asthma or allergic rhinitis 10 mg/day. *PO: Peds: 6–14 yr:* Asthma or allergic rhinitis 5 mg/day. *PO: Peds: 6 months–5 yr:* Asthma or allergic rhinitis 4 mg/day. *PO: Adults: Exercise-induced bronchospasm*—10 mg 2 hr before exercise; **Availability:** *Tabs:* 10 mg. *Chew tabs:* 4, 5 mg. *Granules:* 4 mg/packet; **Monitor:** LFTs, RR, PFTs, S/S asthma/rhinitis; **Notes:** Give in the evening for asthma; give granules directly into mouth or mix in applesauce, mashed carrots, rice, or ice cream. Not for acute asthma attacks.

morphine (Astramorph, Astramorph PF, Avinza, Duramorph, DepoDur, Infumorph, Kadian, MS, MS Contin, MSIR, OMS Concentrate, Oramorph SR, RMS, Roxanol, Roxanol Rescudose, Roxanol-T) **Uses:** Severe pain; Pulmonary edema; Preanesthetic med; **Class:** opioid agonists; **Preg:** C; **CIs:** Hypersensitivity; Current or recent use (within 2 wk) of MAOIs, Head trauma; ↑ ICP; Respiratory depression, Undiagnosed abdominal pain; **ADRs:** <u>confusion</u>, <u>sedation</u>, dizziness, dysphoria, euphoria, hallucinations, HA, blurred vision, diplopia, miosis, respiratory depression, ↓ <u>BP</u>, <u>constipation</u>, N/V, urinary retention, flushing, sweating, physical/psychological dependence, tolerance; **Interactions:** Concurrent MAOI use may result in severe, unpredictable reactions—↓ morphine to 25% of usual dose; ↑ CNS depression with alcohol, sedative/hypnotics, barbiturates, TCAs, and antihistamines, Partial-antagonist opioid analgesics may precipitate withdrawal in physically dependent patients, Buprenorphine, nalbuphine, butorphanol, or pentazocine may ↓ analgesia; May ↑ risk of bleeding with warfarin; **Dose:** *PO: Rect Adults: ≥50 kg Moderate-to-severe pain (opioid-naive)*—30 mg q 3–4 hr *or* once daily opioid requirement is determined, convert to CR, ER, or SR prep by giving total daily dose q 24 hr (as *Kadian, Avinza*), divided q 12 hr (as *Oramorph SR, Kadian, MS Contin*), divided q 8 hr (as *MS Contin*). *Avinza* max: 1600 mg/day. *PO, Rect: Adults and Peds: <50 kg Moderate-to-severe pain (opioid-naive)*—0.3 mg/kg q 3–4 hr. *PO: Peds: >1 mo IR tabs and soln*—0.2–0.5 mg/kg q 4–6 hr prn. *CR tabs*—0.3–0.6 mg/kg q 12 hr. *IM, IV, Subcut: Adults: ≥50 kg Moderate-to-severe pain (opioid-naive)*—4–10 mg q 3–4 hr. *Acute MI pain*—8–15 mg. *IM, IV, Subcut: Adults and Peds: <50 kg Moderate-to-severe pain (opioid-naive)*—0.05–0.2 mg/kg q 3–4 hr (max: 15 mg/dose). *IM, IV, Subcut: Neonates:* 0.05 mg/kg q 4–8 hr (max dose: 0.1 mg/kg) (preservative-free). *IV, Subcut: Adults: Continuous infusion*—15 mg bolus then 0.8–10 mg/hr; rates vary depending on tolerance level. *IV, Subcut: Peds: >1 mo Continuous infusion*—0.01–2.6 mg/kg/hr. *IV: Neonates Continuous infusion*—0.01–0.03 mg/kg/hr. *Epidural: Adults: Intermittent inject*—5 mg/day (initially); if no relief within 60 min, ↑ by 1–2 mg (max: 10 mg/day). *Continuous infusion*—2–4 mg/24 hr; ↑ by 1–2 mg/day (max: 30 mg/day). *Single dose ER liposomal inject*—lower extremity orthopedic surgery: 15 mg; lower abdominal/pelvic surgery: 10–15 mg; C-section: 10 mg (preservative-free). *Epidural: Peds: >1 mo:* 0.03–0.05 mg/kg (max dose: 0.1 mg/kg or 5 mg/24 hr) (preservative-free). *IT: Adults:* 0.2–1 mg (preservative-free). **Availability (G):** *Tabs:* 15, 30 mg. *ER, CR, SR tabs:* 15, 30, 60, 100, 200 mg. *SR caps (Kadian):* 10, 20, 30, 50, 60, 80, 100, 200 mg. *ER caps (Avinza):* 30, 60, 90, 120 mg. *Oral soln:* 10 mg/5 ml, 20 mg/5 ml, 100 mg/5 ml, 20 mg/ml (concentrate). *Supp:* 5, 10, 20, 30 mg. *Inject:* 1 mg/ml, 2 mg/ml, 4 mg/ml, 5 mg/ml, 8 mg/ml, 10 mg/ml, 15 mg/ml, 25 mg/ml, 50 mg/ml. *Epidural inject (preservative-free):* 0.5 mg/ml, 1 mg/ml. *Epidural/IT inject (continuous microinfusion device; preservative-free):* 10 mg/ml, 25 mg/ml. *ER liposome inject for epidural use:* 10 mg/ml. *Inject (PCA device):* 1 mg/ml, 2 mg/ml, 3 mg/ml, 5 mg/ml; **Monitor:** BP, RR, HR, pain, S/S withdrawal/sedation; **Notes:** Schedule II controlled substance. Prevent constipation with ↑ intake of fluids, bulk, and laxatives. Discontinue gradually after long-term use to prevent withdrawal symptoms; use only preservative-free formulations in neonates, and for epidural and IT routes in all patients. Naloxone is antidote. Do not crush ER, CR, or SR products. Kadian and Avinza can be opened and sprinkled on applesauce (do not chew or crush the beads).

M

moxifloxacin (Avelox, Vigamox) Uses: PO, IV: Respiratory tract infections, skin/skin structure infections, and intra-abdominal infections due to susceptible organisms (e.g., *S. pneumo*, *S. aureus*, *S. pyogenes*, *E. faecalis*, *E. coli*, *Klebsiella*, *H. flu*, *M. catarrhalis*, *B. fragilis*, *Enterobacter*, or *Proteus*); **Ophth:** Conjunctivitis; **Class:** fluoroquinolones; **Preg:** C; **CIs:** Hypersensitivity (cross-sensitivity within class may exist); QT interval prolongation; Do not use during pregnancy unless potential benefit outweighs potential fetal risk; Peds (safety not established); **ADRs:** SEIZURES, agitation, anxiety, dizziness, HA, insomnia, QT interval prolongation, PSEUDOMEMBRANOUS COLITIS, abdominal pain, ↑ LFTs, <u>N/V/D</u>, photosensitivity, rash, ↑↓ BG, dyspepsia, tendonitis, tendon rupture, HYPERSENSITIVITY REACTIONS including

ANAPHYLAXIS; **Interactions:** ↑ risk of QT prolongation with other QT-prolonging drugs; Use with antacids, Ca++ supplements, iron salts, zinc, didanosine, or sucralfate may ↓ absorption; May ↑ the effects of warfarin; May ↑ risk of hypoglycemia with sulfonylureas; May ↑ risk of seizures when used with NSAIDs; ↑ risk of tendon rupture with corticosteroids; Absorption ↓ by dairy products; **Dose:** *IV, PO: Adults:* 400 mg/day (× 5–21 days, depending on infection). *Ophth: Adults:* Instill 1 gtt in eye tid × 7 days; **Availability:** *Tabs:* 400 mg. *Inject:* 400 mg. *Ophth soln:* 0.5%; **Monitor:** BP, HR, temp, sputum, U/A, CBC, BG (in DM), rash, tendon pain; **Notes:** Give ≥4 hr before or ≥8 hr after products/foods containing Ca++, Mg++, aluminum, iron, or zinc. Advise patient to use sunscreen.

mupirocin (Bactroban, Bactroban Nasal) **Uses: Topical:** Treatment of: Impetigo, Skin lesions caused by *Staphylococcus aureus* and *Streptococcus pyogenes*; **Intranasal:** Eradication of nasal colonization with MRSA; **Class:** (top); **Preg:** B; **CIs:** Hypersensitivity; **ADRs:** HA, cough, itching, pharyngitis, rhinitis, upper respiratory tract congestion, nausea, altered taste, burning sensation, itching, pain, stinging; **Interactions:** Nasal mupirocin should not be used concurrently with other nasal products; **Dose:** *Top: Adults and Peds: ≥2 mo:* Oint: Apply 3–5 times/day × 5–14 days. *Top: Adults and Peds: ≥3 mo:* Cream: Apply tid × 10 days; *Intranasal: Adults and Peds: ≥1 yr:* Apply small amount nasal oint to each nostril bid–qid × 5–14 days; **Availability (G):** *Oint/Cream:* 2%. *Nasal oint:* 2%; **Monitor:** Resolution of skin lesions; **Notes:** Apply one half of nasal oint to each nostril; after application, close nostrils by pressing together and releasing sides of the nose repeatedly for 1 min.

M

muromonab-CD3 (Orthoclone OKT3) **Uses:** Acute renal, hepatic, or cardiac allograft rejection reactions in transplant patients; **Class:** monoclonal antibodies; **Preg:** C; **CIs:** Hypersensitivity to muromonab-CD3 or murine (mouse) proteins; Fluid overload; **ADRs:** tremor, aseptic meningitis, dizziness, PULMONARY EDEMA, dyspnea, wheezing, CP, N/V/D, CYTOKINE RELEASE SYNDROME, INFECTIONS, chills, fever, hypersensitivity reactions, ↑ risk of lymphoma; **Interactions:** ↑ immunosuppression with other immunosuppressives, Prednisone, cyclosporine, and azathioprine dosages should be ↓ (↑ risk of infection and lymphoproliferative disorders), ↑ CNS reactions with indomethacin, ↓ antibody response to live-virus vaccines; **Dose:** *IV: Adults:* 5 mg/day × 10–14 days (pretreatment with corticosteroids, acetaminophen, and/or antihistamines recommended). *IV: Peds:* 0.1 mg/kg/day × 10–14 days; **Availability:** *Inject:* 1 mg/ml; **Monitor:** CXR, wt, I/Os, edema, CBC, temp, BP, RR, HR, OKT3 levels, S/S anaphylaxis; **Notes:** Target levels should be >0.8 mcg/ml; may give IV push undiluted.

mycophenolate (CellCept, Myfortic) **Uses: Mycophenolate mofetil:** Prevention of rejection in allogenic renal, hepatic, and cardiac transplantation; *Mycophenolic acid:* Prevention of rejection in allogenic renal transplantation; **Class:** immunosuppressants; **Preg:** D; **CIs:** Hypersensitivity to mycophenolate or polysorbate 80 (IV form); Phenylketonuria (oral suspension contains aspartame); Patients with childbearing potential; **ADRs:** PROGRESSIVE MULTIFOCAL LEUKOENCEPHALOPATHY, anxiety, dizziness, HA, insomnia, paresthesia, tremor, edema, HTN, ↓ BP, ↑ HR, rash, hypercholesterolemia, ↑ BG, ↑↓ K+, ↓ Ca++, ↓ Mg++, GI BLEEDING, anorexia, constipation, N/V/D, abdominal pain, renal dysfunction, leukocytosis, leukopenia, thrombocytopenia, anemia, cough, dyspnea, fever, infection, ↑ risk of malignancy; **Interactions:** Combined use with azathioprine is not recommended (effects unknown); Acyclovir and ganciclovir may ↑ toxicity; Mg and aluminum containing antacids, cholestyramine, and colestipol ↓ absorption (avoid concurrent use); May interfere with the action of oral contraceptives (additional contraceptive method should be used); May ↓ the antibody response/↑ risk of ADRs from live-virus vaccines; **Dose:** *Mycophenolate mofetil PO, IV: Adults: Renal transplantation*—1 g bid; IV should be started ≤24 hr after transplantation and switched to PO as soon as possible (IV not recommended for ≥14 days). *PO: Peds: 3 mo–18 yr Renal transplantation*—600 mg/m^2 bid (max: 2 g/day). *PO, IV: Adults: Liver transplantation*—1 g bid IV *or* 1.5 g bid PO. IV should be started ≤24 hr after transplantation and switched to PO as soon as possible (IV not recommended for ≥14 days). *PO, IV: Adults: Heart transplantation*—1.5 g bid; IV should be started ≤24 hr after transplantation and switched to PO as soon as possible (IV not recommended for ≥14 days). *Renal Impairment PO, IV: Adults: CrCl <25 ml/min*—daily dose should not exceed 2 g. *Mycophenolic acid PO: Adults: Renal transplantation*—720 mg bid. *PO: Peds: 5–16 yr and ≥1.19 m^2 Renal transplantation*—400 mg/m^2 bid (max: 720 mg bid); **Availability: Mycophenolate mofetil (Cellcept)** *Caps:* 250 mg. *Tabs:* 500 mg. *Oral susp:* 200 mg/ml. *Powder for inject:* 500 mg. **Mycophenolic acid (Myfortic)** *DR tabs (Myfortic):* 180, 360 mg; **Monitor:** CBC, electrolytes, BG, BUN/SCr, LFTs, BP, Lipid panel, S/S organ rejection; **Notes:** Neutropenia occurs most frequently from 31–180 days post-transplant. If ANC <1000, dose should be ↓ or discontinued. Give on an empty stomach. Caps and DR tabs should not be opened, crushed, or chewed. May be teratogenic; contents of capsules should not be inhaled or come in contact with skin or mucous membranes.

nadolol (Corgard) **Uses:** HTN; Angina; **Class:** beta blockers; **Preg:** C; **CIs:** Hypersensitivity; Decompensated HF; Pulmonary edema; Cardiogenic shock; Bradycardia or ≥2nd-degree heart block (in absence of pacemaker); **ADRs:** fatigue, weakness, depression, dizziness, drowsiness, nightmares, blurred vision, bronchospasm, BRADYCARDIA, HF, PULMONARY EDEMA, ↓ BP, N/V/D, ED, ↓ libido, ↑↓ BG; **Interactions:** ↑ risk of bradycardia with digoxin, diltiazem, verapamil, or clonidine; ↑ effects with other antihypertensives; ↑ risk of hypertensive crisis if concurrent clonidine discontinued; May alter the effectiveness of insulins or oral hypoglycemic agents; May ↓ the effects of $beta_1$ agonists (e.g., dopamine, dobutamine); **Dose:** *PO: Adults: Angina*—40–80 mg/day (max: 240 mg/day). *HTN*—40–80 mg/day (max: 320 mg/day). *Renal Impairment PO: Adults:* ↓ dose if CrCl <40 ml/min; **Availability (G):** *Tabs:* 20, 40, 80, 120, 160 mg; **Monitor:** BP, HR, ECG, S/S HF, edema, wt, S/S angina, BUN/SCr, BG (in DM); **Notes:** Abrupt withdrawal may cause life-threatening arrhythmias, hypertensive crises, or myocardial ischemia. May mask S/S of hypoglycemia (esp. tachycardia) in DM.

nafcillin (Nallpen, Unipen) **Uses:** Osteomyelitis, skin/skin structure infections, bacteremia, and endocarditis due to penicillinase-producing staphylococci; **Class:** penicillinase resistant penicillins; **Preg:** B; **CIs:** Hypersensitivity (cross-sensitivity to other beta-lactam antibiotics may exist); **ADRs:** SEIZURES, PSEUDOMEMBRANOUS COLITIS, N/V/D, ↑ LFTs, interstitial nephritis, rash, urticaria, eosinophilia, leukopenia, ANAPHYLAXIS and SERUM SICKNESS, superinfection; **Interactions:** Probenecid ↓ excretion and ↑ levels; **Dose:** *IM, Adults:* 500 mg q 4–6 hr. *IV: Adults:* 500–2000 mg q 4–6 hr. *IM, IV: Peds: and Infants:* 50–200 mg/kg/day divided q 4–6 hr (max: 12 g/day). *IM, IV: Neonates: <7 days, <2 kg* 50 mg/kg/day divided q 12 hr. *IM, IV: Neonates: <7 days, >2 kg:* 75 mg/kg/day divided q 8 hr. *IM, IV: Neonates: ≥7 days, <2 kg:* 75 mg/kg/day divided q 8 hr. *IM, IV: Neonates: ≥7 days, >2 kg:* 100–140 mg/kg/day divided q 6 hr; **Availability (G):** *Inject:* 1 g, 2 g, 10 g; **Monitor:** BP, HR, temp, sputum, U/A, BUN/SCr, CBC, LFTs; **Notes:** Use with caution in patients with beta-lactam allergy (do not use if history of anaphylaxis or hives). Dilute to a concentration of 2–40 mg/ml and infuse IV over 30–60 min to avoid vein irritation.

nalbuphine (Nubain) **Uses:** Moderate-to-severe pain; Analgesia during labor; Sedation before surgery; Supplement to balanced anesthesia; **Class:** opioid agonists/analgesics; **Preg:** C; **CIs:** Hypersensitivity; Patients physically dependent on opioids; ↑ ICP; Undiagnosed abdominal pain; **ADRs:** dizziness, HA, sedation, confusion, dysphoria, euphoria, hallucinations, respiratory depression, orthostatic hypotension, ↑ HR, dry mouth, N/V, constipation, ileus, urinary urgency, sweating, physical/psychological dependence, tolerance; **Interactions:** Concurrent MAOIs (↓ nalbuphine to 25% of usual dose); ↑ CNS depression with alcohol, antihistamines, and sedative/hypnotics; May precipitate withdrawal in patients who are physically dependent on opioid agonists, opioid analgesic agonists may ↓ analgesic effects; **Dose:** *IM, Subcut, IV: Adults:* 10 mg q 3–6 hr (max: 20 mg/dose or 160 mg/day). *IM, IV, Subcut: Peds:* 0.1–0.2 mg/kg q 3–4 hr prn (max: 20 mg/dose or 160 mg/day). *IV: Adults: Anesthesia supplement*—0.3–3 mg/kg over 10–15 min then 0.25–0.5 mg/kg prn;

N

Availability (G): *Inject:* 10 mg/ml, 20 mg/ml; **Monitor:** Pain, BP, HR, RR, S/S withdrawal; **Notes:** May give IV undiluted at a rate of 10 mg over 3–5 min.

naloxone (Narcan) **Uses:** Reversal of CNS/respiratory depression from opioid overdose; **Class:** opioid antagonists; **Preg:** B; **CIs:** Hypersensitivity; CV disease; Patients physically dependent on opioids; **ADRs:** HTN, ↓ BP, VT/VF, N/V; **Interactions:** Causes withdrawal in patients physically dependent on opioid analgesics; Larger doses may be required to reverse the effects of buprenorphine; butorphanol, nalbuphine, pentazocine, or propoxyphene; Antagonizes postoperative opioid analgesics; **Dose:** *IV: Adults Postoperative opioid-induced respiratory depression*—0.02–0.2 mg q 2–3 min until response; repeat q 1–2 hr if needed. *IV: Peds and Neonates: Postoperative opioid-induced respiratory depression*—0.01 mg/kg; may repeat q 2–3 min until response; repeat q 1–2 hr if needed. *IV, IM, Subcut: Adults: >40 kg Opioid-induced respiratory depression from chronic opioid use (>1 wk)*—0.02–0.04 mg given as small, frequent (q min) boluses or as an infusion titrated to improve respiratory function without reversing analgesia. *IV, IM, Subcut: Adults and Peds: <40 kg Opioid-induced depression from chronic opioid use* (> *1 wk*)—0.005–0.02 mg/dose given as small, frequent (q min) boluses or as an infusion. *IV, IM, Subcut: Adults: Opioid overdoses in patients not suspected of being opioid dependent*—0.4–2 mg; may repeat q 2–3 min. *Patients suspected of being opioid dependent*—0.1–0.2 mg q 2–3 min. *IV, IM, Subcut: Peds: >5 yr or >20 kg Opioid overdose*—2 mg/dose, may repeat q 2–3 min. *IV, IM, Subcut: Infants: <5 yr or <20 kg Opioid overdose*—0.1 mg/kg, may repeat q 2–3 min. *IV: Adults and Peds: Opioid-induced pruritus*—0.25–2 mcg/kg/hr continuous infusion; **Availability (G):** *Inject:* 0.4 mg/ml, 1 mg/ml; **Monitor:** RR, HR, BP, ECG, S/S opioid withdrawal; **Notes:** Lack of response indicates that symptoms are caused by a disease process or other non-opioid CNS depressants not affected by naloxone.

naproxen (Aleve, Anaprox, Anaprox DS, EC-Naprosyn, Naprelan, Naprosyn) **Uses:** Pain/fever; Dysmenorrhea; Gout; OA; RA; **Class:** NSAIDs; **Preg:** C, D (3rd tri); **CIs:** Hypersensitivity to aspirin or NSAIDs; Active bleeding; Perioperative pain from CABG surgery; **ADRs:** HA, dizziness, tinnitus, edema, GI BLEEDING, N/V/D, ↑ SCr, rash; **Interactions:** ↑ adverse GI effects with aspirin and corticosteroids; ↓ effects of aspirin, or antihypertensives; ↑ risk of bleeding with antiplatelet agents or anticoagulants; ↑ nephrotoxicity with cyclosporine; ↑ levels of methotrexate or lithium; **Dose:** *PO: Adults: Anti-inflammatory/Analgesic/Antidysmenorrheal*—Naproxen: 250–500 mg bid (max: 1.5 g/day); DR tabs: 375–500 mg bid; naproxen Na: 275–550 mg bid (max: 1.65 g/day). *Gout*—Naproxen: 750 mg × 1, then 250 mg q 8 hr; naproxen Na: 825 mg × 1, then 275 mg q 8 hr. *PO: Peds: >2 yr Analgesia*—5–7 mg/kg q 8–12 hr. *Inflammatory disease*—10–15 mg/kg/day divided q 12 hr (max: 1000 mg/

day). *Renal Impairment Adults and Peds:* Not recommended for use when CrCl <30 ml/min; **Availability (G):** *Tabs (naproxen):* 250, 375, 500 mg. *CR tabs (naproxen sodium):* 412.5, 550 mg. *DR, EC tabs:* 375, 500 mg. *Tabs (naproxen sodium):* 220, 275, 550 mg. *Oral susp:* 125 mg/5 ml; **Monitor:** Pain, temp, S/S of GI upset/bleeding, BUN/SCr, LFTs, CBC; **Notes:** Avoid use in oliguria/anuria. Give with food. 275 mg naproxen sodium = 250 mg naproxen.

naratriptan (Amerge) **Uses:** Acute treatment of migraines; **Class:** 5–HT_1 agonists; **Preg:** C; **CIs:** Hypersensitivity; CAD or significant CV disease; Uncontrolled HTN; Use of other 5-HT_1 agonists or ergot-type drugs (dihydroergotamine) within 24 hr; Basilar or hemiplegic migraine; Concurrent or recent (within 2 wk) use of MAOIs; CV risk factors (use only if CV status has been determined to be safe and 1st dose is administered under supervision); Severe renal (CrCl <15 ml/min) and hepatic impairment; **ADRs:** dizziness, drowsiness, CORONARY ARTERY VASOSPASM, MI/ISCHEMIA, VT/VF, nausea; **Interactions:** MAOIs ↑ levels (concurrent or recent [within 2 wk] use contraindicated); Use with other 5-HT_1 agonists or ergot-type compounds may ↑ risk of vasospasm (avoid use within 24 hr of each other); Use with SSRIs or SNRIs may ↑ risk of serotonin syndrome; Hormonal contraceptives may ↑ levels/toxicity; **Dose:** *PO: Adults:* 1–2.5 mg initially, may repeat in 4 hr (max: 5 mg in 24 hr). *Renal Impairment PO: Adults:* ↓ dose if CrCl <40 ml/min. *Hepatic Impairment PO: Adults:* Mild-to-moderate hepatic impairment: 1 mg (max 2.5 mg/day); **Availability:** *Tabs:* 1, 2.5 mg; **Monitor:** BP, HR, pain; **Notes:** Do not crush or chew tab. For acute treatment only, not for prophylaxis; administer as soon as migraine symptoms occur.

nateglinide (Starlix) **Uses:** Type 2 DM; **Class:** meglitinides; **Preg:** C; **CIs:** Hypersensitivity; DKA; Type 1 DM; **ADRs:** dizziness, diarrhea, ↑ LFTs, ↑ wt, ↓ BG, arthropathy, ↑ uric acid, flu symptoms; **Interactions:** Beta blockers may mask hypoglycemia, Alcohol, antidiabetic agents, NSAIDs, MAOIs, nonselective beta blockers may ↑ risk of hypoglycemia; Diuretics, corticosteroids, thyroid supplements, or sympathomimetics may ↓ effects; **Dose:** *PO: Adults:* 60–120 mg tid ac; **Availability:** *Tabs:* 60, 120 mg; **Monitor:** A1C, glucose, wt, LFTs, S/S hypoglycemia; **Notes:** Administer 1–30 min ac. Skip dose if NPO.

nesiritide (Natrecor) **Uses:** Acutely decompensated HF; **Class:** vasodilators; **Preg:** C; **CIs:** Hypersensitivity; Cardiogenic shock; SBP <90 mmHg; **ADRs:** dizziness, HA, ↓ BP, N/V, ↑ BUN/SCr, inject site reactions; **Interactions:** ↑ risk of hypotension with antihypertensive agents; **Dose:** *IV: Adults:* 2 mcg/kg bolus followed by 0.01 mcg/kg/min as a continuous infusion. May ↑ by 0.005 mcg/kg/min q 3 hr (max infusion rate: 0.03 mcg/kg/min); **Availability:** *Inject:* 1.5 mg; **Monitor:** BP, HR, ECG, CI, PCWP, CVP, I/Os, peripheral pulses, BUN/SCr, S/S HF;

N

Notes: ↓ dose or discontinue if hypotension develops. Bolus should be drawn from infusion bag. Usually administered for 48 hr.

nevirapine (Viramune) **Uses:** HIV infection (with other antiretrovirals); **Class:** non-nucleoside reverse transcriptase inhibitors; **Preg:** C; **CIs:** Hypersensitivity, Moderate-to-severe hepatic impairment; **ADRs:** HA, HEPATOTOXICITY, ↑ LFTs, N/V/D, abdominal pain, SJS, TEN, rash, myalgia, fever; **Interactions:** CYP3A4 inhibitors may ↑ levels/toxicity; CYP3A4 inducers may ↓ levels/effects; May ↓ levels/effects of CYP2B6 substrates and CYP3A4 substrates; ↑ risk of bleeding with warfarin; May ↑ rifabutin levels; Prednisone may ↑ risk of rash; **Dose:** *PO: Adults:* 200 mg/day × 2 wk, then 200 mg bid. *PO: Peds >15 days:* 150 mg/m^2 daily × 2 wk, then 150 mg/m^2 bid (max: 400 mg/day); **Availability:** *Tabs:* 200 mg. *Oral susp:* 50 mg/5 ml; **Monitor:** CD4 count, viral load, LFTs, S/S rash; **Notes:** Discontinue if rash develops (may progress to TEN or SJS); females with CD4 >250 cells/mm^3 or males with CD4 >400 cells/mm^3 are at ↑ risk of hepatotoxicity.

niCARdipine (Cardene, Cardene SR, Cardene IV) **Uses:** HTN; Chronic stable angina; **Class:** Ca channel blockers; **Preg:** C; **CIs:** Hypersensitivity, Advanced aortic stenosis; **ADRs:** HA, dizziness, peripheral edema, ↓ BP, ↑ angina, ↑ HR, N/V/D, flushing, gingival hyperplasia; **Interactions:** NSAIDs may ↓ effectiveness; May ↑ levels/effects of CYP3A4 substrates; ↑ effects with other antihypertensives; CYP3A4 inhibitors may ↑ levels; CYP3A4 inducers may ↓ levels; **Dose:** *PO: Adults: HTN*—20–40 mg tid (IR) *or* 30–60 mg bid (SR). *Angina*—20–40 mg tid (IR). *IV: Adults: To replace PO use*—0.5–2.2 mg/hr continuous infusion (20 mg tid PO = 0.5 mg/hr IV; 30 mg tid PO = 1.2 mg/hr IV; 40 mg tid PO = 2.2 mg/hr IV). *Hypertensive crises*—5–15 mg/hr; **Availability (G):** *Caps:* 20, 30 mg. *SR caps:* 30, 45, 60 mg. *Inject:* 2.5 mg/ml; **Monitor:** BP, HR, ECG, peripheral edema, S/S angina; **Notes:** Instruct patient to avoid grapefruit juice (may ↑ effects). Do not crush, chew, or open SR caps.

N

nicotine (Nicorette, Commit, Nicotrol Inhaler, Nicotrol NS, Nicoderm CQ Thrive) **Uses:** Management of nicotine withdrawal; **Class:** smoking deterrents; **Preg:** D; **CIs:** Hypersensitivity; Pregnancy, Active temporomandibular joint disease (gum only); Recent MI; Arrhythmias; Severe or worsening angina; **ADRs:** HA, insomnia, dizziness, drowsiness, weakness, pharyngitis, ↑ HR, CP, ↑ BP, ↑ appetite, belching, oral injury, ↑ salivation, sore mouth, abdominal pain, abnormal taste, constipation, dry mouth, dyspepsia, hiccups, N/V/D, dysmenorrhea, jaw ache, arthralgia, back pain, myalgia, paresthesia; **Interactions:** Effects of acetaminophen, caffeine, imipramine, insulin, oxazepam, beta blockers, and theophylline may be ↑ during smoking cessation; dosage ↓ at cessation may be necessary; Doses of adrenergic agonists may need to be ↑ at cessation of smoking; Concurrent use of bupropion may cause treatment-emergent HTN; **Dose:** *Gum: Adults:* <25 cigarettes/day: 2 mg;

≥25 cigarettes/day: 4 mg. Chew one piece q 1–2 hr × 6 wk, then one piece q 2–4 hr × 2 wk, then one piece q 4–8 hr × 2 wk, then discontinue (max: 24 pieces/day). *Inhaln: Adults:* 6–16 cartridges/day × 3 mo, followed by gradual withdrawal over 6–12 wk. *Lozenge: Adults:* If 1st cigarette desired >30 min after awakening, start with 2 mg; if 1st cigarette desired <30 min after awakening, start with 4 mg. One lozenge q 1–2 hr × 6 wk, then one q 2–4 hr × 2 wk, then one q 4–8 hr × 2 wk, then discontinue (max 20 lozenges/day). *Intranasal: Adults:* One spray in each nostril 1–2 ×/hr, up to 5 ×/hr (max of 40 ×/day). *Transdermal: Adults: >10 cigarettes/day*—21 mg/day × 6 wk, then 14 mg/day × 2 wk, then 7 mg/day × 2 wk, then discontinue; *≤10 cigarettes/day*—14 mg/day × 6 wk, then 7 mg/day × 2 wk, then discontinue; **Availability (G):** *Gum*[OTC]*:* 2, 4 mg. *Inhalation:* 10 mg (4 mg nicotine)/cartridge. *Lozenge*[OTC]*:* 2, 4 mg. *Nasal spray:* 10 mg/ml (0.5 mg/spray). *Transdermal patch*[OTC]*:* 7 mg/day, 14 mg/day, 21 mg/day; **Monitor:** BP, HR, S/S nicotine toxicity; **Notes:** Inhalation regimens should consist of frequent, continuous puffing for 20 min; lozenges should be dissolved in the mouth, do not chew or swallow; do not sniff, swallow, or inhale nasal spray through nose during administration; apply patch daily to hairless, dry skin of upper arm or torso.

NIFEdipine (Adalat CC, Afeditab CR, Nifediac CC, Nifedical XL, Procardia, Procardia XL) **Uses:** HTN; Pulmonary HTN; Chronic stable angina or vasospastic (Prinzmetal's) angina; **Class:** Calcium channel blockers; **Preg:** C; **CIs:** Hypersensitivity; Acute MI; Hypertensive crisis (IR); **ADRs:** HA, dizziness, peripheral edema, ↓ BP, ↑ angina, ↑ HR, N/V/D, flushing, gingival hyperplasia; **Interactions:** NSAIDs may ↓ effectiveness; May ↑ levels/effects of CYP3A4 substrates; ↑ effects with other antihypertensives; CYP3A4 inhibitors may ↑ levels; CYP3A4 inducers may ↓ levels; **Dose:** *PO: Adults:* 10–30 mg tid (IR) (max: 180 mg/day) *or* 30–90 mg/day (ER) (max: 180 mg/day). *PO: Peds:* 0.6–0.9 mg/kg/day in 3–4 divided doses. *Hepatic Impairment PO: Adults and Peds:* ↓ dose by 50% (cirrhosis); **Availability (G):** *Caps:* 10, 20 mg. *ER tabs:* 30, 60, 90 mg; **Monitor:** BP, HR, ECG, peripheral edema, S/S angina; **Notes:** Instruct patient to avoid grapefruit juice (may ↑ effects). ER tabs should be used for angina and HTN. Do not crush, chew, or break ER tabs. ER tabs should be given on empty stomach.

nimodipine (Nimotop) **Uses:** Subarachnoid hemorrhage; **Class:** Calcium channel blockers; **Preg:** C; **CIs:** Hypersensitivity; **ADRs:** dizziness, HA, ↓ BP, peripheral edema, abdominal discomfort, diarrhea, ↑ LFTs, rash; **Interactions:** ↑ effects with other antihypertensives; CYP3A4 inhibitors may ↑ levels; CYP3A4 inducers may ↓ levels; **Dose:** *PO: Adults:* 60 mg q 4 hr within 96 hr of subarachnoid hemorrhage × 21 days; *Hepatic Impairment PO: Adults: Hepatic failure*—30 mg q 4 hr; **Availability (G):** *Caps:* 30 mg; **Monitor:** BP, HR, ECG, LFTs, peripheral edema, neurologic status; **Notes:** Have patient avoid grapefruit juice (may ↑ effects).

nisoldipine (Sular) Uses: HTN; **Class:** Calcium channel blockers; **Preg:** C; **CIs:** Hypersensitivity; **ADRs:** HA, dizziness, peripheral edema, ↓ BP, ↑ angina, ↑ HR, N/V/D, flushing, gingival hyperplasia; **Interactions:** NSAIDs may ↓ effectiveness; ↑ effects with other antihypertensives; CYP3A4 inhibitors may ↑ levels; CYP3A4 inducers may ↓ levels; **Dose:** *PO: Adults:* 17 mg/day; may ↑ by 8.5 mg q 7 days (max: 34 mg/day). *Hepatic Impairment PO: Adults:* ↓ starting dose to 8.5 mg/day; **Availability:** *ER tabs:* 8.5, 17, 25.5, 34 mg; **Monitor:** BP, HR, ECG, peripheral edema, S/S angina; **Notes:** Instruct patient to avoid grapefruit juice (may ↑ effects). Give on empty stomach (1 hr ac or 2 hr pc). Do not crush, chew, or break ER tabs.

nitrofurantoin (Furadantin, Macrobid, Macrodantin) Uses: Prevention/treatment of UTIs caused by susceptible organisms; **Class:** antibiotics; **Preg:** B; **CIs:** Hypersensitivity; Oliguria, anuria, or significant renal impairment (CrCl <60 ml/min); Infants <1 mo and pregnancy near term; **ADRs:** dizziness, drowsiness, HA, nystagmus, pneumonitis, CP, PSEUDOMEMBRANOUS COLITIS, anorexia, N/V/D, abdominal pain, ↑ LFTs, photosensitivity, blood dyscrasias, hemolytic anemia (↑ in infants <1 mo), peripheral neuropathy, hypersensitivity reactions; **Interactions:** Antacids ↓ absorption; ↑ neurotoxicity with neurotoxic drugs; ↑ hepatotoxicity with hepatotoxic drugs; ↑ pneumonitis with drugs having pulmonary toxicity; **Dose:** *PO: Adults: Treatment*—50–100 mg q 6–8 hr *or* 100 mg q 12 hr (ER). *Prophylaxis*—50–100 mg at bedtime. *PO: Peds: >1 mo Treatment*—5–7 mg/kg/day divided q 6 hr (max: 400 mg/day). *Prophylaxis*—1–2 mg/kg at bedtime (max: 100 mg/day); **Availability (G):** *Oral susp:* 25 mg/5 ml. *Caps:* 25, 50, 100. *ER caps:* 100 mg; **Monitor:** CBC, U/A, urine culture/sensitivities, BUN/SCr, LFTs; **Notes:** Give with food.

nitroglycerin (Nitro-Time, Tridil, Nitrolingual, Nitro-Bid, Nitrol, Nitrostat, NitroQuick, Minitran, Nitrek, Nitrodisc, Nitro-Dur, Transderm-Nitro) Uses: Acute (translingual and SL) and long-term prophylatic (oral, buccal, transdermal) management of angina pectoris, **PO:** HF; **IV:** Acute MI; Hypertensive crisis; **Class:** nitrates; **Preg:** C; **CIs:** Hypersensitivity; Severe anemia; Pericardial tamponade; Constrictive pericarditis; Concurrent use of phosphodiesterase-5 inhibitors; Head trauma or cerebral hemorrhage; Narrow angle glaucoma; Hypertrophic cardiomyopathy; Hypovolemia (IV); **ADRs:** dizziness, HA, weakness, blurred vision, ↓ BP, ↑ HR, syncope, abdominal pain, N/V, contact dermatitis (transdermal or oint), flushing, tolerance; **Interactions:** Use with sildenafil, tadalafil, and vardenafil ↑ risk for fatal hypotension (contraindicated); ↑ hypotension with antihypertensives, alcohol, haloperidol, or phenothiazines; **Dose:** *SL: Adults:* 0.3–0.6 mg; may repeat q 5 min × 15 min. *Prophytaxis*—0.3–0.6 mg 5–10 min before activities that precipitate attacks. *Lingual Spray: Adults:*

1–2 sprays; may repeat q 5 min × 15 min. Prophylaxis: 1–2 sprays 5–10 min before activities that precipitate attacks. *IV: Adults:* 5 mcg/min; ↑ by 5 mcg/min q 3–5 min to 20 mcg/min, then ↑ by 10–20 mcg/min q 3–5 min; *Transdermal: Adults: Oint*—(1 in. = 15 mg) 1–2 in. q 8 hr (up to 5 in. q 4 hr). *Transdermal patch*—0.1–0.6 mg/hr, up to 0.8 mg/hr × 12–14 hr/day; **Availability (G):** *ER caps:* 2.5, 6.5, 9 mg. *SL tabs:* 0.3, 0.4, 0.6 mg. *Translingual spray:* 400 mcg/spray. *Transdermal systems:* 0.1 mg/hr, 0.2 mg/hr, 0.3 mg/hr, 0.4 mg/hr, 0.6 mg/hr, 0.8 mg/hr. *Transdermal oint:* 2%. *Inject:* 5 mg/ml; **Monitor:** BP, HR, ECG; **Notes: PO:** Give 1 hr ac or 2 hr pc with a full glass of water. Do not crush, break, or chew SR caps; **SL:** Hold under tongue until dissolved. Avoid eating, drinking, or smoking until tablet is dissolved; Place patches/oint onto non-hairy areas of skin. Do not touch oint with hands.

nitroprusside (Nitropress) Uses: Hypertensive crises; Controlled hypotension during anesthesia; Acute decompensated HF; **Class:** vasodilators; **Preg:** C; **CIs:** Hypersensitivity; Treatment of compensatory HTN; High output HF; **ADRs:** dizziness, HA, restlessness, blurred vision, tinnitus, dyspnea, ↓ BP, ↑ HR, abdominal pain, N/V, acidosis, phlebitis at IV site, CYANIDE TOXICITY, thiocyanate toxicity; **Interactions:** ↑ hypotension with ganglionic blocking agents, general anesthetics, and other antihypertensives; Sympathomimetics may ↓ response; **Dose:** *IV: Adults and Peds:* 0.3–4 mcg/kg/min (max: 5 mcg/kg/min in peds and 10 mcg/kg/min in adults); **Availability (G):** *Inject:* 25 mg/ml; **Monitor:** BP, HR, ECG, PCWP, acid/base status, thiocyanate levels (treatment >3 days, >4 mcg/kg/min, or if renal dysfunction), cyanide levels (if hepatic dysfunction); **Notes:** Protect infusion from light.

nizatidine (Axid, Axid AR) Uses: Short-term treatment of duodenal and gastric ulcers; Maintenance therapy for duodenal ulcers; GERD; Heartburn (OTC use); **Class:** histamine H_2 antagonists; **Preg:** B; **CIs:** Hypersensitivity; **ADRs:** confusion, dizziness, drowsiness, hallucinations, HA, ↑ LFTs, N/V/D, anemia, neutropenia, thrombocytopenia, rash; **Interactions:** ↓ absorption of ketoconazole and itraconazole; Antacids and sucralfate ↓ absorption; **Dose:** *PO: Adults: Short-term treatment of active ulcers*—150 mg bid *or* 300 mg at bedtime. *Maintenance treatment of duodenal ulcers*—150 mg at bedtime. *GERD*—150 mg bid. *OTC use*—75 mg 30–60 min before eating foods that cause heartburn. *PO: Peds: <12 yr GERD*—5 mg/kg bid. *Renal Impairment PO, IV: Adults* ↓ dose if CrCl <50 ml/min; **Availability (G):** *Tabs:* 75 mg[OTC]. *Caps:* 150, 300 mg; **Monitor:** S/S GERD/PUD, bleeding, BUN/SCr, CBC, LFTs; **Notes:** Give with meals and/or at bedtime. Should not take OTC for >2 wk.

nortriptyline (Pamelor) Uses: Depression; **Class:** tricyclic antidepressants; **Preg:** D; **CIs:** Hypersensitivity; Concurrent use with MAOIs (within 2 wk); Post-MI, May ↑ risk of suicidal thoughts/behaviors, esp. during early treatment or dose adjustment (risk may be ↑ in peds and

N

adolescents); **ADRs:** confusion, lethargy, sedation, blurred vision, dry mouth, ARRHYTHMIAS, ↓ BP, constipation, ↑ LFTs, ↑ appetite, ↑ wt, urinary retention, ↓ libido, gynecomastia, blood dyscrasias, SUICIDAL THOUGHTS; **Interactions:** CYP2D6 inhibitors may ↑ levels; ↑ risk of hypertensive crises, seizures, or death with MAOIs (discontinue for ≥2 wk); ↑ risk of toxicity with SSRIs; ↑ risk of arrhythmias with other drugs that prolong QT_C interval; ↑ CNS depression with other CNS depressants including alcohol, antihistamines, opioids, and sedative/hypnotics; ↑ risk of anticholinergic effects with other anticholinergic agents; **Dose:** *PO: Adults:* 25 mg tid–qid (max: 150 mg/day). *PO: Geriatric Patients or Adolescents:* 30–50 mg/day in divided doses or as a single dose; **Availability (G):** *Caps:* 10, 25, 50, 75 mg. *Oral soln:* 10 mg/5 ml; **Monitor:** BP, HR, ECG, mental status, suicidal thoughts/behaviors; **Notes:** May take 4–6 wk to see effect. May give entire dose at bedtime. May require tapering to avoid withdrawal. Use with caution in elderly (↑ risk of sedation and anticholinergic effects).

nystatin (Mycostatin, Nilstat, Nystex) **Uses: Loz, oral suspension:** Oropharyngeal candidiasis; Intestinal candidiasis, **Topical:** Cutaneous candidiasis, tinea pedis, tinea cruris, tinea corporis, and tinea versicolor, **Vag:** Vulvovaginal candidiasis; **Class:** antifungals; **Preg:** B, C (oral); **CIs:** Hypersensitivity; **ADRs:** N/V/D, stomach pain, burning sensation, contact dermatitis, itching, local hypersensitivity reactions, redness; **Interactions:** None significant; **Dose:** *PO: Adults and Peds: Oral candidiasis*—400,000–600,000 units as susp qid *or* 200,000–400,000 units 4–5 ×/day as loz. *PO: Infants: Oral candidiasis*—200,000 units as susp qid or 100,000 units as susp to each side of the mouth qid. *PO: Neonates: Oral candidiasis*—100,000 units as susp qid or 50,000 units as susp to each side of the mouth qid. *PO: Adults: Intestinal candidiasis*—500,000–1 million units q 8 hr. *Topical: Adults and Peds:* Apply cream, oint, or powder bid–tid; *Vag: Adults:* 100,000 units daily × 2 wk; **Availability (G):** *Oral susp:* 100,000 units/ml. *Loz, troche:* 200,000 units/troche. *Powder for compounding:* 50, 150, and 500 million units and 1–2 billion units. *Oral tabs:* 500,000 units. *Cream/Oint/Powder:* 100,000 units/g. *Vag tabs:* 100,000 units; **Monitor:** Mucous membranes, resolution of skin infection; **Notes:** Oral susp should be given as a swish and swallow. Loz should be dissolved completely in mouth (do not chew or swallow whole). Avoid tampon use with vag therapy.

octreotide (Sandostatin, Sandostatin LAR) **Uses:** Treatment of symptoms from metastatic carcinoid and vasoactive intestinal peptide tumors (VIPomas); acromegaly; secretory diarrhea; bleeding esophageal varices; **Class:** somatostatin analogues; **Preg:** B; **CIs:** Hypersensitivity; Gallbladder disease; **ADRs:** dizziness, drowsiness, fatigue, HA, weakness, visual disturbances, edema, orthostatic hypotension, palpitations, abdominal pain, cholelithiasis, N/V/D, fat malabsorption, flushing,

↑↓ BG, inject site pain; **Interactions:** May alter requirements for insulin or oral hypoglycemic agents; May ↓ levels of cyclosporine; **Dose:** *Subcut, IV: Adults: Carcinoid tumors*—100–600 mcg/day divided bid–qid (range: 50–1500 mcg/day). *VIPomas*—200–300 mcg/day divided bid–qid (range: 150–750 mcg/day). *Acromegaly*—50 mcg tid, titrate to growth hormone levels (range: 300–1500 mcg/day). *Diarrhea*—50–100 mcg IV q 8 hr (max: 500 mcg q 8 hr). *Bleeding esophageal varices*—25–50 mcg IV bolus then 25–50 mcg/hr infusion. *IM: Adults: Sandostatin LAR*—10–40 mg q 2–4 wk; **Availability (G):** *Inject:* 0.05 mg/ml, 0.1 mg/ml, 0.2 mg/ml, 0.5 mg/ml, 1 mg/ml. *Depot inject (LAR):* 10, 20, 30 mg; **Monitor:** Stool frequency, HR, BP, glucose, growth hormone, 5-HIAA, plasma serotonin, and plasma substance P in patients with carcinoid; plasma VIP in patients with VIPoma; **Notes:** Give IM intragluteally; may give IV undiluted over 3 min.

ofloxacin (Floxin, Floxin Otic, Ocuflox) **Uses:** Respiratory tract infections, skin/skin structure infections, UTIs, and PID due to susceptible organisms (e.g., *S. pneumo*, *S. aureus*, *S. pyogenes*, *Chlamydia*, *E. coli*, *Klebsiella*, *H. flu*, *Enterobacter*, *Citrobacter*, or *Proteus*); **Ophth:** Conjunctivitis/corneal ulcers; **Otic:** Otitis externa/OT; **Class:** FQs; **Preg:** C; **CIs:** Hypersensitivity (cross-sensitivity within class may exist); QT interval prolongation; Do not use during pregnancy unless potential benefit outweighs potential fetal risk; Peds; **ADRs:** SEIZURES, <u>dizziness</u>, <u>HA</u>, <u>insomnia</u>, hepatotoxicity, confusion, PSEUDOMEMBRANOUS COLITIS, abdominal pain, <u>N/V/D</u>, vaginitis, photosensitivity, rash, ↑↓ BG, phlebitis at IV site, tendonitis, tendon rupture, ANAPHYLAXIS; **Interactions:** May ↑ levels/toxicity of CYP1A2 substrates; ↑ risk of QT prolongation with other QT-prolonging drugs; May ↑ theophylline levels/toxicity; if concurrent use cannot be avoided, monitor theophylline levels; Use with antacids, Ca supplements, iron salts, zinc, didanosine, or sucralfate may ↓ absorption; May ↑ the effects of warfarin; May ↑ risk of hypoglycemia with sulfonylureas; May ↑ methotrexate levels/toxicity; May ↑ risk of seizures when used with NSAIDs; ↑ risk of tendon rupture with corticosteroids; Absorption ↓ by dairy products; **Dose:** *PO: Adults:* 200–400 mg q 12 hr. *Ophth: Adults and Peds: ≥1 yr:* 1–2 gtt q 4–6 hr. *Otic Adults:* 10 gtt 1–2 ×/day. *Otic Peds: ≤12 yr:* 5 gtt bid. *Renal Impairment PO: Adults:* ↓ dose if CrCl <20 ml/min; **Availability:** *Tabs:* 200, 300, 400 mg. *Ophth soln:* 0.3%. *Otic soln:* 0.3%; **Monitor:** BP, HR, temp, sputum, U/A, CBC, BG (in DM), rash, tendon pain; **Notes:** Give ≥2 hr before or after products/foods containing Ca, Mg, aluminum, iron, or zinc. Advise patients to use sunscreen.

olanzapine (Zyprexa, Zyprexa Zydis) **Uses:** Bipolar disorder; mania; schizophrenia; **Class:** antipsychotics; **Preg:** C; **CIs:** Hypersensitivity; Dementia-related psychosis; Phenylketonuria (ODTs contain phenylalanine); Suicidal tendency; **ADRs:** NMS, SEIZURES,

O

dizziness, sedation, weakness, insomnia, personality disorder, speech impairment, EPS, amblyopia, ↑ salivation, orthostatic hypotension, cough, SOB, ↑ HR, CP, constipation, dry mouth, abdominal pain, ↑ appetite, ↑ wt, ↑ LFTs, ↓ libido, urinary incontinence, photosensitivity, hyperglycemia, N/V, dyslipidemia, hypertonia, joint pain, tremor, fever, flu-like syndrome; **Interactions:** CYP1A2 inhibitors may ↑ levels/effects; CYP1A2 inducers may ↓ levels/effects; ↑ hypotension with antihypertensives; ↑ CNS depression with alcohol or other CNS depressants; May ↓ effects of levodopa or other dopamine agonists; **Dose:** *PO: Adults: Schizophrenia*—5–10 mg/day (max: 20 mg/day). *Bipolar mania*—10–15 mg/day (max: 20 mg/day). *IM: Adults: Acute agitation*—5–10 mg, repeat q 2 hr × 2; **Availability:** *Tabs:* 2.5, 5, 7.5, 10, 15, 20 mg. *ODTs (Zydis):* 5, 10, 15, 20 mg. *Inject:* 10 mg; **Monitor:** Mental status, BP, HR, lipid panel, glucose, LFTs, wt, BMI, S/S EPS; **Notes:** Give without regard to meals. Advise patient to use sunscreen.

olmesartan (Benicar) **Uses:** HTN; **Class:** angiotensin II receptor antagonists; **Preg:** C (1st tri), D (2nd and 3rd tri); **CIs:** Hypersensitivity; Pregnancy/lactation; **ADRs:** dizziness, ↓ BP, ↑ K+, ↑ SCr, ANGIOEDEMA; **Interactions:** ↑ effects with other antihypertensives; ↑ risk of hyperkalemia with ACEIs, K+ supplements, K+ salt substitutes, K+ sparing diuretics, or NSAIDs; NSAIDs may ↓ effectiveness, ↑ lithium levels; **Dose:** *PO: Adults:* 20–40 mg/day; **Availability:** *Tabs:* 5, 20, 40 mg; **Monitor:** BP, HR, wt, edema, BUN/SCr, K+; **Notes:** Can be used in patients intolerant to ACEI (due to cough); just as likely as ACEI to cause ↑ K+ and ↑ SCr.

O

omega-3-acid ethyl esters (Lovaza) **Uses:** Hypertriglyceridemia (TG ≥500 mg/dl); **Class:** fatty acids; **Preg:** C; **CIs:** Fish allergy; **ADRs:** altered taste, eructation, rash; **Interactions:** May prolong bleeding time with anticoagulants or antiplatelets; **Dose:** *PO: Adults:* 4 g/day as single dose or in 2 divided doses; **Availability:** *Caps:* 1 g; **Monitor:** Lipid panel; **Notes:** Use in conjunction with lipid-lowering diet.

omeprazole (Prilosec) **Uses:** GERD/Erosive esophagitis, PUD, *H. pylori* eradication; Hypersecretory conditions; Heartburn; **Class:** proton pump inhibitors; **Preg:** C; **CIs:** Hypersensitivity; **ADRs:** dizziness, HA, N/V/D, abdominal pain, rash; **Interactions:** May ↑ levels/toxicity of CYP2C9 substrates and CYP2C19 substrates; ↓ absorption of ampicillin, iron, digoxin, ketoconazole, itraconazole, and atazanavir; ↑ risk of bleeding with warfarin; **Dose:** *PO: Adults: GERD/Esophagitis*—20 mg/day. *H. pylori eradication*—20–40 mg/day. *PUD*—20–40 mg/day × 4–8 wk. *Hypersecretory conditions*—60–120 mg daily–tid. *Heartburn (OTC use)*—20 mg/day. *PO: Peds:* ≥2 *yr* <20 kg: 10 mg/day; ≥20 kg: 20 mg/day; **Availability (G):** *Caps:* 10, 20, 40 mg. *Tabs:* 20 mg^{OTC};

Monitor: Hgb/Hct, LFTs, BUN/SCr, S/S abdominal pain/GI bleeding; **Notes:** Capsule contents may be mixed in juice for NG use; mix in Na bicarbonate for NG use.

ondansetron (Zofran) Uses: IV, PO: Prevention of N/V associated with chemotherapy or radiation therapy; **PO, IM, IV:** Prevention of PONV; **Class:** 5-HT_3 antagonists; **Preg:** B; **CIs:** Hypersensitivity; **ADRs:** HA, dizziness, drowsiness, fatigue, weakness, abdominal pain, constipation, diarrhea, dry mouth, ↑ LFTs; **Interactions:** None; **Dose:** *PO: Adults and Peds: ≥12 yr Chemotherapy-induced N/V*—Moderately emetogenic agents: 8 mg 30 min prior to chemotherapy, repeat 8 hr later, then 8 mg q 12 hr × 1–2 days after chemotherapy completed. *PO: Adults: Chemotherapy-induced N/V*—Highly emetogenic agents: 24 mg 30 min prior to chemotherapy. *PONV*—16 mg 1 hr prior to anesthesia. *IV: Adults: Chemotherapy-induced N/V*—32 mg 30 min prior to chemotherapy *or* 0.15 mg/kg 30 min prior to chemotherapy, repeat 4 and 8 hr later. *IM, IV: Adults: PONV*—4 mg prior to anesthesia or postoperatively. *PO: Peds: 4–11 yr:* 4 mg 30 min prior to chemotherapy, repeat 4 and 8 hr later, then 4 mg q 8 hr × 1–2 days after chemotherapy completed. *IV: Peds: 6 mo–18 yr Chemotherapy-induced N/V*—0.15 mg/kg 15–30 min prior to chemotherapy, repeat 4 and 8 hr later. *IV: Peds: 1 mo–12 yr PONV*—≤40 kg: 0.1 mg/kg IV × 1 prior to anesthesia or postoperatively; >40 kg: 4 mg IV × 1 prior to anesthesia or postoperatively. *Hepatic Impairment PO, IM, IV: Adults:* Max: 8 mg/day; **Availability (G):** *ODTs:* 4, 8 mg. *Tabs:* 4, 8 mg. *Oral soln:* 4 mg/5 ml. *Inject:* 2 mg/ml; **Monitor:** BP, HR, N/V, I/Os, LFTs; **Notes:** May give IV undiluted over 2–5 min for PONV.

orlistat (Xenical, Alli) Uses: Obesity management (BMI ≥30 kg/m^2 or ≥27 kg/m^2) in presence of other risk factors [e.g., HTN, D4, dyslipidemia]; **Class:** lipase inhibitors; **Preg:** B; **CIs:** Hypersensitivity; Chronic malabsorption syndrome or cholestasis; **ADRs:** fecal urgency, flatus with discharge, ↑ defecation, oily evacuation, oily spotting, fecal incontinence; **Interactions:** ↓ absorption of cyclosporine and vitamins A, D, E, and K; **Dose:** *PO: Adults and Peds: ≥12 yr:* 60–120 mg tid with a fat-containing meal; **Availability:** *Caps:* 60 mg[OTC]120 mg; **Monitor:** wt; **Notes:** If meal does not contain fat, dose may be omitted. GI side effects ↑ if meal contains >30% fat. Should also give patient multivitamin.

oseltamivir (Tamiflu) Uses: Treatment/prevention of influenza; **Class:** neuramidase inhibitors; **Preg:** C; **CIs:** Hypersensitivity; Peds <1 yr; **ADRs:** delirium, hallucination, self-injurious behavior, abdominal pain, N/V; **Interactions:** Do not give within 2 wk of influenza vaccine nasal spray; **Dose:** *PO: Adults and Peds: ≥13 yr or >40 kg and ≥1 yr Prophylaxis*—75 mg/day × 10 days (6 wk for community outbreak).

Treatment—75 mg bid × 5 days. *PO: Peds: 24–40 kg and ≥1 yr Prophylaxis*—60 mg/day × 10 days. *Treatment*—60 mg bid × 5 days. *PO: Peds: 16–23 kg and ≥1 yr Prophylaxis*—45 mg/day × 10 days. *Treatment*—45 mg bid × 5 days. *PO: Peds: ≤ 15 kg and ≥1 yr Prophylaxis*—30 mg/day × 10 days. *Treatment*—30 mg bid × 5 days. *Renal Impairment: PO: Adults:* ↓ dose if CrCl ≤30 ml/min; **Availability:** *Caps:* 30, 45, 75 mg. *Oral susp:* 12 mg/ml; **Monitor:** S/S influenza, mental status; **Notes:** Give within 2 days of symptom onset (treatment) or exposure (prophylaxis).

oxacillin (Bactocill) **Uses:** Osteomyelitis, skin/skin structure infections, bacteremia, and IE due to penicillinase-producing staphylococci; **Class:** penicillinase-resistant penicillins; **Preg:** B; **CIs:** Hypersensitivity (cross-sensitivity to other beta-lactam antibiotics may exist); **ADRs:** SEIZURES, PSEUDOMEMBRANOUS COLITIS, N/V/D, ↑ LFTs, interstitial nephritis, rash, urticaria, eosinophilia, leukopenia, ANAPHYLAXIS and SERUM SICKNESS, superinfection; **Interactions:** Probenecid ↓ excretion and ↑ levels; **Dose:** *IM, IV: Adults:* 250–2000 mg q 4–6 hr (max: 12 g/day). *IM, IV: Peds:* 100–200 mg/kg/day divided q 6 hr (max: 12 g/day); **Availability (G):** *Inject:* 1 g, 2 g; **Monitor:** BP, HR, temp, sputum, U/A, BUN/SCr, CBC, LFTs; **Notes:** Use with caution in patients with beta-lactam allergy (do not use if history of anaphylaxis or hives). Dilute to a concentration of 0.5–40 mg/ml and give over 10 min.

O

oxaliplatin (Eloxatin) **Uses:** Treatment of advanced colon and rectal CA; **Class:** antineoplastics; **Preg:** D; **CIs:** Prior sensitivity to other platinum compounds; Pregnancy; **ADRs:** fatigue, CP, edema, thromboembolism, PULMONARY FIBROSIS, cough, dyspnea, N/V/D, abdominal pain, anorexia, GERD, stomatitis, ↑ LFTs, ↓ K+, leukopenia, NEUTROPENIA, THROMBOCYTOPENIA, anemia, inject site reactions, back pain, peripheral neuropathy, ANAPHYLAXIS, fever; **Interactions:** Nephrotoxic agents may ↑ toxicity; May ↓ digoxin levels; **Dose:** *IV: Adults:* 85 mg/m² q 2 wk *or* 20–25 mg/m² on Days 1–5 q 3 wk *or* 100–130 mg/m² q 2–3 wk; **Availability:** *Inject:* 5 mg/ml; **Monitor:** CBC, BUN/SCr, LFTs, S/S neuropathy and pulmonary fibrosis; **Notes:** Do not mix with NS; give over 2–6 hr at a concentration of 0.2–0.6 mg/ml.

oxaprozin (Daypro) **Uses:** OA; RA; Juvenile RA; **Class:** NSAIDs; **Preg:** C, D (3rd tri); **CIs:** Hypersensitivity to aspirin or NSAIDs; Active bleeding; Perioperative pain from CABG surgery; **ADRs:** HA, dizziness, tinnitus, edema, GI BLEEDING, ↑ LFTs, N/V/D, ↑ SCr, rash; **Interactions:** ↑ adverse GI effects with aspirin and corticosteroids; ↓ effects of aspirin or antihypertensives; ↑ risk of bleeding with antiplatelet agents or anticoagulants; ↑ risk of nephrotoxicity with cyclosporine; ↑ levels of methotrexate or lithium; **Dose:** *PO: Adults: OA*—600–1200 mg/day. *RA*—1200 mg/day. *PO: Peds:* 600–1200 mg/day (max: 1200 mg/day); **Availability (G):** *Tabs:* 600 mg; **Monitor:**

Pain, S/S of GI upset/bleeding, BUN/SCr, LFTs, CBC; **Notes:** Discontinue 1 wk prior to surgery. Give with food.

oxazepam (Serax) Uses: Anxiety; Alcohol withdrawal; **Class:** benzodiazepines; **Preg:** D; **CIs:** Prior sensitivity to other BZs; Acute narrow-angle glaucoma; Sleep apnea; Severe hepatic/renal/pulmonary impairment; **ADRs:** sedation, HA, ataxia, slurred speech, amnesia, confusion, mental depression, blurred vision, respiratory depression, ↑ LFTs, constipation, N/V/D, rash, physical/psychological dependence, tolerance; **Interactions:** ↑ CNS depression with alcohol, antihistamines, antidepressants, opioid analgesics, and other sedative/hypnotics; ↓ sedative effects when used with theophylline, ↓ effects of levodopa; Oral contraceptives and phenytoin may ↑ clearance; **Dose:** *PO: Adults: Anxiety*—10–30 mg tid–qid. *Sedative/hypnotic/alcohol withdrawal*—15–30 mg tid–qid. *PO: Peds:* 1 mg/kg/day; **Availability (G):** *Caps:* 10, 15, 30 mg. *Tabs:* 15 mg; **Monitor:** HR, BP, RR, LFTs, S/S CNS depression; **Notes:** Elderly may require lower doses. Do not discontinue abruptly.

oxcarbazepine (Trileptal) Uses: Partial seizures; **Class:** anticonvulsants; **Preg:** C; **CIs:** Prior sensitivity to carbamazepine; **ADRs:** ataxia, dizziness, drowsiness, HA, fatigue, vertigo, blurred vision, nystagmus, N/V, SJS, TEN, photosensitivity, pruritis, rash, urticaria, ↓ Na+, tremor; **Interactions:** May ↓ levels/effects of CYP3A4 substrates; ↓ levels/effects of hormonal contraceptives. Phenobarbital, phenytoin, valproic acid, and verapamil ↓ levels; ↑ levels/effects of phenytoin and phenobarbital; **Dose:** *PO: Adults:* 300–600 mg bid (max: 2400 mg/day). *PO: Peds: 2–3 yr Adjunctive therapy*—8–10 mg/kg/day in 2 divided doses initially (max: 600 mg/day); may then titrate up to 20 mg/kg/day. *PO: Peds: 4–16 yr Adjunctive therapy*—8–10 mg/kg/day in 2 divided doses initially (max: 600 mg/day); may then titrate up to target dose (20–29 kg: 900 mg/day; 29.1–39 kg: 1200 mg/day; >39 kg: 1800 mg/day). *Renal Impairment PO: Adults:* ↓ dose if CrCl<30 ml/min; **Availability (G):** *Tabs:* 150, 300, 600 mg. *Oral susp:* 60 mg/ml; **Monitor:** Seizure frequency, Na+, mental status; **Notes:** May give without regard to meals.

oxybutynin (Ditropan, Ditropan XL, Oxytrol) Uses: Overactive bladder with symptoms of urge incontinence, urgency, and frequency; **Class:** anticholinergics; **Preg:** B; **CIs:** Hypersensitivity; Uncontrolled angle-closure glaucoma; Intestinal obstruction or atony; Urinary retention; **ADRs:** dizziness, drowsiness, agitation, confusion, hallucinations, HA, blurred vision, ↑ HR, constipation, dry mouth, nausea, abdominal pain, urinary retention, ↓ sweating: application site reactions (transdermal), hyperthermia; **Interactions:** ↑ anticholinergic effects with other anticholinergic drugs; Additive CNS depression with other CNS depressants, including alcohol, antihistamines, antidepressants, opioids, and sedative/hypnotics; CYP3A4 inhibitors may ↑ levels/effects; **Dose:** *PO: Adults: IR tabs*—5 mg bid–tid (max: 20 mg/day) (may start

O

with 2.5 mg bid–tid in elderly). *ER tabs*—5–10 mg/day; may ↑ by 5 mg/day at weekly intervals (max: 30 mg/day). *PO: Peds: ≥6 yr IR tabs*—5 mg bid–tid (max: 15 mg/day). *ER tabs (*>6 yr)—5 mg/day; may ↑ by 5 mg/day at weekly intervals (max: 20 mg/day). *Transdermal: Adults:* One 3.9-mg system applied twice weekly (q 3–4 days); **Availability (G):** *Tabs:* 5 mg. *ER tabs:* 5, 10, 15 mg. *Syrup:* 5 mg/5 ml. *Transdermal system:* 3.9 mg/day system; **Monitor:** Voiding pattern, I/Os, anticholinergic effects; **Notes:** May give on empty stomach or with meals to prevent gastric irritation. Do not crush ER tabs. Apply patch on same 2 days q wk to hip, abdomen, or buttock in clean, dry area without irritation (avoid reapplication to same site within 7 days).

oxycodone (Oxycontin, OxyFAST, OxyIR, Roxicodone) **Uses:** Moderate-to-severe pain; **Class:** opioid agonists; **Preg:** B, D (high doses at term); **CIs:** Hypersensitivity; Hypercarbia; Acute asthma; Paralytic ileus; **ADRs:** confusion, sedation, dizziness, dysphoria, euphoria, hallucinations, HA, unusual dreams, blurred vision, diplopia, miosis, RESPIRATORY DEPRESSION, orthostatic hypotension, constipation, dry mouth, N/V, urinary retention, flushing, sweating, physical/psychological dependence, tolerance; **Interactions:** ↑ CNS depression with alcohol, antihistamines, and sedative/hypnotics; Partial-antagonist opioid analgesics may precipitate withdrawal; Nalbuphine, buprenorphine, or pentazocine may ↓ analgesia; Phenothiazines may ↑ hypotensive effects; **Dose:** *PO: Adults: ≥50 kg:* 5–10 mg q 3–4 hr prn (CR tabs: divide dose q 12 hr). *PO: Adults: <50 kg or Peds:* 0.2 mg/kg q 3–4 hr prn; **Availability (G):** *Tabs:* 5, 15, 30 mg. *Caps:* 5 mg. *CR tabs:* 10, 20, 40, 60, 80, 160 mg. *Soln:* 5 mg/5 ml. *Concentrated oral soln:* 20 mg/ml; **Monitor:** Pain, BP, RR, S/S CNS or respiratory depression; **Notes:** Schedule II controlled substance. Do not crush CR tabs. Discontinue gradually after long-term use. Naloxone is antidote.

oxycodone/acetaminophen (Percocet, Roxicet, Endocet, Tylox) **Uses:** Moderate-to-severe pain; **Class:** opioid agonists; **Preg:** C, D (high doses at term); **CIs:** Hypersensitivity; Hypercarbia; Acute asthma; Paralytic ileus; **ADRs:** confusion, sedation, dizziness, dysphoria, euphoria, hallucinations, HA, unusual dreams, blurred vision, diplopia, miosis, RESPIRATORY DEPRESSION, orthostatic hypotension, constipation, dry mouth, N/V, urinary retention, flushing, sweating, physical/psychological dependence, tolerance; **Interactions:** ↑ CNS depression with alcohol, antihistamines, and sedative/hypnotics; Partial-antagonist opioid analgesics may precipitate withdrawal; Nalbuphine, buprenorphine, or pentazocine may ↓ analgesia; Phenothiazines may ↑ hypotensive effects; **Dose:** *PO: Adults:* 5–30 mg oxycodone content q 4–6 hr prn (max acetaminophen dose: 4 g/day). *PO: Peds:* 0.05–0.3 mg/kg/dose oxycodone content (max acetaminophen dose: 90 mg/kg/day or 4 g/day); **Availability (G):** *Tabs:* 5 mg oxycodone/325 mg acetaminophen, 7.5/500 mg, 10/650 mg. *Caps:* 5/500 mg. *Caplets:* 5/500 mg. *Soln:* 5 mg oxycodone/325 mg acetaminophen/5 ml; **Monitor:** Pain, BP, RR, S/S CNS or respiratory depression; **Notes:** Schedule II controlled substance. Reduce dose in severe hepatic impairment. Discontinue gradually after long-term use.

oxytocin (Pitocin, Syntocinon) Uses: IV: Induction of labor, Facilitation of abortion; Control of postpartum bleeding; **Intranasal:** Promotion of milk letdown in lactating women; **Class:** oxytocics; **Preg:** X; **CIs:** Hypersensitivity; Conditions under which vag delivery is contraindicated; **ADRs:** NEONATAL SEIZURES, INTRACRANIAL HEMORRHAGE, ↑ BP, arrhythmias, ↓ Na+, water intoxication, uterine rupture, painful contractions, abruptio placentae, postpartum hemorrhage; **Interactions:** Severe HTN with vasopressors; Dinoprostone and misoprostol may ↑ effects; **Dose:** *IV: Adults: Induction of labor*—0.5–1 milliunits/min; ↑ by 1–2 milliunits/min q 15–60 min until desired contraction pattern reached. *Postpartum bleeding*—10 units IM post delivery or 10–40 units IV infusion until uterine atony controlled. *Abortion*—10–20 milliunits/min IV (max: 30 units/12 h). *Intranasal: Adults:* 1 spray in 1 or both nostrils 2–3 min before breastfeeding; **Availability (G):** *Inject:* 10 units/ml. *Nasal spray:* 40 units/ml; **Monitor:** Fetal monitoring, BP, HR, ECG, uterine contraction rate, electrolytes; **Notes:** Dilute 10–40 units in 1000 ml of D5W, NS, or LR for IV infusion.

paclitaxel (Onxol, Taxol, Abraxane) Uses: Paclitaxel: Advanced ovarian CA; Non–small-cell lung CA; Metastatic breast CA; Node-positive breast CA; AIDS-related Kaposi's sarcoma; **Paclitaxel (albumin-bound):** Metastatic breast CA after treatment failure or relapse from anthracycline; **Class:** taxoids; **Preg:** D; **CIs:** Hypersensitivity to paclitaxel or to castor oil; Pregnancy/lactation; ANC $\leq 1500/mm^3$ in patients with ovarian, lung, or breast CA; ANC $\leq 1000/mm^3$ in patients with AIDS-related Kaposi's sarcoma; **ADRs:** ECG changes, ↓ BP, ↓ HR, ↑ LFTs, N/V/D, mucositis, alopecia, anemia, neutropenia, thrombocytopenia, arthralgia, myalgia, peripheral neuropathy, cough, dyspnea, inject site reactions, ANAPHYLAXIS and SJS, TEN; **Interactions:** CYP2C8 inhibitors and CYP3A4 inhibitors may ↑ levels/toxicity; CYP2C8 inducers and CYP3A4 inducers may ↓ levels/effects; ↑ risk of myelosuppression with other antineoplastics or radiation therapy; May ↑ levels/toxicity of doxorubicin; May ↓ antibody response to/↑ risk of adverse reactions from live-virus vaccines; **Dose:** *IV: Adults: Ovarian CA (previously untreated)*—175 mg/m² over 3 hr followed by cisplatin (regimen given q 3 wk) *or* 135 mg/m² over 24 hr followed by cisplatin (regimen given q 3 wk). *Ovarian CA (previously treated)*—135 mg/m² or 175 mg/m² over 3 hr q 3 wk. *Adjuvant treatment of node-positive breast CA*—175 mg/m² over 3 hr q 3 wk × 4 courses administered sequentially to doxorubicin-containing combination chemotherapy. *Failure of initial therapy for metastatic breast CA or relapse*

P

within 6 mo of adjuvant therapy—175 mg/m^2 over 3 hr q 3 wk; *Non–small-cell lung CA*—135 mg/m^2 over 24 hr followed by cisplatin (regimen given q 3 wk). *Kaposi's sarcoma*—135 mg/m^2 over 3 hr q 3 wk *or* 100 mg/m^2 over 3 hr q 2 wk. *IV: Adults: Protein-bound particles*—260 mg/m^2 over 30 min q 3 wk; **Availability (G): Paclitaxel** *Inject:* 6 mg/ml. **Paclitaxel Protein-Bound Particles (albumin-bound) (Abraxane)** *Powder for inject:* 100 mg; **Monitor:** BP, HR, RR, temp, CBC, LFTs, ECG, S/S infection; **Notes:** Monitor for hypersensitivity reactions continuously during the first 30 min of paclitaxel infusion and frequently thereafter. Pretreatment recommended for **all** patients and should include dexamethasone 20 mg PO (10 mg for patients with advanced HIV disease) 12 and 6 hr prior to paclitaxel, diphenhydramine 50 mg IV 30–60 min prior to paclitaxel, and cimetidine 300 mg or ranitidine 50 mg IV 30–60 min prior to paclitaxel. No premedication is required for paclitaxel protein-bound (albumin-bound). The nadir of leukopenia occurs in 11 days, with recovery by days 15–21.

palifermin (Kepivance) **Uses:** Mucositis; **Class:** keratinocyte growth factors; **Preg:** C; **CIs:** Hypersensitivity to *E. coli*-derived proteins; **ADRs:** <u>skin toxicity</u>, <u>oral discoloration</u>, ↑ amylase, ↑ lipase, edema, HTN, <u>arthralgia, dysesthesia</u>; **Interactions:** Binds to and inactivates heparin; **Dose:** *IV: Adults:* 60 mcg/kg/day for 3 days prior to and after myelotoxic therapy; **Availability:** *Inject:* 6.25 mg; **Monitor:** BP, amylase/lipase, oral pain, S/S rash; **Notes:** Do not give within 24 hrs of chemotherapy.

P

paliperidone (Invega) **Uses:** Schizophrenia; **Class:** antipsychotics; **Preg:** C; **CIs:** Hypersensitivity to paliperidone or risperidone; Patients at risk for QT_C prolongation; GI narrowing; Dementia-related psychosis; Suicidal tendency; History of seizures; **ADRs:** NMS, <u>HA</u>, anxiety, confusion, dizziness, extrapyramidal disorders, fatigue, Parkinsonism, tardive dyskinesia, ↑ wt, <u>SOB</u>, ↑ <u>HR</u>, ↑ QT_C interval, <u>abdominal pain</u>, dry mouth, hyperglycemia, orthostatic hypotension, dystonia, akathisia, dyskinesia, tremor; **Interactions:** ↑ CNS depression with CNS depressants, alcohol, antihistamines, sedative/hypnotics, or opioid analgesics; May ↓ effects of levodopa and dopamine agonists; ↑ orthostatic hypotension with antihypertensives and nitrates; ↑ risk of QT_C interval prolongation with antiarrythmics, chlorpromazine, thioridazine, and moxifloxacin; **Dose:** *PO: Adults:* 3–12 mg/day. *Renal:*↓ dose for CrCl <80 ml/min; **Availability:** *ER tabs:* 3, 6, 9 mg; **Monitor:** Mental status, HR, BP, QT_C interval, glucose, wt, S/S extrapyramidal effects; **Notes:** Give in the morning without regard to food. Do not crush tabs.

palonosetron (Aloxi) **Uses:** Prevention of chemotherapy-associated N/V; Prevention of PONV; **Class:** 5–HT_3 antagonists; **Preg:** B; **CIs:** Hypersensitivity; QT interval prolongation; **ADRs:** HA, QT_C prolongation, diarrhea; **Interactions:** None; **Dose:** *IV: Adults:*

Chemotherapy-induced N/V—0.25 mg 30 min prior to chemotherapy. *PONV*—0.075 mg/kg prior to anesthesia; **Availability:** *Inject:* 0.05 mg/ml; **Monitor:** BP, HR, N/V, I/Os, ECG, LFTs, QT_C interval in patients at risk; **Notes:** Give IV over 30 sec (for chemotherapy-induced N/V); 10 sec for PONV.

pamidronate (Aredia) Uses: Hypercalcemia of malignancy; Osteolytic bone lesions from multiple myeloma or breast CA; Paget's disease; **Class:** biphosphonates, hypocalcemics; **Preg:** D; **CIs:** Prior sensitivity to pamidronate or other biphosphonates; Concurrent dental surgery; Severe renal impairment; Pregnancy; **ADRs:** fatigue, arrhythmias, ↑ BP, syncope, ↑ HR, N/V, abdominal pain, anorexia, constipation, ↓ Ca, ↓ K, ↓ Mg, ↓ PO_4, edema, leukopenia, anemia, phlebitis at inject site, jaw osteonecrosis, musculoskeletal pain, fever, generalized pain; **Interactions:** ↑ risk of GI side effects with NSAIDs; ↑ hypocalcemic effects with aminoglycosides and PO_4 supplements; Ca and vitamin D will ↓ effects; **Dose:** *IV: Adults: Hypercalcemia*—60–90 mg × 1; may repeat after 1 wk. *Osteolytic bone lesions*—90 mg q 3–4 wk. *Paget's disease:*—30 mg daily × 3 days; **Availability (G):** *Inject:* 3 mg/ml, 6 mg/ml, 9 mg/ml; **Monitor:** BP, HR, I/Os, CBC, BUN/SCr, electrolytes, S/S hypo/hypercalcemia, pain; **Notes:** Give IV over 4–24 hr; withold dose if SCr rises >0.5–1 mg/dl over baseline; SCr should be monitored before each treatment. Patients at risk for jaw osteonecrosis should be advised to have any needed dental exams and dental work done before receiving pamidronate (dental work should not be done during therapy).

pancrelipase (Lipram, Creon, Pancrease, Ultrase, Viokase) Uses: Replacement therapy in the treatment of malabsorption syndrome caused by pancreatic insufficiency; **Class:** pancreatic enzymes; **Preg:** C; **CIs:** Hypersensitivity to pork proteins; Acute pancreatitis; **ADRs:** dyspnea, wheezing, abdominal pain, N/V/D, stomach cramps, oral irritation, rash, hyperuricemia; **Interactions:** Antacids (Ca carbonate or Mg hydroxide) ↓ effects; May ↓ absorption iron supplements; **Dose:** *PO: Adults and Peds:* 1–3 caps with meals or snacks (up to 8 caps) *or* 1–2 DR caps, *or* 0.7 g powder; **Availability (G):** *Caps:* 8000 units lipase/30,000 units protease and amylase. *DR caps:* 4000 units lipase/12,000 units protease and amylase, 4000 units lipase/25,000 units protease/20,000 units amylase, 5000 units lipase/20,000 units protease and amylase, 10,000 units lipase/30,000 units protease and amylase, 12,000 units lipase/24,000 units protease and amylase, 12,000 units lipase/39,000 units protease and amylase, 16,000 units lipase/48,000 units protease and amylase, 20,000 units lipase/65,000 units protease and amylase, 24,000 units lipase/78,000 units protease and amylase. *Powder:* 16,800 units lipase/70,000 units protease and amylase; **Monitor:** Abdominal symptoms, fecal fat, nutritional intake, uric acid; **Notes:** Capsule contents may be sprinkled on food. Do not chew tabs or enteric-coated beads.

P

pancuronium (Pavulon) Uses: Induction of skeletal muscle paralysis and facilitation of intubation after induction of anesthesia in surgery and compliance during mechanical ventilation; **Class:** neuromuscular blocking agents; **Preg:** C; **CIs:** Hypersensitivity; Situations in which histamine release would be problematic; Myasthenia gravis (small test dose may be used to assess response); **ADRs:** bronchospasm, HTN, ↑ HR, excessive salivation, rash, ANAPHYLAXIS; **Interactions:** Intensity and duration of paralysis may be prolonged by succinylcholine, general anesthesia (inhalation), aminoglycosides, vancomycin, tetracyclines, polymyxin B, colistin, cyclosporine, Ca channel blockers, clindamycin, lidocaine, and other local anesthetics, lithium, quinidine, procainamide, beta blockers, K-losing diuretics, or Mg; Inhalation anesthetics may enhance effects; **Dose:** *IV: Adults and Peds: >12 yr:* 0.15 mg/kg q 20–60 min prn or as a continuous infusion of 0.02–0.04 mg/kg/hr. *IV: Peds: >1 yr* 0.15 mg/kg q 30–60 min prn or as a continuous infusion of 0.03–0.1 mg/kg/hr. *IV: Neonates and Infants:* 0.1 mg/kg q 30–60 min prn or as a continuous infusion of 0.02–0.04 mg/kg/hr; **Availability:** *Inject:* 1 mg/ml, 2 mg/ml; **Monitor:** HR, RR, BP, ECG; **Notes:** BZs and/or analgesics should be given when therapy is used during mechanical ventilation to assure adequate sedation and amnesia. Contains benzyl alcohol, which can cause potentially fatal gasping syndrome in neonates.

panitumumab (Vectibix) Uses: Metastatic colorectal CA that expresses EGFR; **Class:** monoclonal antibodies; **Preg:** C; **CIs:** Hypersensitivity; **ADRs:** fatigue, OCULAR TOXICITY, eyelash growth, PULMONARY FIBROSIS, cough, abdominal pain, constipation, N/V/D, stomatitis, DERMATOLOGIC TOXICITY, paromychia, photosensitivity, edema, ↓ Ca, ↓ Mg, INFUSION REACTIONS; **Interactions:** Concurrent irinotecan, fluorouracil, or leucovorin use ↑ risk for severe diarrhea; **Dose:** *IV: Adults:* 6 mg/kg as a 60-min infusion q 14 days; ↓ infusion rates/dose for infusion reactions and other serious toxicities; **Availability:** *Inject:* 20 mg/ml; **Monitor:** Electrolytes, HR, RR, BP, temp, S/S infusion reactions or dermatologic toxicity; **Notes:** Permanently discontinue if pulmonary fibrosis or severe infusion reaction occurs.

P

pantoprazole (Protonix) Uses: GERD/Erosive esophagitis; Hypersecretory conditions; **Class:** PPIs; **Preg:** B; **CIs:** Hypersensitivity; **ADRs:** HA, abdominal pain, N/V/D, rash, flatulence, ↑ LFTs; **Interactions:** ↓ absorption of ampicillin, iron, digoxin, ketoconazole, itraconazole, and atazanavir; ↑ risk of bleeding with warfarin; **Dose:** *PO, IV: Adults: GERD/Erosive esophagitis*—40 mg/day. *Hypersecretory conditions*—40–120 mg bid PO *or* 80–120 mg IV bid; **Availability (G):** *Tabs:* 20, 40 mg. *Packets for susp:* 40 mg. *Inject:* 40 mg; **Monitor:** Hgb/Hct, LFTs, BUN/SCr, S/S abdominal pain/GI bleeding; **Notes:** Do not crush or chew tabs.

paricalcitol (Zemplar) **Uses:** Secondary hyperparathyroidism in Stage 3 or 4 (PO) or Stage 5 (IV) CKD; **Class:** fat-soluble vitamins; **Preg:** C; **CIs:** Hypersensitivity; Hypercalcemia; Vitamin D toxicity; Patients receiving digoxin; **ADRs:** dizziness, HA, somnolence, weakness, conjunctivitis, photophobia, rhinorrhea, arrhythmias, edema, HTN, ↑ HR, anorexia, constipation, N/V/D, dry mouth, ↑ LFTs, metallic taste, PANCREATITIS, polydipsia, wt loss, albuminuria, azotemia, ↓ libido, pruritus, rash, gout, ↑ Ca, hyperthermia, bone pain, metastatic calcification, muscle pain; **Interactions:** Cholestyramine, colestipol, or mineral oil ↓ absorption; thiazide diuretics ↑ risk of hypercalcemia; Corticosteroids ↓ effects; Digoxin ↑ risk of arrhythmias; Mg-containing drugs may ↑ hypermagnesemia; Ca-containing drugs and vitamin D supplements ↑ hypercalcemia; CYP3A4 inhibitors ↑ levels/effects; **Dose:** *PO: Adults: Baseline intact PTH level ≤500 pg/ml*—1 mcg/day or 2 mcg 3 times weekly. *Baseline intact PTH level >500 pg/ml*—2 mcg/day or 4 mcg 3 times weekly; may adjust q 2–4 wk based on PTH level. *IV: Adults and Peds: ≥5 yr:* 0.04–0.1 mcg/kg 3×/wk during dialysis; may adjust by 2–4 mcg q 2–4 wk based on PTH level; **Availability:** *Caps:* 1, 2, 4 mcg. *Inject:* 2 mcg/ml, 5 mcg/ml; **Monitor:** Ca, PO_4, PTH, LFTs, amylase, lipase; **Notes:** Serum Ca, PO_4, and intact PTH levels should be monitored q 2 wk × 3 mo or following any dosage adjustment, then q mo × 3 mo, then q 3 mo.

paroxetine (Paxil, Paxil CR, Pexeva) **Uses: Paxil, Paxil CR, Pexeva:** Major depressive disorder, panic disorder; **Paxil, Pexeva:** OCD, GAD; **Paxil, Paxil CR:** SAD; **Paxil:** PTSD; **Paxil CR:** PMDD; **Class:** SSRIs; **Preg:** D; **CIs:** Hypersensitivity; Concurrent MAOI, thioridazine, or pimozide therapy; History of seizures; History of bipolar disorder; Pregnancy; Severe renal/hepatic impairment; History of mania/risk of suicide; **ADRs:** anxiety, dizziness, drowsiness, HA, insomnia, weakness, agitation, amnesia, confusion, mental depression, suicidal thoughts/behavior, syncope, blurred vision, rhinitis, cough, pharyngitis, yawning, CP, edema, HTN, ↑ HR, postural hypotension, vasodilation, constipation, N/V/D, dry mouth, abdominal pain, ↓↑ appetite, dyspepsia, flatulence, taste disturbances, ejaculatory disturbance, ↓ libido, genital disorders, urinary disorders, urinary frequency, sweating, photosensitivity, pruritus, rash, ↓↑ wt, back pain, myalgia, myopathy, paresthesia, tremor, chills, fever; **Interactions:** Serious, potentially fatal reactions (hyperthermia, rigidity, myoclonus, autonomic instability, with fluctuating vital signs and extreme agitation, which may proceed to delirium and coma) may occur with concurrent MAOI therapy. Discontinue therapy by at least 2 weeks; May ↓ metabolism/↑ effects of drugs that are metabolized by the liver, including antidepressants, phenothiazines, class Ic antiarrhythmics, risperidone, atomoxetine, theophylline, procyclidine, and quinidine (use with caution); Concurrent use with pimozide or thioridazine may ↑ risk of QT_C interval prolongation and torsades de pointes (use contraindicated);

P

Cimetidine ↑ blood levels; Phenobarbital and phenytoin may ↓ effectiveness; May ↓ the effects of digoxin, May ↑ bleeding risk with warfarin, aspirin, or NSAIDS; Concurrent use with 5-HT_1 agonists (frovatriptan, naratriptan, rizatriptan, sumatriptan, zolmitriptan), linezolid, lithium, or tramadol may ↑ serotonin levels and lead to serotonin syndrome; **Dose:** *PO: Adults: Depression*—20 mg as a single dose in the AM; may be ↑ by 10 mg/day q week (max: 50 mg/day). *CR*—25 mg once daily initially. May ↑ q wk by 12.5 mg (max: 62.5 mg/day). *PO: Geriatric Patients or Debilitated Patients:* 10 mg/day initially; may be slowly ↑ (max: 40 mg/day). *CR*—12.5 mg once daily initially; may be slowly ↑ (max: 50 mg/day). *PO: Adults: OCD*—20 mg/day initially; ↑ by 10 mg/day q wk up to 40 mg (max: 60 mg/day). *PO: Adults: Panic*—10 mg/day initially; ↑ by 10 mg/day q wk up to 40 mg (max: 60 mg/day). *CR*—12.5 mg/day initially; ↑ by 12.5 mg/day q wk (max: 75 mg/day). *PO: Adults: SAD*—20 mg/day. *CR*—12.5 mg/day initially; may ↑ by 12.5 mg/day q wk (max: 37.5 mg/day). *PO: Adults: PTSD*—20 mg once daily initially; ↑ by 10 mg/day q wk (max: 50 mg/day). *PO: Adults: GAD*—20 mg/day initially; may be ↑ by 10 mg/day q wk (max: 50 mg/day). *PO: Adults: PMDD: CR*—12.5 mg once daily throughout menstrual cycle or during luteal phase of menstrual cycle only; may be ↑ to 25 mg/day in one wk. *Hepatic Impairment PO: Adults: Severe hepatic impairment*—10 mg/day initially; may be slowly ↑ (max: 40 mg/day). *CR*—12.5 mg once daily initially; may be slowly ↑ (max: 50 mg/day). *Renal Impairment PO: Adults: Severe renal impairment*—10 mg/day initially; may be slowly ↑ (max: 40 mg/day). *CR*—12.5 mg once daily initially; may be slowly ↑ (max: 50 mg/day); **Availability (G):** *Paroxetine hydrochloride tabs:* 10, 20, 30, 40 mg. *Paroxetine hydrochloride CR tabs:* 12.5, 25, 37.5 mg. *Paroxetine hydrochloride oral susp:* 10 mg/5 ml. *Paroxetine mesylate tabs:* 10, 20, 30, 40 mg; **Monitor:** Mood, mental status, appetite, wt, CBC (with diff), BP, HR; **Notes:** Paroxetine mesylate (Pexeva) cannot be substituted for paroxetine (Paxil or Paxil CR) or generic paroxetine. Instruct patient to avoid alcohol. Do not crush, break, or chew tabs.

pegfilgrastim (Neulasta) **Uses:** To ↓ the incidence of febrile neutropenia in patients with nonmyeloid malignancies receiving myelosuppressive antineoplastics; **Class:** colony-stimulating factors; **Preg:** C; **CIs:** Hypersensitivity to filgrastim or *E. coli*-derived proteins; **ADRs:** ARDS, SPLENIC RUPTURE, <u>splenomegaly</u>, leukocytosis, <u>medullary bone pain</u>, ANAPHYLAXIS; **Interactions:** None; **Dose:** *Subcut: Adults:* 6 mg per chemotherapy cycle; **Availability:** *Inject:* 10 mg/ml; **Monitor:** BP, HR, RR, temp, CBC (with diff) (ANC), bone pain; **Notes:** Avoid use for 14 days before and 24 hr after chemotherapy. May precipitate crisis in patients with sickle cell disease. Bone pain can usually be controlled with nonopioid analgesics (may require treatment with opioid analgesics).

peginterferon alpha-2a (Pegasys) **Uses:** Treatment of: Chronic hepatitis C (alone or with ribavirin), Chronic hepatitis B;

Class: interferons; **Preg:** C; **CIs:** Hypersensitivity to alpha interferons or human serum albumin; Autoimmune hepatitis; Hepatic decompensation (Child-Pugh class B and C) before or during therapy; Severe CV, pulmonary, renal, or hepatic disease; Active infections; Underyling CNS pathology or psychiatric history; Decreased bone marrow reserve or underlying immunosuppression; Current history of chickenpox, herpes zoster, or herpes labialis (may reactivate or disseminate disease); Previous or concurrent radiation therapy; Autoimmune disorders (may ↑ risk of exacerbation); Childbearing potential, pregnancy, lactation, and peds <3 yr (safety not established); **ADRs:** NEUROPSYCHIATRIC DISORDERS, confusion, depression, dizziness, fatigue, HA, insomnia, irritability, anxiety, blurred vision, nose bleeds, rhinitis, ISCHEMIC DISORDERS, arrhythmias, CP, edema, COLITIS, PANCREATITIS, anorexia, abdominal pain, N/V/D, dry mouth, taste disorder, wt loss, drug-induced hepatitis, flatulence, alopecia, dry skin, pruritus, rash, sweating, thyroid disorders, LEUKOPENIA, THROMBOCYTOPENIA, anemia, hemolytic anemia (with ribavirin), arthralgia, myalgia, leg cramps, paresthesia, cough, dyspnea, inject site reactions, AUTOIMMUNE DISORDERS, INFECTIOUS DISORDERS, allergic reactions including ANAPHYLAXIS, chills, fever, flu-like syndrome; **Interactions:** Additive myelosuppression with other antineoplastic agents or radiation therapy; ↑ CNS depression may occur with CNS depressants, alcohol, antihistamines, sedative/hypnotics, and opioids; May ↓ metabolism and ↑ blood levels and toxicity of theophylline and methadone; ↑ risk of adverse reactions with zidovudine; May ↓ effects of immunosuppressant agents; **Dose:** *Subcut: Adults: Chronic hepatitis C*—180 mcg once weekly for 48 wk for Genotypes 1, 4 (24 wk for Genotypes 2, 3). *Chronic hepatitis C co-infected with HIV or chronic hepatitis B*—180 mcg once weekly for 48 wk. *Hepatic/Renal Impairment Adults:* ↓ dose for CrCl <50 ml/min or LFTs increasing; **Availability:** *Inject:* 180 mcg/ml vials. *Prefilled syringes:* 180 mcg/0.5 ml; **Monitor:** CBC, platelets, electrolytes, LFTs, uric acid, TSH, ECG (if history of cardiac disease), S/S infection/bleeding; **Notes:** Should be discontinued if ANC<500/mm^3 or platelet count <25,000/mm^3 and then may be restarted at a lower dose if ANC >1000/mm^3. Discontinue drug therapy in cases of severe infection, pancreatitis, or colitis.

peginterferon alfa-2B (Pegintron) **Uses:** Chronic hepatitis C; **Class:** interferons; **Preg:** C; **CIs:** Hypersensitivity; Autoimmune hepatitis; Decompensated liver disease; Pregnancy; Renal failure (do not use if CrCl <50 ml/min); Previous interferon therapy; Severe psychiatric disorders; **ADRs:** anxiety, depression, dizziness, fatigue, HA, insomnia, aggressive behavior, psychoses, suicidal ideation, cotton wool spots, retinal artery/vein obstruction, retinal hemorrhage, arrhythmias, cardiomyopathy, ↓ BP, ↑ HR, PULMONARY INFILTRATES/PNEUMONITIS, pharyngitis, cough, dyspnea, sinusitis, COLITIS, PANCREATITIS, abdominal pain, anorexia, N/V/D, dyspepsia, alopecia, dry skin, flushing, sweating, pruritus, rash, hyperglycemia, thyroid abnormalities, NEUTROPENIA, THROMBOCYTOPENIA, inject site pain/reactions, wt loss, musculoskeletal pain; ANAPHYLAXIS, flu-like syndrome, fever, rigors; **Interactions:** None currently known; **Dose:** *Subcut: Adults: Without ribavirin*—1 mcg/kg/wk for 1 yr. *With ribavirin*—1.5 mcg/kg/wk for 1 yr; **Availability:** *Inject:* 50, 80, 120, 150 mcg; **Monitor:** Mental status, CBC, platelets, LFTs, amylase, lipase, glucose, TSH, serum HCV RNA levels (after 24 wk); **Notes:** If serious ADRs occur, dose should ↓ by 50%. If persistent intolerance occurs following dose reduction, discontinue therapy.

penicillin G (Bicillin L-A, Bicillin C-R, Bicillin C-R 900/300, Pfizerpen, Wycillin, Permapen) **Uses:** Treatment of infections including: Pneumococcal pneumonia, Streptococcal pharyngitis, Syphilis, Gonorrhea strains; Enterococcal infections; Prevention of rheumatic fever; **Class:** penicillins; **Preg:** B; **CIs:** Hypersensitivity (cross-sensitivity to other beta-lactam antibiotics may exist); **ADRs:** SEIZURES, PSEUDOMEMBRANOUS COLITIS, N/V/D, interstitial nephritis, rash, urticaria, pruritis, allergic reactions including ANAPHYLAXIS, SERUM SICKNESS; **Interactions:** Probenecid ↓ excretion and ↑ levels; **Dose:** *IM, IV: Adults: Most infections*—2–4 million units q 4–6 hr. *IM, IV: Peds:* 25,000–400,000 units/kg/day divided q 4–6 hr (max: 24 million units/day). *IV: Infants:* 50,000–200,000 units/kg/day in divided doses q 6–12 hr. *Group B Streptococcal meningitis*—100,000–300,000 units/kg/day in divided doses q 6 hr. *IM: Adults: Streptococcal infections*—2.4 million units × 1 (Bicillin C-R). *Primary, secondary, and early latent syphilis*—2.4 million units × 1 (Bicillin LA). *Tertiary and late latent syphilis (not neurosyphilis)*—2.4 million units q wk × 3 wk (Bicillin LA). *Prevention of rheumatic fever*—1.2 million units q 3–4 wk (Bicillin LA). *Neurosyphilis*—2.4 million units/day with 500 mg probenecid PO qid × 10–14 days (Wycillin). *IM: Peds: Streptococcal infections*—<14 kg: 600,000 units × 1; 14–27 kg: 900,000–1.2 million units × 1; >27 kg: 2.4 million units × 1 (Bicillin C-R). *Primary, secondary, and early latent syphilis*—up to 2.4 million units × 1. *Late latent or latent syphilis of undetermined duration*—50,000 units/kg q wk × 3 wk. *Prevention of rheumatic fever*—1.2 million units q 2–3 wk; **Availability (G):** Inject (aqueous): 5 million units, 20 million units. *Susp for IM inject (penicillin G procaine) (Wycillin):* 600,000 units/ml. *Susp for IM inject (penicillin G benzathine) (Bicillin LA):* 600,000 units/ml. *Susp for IM inject (penicillin G benzathine/procaine combined-Bicillin C-R):* 600,000 units/1 ml (300,000 units benzathine + 300,000 units procaine), 1.2 million units/2 ml (600,000 units benzathine + 600,000 units procaine), 1.2 million units/2 ml (900,000 units benzathine + 300,000 units procaine), 2.4 million units/4 ml (1.2 million units benzathine + 1.2 million units procaine); **Monitor:** BP, HR, temp, sputum, U/A, CBC, LFTs, BUN/SCr; **Notes:** Do not give IM penicillin G benzathine or penicillin G procaine suspensions IV.

penicillin V (Beepen-VK, Pen-Vee K, Veetids) Uses: Treatment of infections including: Pneumococcal pneumonia, Streptococcal pharyngitis, Syphilis, Gonorrhea strains; Enterococcal infections (with an aminoglycoside); Rheumatic fever/pneumococcal prophylaxis; **Class:** penicillins; **Preg:** B; **CIs:** Hypersensitivity (cross-sensitivity to other beta-lactam antibiotics may exist); **ADRs:** SEIZURES, PSEUDOMEMBRANOUS COLITIS, N/V/D, interstitial nephritis, rash, urticaria, pruritis, allergic reactions including ANAPHYLAXIS, SERUM SICKNESS; **Interactions:** Probenecid ↓ excretion and ↑ levels; **Dose:** *PO: Adults and Peds: ≥12 yr*—125–500 mg q 6–8 hr. *Rheumatic fever/pneumococcal prophylaxis*—125–250 mg q 12 hr. *PO: Peds: <12 yr* 25–50 mg/kg/day in 3–4 divided doses (max 3 g/day). *Renal Impairment Adults and Peds:* ↓ dose if CrCl <50 ml/min; **Availability:** *Tabs:* 250, 500 mg. *Oral soln:* 125 mg/5 ml, 250 mg/5 ml; **Monitor:** BP, HR, temp, sputum, U/A, CBC, LFTs, BUN/SCr; **Notes:** Use with caution in patients with beta-lactam allergy (do not use if history of anaphylaxis or hives). Give around the clock without regard for meals.

pentamidine (NebuPent, Pentacarinat Pentam 300) Uses: IV: Treatment of PCP; **Inhaln:** Prevention of PCP in AIDS or HIV+ patients; **Class:** antibiotics; **Preg:** C; **CIs:** History of previous anaphylactic reaction to pentamidine; **ADRs:** anxiety, HA, confusion, dizziness, hallucinations, burning in throat, bronchospasm, cough, ARRHYTHMIAS, ↓ BP, PANCREATITIS, abdominal pain, anorexia, ↑ LFTs, N/V, metallic taste, ↑ BUN/SCr, pallor, rash, HYPOGLYCEMIA, hyperglycemia, ↑ K, ↓ Ca, anemia, leukopenia, thrombocytopenia, phlebitis, pruritus, sterile abscesses at IM sites, ANAPHYLAXIS, SJS, chills; **Interactions:** Concurrent use with erythromycin IV ↑ risk of fatal arrhythmias; ↑ nephrotoxicity with aminoglycosides, amphotericin B, and vancomycin; ↑ bone marrow depression with antineoplastics or previous radiation therapy; ↑ pancreatitis with didanosine; ↑ risk of nephrotoxicity, hypocalcemia, and hypomagnesemia with foscarnet; **Dose:** *IV: Adults and Peds:* 4 mg/kg once daily × 14–21 days. *Renal Impairment IV: Adults and Peds:* ↓ dose for CrCl <50 ml/min. *Inhaln: Adults and Peds: >5 yr NebuPent, Pentacarinat*—300 mg q 4 wk, using a Respirgard II jet nebulizer (150 mg q 2 wk has also been used); **Availability (G):** *Inject:* 300 mg. *Soln for aerosol use (NebuPent, Pentacarinat):* 300 mg; **Monitor:** WBC, CBC, platelets, BUN/SCr, LFTs, electrolytes, glucose, amylase, lipase, temp, cultures/sensitivity, BP, HR, ECG (with IV); **Notes:** *Inhaln:* If using inhaln bronchodilator, administer bronchodilator 5–10 min prior to administration; **IV:** Give over 1–2 hr at a concentration not to exceed 6 mg/ml.

pentoxifylline (Trental) Uses: Intermittent claudication; **Class:** Xanthine derivatives; **Preg:** C; **CIs:** Prior sensitivity to pentoxifylline or other xanthine derivatives; Recent cerebral/retinal hemorrhage;

P

ADRs: dizziness, drowsiness, HA, insomnia, blurred vision, dyspnea, angina, edema, flushing, ↓ BP, abdominal discomfort, N/V/D, dyspepsia, flatus, tremor; **Interactions:** ↑ hypotension with antihypertensives and nitrates; ↑ bleeding with warfarin, heparin, aspirin, NSAIDs, cefoperazone, cefotetan, valproic acid, clopidogrel, ticlopidine, eptifibatide, tirofiban, or thrombolytic agents; ↑ risk of theophylline toxicity; **Dose:** *PO: Adults:* 400 mg tid; if GI or CNS side effects, ↓ to 400 mg bid; **Availability (G):** *CR tabs:* 400 mg. *ER tabs:* 400 mg; **Monitor:** BP, claudication symptom improvement; **Notes:** Give with food. Do not crush tabs.

perindopril (Aceon) **Uses:** HTN; Stable CAD; **Class:** ACEIs; **Preg:** C (1st tri), D (2nd and 3rd tri); **CIs:** Previous sensitivity/intolerance to ACEIs; **ADRs:** dizziness, cough, ↓ BP, ↑ SCr, ↑ K, ANGIOEDEMA; **Interactions:** ↑ effects with other antihypertensives; ↑ risk of hyperkalemia with ARBs, K supplements, K salt substitutes, K sparing diuretics, or NSAIDs; NSAIDs may ↓ effectiveness; ↑ lithium levels; **Dose:** *PO: Adults: HTN*—4–8 mg/day (max: 16 mg/day). *Stable CAD*—4–8 mg/day. *Renal Impairment PO: Adults:* ↓ dose if CrCl <60 ml/min; **Availability:** *Tabs:* 2, 4, 8 mg; **Monitor:** BP, HR, wt, edema, BUN/SCr, K; **Notes:** Correct volume depletion. Advise patient on S/S angioedema and avoidance of K salt substitutes.

phenazopyridine (Azo-Standard, Baridium, Pyridium, Uristat, ReAzo, UTI Relief) **Uses:** Relief from the following UTI symptoms: pain, itching, burning, urgency, frequency; **Class:** urinary tract analgesics; **Preg:** B; **CIs:** Hypersensitivity; Severe hepatitis, uremia, or renal failure (CrCl <50 ml/min); **ADRs:** HA, vertigo, ↑ LFTs, nausea, bright-orange urine, ↑ BUN/SCr, rash, hemolytic anemia, methemoglobinemia; **Interactions:** None significant; **Dose:** *PO: Adults:* 200 mg tid × 2 days. *PO: Peds:* 4 mg/kg tid × 2 days; **Availability (G):** *Tabs:* 95, 100, 200 mg; **Monitor:** Urinary symptom relief, BUN/SCr, LFTs, CBC; **Notes:** Do not crush tabs. Red-orange discoloration of urine may stain fabric. Does not treat infection.

P

phenelzine (Nardil) **Uses:** Treatment of neurotic or atypical depression; **Class:** MAOIs; **Preg:** C; **CIs:** Hypersensitivity; Liver disease; Cerebrovascular disease; CV disease; HTN; Pheochromocytoma; History of HA; Concurrent use of meperidine, SSRI antidepressants, CNS depressants, bupropion, buspirone, sympathomimetics, MAOIs, dextromethorphan, alcohol, general anesthetics, or antihistamines; Foods high in tyramine; Suicidal tendency; **ADRs:** SEIZURES, confusion, dizziness, HA, hallucinations, insomnia, abnormal thinking, nausea, abdominal pain, CP, orthostatic hypotension, dry mouth, HYPERTENSIVE CRISIS, edema, ↑ HR, ↑ LFTs, sexual dysfunction, urinary retention, AGRANULOCYTOSIS, leukopenia, thrombocytopenia, alopecia, rash, muscle spasm; **Interactions:** Serotonin syndrome with cyclobenzaprine, anorexiants, TCAs, or SSRI antidepressants; Hypertensive crisis may occur with amphetamines, methyldopa, buspirone, levodopa, dopamine, epinephrine, norepinephrine, reserpine, methylphenidate, or vasoconstrictors; HTN or hypotension, coma, seizures, resp depression, and death may occur with meperidine (avoid use within 2–3 wk); ↑ hypotension with antihypertensives, spinal anesthesia, opioids, or barbiturates; ↑ hypoglycemia with insulins or oral hypoglycemic agents; Risk of seizures may be ↑ with tramadol; **Dose:** *PO: Adults:* 15 mg tid; ↑ to 60–90 mg/day in divided doses; gradually reduce to smallest effective dose (15 mg/day or every other day); **Availability:** *Tabs:* 15 mg; **Monitor:** Mental status, mood, LFTs, CBC, BP, HR, wt, I/Os; **Notes:** Avoid tyramine-containing foods, tryptophan, alcohol, and caffeine; do not give in the evening due to psychomotor stimulating effects. Abrupt discontinuation may precipitate withdrawal.

phenobarbital (Luminal) **Uses:** Anticonvulsant for tonic-clonic, partial, and febrile seizures; Sedation; Hypnotic (short-term); Hyperbilirubinemia; **Class:** barbiturates; **Preg:** D; **CIs:** Hypersensitivity; Pre-existing CNS depression; Severe resp disease with dyspnea or obstruction; Uncontrolled severe pain; Hepatic dysfunction; Severe renal impairment; Suicidal tendency; **ADRs:** hangover, delirium, depression, drowsiness, lethargy, vertigo, resp depression, LARYNGOSPASM, ↑ LFTs, ↓ BP, constipation, N/V/D, photosensitivity, rash, urticaria, arthralgia, myalgia, neuralgia, physical/psychological dependence; **Interactions:** ↑ CNS depression with CNS depressants, alcohol, antihistamines, opioid analgesics, and other sedative/hypnotics; May induce hepatic enzymes that ↓ effects of hormonal contraceptives, warfarin, chloramphenicol, cyclosporine, dacarbazine, corticosteroids, TCAs, felodipine, clonazepam, carbamazepine, verapamil, theophylline, metronidazole, and quinidine; ↑ hepatic toxicity of acetaminophen; MAOIs and valproates ↓ metabolism/ ↑ sedation; Rifampin may ↑ metabolism ↓ effects; **Dose:** *IV: Adults, Peds, and Neonates: Status epilepticus*—15–20 mg/kg in 1–2 divided doses. *IV, PO: Adults and Peds: >12 yr Anticonvulsant maintenance*—1–3 mg/kg/day in 1–2 divided doses. *IV, PO: Peds: 5–12 yr:* 4–6 mg/kg/day in 1–2 divided doses. *IV, PO: Peds: 1–5 yr:* 6–8 mg/kg/day in 1–2 divided doses. *IV, PO: Infants:* 5–6 mg/kg/day in 1–2 divided doses. *IV, PO: Neonates:* 3–5 mg/kg/day once daily. *PO, IM: Adults: Sedation*—30–120 mg/day in 2–3 divided doses. *Preop*—100–200 mg IM 1–1.5 hrs before the procedure. *PO: Peds:* 2 mg/kg tid. *Preoperative*—1–3 mg/kg PO/IM/IV 1–1.5 hrs before the procedure. *PO, Subcut, IV, IM: Adults: Hypnotic*—100–320 mg at bedtime. *IV, IM, Subcut: Peds:* 3–5 mg/kg at bedtime. *PO: Adults: Hyperbilirubinemia*—90–180 mg/day in 2–3 divided doses. *PO: Peds: <12 yr:* 3–8 mg/kg/day in 2–3 divided doses (max 12 mg/kg/day); **Availability (G):** *Tabs:* 15, 30, 60, 100 mg. *Elixir:* 20 mg/5 ml. *Injection:* 30 mg/ml, 60 mg/ml, 65 mg/ml, 130 mg/ml; **Monitor:** RR,

HR, BP, LFTs, CBC, BUN/SCr, bilirubin, seizure frequency, level of sedation; **Notes:** Therapeutic blood levels are 10–40 mcg/ml. Tabs may be crushed and mixed with food or fluids. Abrupt withdrawal may precipitate seizures or status epilepticus.

phentolamine (Regitine) **Uses:** BP control during surgical removal of pheochromocytoma; Prevention/treatment of extravasation injury from norepinephrine, phenylephrine, or dopamine; **Class:** alpha-adrenergic blockers; **Preg:** C; **CIs:** Hypersensitivity; Coronary or cerebral arteriosclerosis; *Renal impairment;* Concurrent use of PDE-5 inhibitors (sildenafil, tadalafil, vardenafil) causes severe ↓ BP; **ADRs:** CEREBROVASCULAR SPASM, dizziness, weakness, nasal stuffiness, ↓ BP, MI, <u>angina</u>, <u>arrhythmias</u>, ↑ <u>HR</u>, <u>abdominal pain</u>, <u>N/V/D</u>, aggravation of peptic ulcer, flushing; **Interactions:** Antagonizes effects of alpha-adrenergic stimulants; ↓ pressor response to ephedrine or phenylephrine; ↑ hypotension with epinephrine or methoxamine; ↓ peripheral vasoconstriction from high-dose dopamine; **Dose:** *IV: Adults:* 5 mg given 1–2 hr preop, repeat prn; 0.5–1 mg/min infusion during surgery. *IV, IM: Peds:* 1 mg or 0.1 mg/kg given 1–2 hr preop, repeat prn during surgery. *Infiltrate: Adults:* Dilute 5–10 mg in 10 ml NS and infiltrate area within 12 hr of extravasation. *Infiltrate: Peds:* 0.1–0.2 mg/kg diluted in 10 ml NS within 12 hr of extravasation; **Availability (G):** *Inject:* 5 mg; **Monitor:** BP, HR, ECG, area of extravasation; **Notes:** May add 10 mg/1000 ml of fluid containing norepinephrine for prevention of dermal necrosis and sloughing; does not affect pressor effect of norepinephrine.

P

phenytoin (Dilantin) **Uses:** Treatment/prevention of tonic-clonic (grand mal) seizures and complex partial seizures; **Class:** anticonvulsants; **Preg:** D; **CIs:** Hypersensitivity to phenytoin or propylene glycol (inject only); Sinus bradycardia, SA block, 2nd- or 3rd-degree heart block, or Stokes-Adams syndrome (inject only); Severe cardiac or resp disease (inject only); Neonates (susp contains Na benzoate, a metabolite of benzyl alcohol that can cause potentially fatal gasping syndrome); **ADRs:** <u>dizziness</u>, <u>drowsiness</u>, <u>nystagmus</u>, agitation, HA, stupor, vertigo, amblyopia, diplopia, tinnitus, ↓ BP (with rapid IV administration), ↑ HR, dry mouth, N/V, taste perversion, tongue disorder, <u>pruritus</u>, rash, SJS, <u>ataxia</u>, dysarthria, extrapyramidal syndrome, incoordination, paresthesia, tremor; **Interactions:** CYP2C9 inhibitors or CYP2C19 inhibitors may ↑ levels/toxicity; CYP2C9 inducers or CYP2C19 inducers may ↓ levels/effects; May ↓ levels/effects of CYP2C9 substrates, CYP2C19 substrates, and CYP3A4 substrates; IV phenytoin and dopamine may cause additive hypotension; ↑ CNS depression with other CNS depressants, alcohol, antihistamines, antidepressants, opioids, and sedative/hypnotics; Antacids may ↓ absorption of PO phenytoin; ↑ systemic clearance of antileukemic drugs (teniposide and methotrexate), which has been associated with a worse event-free survival, phenytoin use is not recommended in children undergoing chemotherapy for acute lymphocytic leukemia; Ca and sucralfate ↓ phenytoin absorption; Phenytoin may ↓ absorption of folic acid; Concurrent administration of enteral tube feedings may ↓ phenytoin absorption; **Dose:** *PO: Adults:* LD 15–20 mg/kg as ER caps in 3 divided doses given every 2–4 hr; MD 5–6 mg/kg/day given in 1–3 divided doses (range: 200–1200 mg/day). *PO: Peds: 10–16 yr:* 6–7 mg/kg/day in 2–3 divided doses. *PO: Peds: 7–9 yr:* 7–8 mg/kg/day in 2–3 divided doses. *PO: Peds: 4–6 yr:* 7.5–9 mg/kg/day in 2–3 divided doses. *PO: Peds: 0.5–3 yr:* 8–10 mg/kg/day in 2–3 divided doses. *PO: Neonates ≤ 6 months:* 5–8 mg/kg/day in 2 divided doses; may require q 8 hr dosing. *IV: Adults: Status epilepticus LD*—15–20 mg/kg at a rate not to exceed 25–50 mg/min. *MD*—same as PO dosing above. *IV: Peds: Status epilepticus LD*—15–20 mg/kg at a rate not to exceed 1–3 mg/kg/min. *MD*—same as PO dosing above. *Renal/Hepatic Impairment Adults and Peds:* ↓ dose for cirrhosis and CrCl <10 ml/min; **Availability (G):** *Chew tabs:* 50 mg. *Oral susp:* 125 mg/5 ml. *ER caps:* 30, 100, 200, 300 mg. *Inject:* 50 mg/ml; **Monitor:** BP, HR, RR, seizure activity, mental status, ECG, CBC, LFTs, phenytoin levels; **Notes:** Shake susp well. Space doses at least 2 hr from tube feeds. Therapeutic phenytoin levels = 10–20 mcg/ml (unbound = 1–2 mcg/ml); total levels need adjusting for low albumin and CrCl <10 ml/min. Do not give faster than 50 mg/min (to ↓ risk of hypotension). Advise females to use additional nonhormonal method of contraception during therapy.

phytonadione (AquaMEPHYTON, Mephyton, vitamin K) Uses: Hypoprothrombinemia; Hemorrhagic disease of the newborn; **Class:** fat-soluble vitamins; **Preg:** C; **CIs:** Hypersensitivity to vitamin K or benzyl alcohol (IV form); Impaired liver function; **ADRs:** gastric upset, unusual taste, flushing, rash, urticaria, hemolytic anemia, erythema, pain at inject site, swelling, allergic reactions, hyperbilirubinemia, kernicterus; **Interactions:** ↓ effects of warfarin; Bile acid sequestrants, mineral oil, and sucralfate may ↓ absorption; **Dose:** *Adults:* 2.5–25 mg/day PO or 10 mg subcut/IM/IV. *Peds:* 2.5–5 mg PO or 0.5–5 mg SC/IM/IV. *Neonates:* Prophylaxis—0.5–1 mg IM w/in 1 hr of birth; Treatment—1 mg/day; **Availability:** *Tabs:* 5 mg. *Inject:* 2 mg/ml, 10 mg/ml; **Monitor:** CBC, bilirubin, PT, INR, S/S bleeding; **Notes:** Give by slow IV injection (1 mg/min); rapid IV administration may cause anaphylaxis.

P

pilocarpine (oral) (Salagen) Uses: Xerostomia from head/neck CA or Sjögren's syndrome; **Class:** cholinergics; **Preg:** C; **CIs:** Hypersensitivity; Uncontrolled asthma; Angle-closure glaucoma; Severe hepatic impairment; **ADRs:** dizziness, HA, weakness, amblyopia, epistaxis, rhinitis, edema, HTN, ↑ HR, <u>N/V</u>, dyspepsia, dysphagia, urinary frequency, <u>flushing</u>, <u>sweating</u>, tremors, chills, voice change; **Interactions:** Anticholinergics ↓ effects of pilocarpine; Bethanechol or ophthalmic cholinergics may ↑ cholinergic effects; Beta blockers ↑ CV reactions (conduction disturbances); **Dose:** *PO: Adults: Head/neck CA*—5 mg tid initially, titrated to usual range 15–30 mg/day (max 10 mg/dose). *PO: Adults: Sjögren's syndrome*—5 mg qid; **Availability:** *Tabs:* 5, 7.5 mg; **Monitor:** S/S xerostomia; **Notes:** Give adequate daily fluids (1500–2000 ml/day) to avoid dehydration.

pimecrolimus (Elidel) **Uses:** Short-term treatment of atopic dermatitis unresponsive to conventional treatment; **Class:** immunosuppressants (top); **Preg:** C; **CIs:** Hypersensitivity; Active cutaneous viral infections (↑ risk of dissemination); Netherton's syndrome (↑ absorption); Malignant or premalignant skin lesions; Peds <2 yr (safety not established); **ADRs:** burning sensation, ↑ risk of lymphoma/skin CA; **Interactions:** None significant; **Dose:** *Topical: Adults and Peds: ≥2 yr:* Apply bid; **Availability:** *Cream:* 1%; **Monitor:** Skin lesions; **Notes:** Do not use as 1st-line therapy; discontinue upon resolution of symptoms; do not use with occlusive dressings. Advise patient to avoid sunlight exposure.

pioglitazone (Actos) **Uses:** NIDDM; **Class:** antidiabetics; **Preg:** C; **CIs:** Hypersensitivity; DKA; Active liver disease or ↑ ALT (>2.5 × ULN); IDDM; Moderate-to-severe HF; Hepatic impairment; **ADRs:** edema, hepatitis, ↑ LFTs, anemia, fractures (arm, hand, foot) in female patients; **Interactions:** ↓ efficacy of hormonal contraceptives; Ketoconazole ↑ effects; Use with insulin may ↑ risk of HF; **Dose:** *PO: Adults:* 15–45 mg/day; **Availability:** *Tabs:* 15, 30, 45 mg; **Monitor:** CBC, A1C, serum glucose, LFTs, fluid status, S/S HF and hypoglycemia; **Notes:** May be given without regard to meals. Do not use if LFTs >2.5 × ULN.

P

piperacillin/tazobactam (Zosyn) **Uses:** Appendicitis/peritonitis, skin/skin structure infections, PID, or resp tract infections due to susceptible organisms (e.g., *S. aureus*, *E. coli*, *B. fragilis*, *H. flu*, *Acinetobacter*, *Klebsiella*, *Pseudomonas*); **Class:** extended spectrum penicillins; **Preg:** B; **CIs:** Hypersensitivity (cross-sensitivity to other beta-lactam antibiotics may exist); **ADRs:** SEIZURES, HA, PSEUDOMEMBRANOUS COLITIS, N/V/D, ↑ LFTs, ↑ BUN/SCr, rash, urticaria, pruritis, thrombocytopenia, phlebitis, allergic reactions including ANAPHYLAXIS, SERUM SICKNESS; **Interactions:** Probenecid ↓ excretion and ↑ levels; **Dose:** *IV: Adults and Peds: >40 kg Most infections*—3.375 g q 6 hr. *Nosocomial pneumonia*—4.5 g q 6 hr. *IV: Peds: ≥9 mo and ≤40 kg Appendicitis/peritonitis*—100 mg piperacillin/12.5 mg tazobactam per kg dosing for peds q 8 hr. *IV: Peds: 2–8 mo Appendicitis/peritonitis*—80 mg piperacillin/10 mg tazobactam per kg dosing for peds q 8 hr. *Renal Impairment IV: Adults:* ↓ dose if CrCl ≤40 ml/min; **Availability:** *Inject:* 2 g piperacillin/0.25 g tazobactam, 3 g piperacillin/0.375 g tazobactam, 4 g piperacillin/0.5 g tazobactam;

Monitor: BP, HR, temp, sputum, U/A, CBC, LFTs, BUN/SCr; **Notes:** Use with caution in patients with beta-lactam allergy (do not use if history of anaphylaxis or hives).

piroxicam (Feldene) Uses: OA; RA; **Class:** NSAIDs; **Preg:** C, **D** (3rd tri); **CIs:** Hypersensitivity to aspirin or NSAIDs; Active bleeding; Perioperative pain from CABG surgery; **ADRs:** HA, dizziness, tinnitus, edema, GI BLEEDING, N/V/D, ↑ LFTs, ↑ SCr, rash; **Interactions:** ↑ adverse GI effects with aspirin and corticosteroids; ↓ effects of aspirin, diuretics or antihypertensives; ↑ risk of bleeding with drugs affecting platelet function; ↑ risk of nephrotoxicity with cyclosporine; ↑ levels of methotrexate, lithium, aminoglycosides and vancomycin; **Dose:** *PO: Adults:* 10–20 mg daily. *PO: Peds:* 0.2–0.3 mg/kg/day (max: 15 mg/day); **Availability (G):** *Caps:* 10 mg, 20 mg; **Monitor:** Pain, temp, S/S of GI upset/bleeding, BUN/SCr, CBC; **Notes:** Avoid use in oliguria/anuria. Give with food.

polyethylene glycol (MiraLax) Uses: Treatment of constipation; **Class:** osmotics; **Preg:** C; **CIs:** GI obstruction; Gastric retention; Toxic colitis; Megacolon; Abdominal pain of unknown cause; **ADRs:** abdominal bloating, cramping, flatulence, nausea; **Interactions:** None significant; **Dose:** *PO: Adults:* 17 g in 8 oz of water for up to 2 wk; *PO: Peds: >4 yrs:* 0.7–1.5 g/kg daily (max: 17 g/day); **Availability (G):** *Powder:* 14 oz, 16 oz, 24 oz, 26 oz, 17-g (single-dose) packets; **Monitor:** Stool frequency/consistency; **Notes:** 2–4 days may be required to produce a bowel movement.

P

posaconazole (Noxafil) Uses: Prevention of invasive *Aspergillus* and *Candida* infections in severely immunocompromised patients; Treatment of oropharyngeal candidiasis; **Class:** triazoles; **Preg:** C; **CIs:** Prior sensitivity to posaconazole or other azole antifungals; Concurrent use of pimozide, quinidine, sirolimus, or ergot derivatives; **ADRs:** HA, QT prolongation, HEPATOTOXICITY, N/V/D, ↓ K, neutropenia, thrombocytopenia, ALLERGIC REACTIONS; **Interactions:** May ↑ levels/toxicity of CYP3A4 substrates; Rifabutin, phenytoin, cimetidine, and efavirenz ↓ levels/effects; ↑ cyclosporine, sirolimus, and tacrolimus levels/toxicity (concurrent use with sirolimus contraindicated); ↑ risk of arrhythmias with pimozide and quinidine (contraindicated); ↑ rifabutin levels; ↑ levels/toxicity from ergot derivatives (contraindicated); ↑ levels/toxicity of HMG CoA reductase inhibitors (statins); ↑ levels/CV reactions to Ca channel blockers; ↑ digoxin levels; **Dose:** *PO: Adults: Prophylaxis*—200 mg tid. *Oropharyngeal candidiasis treatment*—100 mg bid × 1 day, then 100 mg/day × 13 days. *Oropharyngeal candidiasis refractory to itraconazole or fluconazole*—400 mg bid; **Availability:** *Oral susp:* 40 mg/ml; **Monitor:** BP, HR, temp, sputum, U/A, CBC, LFTs, K; **Notes:** Give with a full meal to ↑ absorption.

potassium and sodium phosphates (K-Phos M.F., K-Phos Neutral, K-Phos No. 2, Neutra-Phos, Uro-KP Neutral) **Uses:** Treatment/prevention PO_4 depletion; Adjunct therapy of UTIs with methenamine hippurate or mandelate; Prevention of Ca urinary stones; **Class:** minerals/electrolytes; **Preg:** C; **CIs:** Hyperkalemia (K salts); Hyperphosphatemia; Hypocalcemia; Severe renal impairment; Untreated Addison's disease (K salts); Hyperparathyroidism; Cardiac disease; Hypernatremia ($NaPO_4$ only); HTN ($NaPO_4$ only); Renal impairment; **ADRs:** confusion, dizziness, HA, weakness, ARRHYTHMIAS, CARDIAC ARREST, ↓ HR, ECG changes, edema, N/V/D, abdominal pain, ↑ K, ↑ Na, ↑ PO_4, ↓ Ca, ↓ Mg, muscle cramps, flaccid paralysis, heaviness of legs, paresthesias, tremors; **Interactions:** K-sparing diuretics, ACEIs, or ARBs may ↑ hyperkalemia; Corticosteroids may ↑ hypernatremia; Ca-, Mg-, and aluminum-containing compounds ↓ absorption of phosphates; **Dose:** *PO: Adults and Peds: >4 yr:* 250–500 mg (8–16 mmol) phosphorus qid. *PO: Peds: <4 yr* 250 mg (8 mmol) phosphorus qid; **Availability:** *Tabs (K-Phos MF):* elemental PO_4 125.6 mg (4 mmol), Na 67 mg (2.9 mEq), and K 44.5 mg (1.1 mEq). *Tabs (K-Phos Neutral):* elemental PO_4 250 mg (8 mmol), Na 298 mg (13 mEq), and K 45 mg (1.1 mEq). *Tabs (K-Phos No.2):* elemental PO_4 250 mg (8 mmol), Na 134 mg (5.8 mEq), and K 88 mg (2.3 mEq). *Tabs (Uro-KP Neutral):* elemental PO_4 258 mg, Na 262.4 mg (10.8 mEq), and K 49.4 mg (1.3 mEq). *Powder for oral soln (Neutra-Phos):* elemental PO_4 250 mg (8 mmol), Na 164 mg (7.1 mEq), and K 278 mg (7.1 mEq)/packet; **Monitor:** Electrolytes, BUN/SCr, urinary pH; **Notes:** Dissolve tabs in a full glass of water; give after meals to ↓ gastric irritation and laxative effect; do not give simultaneously with antacids containing aluminum, Mg, or Ca.

potassium chloride (Kaon-Cl, Kay Ciel, KCl, K-Dur, Klor-Con, Klotrix, K-Tab, Micro-K, Slow-K) **Uses:** Treatment/prevention of K depletion; **Class:** minerals/electrolytes; **Preg:** C; **CIs:** Hyperkalemia; Severe renal impairment; GI hypomotility including dysphagia or esophageal compression (tabs, caps); **ADRs:** confusion, restlessness, weakness, ARRHYTHMIAS, ECG changes, abdominal pain, flatulence, N/V/D, GI ulceration, stenotic lesions, paralysis, paresthesia, irritation at IV site; **Interactions:** ↑ risk of hyperkalemia with ACEIs, ARBs, K salt substitutes, K-sparing diuretics, or NSAIDs, Anticholinergics may ↑ GI mucosal lesions in patients taking wax-matrix KCl preparations; **Dose:** *PO: IV: Adults: Normal daily requirements*—40–80 mEq/day. *PO: Adults: Prevention of hypokalemia during diuretic therapy*—20–40 mEq/day in 1–2 divided doses (max dose: 20 mEq). *Treatment of hypokalemia*—40–100 mEq/day in divided doses. *PO, IV: Peds: Normal daily requirements*—2–3 mEq/kg/day. *PO, IV: Neonates: Normal daily requirements*—2–6 mEq/kg/day. *PO: Neonates, Infants, and Peds Prevention of hypokalemia during diuretic* *therapy*—1–2 mEq/kg/day in 1–2 divided doses. *Treatment of hypokalemia*—2–5 mEq/kg/day in divided doses; *IV: Neonates, Infants, and Peds Treatment of hypokalemia:* 0.5–1 mEg/kg/dose (max: 40 mEG/dose); **Availability (G):** *ER tabs:* 8 mEq, 10 mEq, 15 mEq, 20 mEq. *ER caps:* 8 mEq, 10 mEq. *Oral soln:* 20 mEq/15 ml, 40 mEq/ 15 ml. *Powder for oral soln:* 20-mEq packet, 25-mEq packet. *Inject:* 2 mEq/ml; **Monitor:** S/S hypo/hyperkalemia, ECG, BUN/SCr, K, Mg; **Notes:** Hypomagnesemia should be corrected to facilitate effectiveness of K replacement. Hyperkalemia may be treated with Na polystyrene sulfonate. Do not chew or crush EC or ER tabs or caps. **High Alert:** Medication errors involving IV administration of KCl have resulted in fatalities. Never administer K IV push or bolus. Do not administer undiluted. Dilute to 80 mEq/L via peripheral line and to a max of 200 mEq/L via central line. Infuse slowly, at a rate up to 10 mEq/hr in adults or 0.5 mEq/kg/hr in peds in general care areas. Check hospital policy for maximum infusion rates (usual max rate in monitored setting: 40 mEq/hr in adults or 1 mEq/kg/hr in peds). Use an infusion pump.

potassium iodide (Iosat, SSKI, Thyrosafe, Thyroshield) **Uses:** Expectorant for mucus caused by chronic pulmonary diseases; Reduction of thyroid vascularity prior to thyroidectomy; Thyrotoxic crisis; Block thyroidal uptake of radioactive iodine; **Class:** antithyroid agents; **Preg:** D; **CIs:** Hypersensitivity to iodine; Hyperkalemia; Pregnancy; Impaired renal function; Hyperthyroidism; Pulmonary edema; Iodine-induced goiter; **ADRs:** confusion, tiredness, fever, irregular heartbeat, <u>N/V/D</u>, abdominal pain, <u>goiter</u>, rash, neck/throat swelling, numbness, tingling; **Interactions:** Use with K-sparing diuretics, ACEIs, K supplements, or ARBs may lead to hyperkalemia; Lithium may ↑ hypothyroid effects; **Dose:** *PO: Adults: Expectorant*—300–600 mg tid–qid (SSKI). *PO: Adults and Peds: Preop thyroidectomy*—50–250 mg (1–5 gtt SSKI) tid for 10 days prior to surgery. *PO: Adults and Peds: Thyrotoxic crisis*—300–500 mg (6–10 gtt SSKI) tid. *PO: Infants <1 yr Thyrotoxic crisis*—150–250 mg (3–5 gtt SSKI) tid. *PO: Adults and Peds: >68 kg Radiation protectant*—130 mg/day until risk of exposure has passed. *PO: Peds: 3–18 yr and ≤68 kg Radiation protectant*—65 mg/day until risk of exposure has passed. *PO: Peds: 1 mo–3 yr Radiation protectant*—32.5 mg/day until risk of exposure has passed. *PO: Infants <1 mo:* 16.25 mg daily until risk of exposure has passed; **Availability:** *Tabs:* 65, 130 mg. *Oral soln:* 65 mg/ml (Thyroshield), 1 g/ml (SSKI); **Monitor:** TFTs, S/S hyperthyroidism; **Notes:** 10 gtt of SSKI = 500 mg potassium iodide. When used as an expectorant, take with a full glass of water. Dilute SSKI in a full glass of water, juice, or milk. Give with food to minimize GI upset.

pramipexole (Mirapex) **Uses:** Parkinson's disease; Restless legs syndrome; **Class:** dopamine agonists; **Preg:** C; **CIs:** Hypersensitivity;

P

ADRs: SLEEP ATTACKS, amnesia, dizziness, drowsiness, hallucinations, weakness, abnormal dreams, confusion, dyskinesia, extrapyramidal effects, HA, insomnia, postural hypotension, constipation, dry mouth, dyspepsia, nausea, urinary frequency, leg cramps, hypertonia, unsteadiness/falling; **Interactions:** Concurrent levodopa ↑ risk of hallucinations and dyskinesia; Effects ↑ by cimetidine; Effects ↓ by butyrophenones, metoclopramide, phenothiazines, or thioxanthenes; **Dose:** *PO: Adults: Parkinson's disease*—0.125 mg tid initially; may ↑ q 5–7 days (range: 1.5–4.5 mg/day). *Restless legs syndrome*—0.125 mg once daily 1–3 hrs before bedtime. May ↑ q 4–7 days to 0.25 mg, then up to 0.5 mg. *Renal Impairment PO: Adults:* ↓ dose for CrCl <60 ml/min; **Availability:** *Tabs:* 0.125, 0.25, 0.5, 0.75, 1, 1.5 mg; **Monitor:** BP, HR, ECG, wt, sleep patterns, S/S Parkinson's disease; **Notes:** Administer with meals to minimize nausea. Sleep attacks during activities that require active participation may occur without warning.

pramlintide (Symlin) Uses: Used with mealtime insulin in the management of diabetics; **Class:** hormones; **Preg:** C; **CIs:** Hypersensitivty; Inability to identify hypoglycemia; Gastroparesis; A1C >9%; Recurring severe hypoglycemia, requiring treatment; **ADRs:** dizziness, fatigue, HA, cough, N/V, abdominal pain, anorexia, HYPOGLYCEMIA, local allergy, arthralgia, systemic allergic reactions; **Interactions:** ↑ hypoglycemia with short-acting insulin; reduce dose of short-acting pre-meal insulin by 50%; Avoid use with agents that ↓ GI motility, including atropine and other anticholinergics; Avoid use with agents that ↓ GI absorption of nutrients, including alpha-glucosidase inhibitors including acarbose and miglitol; May delay absorption of concurrently administered drugs; give 1 hr before or 2 hr after; **Dose:** *Subcut: Adults: NIDDM*—60 mcg, immediately prior to major meals; if no significant nausea occurs, may ↑ to 120 mcg. *Subcut: Adults: IDDM*—15 mcg immediately prior to major meals; if no significant nausea occurs, may ↑ by 15 mcg q 3 days up to 60 mcg; **Availability:** *Inject:* 0.6 mg/ml; **Monitor:** A1C, glucose, wt, urine ketones, electrolytes, S/S hypoglycemia; **Notes:** Give pramlintide and insulin separately; do not mix.

P

pravastatin (Pravachol) Uses: Hyperlipidemia; Primary and secondary prevention of CV disease; **Class:** HMG-CoA reductase inhibitors; **Preg:** X; **CIs:** Hypersensitivity; Liver disease; Pregnancy/lactation; **ADRs:** HA, abdominal cramps, constipation, diarrhea, dyspepsia, flatulence, ↑ LFTs, nausea, rash, RHABDOMYOLYSIS, myalgia; **Interactions:** ↑ risk of myopathy with gemfibrozil or niacin (≥1 g/day); **Dose:** *PO: Adults:* 10–80 mg/day in the evening. *Concurrent cyclosporine therapy*—10–20 mg/day. *PO: Peds: ≥8 yr:* 20–40 mg/day. *Hepatic/Renal Impairment PO: Adults:* Start with 10 mg/day; **Availability (G):** *Tabs:* 10, 20, 40, 80 mg; **Monitor:** Lipid panel, LFTs, CK (if symptoms); **Notes:** Discontinue if LFTs persistently >3 × ULN.

prazosin (Minipress) Uses: HTN; **Class:** peripherally acting antiadrenergics; **Preg:** C; **CIs:** Hypersensitivity; Concurrent use with PDE-5 inhibitors (sildenafil, tadalafil, or vardenafil); **ADRs:** dizziness, HA, drowsiness, blurred vision, first-dose orthostatic hypotension, edema, palpitations, diarrhea, dry mouth, nausea; **Interactions:** ↑ effects with other antihypertensives and PDE-5 inhibitors; **Dose:** *PO: Adults:* 1 mg bid–tid; may ↑ gradually to 6–15 mg/day in 2–3 divided doses (max: 20 mg/day); **Availability (G):** *Caps:* 1, 2, 5 mg; **Monitor:** BP (sitting, standing), HR, I/Os, wt, edema; **Notes:** First-dose orthostatic hypotension most frequently occurs 30–90 min after initial dose; give 1st dose at bedtime.

prednisoLONE (Orapred, Orapred-ODT, Pediapred, Prelone) Uses: Treatment of chronic diseases including: Inflammatory, Allergic, Hematologic, Neoplastic, Autoimmune disorders; Replacement therapy in adrenal insufficiency; **Class:** corticosteroids; **Preg:** C; **CIs:** Active untreated infections; **ADRs:** depression, euphoria, HA, ↑ ICP, psychoses, cataracts, ↑ IOP, HTN, PEPTIC ULCERATION, anorexia, N/V, acne, ↓ wound healing, ecchymoses, fragility, hirsutism, petechiae, adrenal suppression, hyperglycemia, fluid retention, ↓ K, alkalosis, THROMBOEMBOLISM, thrombophlebitis, ↑ wt, muscle wasting, osteoporosis, cushingoid appearance, ↑ susceptibility to infection; **Interactions:** ↑ hypokalemia with thiazide and loop diuretics, or amphotericin B; ↑ requirement for insulin or oral hypoglycemic agents; Phenytoin, phenobarbital, and rifampin stimulate metabolism/may ↓ effects; ↑ GI effects with NSAIDs and aspirin; ↓ response/↑ ADRs from live-virus vaccines; ↑ risk of tendon rupture from FQs; **Dose:** *PO: Adults: Most uses*—5–60 mg/day single dose or divided doses. *Multiple sclerosis*—200 mg/day × 7 days, then 80 mg every other day × 1 mo. *Asthma exacerbations*—120–180 mg/day in divided doses 3–4 ×/day × 48 hrs, then 60–80 mg/day divided bid. *PO: Peds: Anti–inflammatory/Immunosuppressive*—0.1–2 mg/kg/day in 1–4 divided doses. *Nephrotic syndrome*—2 mg/kg/day in 1–3 divided doses (max: 80 mg/day) until urine is protein free for 4–6 wk. MD: 2 mg/kg every other day in the AM; gradually taper off after 4–6 wk. *Asthma exacerbation*—1–2 mg kg/day divided bid (max: 60 mg/day) divided bid; **Availability (G):** *Tabs:* 5 mg. *ODT:* 10, 15, 30 mg. *Syrup/Soln:* 5 mg/5 ml, 15 mg/5 ml; **Monitor:** CBC, electrolytes, glucose, BP, wt, I/Os, growth (peds), S/S adrenal insufficiency; **Notes:** Give with food. Use lowest possible dose to treat condition.

predniSONE (Deltasone, Sterapred) Uses: Treatment of chronic diseases including: Inflammatory, Allergic, Hematologic, Neoplastic, Autoimmune disorders; **Class:** corticosteroids; **Preg:** C; **CIs:** Active untreated infections; **ADRs:** depression, euphoria, HA, ↑ ICP, psychoses, cataracts, ↑ IOP, HTN, PEPTIC ULCERATION, anorexia,

P

N/V, acne, ↓ wound healing, ecchymoses, fragility, hirsutism, petechiae, adrenal suppression, hyperglycemia, fluid retention, ↓ K, alkalosis, THROMBOEMBOLISM, thrombophlebitis, ↑ wt, muscle wasting, osteoporosis, cushingoid appearance, ↑ susceptibility to infection; **Interactions:** ↑ hypokalemia with thiazide and loop diuretics, or amphotericin B; ↑ requirement for insulin or oral hypoglycemic agents; Phenytoin, phenobarbital, and rifampin stimulate metabolism/may ↓ effects; ↑ GI effects with NSAIDs and aspirin; ↓ response/↑ ADRs from live-virus vaccines; ↑ risk of tendon rupture from FQs; **Dose:** *PO: Adults: Most uses*—5–60 mg/day single dose or divided doses. *Multiple sclerosis*—200 mg/day × 1 wk, then 80 mg every other day × 1 mo. *Adjunctive therapy of PCP in HIV patients*—40 mg bid × 5 days, then 40 mg once daily × 5 days, then 20 mg once daily × 10 days. *PO: Peds: Nephrotic syndrome*—2 mg/kg/day in 1–3 divided doses (max: 80 mg/day) until urine is protein free for 4–6 wk. *MD:* 2 mg/kg/day every other day in the AM; gradually taper off after 4–6 wk. *Asthma exacerbation*—1–2 mg/kg/day (max: 60 mg/day) divided bid; **Availability (G):** *Tabs:* 1, 2.5, 5, 10, 20, 50 mg. *Oral soln:* 1 mg/ml, 5 mg/ml; **Monitor:** CBC, electrolytes, glucose, BP, wt, I/Os, growth (peds), S/S adrenal insufficiency; **Notes:** Give with food. Use lowest possible dose to treat condition.

pregabalin (Lyrica) **Uses:** Pain due to: Diabetic peripheral neuropathy, Postherpetic neuralgia, Fibromyalgia; Partial-onset seizures; **Class:** GABA analogues, nonopioid analgesics; **Preg:** C; **CIs:** Myopathy (known/suspected); HF (↑ risk of edema); **ADRs:** dizziness, drowsiness, impaired attention/concentration/thinking, edema, blurred vision, dry mouth, abdominal pain, constipation, ↑ appetite, vomiting, ↓ platelet count, ↑ wt, allergic reactions, fever; **Interactions:** Concurrent use with pioglitazone and rosiglitazone ↑ fluid retention; ↑ CNS depression with CNS depressants, opioids, alcohol, BZs, or other sedatives/hypnotics; **Dose:** *PO: Adults: Diabetic neuropathic pain*—50 mg tid, ↑ over 7 days up to 100 mg tid. *Partial onset seizures*—150 mg/day initially in 2–3 divided doses, may ↑ to 600 mg/day. *Post-herpetic neuralgia*—75 mg bid *or* 50 mg tid initially; may ↑ over 7 days to 300 mg/day, after 2–4 wk may ↑ to 600 mg/day. *Renal Impairment PO: Adults:* ↓ dose for CrCl <60 ml/min; **Availability:** *Caps:* 25, 50, 75, 100, 150, 200, 225, 300 mg; **Monitor:** Pain, seizure activity, CK, platelets, wt, fluid status; **Notes:** Give without regard to meals. Do not discontinue abruptly.

probenecid (Probalan) **Uses:** Prevention of hyperuricemia associated with gouty arthritis or thiazide therapy; Prolongation and elevation of beta-lactam levels, anti-infectives; **Class:** uricosurics; **Preg:** B; **CIs:** Hypersensitivity; Chronic high-dose salicylate therapy; Peds <2 yr; Blood dyscrasias; Renal impairment (avoid use if CrCl <30 ml/min); Uric acid kidney stones; **ADRs:** HA, dizziness, N/V/D, abdominal pain, drug-induced hepatitis, sore gums, uric acid stones, urinary frequency,

P

flushing, rash, APLASTIC ANEMIA, anemia; **Interactions:** ↑ levels of acyclovir, allopurinol, barbiturates, BZs, beta-lactams, clofibrate, dapsone, methotrexate, NSAIDs, pantothenic acid, penicillamine, rifampin, sulfonamides, sulfonylurea oral hypoglycemic agents, or zidovudine; Large doses of salicylates ↓ uricosuric activity; **Dose:** *PO: Adults and Peds: >50 kg Hyperuricemia*—250 mg bid × 1 wk; ↑ to 500 mg bid, then ↑ by 500 mg/day q 4 wk (max: 3 g/day). *Augmentation of beta-lactams*—500 mg qid. *Single-dose therapy of gonorrhea*—1 g with amoxicillin or penicillin. *PO: Peds: 2–14 yr and ≤50 kg:* 25 mg/kg initially; then 10 mg/kg qid (max: 500 mg/dose); **Availability:** *Tabs:* 500 mg; **Monitor:** Uric acid, BUN/SCr, LFTs, CBC, I/Os, joint pain; **Notes:** Administer with food or antacid to minimize GI irritation. Fluids should be encouraged to prevent urate stone formation.

procainamide (Pronestyl) **Uses:** Treatment of VT, PVCs, PAT, and AF; Prevention of recurrence of VT, PSVT, AF, and atrial flutter; **Class:** antiarrhythmics (class Ia); **Preg:** C; **CIs:** Hypersensitivity; 2nd- or 3rd-degree heart block (in absence of pacemaker); SLE; QT prolongation; **ADRs:** SEIZURES, confusion, dizziness, ASYSTOLE, HEART BLOCK, TORSADES DE POINTES, VENTRICULAR ARRHYTHMIAS, ↓ BP, N/V/D, rash, AGRANULOCYTOSIS, leukopenia, thrombocytopenia, chills, drug-induced lupus syndrome, fever; **Interactions:** CYP2D6 inhibitors may ↑ levels; Antihypertensives and nitrates may ↑ hypotensive effect; ↑ risk of QT_C prolongation with other QT_C prolonging drugs; **Dose:** *IM: Adults:* 50 mg/kg/day in divided doses q 3–6 hr. *IV: Adults:* 100 mg q 5 min until arrhythmia is abolished or 1000 mg has been given *or* loading infusion of 500–600 mg over 30–60 min followed by maintenance infusion of 1–4 mg/min; **Availability:** *Inject:* 100 mg/ml, 500 mg/ml; **Monitor:** BP, HR, ECG, CBC, ANA, electrolytes, I/Os, S/S HF; **Notes:** discontinue if any of the following occur: arrhythmia resolves, QRS complex widens by 50%, prolonged PR interval, BP ↓ >15 mmHg, or toxic side effects develop. Max IV rate 25 mg/min; therapeutic blood level is 4–8 mcg/ml.

procarbazine (Matulane) **Uses:** Hodgkin's disease; **Class:** alkylating agents; **Preg:** D; **CIs:** Hypersensitivity; Pregnancy or lactation; Alcoholism; Tyramine-containing foods/beverages; HF; Decreased bone marrow reserve; **ADRs:** SEIZURES, confusion, dizziness, drowsiness, hallucinations, HA, mania, depression, psychosis, tremor, nystagmus, photophobia, retinal hemorrhage, cough, pleural effusion, edema, ↓ BP, ↑ HR, N/V/D, anorexia, dry mouth, dysphagia, ↑ LFTs, stomatitis, gonadal suppression, alopecia, photosensitivity, pruritus, rash, gynecomastia, anemia, leukopenia, thrombocytopenia, neuropathy, paresthesia, ascites, secondary malignancy; **Interactions:** Concurrent use (within 14 days) of sympathomimetics including methylphenidate may produce life-threatening HTN; ↑ bone marrow depression with antineoplastics or radiation therapy; Seizures and hyperpyrexia may occur with concurrent use of MAOIs, TCAs, SSRI antidepressants (do not use within 5 wk of fluoxetine), or carbamazepine; ↓ serum digoxin levels; Concurrent use with levodopa ↑ flushing and HTN; ↑ CNS depression with other CNS depressants, including alcohol, antidepressants, antihistamines, opioid analgesics, phenothiazines, and sedative/hypnotics; Disulfiram-like reaction with alcohol; **Dose:** *PO: Adults:* 2–4 mg/kg/day × 1 wk, then 4–6 mg/kg/day until response is obtained; then MD of 1–2 mg/kg/day. Round to the nearest 50 mg. *PO: Peds:* 50 mg/m²/day × 7 days, then 100 mg/m²/day; MD of 50 mg/m²/day; **Availability:** *Caps:* 50 mg; **Monitor:** CBC, LFTs, BP, HR, RR, wt, S/S bleeding/infection; **Notes:** Administer with food or fluids if GI irritation occurs; avoid tyramine-rich foods (e.g., chocolate, blue cheese), caffeine, and alcohol. Nadir of leukopenia and thrombocytopenia occurs in 2–8 wk, with recovery in about 6 wk.

prochlorperazine (Compazine, Ultrazine) Uses: Management of N/V; Treatment of psychoses; Treatment of anxiety; **Class:** phenothiazines; **Preg:** C; **CIs:** Prior sensitivity to other phenothiazines; Narrow-angle glaucoma; Severe liver or CV disease; CNS depression; **ADRs:** NMS, <u>extrapyramidal reactions</u>, sedation, tardive dyskinesia, <u>blurred vision</u>, <u>dry eyes</u>, lens opacities, ECG changes, ↓ BP, ↑ HR, <u>constipation</u>, <u>dry mouth</u>, anorexia, ↑ LFTs, ileus, urinary retention, photosensitivity, pigment changes, rash, galactorrhea, AGRANULOCYTOSIS, leukopenia, hyperthermia, allergic reactions; **Interactions:** ↑ hypotension with antihypertensives, nitrates, or alcohol; ↑ CNS depression with CNS depressants, alcohol, antidepressants, antihistamines; opioid analgesics, sedative/hypnotics, or general anesthetics; ↑ anticholinergic effects with drugs possessing anticholinergic properties; Lithium ↑ risk of extrapyramidal reactions; ↑ risk of agranulocytosis with antithyroid agents; ↓ effects of levodopa; Antacids may ↓ absorption; **Dose:** *PO: Adults and Peds: ≥12 yr Antiemetic*—5–10 mg tid–qid (max: 40 mg/day). *Antipsychotic*—5–10 mg tid–qid (max: 150 mg/day). *PO: Peds: 2–12 yr Antipsychotic*—2.5 mg tid–qid (max: 25 mg/day). *PO, Rect: Peds: 2–12 yr Antiemetic*—0.4 mg/kg/day in 3–4 divided doses. *IM: Adults and Peds: ≥12 yr:* 5–10 mg q 3–4 hr prn. *IM, IV: Peds: 2–12 yr:* 0.1–0.15 mg/kg/dose q 8–12 hr (max: 40 mg/day). *IV: Adults and Peds: ≥12 yr:* 2.5–10 mg (max: 40 mg/day). *Rect: Adults:* 25 mg bid. *IM: Adults: Antipsychotic*—10–20 mg q 2–4 hr × 4 doses, then 10–20 mg q 4–6 hr (max 200 mg/day). *Rect: Adults:* 10 mg tid–qid; may ↑ by 5–10 mg q 2–3 days prn. *PO: Adults and Peds: ≥12 yr: Antianxiety*—5 mg tid–qid (max: 20 mg/day or longer than 12 wk). *IM: Adults and Peds: ≥12 yr:* 5–10 mg q 3–4 hr prn (max: 40 mg/day). *IV: Adults:* 2.5–10 mg (max: 40 mg/day); **Availability (G):** *Tabs:* 5, 10 mg. *Inject:* 5 mg/ml. *Supp:* 25 mg; **Monitor:** BP, HR, RR, ECG, CBC, LFTs, S/S extrapyramidal reactions, N/V, eye exams (chronic use), mental status; **Notes:** Give with food, milk, or a full glass of water to minimize gastric irritation.

P

promethazine (Phenergan, Promethacon) Uses: Treatment of allergic conditions and motion sickness; Preoperative sedation; Treatment and prevention of N/V; Adjunct to anesthesia and analgesia; **Class:** phenothiazines; **Preg:** C; **CIs:** Hypersensitivity; Comatose patients; Peds <2 yr (may cause fatal resp depression); **ADRs:** NMS, confusion, disorientation, sedation, dizziness, extrapyramidal reactions, fatigue, insomnia, nervousness, blurred vision, diplopia, tinnitus, ↓ HR, HTN, ↓ BP, ↑ HR, constipation, ↑ LFTs, dry mouth, severe tissue necrosis upon infiltration at IV site, rash; **Interactions:** ↑ CNS depression with other CNS depressants, including alcohol, antihistamines, opioid analgesics, and sedative/hypnotics; NMS can occur when used with antipsychotics; ↑ risk of anticholinergic effects with other anticholinergic agents; May precipitate seizures when used with drugs that lower seizure threshold; Concurrent use with MAOIs may result in ↑ sedation and anticholinergic side effects; **Dose:** *PO: Adults: Antihistamine*—6.25–12.5 mg tid and 25 mg at bedtime. *Motion sickness*—25 mg 30–60 min before departure; may repeat in 8–12 hr. *IM, IV, Rect: Adults: Antihistamine*—25 mg; may repeat in 2 hr. *PO, Rect, IM, IV, Adults: Sedation*—25–50 mg; may repeat q 4–6 hr if needed. *Antiemetic*—12.5–25 mg q 4 hr prn. *PO: Peds: ≥2 yr: Antihistamine*—0.1 mg/kg/dose (max: 12.5 mg/dose) q 6 hr during the day and 0.5 mg/kg/dose (max: 25 mg/dose) at bedtime. *Rect: Peds: ≥2 yr: Antihistamine*—0.125 mg/kg q 4–6 hr *or* 0.5 mg/kg at bedtime. *PO, Rect: Peds: ≥2 yr: Motion sickness*—0.5 mg/kg (max: 25 mg) 30–60 min before departure; may be given q 12 hr prn. *PO, Rect, IM: Peds: ≥2 yr Sedation*—0.5–1 mg/kg (max: 50 mg) q 6 hr prn. *PO, Rect, IM, IV: Peds: ≥2 yr Antiemetic*—0.25–1 mg/kg (max: 25 mg) q 4–6 hr; **Availability (G):** *Tabs:* 12.5, 25, 50 mg. *Syrup:* 6.25 mg/5 ml. *Inject:* 25 mg/ml, 50 mg/ml. *Supp:* 12.5, 25, 50 mg; **Monitor:** BP, HR, RR, CBC, level of sedation, extrapyramidal effects, anticholinergic effects; **Notes:** Use lowest effective dose in peds >2 yr. Avoid concurrent use with resp depressants.

P

propafenone (Rythmol) Uses: Ventricular arrhythmias; Paroxysmal atrial arrhythmias, including paroxysmal AF/AFl and PSVT; **Class:** antiarrhythmics (class Ic); **Preg:** C; **CIs:** Hypersensitivity; Cardiogenic shock; Sick sinus syndrome and AV block (without a pacemaker); Bradycardia; Severe hypotension; Concurrent ritonavir; Nonallergic bronchospasm; Electrolyte disturbances; Uncontrolled HF; **ADRs:** dizziness, weakness, blurred vision, ARRHYTHMIAS, conduction disturbances, angina, ↓ HR, ↓ BP, altered taste, constipation, N/V, dry mouth, rash; **Interactions:** CYP2D6 inhibitors may ↑ levels; ↑ risk of bradycardia with digoxin, diltiazem, verapamil, or beta blockers, ↑ effects of warfarin; **Dose:** *PO: Adults: IR*—150 mg q 8 hr; may ↑ q 4–5 days to 300 mg q 8–12 hr. *ER*—225 mg q 12 hr; may ↑ q 6 days to 325 mg q 12 hr, and then to 425 mg q 12 hr. *Single-dose treatment of AF (unlabeled)*—450 (<70 kg) or 600 mg (≥70 kg); **Availability (G):** *IR* *tabs:* 150, 225, 300 mg. *ER caps:* 225, 325, 425 mg; **Monitor:** BP, HR, ECG, electrolytes, I/Os, S/S HF; **Notes:** Should initiate therapy during cardiac rhythm monitoring; proarrhythmic effects usually seen within 1st 2 wk. Correct electrolyte disturbances prior to therapy. Do not crush or chew caps.

propofol (Diprivan) Uses: General anesthesia induction in peds >3 yr and adults; Maintenance of balanced anesthesia in peds >2 months and adults; Initiation and maintenance of MAC sedation of intubated, mechanically ventilated patients; **Class:** anesthetic; **Preg:** B; **CIs:** Hypersensitivity to propofol, soybean oil, egg lecithin, or glycerol; Labor and delivery; CV disease; Lipid disorders (emulsion may have detrimental effect); ↑ ICP; Cerebrovascular disorders; **ADRs:** dizziness, HA, APNEA, cough, ↓ HR, ↓ BP, HTN, abdominal cramping, hiccups, N/V, flushing, burning sensation, pain, stinging, coldness, numbness, tingling at IV site, involuntary muscle movements, perioperative myoclonia, green urine; **Interactions:** ↑ CNS and resp depression with alcohol, antihistamines, opioid analgesics, and sedative/hypnotics; Theophylline may antagonize the CNS effects of propofol; ↑ levels of alfentanil; Cardiorespiratory instability with acetazolamide; Serious bradycardia with fentanyl in peds; ↑ risk of hypertriglyceridemia with IV fat emulsion; **Dose:** *IV: Adults: <55 yr Induction*—40 mg q 10 sec until induction achieved (2–2.5 mg/kg total). *Maintenance*—100–200 mcg/kg/min. *IV: Geriatric Patients, Cardiac Patients, Debilitated Patients, or Hypovolemic Patients Induction*—20 mg q 10 sec until induction achieved (1–1.5 mg/kg total). *Maintenance*—50–100 mcg/kg/min. *IV: Adults: Undergoing Neurosurgical Procedures Induction*—20 mg q 10 sec until induction achieved (1–2 mg/kg total). *Maintenance*—100–200 mcg/kg/min. *IV: Peds: ≥3 yr–16 yr Induction*—2.5–3.5 mg/kg; use lower dose for peds ASA III or IV. *IV: Peds: 2 mo–16 yr Maintenance*—125–300 mcg/kg/min *IV: Adults: <55 yr MAC Sedation: Initiation*—100–150 mcg/kg/min infusion *or* 0.5 mg/kg as slow inject. *Maintenance*—25–75 mcg/kg/min infusion or incremental boluses of 10–20 mg. *IV: Geriatric Patients, Debilitated Patients, or ASA III/IV Patients Initiation*—Same doses as adults with slower infusion rates. *Maintenance*—20% less than the usual adult infusion dose; rapid/repeated bolus dosing should be avoided. *IV: Adults: ICU sedation*—5–50 mcg/kg/min; **Availability (G):** *Inject:* 10 mg/ml; **Monitor:** RR, HR, BP, TGs, level of sedation; **Notes:** Contains 1.1 kcal/ml (0.1 g fat/ml); give undiluted; wean gradually.

propoxyphene (Darvon, Darvon N) Uses: Mild-to-moderate pain; **Class:** opioid agonists; **Preg:** C; **CIs:** Hypersensitivity; Head trauma; ↑ ICP; **ADRs:** disorientation, dizziness, weakness, dysphoria, euphoria, HA, insomnia, paradoxical excitement, sedation, blurred vision, ↓ BP, N/V, abdominal pain, constipation, rash, psychological/physical dependence, tolerance; **Interactions:** MAOIs may cause fatal reactions—↓ initial dose to 25% of usual dose; ↑ CNS depression with alcohol, antidepressants, and sedative/hypnotics; Administration of partial-antagonist opioid analgesics may precipitate withdrawal in physically dependent patients; Nalbuphine, buprenorphine, or pentazocine may ↓ analgesia; **Dose:** *PO: Adults: Hydrochloride*—65 mg q 4 hr prn (max: 390 mg/day). *PO: Adults: Napsylate*—100 mg q 4 hr prn (max: 600 mg/day). *Renal Impairment Adults:* Avoid use if CrCl <10 ml/min; **Availability (G):** *Caps (Darvon):* 65 mg (hydrochloride). *Tabs (Darvon-N):* 100 mg (napsylate); **Monitor:** Pain, BP, HR, RR, LFTs, S/S CNS depression; **Notes:** 100 mg propoxyphene napsylate = 65 mg propoxyphene hydrochloride. Discontinue gradually after long-term use to prevent withdrawal.

propoxyphene napsylate/acetaminophen (Darvon A500, Darvocet-N 50, Darvocet-N 100) **Uses:** Mild-to-moderate pain with or without fever; **Class:** opioid agonists, opioid agonists/nonopioid analgesic combinations; **Preg:** C; **CIs:** Hypersensitivity; Head trauma; Increased ICP; **ADRs:** disorientation, dizziness, weakness, dysphoria, euphoria, HA, insomnia, paradoxical excitement, sedation, blurred vision, ↓ BP, N/V, abdominal pain, constipation, rash, psychological/physical dependence, tolerance; **Interactions:** MAOIs may cause fatal reactions—↓ initial dose to 25% of usual dose; ↑ CNS depression with alcohol, antidepressants, and sedative/hypnotics; Administration of partial-antagonist opioid analgesics may precipitate withdrawal in physically dependent patients; Nalbuphine, buprenorphine, or pentazocine may ↓ analgesia; **Dose:** *PO: Adults:* 50–100 mg propoxyphene q 4 hr prn (max: 600 mg propoxyphene napsylate/day; 390 mg propoxyphene hydrochloride/day); **Availability (G):** *Tabs:* propoxyphene napsylate 50 mg/acetaminophen 325 mg, propoxyphene hydrochloride 65 mg/acetaminophen 650 mg, propoxyphene napsylate 100 mg/acetaminophen 325 mg, propoxyphene napsylate 100 mg/acetaminophen 500 mg, propoxyphene napsylate 100 mg/acetaminophen 650 mg, propoxyphene hydrochloride 100 mg/acetaminophen 500 mg; **Monitor:** Pain, BP, HR, RR, LFTs, S/S CNS depression; **Notes:** Discontinue gradually after long-term use to prevent withdrawal. Do not exceed max dose of acetaminophen (4 g/day).

P

propranolol (Inderal, Inderal LA, InnoPran XL) **Uses:** HTN; Angina/MI; AF; Essential tremor; Hypertrophic subaortic stenosis; Pheochromocytoma; Migraine prophylaxis; **Class:** beta blockers; **Preg:** C; **CIs:** Hypersensitivity; Decompensated HF; Pulmonary edema; Cardiogenic shock; Bradycardia or ≥2nd-degree heart block (in absence of pacemaker); **ADRs:** fatigue, weakness, depression, dizziness, drowsiness, nightmares, blurred vision, bronchospasm, BRADYCARDIA, HF, PULMONARY EDEMA, ↓ BP, N/V/D, ED, ↓ libido, ↑ BG, ↓ BG; **Interactions:** ↑ risk of bradycardia with digoxin, diltiazem, verapamil, or clonidine; ↑ effects with other antihypertensives; ↑ risk of hypertensive crisis if concurrent clonidine is discontinued; May alter the effectiveness of insulins or oral hypoglycemic agents; May ↓ the effects of $beta_1$ agonists (e.g., dopamine or dobutamine); **Dose:** *PO: Adults: Angina*—80–320 mg/day in 2–4 divided doses (IR) or once daily (ER). *HTN*—80–240 mg/day in 2 divided doses (IR) (max: 640 mg/day) *or* 80–120 mg once daily (ER) (max: 640 mg/day; max for InnoPran XL is 120 mg/day). *AF*—10–30 mg tid–qid (IR). *Post-MI*—180–240 mg/day in 3 divided doses (IR). *Hypertrophic subaortic stenosis*—20–40 mg tid–qid (IR) *or* 80–160 mg once daily (ER). *Pheochromocytoma*—20 mg tid started 3 days before surgery is planned (IR) (used concurrently with alpha-blocking therapy). *Migraine prophylaxis*—80–240 mg/day in 3–4 divided doses (IR) or once daily (ER). *Essential tremor*—40-160 mg bid (IR). *PO: Peds: HTN/Arrhythmias*—0.5–4 mg/kg/day in 2–4 divided doses. *IV: Adults: Arrhythmias*—1–3 mg; may repeat in 2 min and again in 4 hr. *IV: Peds: Arrhythmias*—0.01–0.1 mg/kg (max: 1 mg/dose); may repeat q 6–8 hr; **Availability (G):** *Oral soln:* 4 mg/ml, 8 mg/ml. *Tabs:* 10, 20, 40, 60, 80 mg. *SR caps (Inderal LA):* 60, 80, 120, 160 mg. *ER caps (InnoPran XL):* 60, 80, 120, 160 mg. *Inject:* 1 mg/ml; **Monitor:** BP, HR, ECG, S/S HF, edema, wt, S/S angina, BG (in DM), HA frequency/intensity; **Notes:** Abrupt withdrawal may cause life-threatening arrhythmias, hypertensive crises, or myocardial ischemia. May mask S/S of hypoglycemia (esp. tachycardia) in DM. Do not open/crush ER caps. Give InnoPran XL dose once daily at bedtime.

propylthiouracil (PTU) **Uses:** Hyperthyroidism; Preparation for thyroidectomy or radioactive iodine therapy; **Class:** antithyroid agents; **Preg:** D; **CIs:** Hypersensitivity; Decreased bone marrow reserve; **ADRs:** drowsiness, HA, vertigo, N/V/D, ↑ LFTs, loss of taste, rash, skin discoloration, urticaria, hypothyroidism, AGRANULOCYTOSIS, leukopenia, thrombocytopenia, arthralgia, fever, lymphadenopathy, parotitis; **Interactions:** ↑ bone marrow depression with antineoplastics or radiation therapy; ↑ antithyroid effects with lithium, K iodide, or Na iodide; ↑ agranulocytosis with phenothiazines; **Dose:** *PO: Adults: Thyrotoxic crisis*—200–400 mg q 4 hr during the first 24 hr. *Hyperthyroidism*—300–900 mg once daily or divided bid–qid (max: 1.2 g/day); MD 50–600 mg/day. *PO: Peds: >10 yr:* 50–300 mg/day once daily or divided bid–qid. *PO: Peds: 6–10 yr:* 50–150 mg/day once daily or divided bid–qid. *PO: Neonates:* 10 mg/kg/day in divided doses; **Availability (G):** *Tabs:* 50 mg; **Monitor:** TFTs, CBC, LFTs; **Notes:** Administer at same time in relation to meals every day.

protamine sulfate **Uses:** Acute management of heparin or LMWH overdosage; Used to neutralize heparin received during dialysis, cardiopulmonary bypass, and other procedures; **Class:** antiheparins; **Preg:** C; **CIs:** Hypersensitivity to protamine or fish; Patients who have received previous protamine-containing insulin or vasectomized men (↑ risk of hypersensitivity reactions); **ADRs:** dyspnea, ↓ HR, HTN,

↓ BP, pulmonary HTN, N/V, flushing, warmth, bleeding, back pain, ANAPHYLAXIS, ANGIOEDEMA, and PULMONARY EDEMA; **Interactions:** None significant; **Dose:** *IV: Adults and Peds: Heparin overdose*—1 mg/100 units of heparin. If given >30 min after heparin, give 0.5 mg/100 units of heparin (max: 100 mg/2 hr). If heparin was administered subcut, use 1–1.5 mg/100 units of heparin, give 25–50 mg of the protamine dose slowly followed by a continuous infusion over 8–16 hours. *Enoxaparin overdose*—1 mg/each mg of enoxaparin to be neutralized (unlabeled). *Dalteparin overdose*—1 mg/100 anti-Xa units of dalteparin. A 2nd dose of 0.5 mg/100 anti-Xa units of dalteparin may be given 2–4 hr later if needed (unlabeled); **Availability (G):** *Inject:* 10 mg/ml; **Monitor:** Clotting factors, aPTT, ACT, TT, S/S bleeding; **Notes:** Correct hypovolemia prior to therapy.

pseudoephedrine (Sudafed) **Uses:** Nasal congestion; **Class:** decongestant; **Preg:** B; **CIs:** Hypersensitivity to sympathomimetic amines; HTN; CAD; Concurrent MAOI therapy; **ADRs:** dizziness, drowsiness, excitability, hallucinations, HA, insomnia, weakness, palpitations, HTN, ↑ HR, N/V; **Interactions:** ↑ BP with MAOIs and beta blockers; ↑ effects with adrenergics; ↓ effects of methlydopa and reserpine; **Dose:** *PO: Adults:* 30–60 mg q 4–6 h or SR 120 mg q 12 h. *PO: Peds:* 4 mg/kg/day divided q 6 h (max: 60 mg/day in <5 yr, 120 mg/day in >5 yr); **Availability (G):** *Tabs:* 30, 60 mg. *ER tabs:* 120, 240 mg. *Liquid:* 15 mg/5 ml, 30 mg/5 ml. *Drops:* 7.5 mg/0.8 ml [OTC]; **Monitor:** BP, HR, S/S nasal congestion; **Notes:** Take with food. Do not crush ER products.

pyrazinamide **Uses:** Active TB; **Class:** antituberculars; **Preg:** C; **CIs:** Hypersensitivity; Severe liver impairment; Concurrent use with rifampin; Gout; DM; Acute intermittent porphyria; **ADRs:** HEPATOTOXICITY, anorexia, N/V/D, dysuria, acne, itching, photosensitivity, skin rash, anemia, thrombocytopenia, ↑ uric acid, arthralgia, gouty arthritis; **Interactions:** Use with rifampin may result in life-threatening hepatoxicity; ↓ levels/effects of cyclosporine or antigout agents; **Dose:** *PO: Adults and Peds:* 15–30 mg/kg/day as a single dose. Up to 60 mg/kg/day has been used in isoniazid-resistant TB (max: 2 g/day as a single dose or 3 g/day in divided doses) *or* 50–70 mg/kg 2–3×/wk (max: 3 g/dose for 3 ×/wk regimen or 4 g/dose for 2×/wk regimen). *Patients with HIV*—20–30 mg/kg/day × 2 mo; further dosing depends on regimen employed. *Hepatic/Renal Impairment Adults and Peds:* ↓ dose for CrCl <50 ml/min and for hepatic impairment; **Availability (G):** *Tabs:* 500 mg; **Monitor:** CBC, LFTs, CXR, cultures for TB, uric acid; **Notes:** Treatment must continue even after symptoms subside. Advise patient to use sunscreen.

quetiapine (Seroquel, Seroquel XR) **Uses:** Schizophrenia; Depression with bipolar disorder; Bipolar mania; **Class:** antipsychotics;

Q

Preg: C; **CIs:** Hypersensitivity; Bone marrow suppression; Dementia-related psychoses; Severe CNS depression; Severe hepatic impairment, Blood dyscrasias; Coma; **ADRs:** dizziness, cognitive impairment, EPS, sedation, tardive dyskinesia, ↑ TGs, agitation, HA, ↑ LFTs, ↑ cholesterol, palpitations, peripheral edema, postural hypotension, anorexia, constipation, dry mouth, dyspepsia, sweating, leukopenia, ↑ wt, flu-like syndrome; **Interactions:** ↑ CNS depression with alcohol, antihistamines, opioid analgesics, and sedative/hypnotics; ↑ hypotension with alcohol or antihypertensives; Phenytoin, carbamazepine, barbiturates, rifampin, corticosteroids, thioridazine ↑ clearance/↓ effectiveness; Effects ↑ by azole antifungals, or erythromycin, and other CYP3A4 enzyme inhibitors; **Dose:** *PO: Adults: Schizophrenia*—25 mg bid, ↑ by 25–50 mg bid–tid over 3 days, up to 300–400 mg/day by Day 4 (max: 800 mg/day) *or* 300 mg XR once daily, ↑ by 300 mg/day, up to 400–800 mg/day (max: 800 mg/day). *Bipolar mania*—50 mg bid Day 1, ↑ dose by 100 mg/day up to 400 mg/day by Day 4, then may ↑ by 200 mg/day up to 800 mg/day on Day 6. *Bipolar depression*—50 mg daily at bedtime, then double dose daily until 300 mg by Day 4; **Availability:** *Tabs:* 25, 50, 100, 200, 300, 400 mg. *ER tabs:* 200, 300, 400 mg; **Monitor:** Mental status, BP, wt, BMI, lipid profile, LFTs, CBC, S/S extrapyramidal effects; **Notes:** Elderly require lower doses and slower titration. Instruct patient to avoid alcohol. Do not crush ER tabs.

quinapril (Accupril) **Uses:** HTN; HF; **Class:** ACEIs; **Preg:** C (1st tri), D (2nd and 3rd tri); **CIs:** Previous sensitivity/intolerance to ACEIs; **ADRs:** dizziness, cough, ↓ BP, ↑ SCr, ↑ K, ANGIOEDEMA; **Interactions:** ↑ effects with other antihypertensives; ↑ risk of hyperkalemia with ARBs, K supplements, K salt substitutes, K-sparing diuretics, or NSAIDs; NSAIDs may ↓ effectiveness; ↑ lithium levels; **Dose:** *PO: Adults: HTN*—10–20 mg/day (max: 40 mg/day). *HF*—5 mg daily–bid; may ↑ weekly up to 20 mg bid. *Renal Impairment PO: Adults:* ↓ dose if CrCl <60 ml/min; **Availability (G):** *Tabs:* 5, 10, 20, 40 mg; **Monitor:** BP, HR, wt, edema, BUN/SCr, K; **Notes:** Correct volume depletion. Advise patient on S/S angioedema avoidance of K salt substitutes.

Q

quinidine **Uses:** Restoration and maintenance of sinus rhythm in patients with AF or AFl; Prevention of recurrent ventricular arrhythmias; Treatment of malaria; **Class:** antiarrhythmics (class Ia); **Preg:** C; **CIs:** Hypersensitivity; 2nd- or 3rd-degree heart block (in absence of a pacemaker); Myasthenia gravis; Hypokalemia or hypomagnesemia (↑ risk of torsades de pointes); Bradycardia (↑ risk of torsades de pointes); **ADRs:** dizziness, confusion, fatigue, HA, syncope, vertigo, blurred vision, diplopia, tinnitus, ARRHYTHMIAS, HYPOTENSION, TORSADES DE POINTES, palpitations, ↑ HR, anorexia, abdominal cramping, N/V/D, ↑ LFTs, rash, AGRANULOCYTOSIS, hemolytic anemia, thrombocytopenia, ataxia, tremor, fever; **Interactions:** ↑ risk of QT_C

prolongation with other QT_C-prolonging drugs; CYP3A4 inhibitors may ↑ levels/toxicity; May ↑ levels/toxicity of CYP2D6 substrates and CYP3A4 substrates; ↑ serum digoxin levels/toxicity (dose ↓ recommended); Excretion is delayed/effects ↑ by drugs and foods that alkalinize the urine; May ↑ the risk of bleeding with warfarin; ↑ hypotension with antihypertensives, nitrates, and alcohol; May antagonize anticholinesterase therapy in myasthenia gravis; ↑ anticholinergic effects may occur with agents having anticholinergic properties; **Dose:** Dose expressed in terms of salt *PO: Adults: Atrial/ventricular arrhythmias*—100–600 mg sulfate q 4–6 hr; may ↑ to achieve therapeutic response (max: 3–4 g/day); 324–972 mg gluconate q 8–12 hr. *IV: Adults:* 200–400 mg gluconate given at a rate ≤10 mg/min until arrhythmia is suppressed, QRS complex widens, bradycardia or hypotension occurs. *PO: Peds:* 15–60 mg/kg/day sulfate in 4–5 divided doses. *Renal Impairment PO: Adults and Peds:* ↓ dose if CrCl <10 ml/min; **Availability (G):** Quinidine Gluconate *ER tabs:* 324 mg. *Inject:* 80 mg/ml. Quinidine Sulfate *Tabs:* 200, 300 mg. *ER tabs:* 300 mg; **Monitor:** BP, HR, ECG, CBC, BUN/SCr, LFTs, serum quinidine levels; **Notes:** 267 mg quinidine gluconate = 200 mg quinidine sulfate; therapeutic range: 2–7 mcg/ml. Discontinue IV if any of the following occur: arrhythmia is resolved, QRS complex widens by 50%, PR or QT_C intervals are prolonged, or frequent ventricular ectopic beats or tachycardia, bradycardia, or hypotension develops; patient should remain supine throughout IV administration to ↓ hypotension.

quinine (Qualaquin) **Uses:** Chloroquine-resistant malaria; **Class:** antimalarials; **Preg:** C; **CIs:** Prior sensitivity to quinine, quinidine, or mefloquine; QT_C prolongation; G6PD deficiency; Myasthenia gravis; Optic neuritis; Thrombocytopenic purpura; **ADRs:** ARRHYTHMIAS, ↑ BUN/SCr, N/V/D, ↑ LFTs, rash, hypoglycemia, bleeding, blood dyscrasias, thrombotic thrombocytopenic pupura, thrombocytopenia, ANAPHYLAXIS, HEMOLYTIC UREMIC SYNDROME, SJS; **Interactions:** Class IA or III antiarrhythmics, mefloquine, pimozide, or macrolides ↑ risk of arrhythmias; Cimetidine, rifampin, and rifabutin ↓ metabolism/↑ effects; ↑ effects of neuromuscular blocking agents; ↑ digoxin levels; ↑ bleeding with warfarin; Mefloquine ↑ risk of seizures and CV effects; Urinary alkalinizers may ↑ blood levels; may ↑ levels of carbamazepine, phenobarbital, and phenytoin; **Dose:** *PO: Adults:* 648 mg q 8 hr × 7 days. *Peds:* 10 mg/kg q 8 h. *Renal Impairment PO: Adults:* ↓ dose for CrCl <50 ml/min; **Availability:** *Caps:* 324 mg; **Monitor:** CBC with platelets, LFTs, glucose, eye exam; **Notes:** Give with food. Instruct patients to avoid antacids.

quinupristin/dalfopristin (Synercid) **Uses:** Serious or life-threatening infections caused by VRE or skin/skin structure infections caused by MSSA or methicillin-susceptible *Streptococcus pyogenes*; **Class:** streptogramins; **Preg:** B; **CIs:** Hypersensitivity; **ADRs:** HA,

Q

thrombophlebitis, PSEUDOMEMBRANOUS COLITIS, ↑ bilirubin, N/V/D, pruritus, rash, arthralgia, myalgia, edema/inflammation/pain at infusion site, infusion site reactions, ANAPHYLAXIS; **Interactions:** May ↑ cyclosporine levels; **Dose:** *IV: Adults: VRE*—7.5 mg/kg q 8 hr. *Skin/skin structure infections*—7.5 mg/kg q 12 hr; **Availability:** *Inject:* 500 mg (150 mg quinupristin/350 mg dalfopristin), 600 mg (180 mg quinupristin/420 mg dalfopristin); **Monitor:** BP, HR, WBC, temp, cultures, resolution of infection, S/S rash, bilirubin; **Notes:** Infuse over 60 min in D5W.

rabeprazole (Aciphex) **Uses:** GERD/Erosive esophagitis; Duodenal ulcers; *H. pylori* eradication; Hypersecretory conditions; **Class:** PPIs; **Preg:** B; **CIs:** Hypersensitivity; **ADRs:** dizziness, HA, N/V/D, abdominal pain, rash; **Interactions:** May ↑ levels/toxicity of CYP2C19 substrates; CYP2C19 inducers may ↓ levels/effects; ↓ absorption of ampicillin, iron, digoxin, ketoconazole, itraconazole, and atazanavir; ↑ risk of bleeding with warfarin; **Dose:** *PO: Adults: GERD/Duodenal ulcers*—20 mg/day. *H. pylori eradication*—20 mg bid. *Hypersecretory conditions*—60–120 mg/day; **Availability:** *Tabs:* 20 mg; **Monitor:** Hgb/Hct, LFTs, BUN/SCr, S/S abdominal pain/GI bleeding; **Notes:** Do not crush or chew tabs.

raloxifene (Evista) **Uses:** Prevention/treatment of osteoporosis in postmenopausal women; Reduction of the risk of breast CA in postmenopausal women; **Class:** selective estrogen receptor modulators; **Preg:** X; **CIs:** Hypersensitivity; Active or history of venous thromboembolic events; Pregnancy/lactation; **ADRs:** STROKE, DVT, PE, peripheral edema, retinal vein thrombosis, leg cramps, ↑ TGs, hot flashes; **Interactions:** Cholestyramine ↓ absorption; May alter effects of warfarin and other highly protein-bound drugs; **Dose:** *PO: Adults:* 60 mg once daily; **Availability:** *Tabs:* 60 mg; **Monitor:** BMD, CBC, lipid profile; **Notes:** Supplemental Ca or vitamin D may be required.

ramelteon (Rozerem) **Uses:** Insomnia; **Class:** sedative/hypnotics; **Preg:** C; **CIs:** Hypersensitivity; Severe hepatic impairment; Concurrent fluvoxamine; Severe COPD; **ADRs:** abnormal thinking, behavior changes, dizziness, fatigue, HA, insomnia (worsened), sleep driving, nausea; **Interactions:** Fluvoxamine ↑ levels/toxicity (contraindicated); CYP1A2 inhibitors may ↑ levels/toxicity; CYP1A2 inducers may ↓ levels/effects; ↑ CNS depression with alcohol, BZs, opioids, and other sedative/hypnotics; **Dose:** *PO: Adults:* 8 mg within 30 min of going to bed; **Availability:** *Tabs:* 8 mg; **Monitor:** Mental status, sleep patterns, abnormal behaviors; **Notes:** Do not give with a high-fat meal.

ramipril (Altace) **Uses:** HTN; HF post-MI; Reduction of risk of MI, stroke, or death from CV causes in patients at increased risk for these events; **Class:** ACEIs; **Preg:** C (1st tri), D (2nd and 3rd tri); **CIs:** Previous sensitivity/intolerance to ACEIs; **ADRs:** dizziness, cough, ↓ BP, ↑ SCr, ↑ K, ANGIOEDEMA; **Interactions:** ↑ effects with other antihypertensives; ↑ risk of hyperkalemia with ARBs, K supplements, K salt substitutes, K- sparing diuretics, or NSAIDs; NSAIDs may ↓ effectiveness; ↑ lithium levels; **Dose:** *PO: Adults: HTN*—2.5–5 mg/day (max: 10 mg/day). *HF post-MI*—2.5 mg bid; may ↑ to 5 mg bid. *Reduce risk of MI, stroke, and death from CV causes in high-risk patients*—2.5 mg/day × 1 wk, then 5 mg/day × 3 wk, then 10 mg/day. *Renal Impairment PO: Adults:* ↓ dose if CrCl <40 ml/min; **Availability (G):** *Caps:* 1.25, 2.5, 5, 10 mg; **Monitor:** BP, HR, wt, edema, BUN/SCr, K; **Notes:** Correct volume depletion. Advise patient on S/S angioedema and avoidance of K salt substitutes.

ranitidine (Zantac, Zantac 75) **Uses:** Treatment of duodenal and gastric ulcers; Gastric hypersecretory states (Zollinger-Ellison syndrome); Erosive esophagitis; GERD; Heartburn; acid indigestion, and sour stomach (OTC use); Stress ulcer treatment/prophylaxis in critically ill patients; **Class:** H_2 antagonists; **Preg:** B; **CIs:** Hypersensitivity; Phenylketonuria (effervescent tabs); Acute porphyria; **ADRs:** dizziness, drowsiness, confusion, hallucinations, HA, pancreatitis, anemia, leukopenia, thrombocytopenia, ↑ LFTs, rash; **Interactions:** ↓ absorption of ketoconazole and itraconazole; Antacids and sucralfate ↓ absorption; Clarithromycin ↑ levels; **Dose:** *PO: Adults:* 75–150 mg daily–qid. *PO: Peds:* 2–10 mg/kg/day divided bid (max: 600 mg/day). *PO: Neonates* 2 mg/kg/day divided q 12 hr. *IV, IM: Adults:* 50 mg q 6–8 hr. *Continuous IV infusion*—1 mg/kg/hr; may ↑ by 0.5 mg/kg/hr (max: 2.5 mg/kg/hr). *IV, IM: Peds:* 2–4 mg/kg/day divided q 6–8 hr (max: 200 mg/day). *Continuous infusion*—1 mg/kg/dose followed by 0.08–0.17 mg/kg/hr. *IV: Neonates:* 1.5 mg/kg/dose, then in 12 hr 1.5–2 mg/kg/day divided q 12 hr. *Continuous IV infusion*—1.5 mg/kg/dose followed by 0.04–0.08 mg/kg/hr. *Renal Impairment PO: Adults:* ↓ dose for CrCl <50 ml/min; **Availability (G):** *Tabs:* 75, 150, 300 mg. *Effervescent tabs:* 25, 150 mg. *Caps:* 150, 300 mg. *Syrup:* 15 mg/ml. *Inject:* 25 mg/ml; **Monitor:** Gastric pH, BUN/SCr, LFTs, CBC, platelets, S/S PUD, and GI bleeding; **Notes:** Give with meals and/or at bedtime. Effervescent tabs contain phenylalanine and should be dissolved in water before taking.

R

ranolazine (Ranexa) **Uses:** Chronic angina pectoris; **Class:** antianginal; **Preg:** C; **CIs:** Hypersensitivity; Patents at risk for QT_C prolongation; Concurrent use with CYP3A4 inhibitors (ketoconazole, verapamil, diltiazem); Hepatic impairment; VT; **ADRs:** dizziness, HA, syncope, palpitations, QT_C prolongation, ↑ SCr, abdominal pain, constipation, dry mouth, peripheral edema, N/V; **Interactions:** ↑ levels of simvastatin; CYP3A4 inhibitors ↑ effects; CYP3A4 inducers ↓ effects; ↑ effects with agents that prolong the QT_C interval; ↑ digoxin levels; **Dose:** *PO: Adults:* 500–1000 mg bid; **Availability:** *ER tabs:* 500 mg;

Monitor: ECG, BP, K, SCr; **Notes:** Hypokalemia may predispose to QT_C interval prolongation. Do not give with grapefruit juice.

rasagiline (Azilect) **Uses:** Parkinson's disease; **Class:** monoamine oxidase type B inhibitors; **Preg:** C; **CIs:** Hypersensitivity; Concurrent meperidine, tramadol, propoxyphene, methadone, sympathomimetic amines, dextromethorphan, mirtazapine, cyclobenzaprine, MAOIs, or St. John's wort; Elective surgery requiring general anesthesia; Pheochromocytoma; **ADRs:** depression, dizziness, hallucinations, ↑ LFTs, vertigo, conjunctivitis, rhinitis, asthma, CP, postural hypotension, syncope, anorexia, dizziness, dyspepsia, gastroenteritis, N/V/D, albuminuria, alopecia, ecchymosis, ↑ melanoma risk, rash, wt loss, leukopenia, arthralgia, arthritis, neck pain, dyskinesia, paresthesia, flu-like syndrome; **Interactions:** ciprofloxacin and other CYP1A2 inhibitors ↑ levels; Hypertensive crisis with sympathomimetic amines, amphetamines, MAOIs, cold products, and products containing pseudoephedrine, phenylephrine, or ephedrine; CNS toxicity is ↑ with TCAs, SSRIs, SNRIs, and other MAOIs; **Dose:** *PO: Adults: Monotherapy*—1 mg/day. *Adjunct therapy*—0.5 mg/day, may ↑ to 1 mg/day. *Concurrent CYP1A2 inhibitors*—0.5 mg/day. *Hepatic Impairment PO: Adults: Mild hepatic impairment*—0.5 mg daily; **Availability:** *Tabs:* 0.5, 1 mg; **Monitor:** BP, S/S Parkinson's disease, mood, behavior, LFTs; **Notes:** Avoid tyramine-rich foods/beverages (may precipitate a hypertensive crisis).

repaglinide (Prandin) **Uses:** Type 2 DM; **Class:** meglitinides; **Preg:** C; **CIs:** Hypersensitivity; DKA; Type 1 DM; Concurrent use of gemfibrozil; **ADRs:** HA, angina, CP, diarrhea, ↓ BG; **Interactions:** CYP2C8 inhibitors and CYP3A4 inhibitors may ↑ levels/↑ risk of hypoglycemia (concurrent use of gemfibrozil should be avoided); CYP2C8 inducers and CYP3A4 inducers may ↓ levels/effects; Beta blockers may mask hypoglycemia; Alcohol, antidiabetic agents, NSAIDs, MAOIs, and nonselective beta blockers may ↑ risk of hypoglycemia; Diuretics, corticosteroids, thyroid supplements, or sympathomimetics may ↓ effects; **Dose:** *PO: Adults: A1C <8% or not previously treated*—0.5 mg tid ac. *Previously treated and A1C ≥8%*—1–2 mg tid ac (max: 16 mg/day). *Renal Impairment PO: Adults:* ↓ dose if CrCl ≤40 ml/min; **Availability:** *Tabs:* 0.5, 1, 2 mg; **Monitor:** A1C, glucose, wt, LFTs, S/S hypoglycemia; **Notes:** Give 15–30 min ac; skip doses if NPO.

R

reteplase (Retavase) **Uses:** Acute MI; **Class:** plasminogen activators; **Preg:** C; **CIs:** Active bleeding; History of CVA; Recent (within 2 mo) intracranial or intraspinal injury/trauma; Intracranial neoplasm, AVM, or aneurysm; Severe uncontrolled HTN; Hypersensitivity; Recent (within 10 days) major surgery, trauma, GI/GU bleeding; Concurrent anticoagulant therapy; **ADRs:** INTRACRANIAL HEMORRHAGE, reperfusion arrhythmias, ↓ BP, BLEEDING, N/V, flushing, urticaria, allerigic reactions including ANAPHYLAXIS; **Interactions:** Aspirin, clopidogrel, ticlopidine, dipyridamole, NSAIDs, GP IIb/IIIa inhibitors, warfarin, heparin, and LMWHs ↑ risk of bleeding; **Dose:** *IV: Adults:* 10 units, followed 30 min later by an additional 10 units; **Availability:** *Inject:* 10.4 units (18.1 mg)/vial; **Monitor:** BP, HR, RR, ECG, cardiac enzymes, CBC, aPTT, INR, CP, bleeding, neurologic status; **Notes:** If local bleeding occurs, apply pressure to site. If severe or internal bleeding occurs, discontinue.

Rh_o (D) immune globulin (HyperRHO S/D Full Dose, RhoGAM, HyperRHO S/D Mini-Dose, MICRhoGAM, WinRho SDF, Rhophylac) **Uses: IM, IV:** Administered to Rh_o (D)-negative patients who have been exposed to Rh_o (D)-positive blood by: Pregnancy or delivery of a Rh_o (D)-positive infant, Abortion of a Rh_o (D)-positive fetus, Fetal-maternal hemorrhage while carrying a Rh_o (D)-positive fetus, Transfusion of Rh_o (D)-positive blood or blood products to a Rh_o (D)-negative patient. **IV:** Management of ITP; **Class:** immune globulins; **Preg:** C; **CIs:** Prior hypersensitivity reaction to human immune globulin, Prior sensitization to Rh_o(D); **ADRs:** dizziness, HA, HTN, ↓ BP, rash, N/V/D, anemia, intravascular hemolysis, arthralgia, myalgia, pain at inject site, fever; **Interactions:** May ↓ antibody response to some live-virus vaccines (measles, mumps, rubella); **Dose:** *IM: Adults: After delivery (HyperRHO S/D Full Dose, RhoGAM)*—1-vial standard dose (300 mcg) within 72 hr of delivery. *IM: Adults: Prior to delivery (HyperRHO S/D Full Dose, RhoGAM)*—1-vial standard dose (300 mcg) at 26–28 wk. *IM: Adults: Termination of pregnancy (<13 wk gestation) (Hyper RHO S/D Mini-Dose, MICRhoGAM)*—1 vial of microdose (50 mcg) within 72 hr. *IM: Adults: Termination of pregnancy (>13 wk gestation) (RhoGAM)*—1-vial standard dose (300 mcg) within 72 hr. *IM: Adults: Transfusion accident (HyperRHO S/D Full Dose, RhoGAM)*—Volume of Rh-positive blood administered × Hct of donor blood)/15 = number of vials of standard dose (300 mcg) preparation (round to next whole number of vials). *IM, IV: Adults: After delivery (WinRho SDF)*—600 units (120 mcg) within 72 hr of delivery. *Rhophylac*—1500 units (300 mcg) within 72 hr of delivery. *IM, IV: Adults: Prior to delivery (WinRho SDF, Rhophylac)*—1500 units (300 mcg) at 28 wk; if initiated earlier in pregnancy, repeat q 12 wk. *IM, IV: Adults: Following amniocentesis or chorionic villus sampling (WinRho SDF<34 wk gestation)*—1500 units (300 mcg) immediately; repeat q 12 wk during pregnancy. *Rhophylac*—1500 units (300 mcg) within 72 hr of procedure. *IM: Adults: Fetal-Maternal Hemorrhage/Transfusion accident (WinRho SDF)*—6000 units (1200 mcg) q 12 hr until total dose is given (total dose determined by amount of blood loss/hemorrhage). *IV: Adults:* 3000 units (600 mcg) q 8 hr until total dose is given (total dose determined by amount of blood loss/hemorrhage). *IV: Adults and Peds: ITP (WinRho SDF,*

R

Rhophylac)—50 mcg (250 units)/kg initially (if Hgb <10 g/dl, ↓ dose to 25–40 mcg [125–200 units]/kg); further dosing/frequency determined by clinical response (range: 25–60 mcg [125–300 units]/kg). Each dose may be given as a single dose or in 2 divided doses on separate days; **Availability:** Rh_o (D) Immune Globulin (for IM Use) *Inject:* 50 mcg/vial (microdose: MICRhoGAM, HyperRHO S/D Mini-Dose), 300 mcg/vial (standard dose: RhoGAM, HyperRHO S/D Full Dose). Rh_o (D) Immune Globulin Intravenous (for IM or IV Use) *Inject:* 600 units (120 mcg)/vial, 1500 units (300 mcg)/vial, 2500 units (500 mcg)/vial, 5000 units (1000 mcg)/vial, 15,000 units (3000 mcg)/vial. *Prefilled syringes:* 1500 units (300 mcg/2 ml); **Monitor:** S/S intravascular hemolysis or infusion reactions, CBC, platelets, BUN/SCr, LFTs; **Notes:** Do not give to infant, to Rh_o (D)-positive individual, or to Rh_o (D)-negative individual previously sensitized to the Rh[info](D) antigen. IV products may be given IM; IM products may NOT be given IV. Administer IM into the deltoid muscle.

ribavirin (Copegus, Rebetol, Virazole) **Uses: Inhaln:** Treatment of RSV infection; **PO:** *Rebetol*—with interferon alfa-2b or peginterferon alfa-2b in the treatment of chronic hepatitis C; **PO:** *Copegus*—with peginterferon alfa-2a in the treatment of chronic hepatitis C; **Class:** nucleoside analogues; **Preg:** X; **CIs:** Hypersensitivity; **Inhalation:** Patients receiving mechanically assisted ventilation; **Oral:** Pregnancy or lactation; Male partners of pregnant patients; CrCl <50 ml/min; Severe CV disease; Hemoglobinopathies; Autoimmune hepatitis; Anemia; **ADRs:** dizziness, faintness, blurred vision, conjunctivitis, erythema of the eyelids, ocular irritation, photosensitivity, CARDIAC ARREST, ↓ BP, rash, <u>hemolytic anemia</u>, reticulocytosis, emotional lability, fatigue, impaired concentration, insomnia, irritability, dry mouth, dyspnea, anorexia, ↑ LFTs, vomiting, pruritus, arthralgia, fever; **Interactions:** *Oral:* ↓ the antiretroviral action of stavudine and zidovudine; ↑ hematologic toxicity of zidovudine; ↑ levels/toxicity of didanosine; Use with interferon alpha 2b ↑ risk of hemolytic anemia; **Dose:** *Inhaln: (Infants and Young Peds RSV*—6 g/300 ml via continuous aerosol × 12–18 hr/day. *PO: Adults: >75 kg Chronic hepatitis C (Rebetol)*—600 mg in the AM, then 600 mg in the PM for 6 mo. *PO: Adults: ≤75 kg and Peds >61 kg:* 400 mg in the AM, then 600 mg in the PM × 6 mo. *PO: Peds: 50–61 kg:* 400 mg bid. *PO: Peds: 37–49 kg:* 200 mg in the AM and 400 mg in the PM. *PO: Peds: 25–36 kg:* 200 mg bid. *PO: Peds: <25 kg:* 15 mg/kg/day divided bid. *PO: Adults: ≥75 kg Chronic hepatitis C (Copegus)*—600 mg bid × 48 wk. *PO: Adults: <75 kg:* 500 mg bid × 48 wk. *PO: Adults: Coinfection with HIV*—400 mg bid × 48 wk; **Availability:** *Powder for aerosol:* 6 g. *Caps (Rebetol):* 200 mg. *Tabs (Copegus):* 200, 400 mg; **Monitor:** Resp function, BP, culture for RSV, CBC, retic count, LFTs; **Notes:** Ribavirin aerosol should be administered using the Viratek SPAG model SPAG-2 only. Do not crush oral dosage forms.

rifabutin (Mycobutin) Uses: Prevention of disseminated MAC disease; **Class:** antituberculars; **Preg:** B; **CIs:** Hypersensitivity or prior sensitivity to rifamycins; Active TB; WBC <1,000/mm^3 or platelets <50, 000/mm^3; **ADRs:** orange discoloration of body fluids, ocular disturbances, dyspnea, CP, chest pressure, altered taste, ↑ LFTs, rash, skin discoloration, hemolysis, neutropenia, thrombocytopenia, arthralgia, myositis, flu-like syndrome; **Interactions:** ↓ effects of amprenavir, efavirenz, indinavir, nelfinavir, nevirapine, saquinavir, delavirdine, corticosteroids, disopyramide, quinidine, opioid analgesics, oral hypoglycemic agents, warfarin, estrogens, phenytoin, verapamil, fluconazole, quinidine, tocainide, theophylline, zidovudine, and chloramphenicol; Ritonavir and efavirenz ↑ levels nevirapine; **Dose:** *PO: Adults:* 300 mg once daily or 150 mg bid. *Concurrent nelfinavir, amprenavir, indinavir*—150 mg/day. *PO: Peds:* 5 mg/kg/day; **Availability:** *Caps:* 150 mg; **Monitor:** LFTs, CBC, platelets, cultures for TB; **Notes:** May be administered without regard to meals. May discolor contact lenses.

rifampin (Rifadin, Rimactane) Uses: Active TB; Elimination of meningococcal carriers; *H. flu*-type b infection prophylaxis; **Class:** antituberculars; **Preg:** C; **CIs:** Hypersensitivity; Concurrent indinavir, nelfinavir, pyrazinamide, or saquinavir; **ADRs:** ataxia, confusion, drowsiness, fatigue, HA, weakness, abdominal pain, flatulence, ↑ BUN/SCr, N/V/D, ↑ LFTs, hemolytic anemia, thrombocytopenia, arthralgia, myalgia, red discoloration of body fluids, flu-like syndrome; **Interactions:** ↑ hepatotoxicity with hepatotoxic agents, including alcohol, ketoconazole, isoniazid, pyrazinamide; ↓ levels of delavirdine, indinavir, nelfinavir, and saquinavir; ↓ effects of ritonavir, nevirapine, efavirenz, corticosteroids, disopyramide, quinidine, opioid analgesics, oral hypoglycemic agents, warfarin, estrogens, phenytoin, verapamil, fluconazole, ketoconazole, itraconazole, tocainide, theophylline, and chloramphenicol; **Dose:** *PO, IV: Adults: TB*—600 mg/day or 10 mg/kg/day (max: 600 mg/day) or may give 2–3 ×/wk. *PO, IV: Peds:* 10–20 mg/kg/day (max: 600 mg/day) or may give 2–3 ×/week. *PO, IV: Adults: Meningitis prophylaxis*—600 mg q 12 hr × 2 days. *PO, IV: Peds: ≥1 mo Meningococcal meningitis prophylaxis*—10 mg/kg q 12 hr × 2 days. *PO: Infants <1 mo:* 5 mg/kg q 12 hr × 2 days. *PO: Adults: H. flu prophylaxis*—600 mg/day × 4 days. *PO: Peds:* 20 mg/kg/day × 4 days; **Availability (G):** *Caps:* 150, 300 mg. *Inject:* 600 mg; **Monitor:** LFTs, CBC, BUN/SCr, platelets, sputum, cultures for TB; **Notes:** Give on an empty stomach. May discolor contact lenses.

R

risedronate (Actonel) Uses: Treatment and prevention of postmenopausal and corticosteroid-induced osteoporosis; Treatment of osteoporosis in men; Treatment of Paget's disease; **Class:** biphosphonates; **Preg:** C; **CIs:** Esophageal disease (that may delay emptying); Unable to stand or sit upright for ≥30 min; At risk for aspiration; Hypocalcemia; Severe renal insufficiency (CrCl <30 ml/min); **ADRs:** HA, abdominal pain, constipation, dyspepsia, dysphagia, esophagitis, flatulence, gastritis, N/V/D, musculoskeletal pain, osteonecrosis (of jaw); **Interactions:** Antacids, Ca, iron, and Mg ↓ absorption; ↑ risk of GI effects with NSAIDs; Food, coffee, and orange juice ↓ absorption; **Dose:** *PO: Adults: Postmenopausal osteoporosis*—5 mg/day *or* 35 mg 1 ×/wk *or* 75 mg taken on 2 consecutive days 1 ×/mo *or* 150 mg 1 ×/mo. *Osteoporosis in men*—35 mg 1 ×/wk. *Glucocorticoid-induced osteoporosis*—5 mg/day. *Paget's disease*—30 mg/day × 2 mo; retreatment may be considered after 2 mo off therapy; **Availability:** *Tabs:* 5, 30, 35, 75, 150 mg; **Monitor:** BMD, S/S Paget's (bone pain, HA), Ca, alk phos (for Paget's); **Notes:** Take first thing in AM with 6–8 oz plain water ≥30 min before other meds, beverages, or food. Remain upright for ≥30 min after dose and after eating. Ca and vitamin D supplements recommended. Avoid dental procedures during therapy.

risperidone (Risperdal, Risperdal M-TAB, Risperdal Consta) Uses: Schizophrenia; Bipolar mania; Treatment of irritability associated with autistic disorder; **Class:** antipsychotics; **Preg:** C; **CIs:** Hypersensitivity; History of seizures; Suicidal tendency; Dementia-related psychoses; **ADRs:** NMS, aggressive behavior, dizziness, extrapyramidal reactions, HA, insomnia, sedation, tardive dyskinesia, pharyngitis, rhinitis, visual disturbances, cough, orthostatic hypotension, ↑ HR, constipation, dry mouth, N/V/D, abdominal pain, ↑ salivation, ↑ wt, polydipsia, sexual dysfunction, dysmenorrhea/menorrhagia, difficulty urinating, polyuria, itching/skin rash, ↑ pigmentation, sweating, photosensitivity, seborrhea, galactorrhea, hyperglycemia, arthralgia, ↑ cholesterol/TGs; **Interactions:** ↓ effects of levodopa or other dopamine agonists; Carbamazepine, phenytoin, rifampin, phenobarbital, and other enzyme inducers ↓ effects; Fluoxetine, clozapine, and paroxetine ↑ effects; ↑ CNS depression with CNS depressants, alcohol, antihistamines, sedative/hypnotics, or opioid analgesics; **Dose:** *PO: Adults: Schizophrenia*—1 mg bid, ↑ by 2 mg/day q 24 hr to 4–8 mg/day. *PO: Peds: 13–17 yr:* 0.5 mg daily–bid, then ↑ q 24 hr to 2–6 mg/day. *IM: Adults:* 25–50 mg q 2 wk. *PO: Adults: Bipolar disorder*—2–3 mg/day, may ↑ by 1 mg/day to 6 mg/day. *PO: Peds: 13–17 yr:* 0.5–3 mg once daily. *PO: Geriatric Patients:* 0.5 mg bid; ↑ by 0.5 mg bid, up to 1.5 mg bid. *PO: Peds: 5–16 yr: <20 kg: Autism*—0.25 mg/day then ↑ to 0.5 mg/day after 4 days. *PO: Peds: 5–16 yr: >20 kg* 0.5 mg/day then ↑ to 1 mg/day after 4 days. *Renal Impairment/Hepatic Impairment PO: Adults:* 0.5 mg bid; **Availability:** *Tabs:* 0.25, 0.5, 1, 2, 3, 4 mg. *ODT (Risperdal M-Tabs):* 0.5, 1, 2, 3, 4 mg. *Oral soln:* 1 mg/ml. *Inject:* 12.5, 25, 37.5, 50 mg; **Monitor:** Mental status, BP, HR, glucose, cholesterol, TGs, CBC, wt, S/S extrapyramidal effects; **Notes:** Do not mix oral soln with cola or tea; may give without regard to meals. Give IM intragluteally.

ritonavir (Norvir) Uses: HIV infection; **Class:** protease inhibitors; **Preg:** B; **CIs:** Hypersensitivity; Concurrent use of alfuzosin, amiodarone, ergot derivatives, flecainide, midazolam, pimozide, propafenone, quinidine, triazolam, or voriconazole; **ADRs:** weakness, dizziness, pharyngitis, ANGIOEDEMA, orthostatic hypotension, abdominal pain, altered taste, anorexia, N/V/D, ↑ LFTs, ↑ BUN/SCr, rash, ↓ WBC, urticaria, ↑ uric acid, ↑ cholesterol/TGs, ↑ CK, myalgia, paresthesias, fever; **Interactions:** ↑ levels/effects of bupropion, clozapine, fluticasone (inhalation), meperidine, piroxicam, propoxyphene, and rifabutin; ↑ sedation and/or resp depression from BZs and zolpidem; ↑ levels/effects of alfentanil, fentanyl, hydrocodone, oxycodone, tramadol, diclofenac, ibuprofen, indomethacin, disopyramide, lidocaine, mexiletine, clarithromycin, erythromycin, amitriptyline, clomipramine, desipramine, imipramine, nortriptyline, nefazodone, sertraline, trazodone, fluoxetine, paroxetine, venlafaxine, dronabinol, ondansetron, metoprolol, pindolol, propranolol, timolol, Ca channel blockers, etoposides, paclitaxel, tamoxifen, vinblastine, vincristine, dexamethasone, prednisone, HMG CoA reductase inhibitors, cyclosporine, tacrolimus, chlorpromazine, haloperidol, perphenazine, risperidone, thioridazine, saquinavir, methamphetamine, and warfarin. Dosage ↓ may be necessary; ↓ levels/effects of hormonal contraceptives, zidovudine, and theophylline. Dose adjustment may be necessary; Levels ↑ by clarithromycin or fluoxetine; **Dose:** *PO: Adults:* 300 mg bid × 1 day, then 400 mg bid × 3 days, then 500 mg bid × 1 day, then 600 mg bid as maintenance. *PO: Peds:* 250 mg/m^2 bid; then ↑ by 50 mg/m^2 bid q 2–3 days up to 400 mg/m^2 bid; **Availability:** *Caps:* 100 mg. *Oral soln:* 80 mg/ml; **Monitor:** Viral load, CD4 count, CBC, LFTs, cholesterol, TGs, CK, uric acid, glucose; **Notes:** Give with food. May be used as a pharmacokinetic booster for other protease inhibitors at doses of 100–400 mg/day.

rituximab (Rituxan) **Uses:** Treatment of CD20–positive, B-cell non-Hodgkin's lymphoma; RA; **Class:** monoclonal antibodies; **Preg:** C; **CIs:** Hypersensitivity to mouse proteins; **ADRs:** HA, bronchospasm, cough, dyspnea, ARRHYTHMIAS, ↓ BP, peripheral edema, abdominal pain, altered taste, dyspepsia, flushing, urticaria, hyperglycemia, ↓ Ca, ANEMIA, NEUTROPENIA, THROMBOCYTOPENIA, arthralgia, back pain, ANAPHYLAXIS and ANGIOEDEMA, infections, INFUSION REACTIONS, TUMOR LYSIS SYNDROME, fever/chills/rigors; **Interactions:** Antihypertensives may cause additive hypotension; Do not give with live-virus vaccines; **Dose:** *IV: Adults: non-Hodgkin's lymphoma*—375 mg/m^2 once weekly × 4–8 doses. *IV: Adults: RA*—2 doses of 1000 mg on Days 1 and 15; **Availability:** *Inject:* 10 mg/ml; **Monitor:** BP, HR, RR, CBC, platelets, CD20 cells, BUN/SCr, LFTs, S/S infusion reactions and tumor lysis; **Notes:** Give at an initial rate of 50 mg/hr; if tolerated, rate may ↑ by 50 mg/hr q 30 min to a max of 400 mg/hr. Premedication with IV methylprednisolone may ↓ risk of infusion reactions.

rivastigmine (Exelon, Exelon Patch) **Uses:** Treatment of mild-to-moderate dementia from AD and Parkinson's disease; **Class:** cholinergics; **Preg:** B; **CIs:** Hypersensitivity to rivastigmine or other

R

carbamates; Sick sinus syndrome or other supraventricular cardiac conduction abnormalities; **ADRs:** weakness, dizziness, drowsiness, HA, sedation, edema, HF, hypotension, anorexia, dyspepsia, N/V/D, abdominal pain, flatulence, tremor, fever, wt loss; **Interactions:** Nicotine ↑ metabolism/↓ levels; **Dose:** *PO: Adults:* 1.5 mg bid; after 2 wk, may ↑ to 3 mg bid, up to 6 mg bid. *Transdermal: Adults:* 4.6 mg/24 hr; after 4 wk may ↑ to 9.5 mg/24 hr; **Availability:** *Caps:* 1.5, 3, 4.5, 6 mg. *Oral soln:* 2 mg/ml. *Transdermal patch:* 4.6 mg/24 hr, 9.5 mg/24 hr; **Monitor:** Cognitive function, S/S GI distress, wt; **Notes:** Apply patch to clean, dry, hairless skin (upper or lower back, arm, or chest). When switching from PO doses of <6 mg to patch, use 4.6 mg/24 hr; for PO doses >6 mg, use 9.5 mg/24 hr patch.

rizatriptan (Maxalt, Maxalt-MLT) **Uses:** Acute treatment of migraines; **Class:** 5-HT_1 agonists; **Preg:** C; **CIs:** Hypersensitivity; CAD or significant CV disease; Uncontrolled HTN; Use of other 5-HT_1 agonists or ergot-type drugs (dihydroergotamine) within 24 hr; Basilar or hemiplegic migraine; Concurrent or recent (within 2 wk) use of an MAOI; CV risk factors (use only if CV status has been determined to be safe and 1st dose is administered under supervision); **ADRs:** dizziness, drowsiness, CORONARY ARTERY VASOSPASM, MI/ISCHEMIA, VT/VF, nausea; **Interactions:** MAOIs ↑ levels (concurrent or recent [within 2 wk] use contraindicated); Use with other 5-HT_1 agonists or ergot-type compounds may ↑ risk of vasospasm (avoid use within 24 hr of each other); Use with SSRIs or SNRIs may ↑ risk of serotonin syndrome; Propranolol ↑ levels; **Dose:** *PO: Adults:* 5–10 mg initially, may repeat in 2 hr (not to exceed 30 mg in 24 hr) (use 5-mg dose if receiving propranolol; max: 15 mg/24 hr); **Availability:** *Tabs:* 5, 10 mg. *ODT:* 5, 10 mg; **Monitor:** BP, HR, HA pain; **Notes:** ODTs contain phenylalanine. For acute treatment only, not for prophylaxis; give as soon as migraine symptoms occur.

ropinirole (Requip) **Uses:** Parkinson's disease; Restless legs syndrome; **Class:** dopamine agonists; **Preg:** C; **CIs:** Hypersensitivity; Patients at risk for hypotension; **ADRs:** DAYTIME SOMNOLENCE, dizziness, syncope, confusion, hallucinations, HA, dyskinesia, weakness, abnormal vision, orthostatic hypotension, peripheral edema, constipation, dry mouth, dyspepsia, N/V, sweating; **Interactions:** Effects ↑ by estrogens, quinolones, ketoconazole, and fluvoxamine; Effects ↓ by phenothiazines, butyrophenones, thioxanthenes, or metoclopramide; ↑ effects of levodopa; **Dose:** *PO: Adults: Parkinson's disease*—0.25 mg tid × 1 wk, then 0.5 mg tid × 1 wk, then 0.75 mg tid × 1 wk, then 1 mg tid × 1 wk; then ↑ by 1.5 mg/day q wk, up to 9 mg/day; then ↑ by 3 mg/day q wk up to 24 mg/day. *Restless legs syndrome*—0.25 mg/day, 1 to 3 hr before bedtime × 2 days, then ↑ to 0.5–1 mg/day by the end of 1st wk, then ↑ by 0.5 mg q wk, up to 4 mg/day; **Availability:** *Tabs:* 0.25, 0.5, 1, 2, 3, 4,

5 mg; **Monitor:** BP, daytime alertness, S/S Parkinson's disease; **Notes:** Daytime sleepiness may occur without warning.

ropivacaine (Naropin) Uses: Local or regional anesthesia for surgery; Postoperative pain management; **Class:** local anesthetic; **Preg:** B; **CIs:** Prior sensitivity to other amide local anesthetics; **ADRs:** dizziness, HA, rigors, ↓ HR, CP, ↑ BP, ↓ BP, ↑ HR, N/V, urinary retention, pruritus, ↓ K, anemia, paresthesia, dyspnea; **Interactions:** ↑ toxicity with other amide local anesthetics; Fluvoxamine, amiodarone, ciprofloxacin, and propofol ↑ effects; **Dose:** *Epidural: Adults: Lumbar epidural*—15–30 ml of 0.5%–1% soln. *Lumbar epidural for cesarean section*—20–30 ml of 0.5% soln or 15–20 ml of 0.75% soln. *Thoracic epidural*—5–15 ml of 0.5–0.75% soln. *Major nerve block: Adults:* 35–50 ml of 0.5% soln or 10–40 ml of 0.75% soln. *Field block: Adults:* 1–40 ml of 0.5% soln. *Epidural: Adults: Lumbar epidural*—10–20 ml of 0.2% soln, then continuous infusion of 6–14 ml/hr of 0.2% soln with incremental inject of 10–15 ml/hr of 0.2% soln. *Epidural: Adults: Lumbar or thoracic epidural*—Continuous infusion of 6–14 ml/hr of 0.2% soln. *Infiltration (minor nerve block): Adults:* 1–100 ml of 0.2% soln or 1–40 ml of 0.5% soln; **Availability:** *Inject (preservative-free):* 0.2%, 0.5%, 0.75%, 1%; **Monitor:** HR, BP, ECG, loss of sensation; **Notes:** Assess patient for systemic toxicity and for return of sensation after procedure.

rosiglitazone (Avandia) Uses: NIDDM; **Class:** thiazolidinediones; **Preg:** C; **CIs:** Hypersensitivity; Jaundice from previous troglitazone therapy; Active liver disease; **ADRs:** HF, edema, macular edema, urticaria, ↑ LFTs, anemia, LACTIC ACIDOSIS, ↑ total cholesterol, LDL, and HDL, ↑ wt fractures (arm, hand, foot) in females; **Interactions:** Gemfibrozil ↑ levels/risk of hypoglycemia; CYP2C8 inducers ↓ levels; CYP2C8 inhibitors ↑ levels; **Dose:** *PO: Adults:* 4 mg once daily or 2 mg bid; after 8 wk, may ↑ to 8 mg once daily or 4 mg bid; **Availability:** *Tabs:* 2, 4, 8 mg; **Monitor:** A1C, serum glucose, LFTs, cholesterol, lipid profile, fluid status, S/S HF and hypoglycemia; **Notes:** May be given without regard to meals. Do not use if LFTs >2.5 × ULN.

R

rosuvastatin (Crestor) Uses: Hypercholesterolemia; **Class:** HMG-CoA reductase inhibitors; **Preg:** X; **CIs:** Hypersensitivity; Liver disease, Pregnancy/lactation; **ADRs:** HA, abdominal cramps, constipation, diarrhea, dyspepsia, flatulence, ↑ LFTs, nausea, rash, RHABDOMYOLYSIS, myalgia; **Interactions:** ↑ risk of myopathy with cyclosporine, gemfibrozil, erythromycin, clarithromycin, protease inhibitors, niacin (≥1 g/day), and azole antifungals; May ↑ effects of warfarin; **Dose:** *PO: Adults:* 5–40 mg/day. *Patients with Asian ancestry or concurrent cyclosporine therapy*—Max dose: 5 mg/day. *Concurrent gemfibrozil or lopinavir/ritonavir therapy*—Max dose: 10 mg/day. *Renal Impairment PO: Adults:* ↓ dose if CrCl <30 ml/min; **Availability:** *Tabs:* 5, 10, 20, 40 mg; **Monitor:** Lipid panel, LFTs, CK (if symptoms); **Notes:** Instruct patients to avoid grapefruit juice. Patients of Asian descent have ↑ risk of myopathy. Discontinue if LFTs persistently >3 × ULN.

salmeterol (Serevent) **Uses:** Asthma; COPD; **Class:** adrenergics; **Preg:** C; **CIs:** Prior sensitivity to salmeterol or other adrenergic amines; Acute relief of bronchospasm; CV disease; **ADRs:** HA, nervousness, palpitations, ↑ HR, abdominal pain, diarrhea, nausea, muscle cramps/soreness, trembling, paradoxical bronchospasm, cough; **Interactions:** Beta blockers may ↓ effects; MAOIs and TCAs ↑ CV effects; **Dose:** *Inhaln: Adults and Peds: ≥4 yr:* 50 mcg (1 inhaln) bid. *Exercise-induced bronchospasm*—50 mcg (1 inhaln) 30–60 min before exercise. **Availability:** *Powder for inhaln (Diskus):* 50 mcg/blister; **Monitor:** Peak flow, PFTs, BP, HR, serum glucose, K; **Notes:** Not for acute relief of bronchospasm. Discard blister pack 6 wk after foil is removed.

saquinavir (Invirase) **Uses:** HIV infection; **Class:** protease inhibitors; **Preg:** B; **CIs:** Hypersensitivity; Concurrent use with amiodarone, ergot derivatives, flecainide, midazolam, pimozide, propafenaone, quinidine, rifampin, and triazolam; Severe hepatic impairment; **ADRs:** SEIZURES, confusion, HA, mental depression, psychic disorders, weakness, thrombophlebitis, abdominal discomfort, N/V/D, ↑ LFTs, jaundice, photosensitivity, severe cutaneous reactions, hyperglycemia, acute myeloblastic leukemia, hemolytic anemia, thrombocytopenia, ataxia, SJS; **Interactions:** Lovastatine and simvastatin ↑ risk of myopathy; Clarithromycin ↑ saquinavir levels and ↓ clarithromycin levels; Levels ↑ by indinavir, delavirdine, nelfinavir, ritonavir, PPIs, and ketoconazole; Carbamazepine, phenobarbital, phenytoin, nevirapine, and dexamethasone may ↓ levels; May ↑ serum trazodone levels; Grapefruit juice ↑ levels/effects; **Dose:** *PO: Adults:* 600 mg tid or 1000 mg bid; **Availability:** *Caps:* 200 mg. *Tabs:* 500 mg; **Monitor:** Viral load, CD4 count, glucose, CBC, LFTs, S/S opportunistic infections; **Notes:** Give within 2 hrs of a meal. Instruct patient to avoid direct sunlight and to use sunscreen.

scopolamine (Isopto Hyoscine, Transderm-Scop) **Uses:** **Transdermal:** Motion sickness; N/V; *IM: IV: Subcut:* Preop to produce amnesia and ↓ salivary and respiratory secretions; **Class:** anticholinergics; **Preg:** C; **CIs:** Hypersensitivity; Narrow-angle glaucoma; Acute hemorrhage; Thyrotoxicosis; Paralytic ileus; GI/GU obstruction; Tachycardia from cardiac insufficiency; Myasthenia gravis; **ADRs:** drowsiness, confusion, blurred vision, mydriasis, photophobia, ↑ HR, dry mouth, constipation, urinary hesitancy, urinary retention, decreased sweating; **Interactions:** ↑ anticholinergic effects with antihistamines, antidepressants, quinidine, or disopyramide; ↑ CNS depression with alcohol, antidepressants, antihistamines, opioid analgesics, or sedative/hypnotics; ↑ GI mucosal lesions with wax-matrix oral KCl preparations; **Dose:** *Transdermal: Adults: Motion sickness:* 1.5 mg patch q 72 hr; *Recovery from anesthesia/surgery*—1.5 mg patch evening before surgery or 1 hr prior to C-section. *IM: IV: Subcut:*

Adults: Antiemetic/anticholinergic—0.3–0.6 mg; *Antisecretory*—0.2–0.6 mg; *Amnestic*—0.32–0.65 mg; *Sedation*—0.6 mg tid-qid. *IM, IV, Subcut: Peds: Antiemetic/anticholinergic*—6 mcg/kg (max 0.3 mg/dose). *IM: Peds: 8–12 yr Antisecretory*—0.3 mg. *IM: Peds: 3–8 yr Antisecretory*—0.2 mg. *IM: Peds: 7 mo–3 yr Antisecretory*—0.15 mg. *IM: Peds: 4–7 mo Antisecretory*—0.1 mg; **Availability (G):** *Transdermal patch:* 1.5 mg (releases 1 mg scopolamine over 3 days). *Inject:* 0.4 mg/ml; **Monitor:** S/S anticholinergic effects, relief of N/V; **Notes:** Apply patch at least 4 hr before travel to prevent motion sickness.

selegiline (Eldepryl, Emsam, Zelapar) **Uses:** **PO:** Parkinson's disease; **Transdermal:** Major depressive disorder; **Class:** monoamine oxidase type b inhibitors; **Preg:** C; **CIs:** Hypersensitivity; Concurrent dextromethorphan, MAOIs, tramadol, bupropion, SSRIs, SNRIs, TCAs, sympathomimetics, St. John's wort, mirtazapine, cyclobenzaprine, carbamazepine, oxcarbazepine, or opioid analgesic therapy; Pheochromocytoma; Foods high in tyramine; **ADRs:** abnormal thinking, confusion, dizziness, hallucinations, HA, insomnia, CP, orthostatic hypotension, nausea, abdominal pain, dry mouth; **Interactions:** Concurrent therapy with SSRIs, SNRIs, TCAs, carbamazepine, oxcarbazepine, bupropion, meperidine, tramadol, methadone, propoxyphene, dextromethorphan, mirtazapine, cyclobenzaprine, sympathomimetics, St. John's wort, or other MAOIs may ↑ risk of hypertensive crisis (contraindicated), ↑ risk of side effects from levodopa/carbidopa (may need to ↓ dosage of levodopa/carbidopa by 10–30%); **Dose:** *PO: Adults:* 5 mg bid or 2.5 mg qid; *ODT*—1.25 mg/day × 6 wk, may ↑ to 2.5 mg/day. *Transdermal: Adults:* 6 mg/24 hr daily, may ↑ q 2 wk by 3 mg, up to 12 mg/24 hr; **Availability (G):** *Caps:* 5 mg. *Tabs:* 5 mg. *ODT:* 1.25 mg. *Transdermal patch:* 6 mg/24 hr, 9 mg/24 hr, 12 mg/24 hr; **Monitor:** Mental status, mood, S/S Parkinson's disease, BP; **Notes:** Instruct patient to avoid tyramine-containing foods.

S

sertraline (Zoloft) **Uses:** Major Depressive Disorder; Panic disorder; OCD; PTSD; SAD; PMDD; **Class:** SSRIs; **Preg:** C; **CIs:** Hypersensitivity; Concurrent MAOI therapy; Concurrent pimozide; **ADRs:** drowsiness, fatigue, insomnia, SUICIDAL THOUGHTS, agitation, anxiety, HA, yawning, tinnitus, visual abnormalities, CP, ↑ HR, dry mouth, N/V/D, abdominal pain, altered taste, anorexia, constipation, flatulence, ↑ appetite, ↓ libido, menstrual disorders, ↑ wt, sweating, rash, back pain, myalgia, tremor, hypertonia, paresthesia; **Interactions:** MAOIs should be spaced at least 14 days from sertraline therapy; ↑ pimozide levels/risk of CV toxicity; ↑ sensitivity to adrenergics and ↑ risk of serotonin syndrome; May ↑ levels/effects of warfarin, phenytoin, TCAs, alprazolam, cloazapine, or tolbutamide; Cimetidine ↑ levels and effects; **Dose:** *PO: Adults: Depression/OCD*—50–200 mg/day. *PO: Peds: 13–17 yr OCD*—50 mg once daily (max: 200 mg/day). *PO: Peds: 6–12 yr*

OCD—25 mg once daily (max: 200 mg/day). *PO: Adults: Panic disorder/PTSD*—25 mg once daily × 1 wk, then 50 mg/day; then may ↑ q wk to 200 mg/day. *PO: Adults: PMDD*—50 mg daily or daily during luteal phase of cycle. May be titrated in 50-mg increments at the beginning of a cycle. In luteal-phase-only dosing, a 50-mg/day titration step for 3 days at the beginning of each luteal-phase dosing period should be used (range: 50–150 mg/day); **Availability (G):** *Tabs:* 25, 50, 100 mg. *Oral concentrate:* 20 mg/ml; **Monitor:** Mental status, suicidal thoughts/behaviors, wt; **Notes:** Do not confuse sertraline with selegiline. Instruct patient to avoid alcohol.

sevelamer (Renagel) **Uses:** Hyperphosphatemia w/ESRD; **Class:** Phosphate binders; **Preg:** C; **CIs:** Hypophosphatemia; Bowel obstruction; **ADRs:** N/V/D, dyspepsia, constipation, flatulence; **Interactions:** ↓ absorption of anticonvulsants or antiarrhythmics; give 1 hr before or 3 hr after; ↓ bioavailability of ciprofloxacin by 50%; **Dose:** *PO: Adults:* 800–1600 mg with each meal; **Availability:** *Tabs:* 400, 800 mg; **Monitor:** Serum phosphorous, Ca, bicarbonate, chloride; **Notes:** Give with food.

sibutramine (Meridia) **Uses:** Treatment of obesity (BMI ≥30 kg/m^2 or ≥27 kg/m^2 in patients with other risk factors); **Class:** appetite suppressants; **Preg:** C; **CIs:** Hypersensitivity; Anorexia or bulimia nervosa; Concurrent use of appetite suppressants or MAOIs within 2 weeks; Uncontrolled HTN; CAD, HF, arrhythmias, or stroke; **ADRs:** SEIZURES, HA, insomnia, dizziness, drowsiness, emotional lability, pharyngitis, rhinitis, sinusitis, ↑ BP, ↑ HR, vasodilation, anorexia, constipation, dry mouth, altered taste, dyspepsia, ↑ appetite, nausea, ↑ LFTs, sweating, rash; **Interactions:** Concurrent use of centrally acting appetite suppressants, MAOIs, SSRIs, serotonin agonists, ergot derivatives, dextromethorphan, meperidine, pentazocine, fentanyl, lithium, or tryptophan may result in serotonin syndrome; Concurrent use of decongestants ↑ risk of HTN; CYP3A4 inhibitors ↑ effects; ↑ levels of TCAs; CYP3A4 inducers ↓ effects; **Dose:** *PO: Adults:* 5–10 mg once daily; may ↑ to 15 mg/day after 4 wk; **Availability:** *Caps:* 5, 10, 15 mg; **Monitor:** Wt, BMI, BP, HR; **Notes:** Increases in BP or HR may require dose ↓ or discontinuation.

S

sildenafil (Revatio, Viagra) **Uses:** ED (Viagra); Pulmonary HTN (Revatio); **Class:** PDE-5 inhibitors; **Preg:** B; **CIs:** Hypersensitivity; Concurrent use of nitrates; Uncontrolled HTN (BP >170/110 mmHg), hypotension (BP <90/50 mmHg), angina during intercourse, HF, or CAD; Life-threatening arrhythmias, stroke, or MI within 6 mo; **ADRs:** HA, hearing loss, nasal congestion, abnormal vision, ↓ BP, dyspepsia, priapism, flushing, back pain, myalgia; **Interactions:** CYP3A4 inhibitors may ↑ levels/toxicity; CYP3A4 inducers may ↓ levels/effects; Nitrates and alpha-adrenergic blockers may cause serious, life-threatening hypotension; **Dose:** *PO: Adults: ED (Viagra)*—25–50 mg taken 30 min–4 hr before sexual activity (should not be given more than once daily) (max: 100 mg/dose). *Pulmonary arterial HTN*—20 mg tid. *Concurrent use of alpha-blockers (with Viagra)*—Initial dose: 25 mg. *Concurrent use of erythromycin, itraconazole, ketoconazole, or saquinavir (with Viagra)*—Initial dose: 25 mg. *Concurrent use of ritonavir (with Viagra)*—Max dose of 25 mg q 48 hr. *PO: Peds: ≥1 mo Pulmonary arterial HTN*—0.25–0.5 mg/kg q 4–6 hr; may ↑ up to 2 mg/kg/dose. *Renal Impairment PO: Adults:* Initial dose of 25 mg if CrCl <30 ml/min (for Viagra); **Availability:** *Tabs (Viagra):* 25, 50, 100 mg. *Tabs (Revatio):* 20 mg; **Monitor:** Response, exercise tolerance, ADRs; **Notes:** Give without regard to meals. Patients should be on stable dose of alpha-blocker therapy before starting therapy with sildenafil.

simethicone (Gas-X, Mylicon) **Uses:** Gas pain relief; **Class:** Antiflatulent; **Preg:** UK; **CIs:** Abdominal pain of unknown cause; **ADRs:** None; **Interactions:** None; **Dose:** *PO: Adults:* 40–125 mg qid (max: 500 mg/day). *PO: Peds:* 20–40 mg qid (max: 240 mg/day); **Availability (G):** *Chew tabs:* 80 mg^{OTC}, 125 mg^{OTC}. *Softgels:* 125 mg^{OTC}, 180 mg^{OTC}. *Gtt:* 40 mg/0.6 ml^{OTC}; **Monitor:** Relief of gas pain symptoms; **Notes:** Give with meals and at bedtime.

simvastatin (Zocor) **Uses:** Hyperlipidemia; Secondary prevention of CV disease; **Class:** HMG-CoA reductase inhibitors; **Preg:** X; **CIs:** Hypersensitivity; Liver disease; Pregnancy/lactation; **ADRs:** HA, abdominal cramps, constipation, diarrhea, dyspepsia, flatulence, ↑ LFTs, nausea, rash, RHABDOMYOLYSIS, myalgia; **Interactions:** CYP3A4 inhibitors may ↑ levels/toxicity; CYP3A4 inducers may ↓ levels/effects; ↑ risk of myopathy with amiodarone, cyclosporine, gemfibrozil, erythromycin, clarithromycin, protease inhibitors, nefazodone, niacin (≥1 g/day), verapamil, and azole antifungals; May ↑ effects of warfarin; **Dose:** *PO: Adults:* 5–80 mg/day in the evening. *Dosing with concomitant meds*—5–10 mg/day if on cyclosporine or danazol; max dose of 10 mg/day with gemfibrozil; max dose of 20 mg/day with amiodarone or verapamil. *PO: Peds: ≥10 yr:* 10–40 mg/day; **Availability (G):** *Tabs:* 5, 10, 20, 40, 80 mg; **Monitor:** Lipid panel, LFTs, CK (if symptoms); **Notes:** Discontinue if LFTs persistently >3× ULN. Instruct patient to avoid grapefruit juice.

sirolimus (Rapamune) **Uses:** Prevention of organ rejection in kidney transplantation; **Class:** immunosuppressants; **Preg:** C; **CIs:** Hypersensitivity; Liver/lung transplant patients (use not recommended); **ADRs:** insomnia, interstitial lung disease, edema, ↓ BP, ↑ LFTs, ↑ BUN/SCr, acne, rash, thrombocytopenic purpura, ↓ K, leukopenia, thrombocytopenia, anemia, hyperlipidemia, arthralgias, tremor, ↑ infection risk, ↑ lymphoma risk, ↓ wound healing, lymphocele; **Interactions:** Cyclosporine ↑ levels (give 4 hr after cyclosporine); CYP3A4 inhibitors

S

↑ levels/risk of toxicity; CYP3A4 inducers ↓ levels; Risk of renal impairment ↑ with nephrotoxic agents; Concurrent use with tacrolimus and corticosteroids in liver transplantation ↑ risk of hepatic artery thrombosis and ↑ risk of anastamotic dehiscence in lung transplantation; ↓ response to live-virus vaccines; **Dose:** *PO: Adults and Peds: ≥13 yr and >40 kg:* 6 mg LD, then 2 mg/day MD. *PO: Adults and Peds: ≥13 yr and <40 kg:* 3 mg/m^2 LD, followed by 1 mg/m^2/day MD. *Dosing following cyclosporine withdrawal*—Sirolimus dose should be titrated to maintain a blood trough level of 12–14 ng/ml; changes can be made at 7–14 day intervals. Sirolimus MD = current dose × (target concentration/current concentration). If needed, a LD may be calculated by: sirolimus LD = 3 × (new MD − current MD). LDs >40 mg should be given over 2 days. *Hepatic Impairment PO: Adults and Peds: ≥13 yr and <40 kg:* ↓ MD by 33%; LD is unchanged; **Availability:** *Tabs:* 1, 2 mg. *Oral soln:* 1 mg/ml; **Monitor:** Sirolimus levels, BUN/SCr, LFTs, CBC, K, cholesterol, TGs, BP; **Notes:** Instruct patient to avoid grapefruit juice; solution may be diluted with water or orange juice only.

sitagliptin (Januvia) Uses: NIDDM; **Class:** antidiabetics; **Preg:** B; **CIs:** Type 1 DM; DKA; Hypersensitivity; **ADRs:** HA, nausea, diarrhea, upper resp tract infection, nasopharyngitis, rash, hypoglycemia; **Interactions:** ↑ digoxin levels; **Dose:** *PO: Adults:* 100 mg once daily. *Renal Impairment PO: Adults:* ↓ dose for CrCl <50 ml/min; **Availability:** *Tabs:* 25, 50, 100 mg; **Monitor:** A1C, glucose, BUN/SCr, S/S hypoglycemia; **Notes:** May give without regard to meals.

sodium bicarbonate (Baking Soda) Uses: PO, IV: Metab acidosis; Urinary alkalinization; Hyperkalemia; **PO:** Antacid; **Class:** alkalinizing agents; **Preg:** C; **CIs:** Metab or resp alkalosis; Hypocalcemia; Hypernatremia; Severe pulmonary edema; **ADRs:** edema, flatulence, gastric distention, <u>metab alkalosis</u>, ↑ Na, ↓ Ca, ↓ K, water retention, irritation at IV site, tetany; **Interactions:** ↓ absorption of ketoconazole; Ca containing antacids may lead to milk-alkali syndrome; ↑ levels of quinidine, ephedrine, pseudoephedrine, flecainide, or amphetamines; ↓ levels of lithium, chlorpropamide, and salicylates; **Dose:** *PO: Adults: Chronic renal failure*—20–36 mEq/day in divided doses. *Renal tubular acidosis*—0.5–2 mEq/kg/day in divided doses. *Urinary alkalinization*—48 mEq, then 12–24 mEq q 4 hr, titrate to desired urinary pH. *PO: Peds: Chronic renal failure*—1–3 mEq/kg/day. *Renal tubular acidosis*—2–3 mEq/kg/day. *Urinary alkalinization*—1–10 mEq divided q 4–6 hr, titrate to desired urinary pH. *PO: Adults: Antacid*—325 mg–2 g 1–4 times daily. *IV: Adults and Peds: Cardiac arrest*—1 mEq/kg; may repeat 0.5 mEq/kg q 10 min. *Hyperkalemia*—1 mEq/kg over 5 min; **Availability (G):** *Oral powder:* 30 mEq Na/½ tsp^OTC^. *Tabs:* 325 mg (3.8 mEq Na), 650 mg (7.7 mEq Na). *Inject:* 4.2% (0.5 mEq/ml), 7.5% (0.9 mEq/ml), 8.4% (1 mEq/ml); **Monitor:** Electrolytes, acid/base status, fluid status, BUN/SCr, urine pH; **Notes:** May cause premature dissolution of EC tabs in the stomach.

sodium chloride (Slo-Salt) **Uses:** **PO, IV:** Hydration and provision of NaCl in deficiency states; **Class:** electrolyte; **Preg:** C; **CIs:** Fluid retention or hypernatremia; **ADRs:** HF, PULMONARY EDEMA, ↑ Na, hypervolemia, ↓ K, extravasation, irritation at IV site; **Interactions:** May ↓ effects of antihypertensives; Corticosteroids may ↑ Na retention; **Dose:** *IV: Adults: 0.9% NaCl*—1 L (154 mEq Na/L), rate and amount determined by condition. *0.45% NaCl* —1–2 L (77 mEq Na/L), rate and amount determined by condition. *3%, 5% NaCl*—100 ml over 1 hr (3% contains 513 mEq Na/L; 5% contains 855 mEq Na/L). *PO: Adults:* 1–2 g tid. *IV: PO: Peds:* 2–4 mEq/kg/day; **Availability (G):** *IV soln:* 0.45%, 0.9%, 3%, 5%. *Concentrate for dilution:* 14.6%, 23.4%. *Tabs:* 650 mg^{OTC}; **Monitor:** Na, K, Cl, bicarbonate, fluid status; **Notes:** Do not confuse concentrated NaCl (23.4%) with normal saline (0.9%).

sodium citrate and citric acid (Bicitra, Oracit) **Uses:** Management of metab acidosis; Alkalinization of urine; **Class:** alkalinizing agents; **Preg:** C; **CIs:** Severe renal insufficiency; Severe Na restriction; **ADRs:** N/V/D, ↑ K, ↑ Na, metab alkalosis, tetany; **Interactions:** ↓ levels of lithium, chlorpropamide, and salicylates; ↑ levels of quinidine, ephedrine, pseudoephedrine, flecainide, or amphetamines; **Dose:** *PO: Adults:* 10–30 ml qid. *PO: Peds:* 2–3 mEq/kg/day or 5–15 ml qid. *PO: Adults:* 10–30 ml soln diluted in water qid. *PO: Adults:* 15–30 ml soln diluted in 15–30 ml of water; **Availability:** *Oral soln:* 500 mg Na citrate/334 mg citric acid/5 ml (Bicitra), 490 mg Na citrate/640 mg citric acid/5 ml (Oracit); **Monitor:** Electrolytes, urine pH, fluid status, BUN/SCr; **Notes:** Give after meals; dilute doses with 30–90 ml water.

sodium ferric gluconate complex (Ferrlecit) **Uses:** Iron deficiency anemia; **Class:** iron supplements; **Preg:** B; **CIs:** Anemia not due to iron deficiency; Hemochromatosis, hemosiderosis, or other evidence of iron overload; Prior sensitivity to injectable iron; **ADRs:** dizziness, HA, syncope, ↓ <u>BP</u>, CP, N/V/D, <u>flushing</u>, urticaria, pain or erythema at inject, arthralgia, myalgia, allergic reactions including ANAPHYLAXIS, fever, lymphadenopathy; **Interactions:** Chloramphenicol and vitamin E may ↓ response; **Dose:** *IV: Adults:* 125 mg elemental iron repeated during 8 sequential dialysis treatments to a total dose of 1 g; **Availability:** *Inject:* 62.5 mg/5 ml; **Monitor:** CBC, retic count, serum ferritin and iron, S/S anaphylaxis; **Notes:** Give a test dose of 25 mg of elemental iron in 50 ml of NS over 60 min; if tolerated, give full dose over 1 hr. Discontinue PO iron prior to IV therapy.

S

sodium polystyrene sulfonate (Kayexalate, SPS) **Uses:** Hyperkalemia; **Class:** cationic exchange resins; **Preg:** C; **CIs:** Hypersensitivity; Bowel obstruction; Hypokalemia; Hypernatremia; **ADRs:** <u>constipation</u>, <u>fecal impaction</u>, anorexia, gastric irritation, N/V, ↓ Ca, ↓ K, ↑ Na, ↓ Mg; **Interactions:** Ca- or Mg-containing antacids may ↓ effects and

↑ systemic alkalosis; Hypokalemia may ↑ digoxin toxicity; **Dose:** *PO: Adults:* 15–40 g 1–4 × daily. *Rect Adults:* 30–50 g as a retention enema; repeat q 6 hr prn. *PO: Rect Peds:* 1 g/kg/dose q 6 hr; **Availability (G):** *Susp:* 15 g/60 ml. *Powder:* 15 g/4 level tsp; **Monitor:** Electrolytes, ECG; **Notes:** Susp contains sorbitol; for retention enema, add powder to 100 ml of sorbitol or 20% dextrose in water and retain for 30–60 min.

solifenacin (VESIcare) **Uses:** Overactive bladder; **Class:** anticholinergics; **Preg:** C; **CIs:** Hypersensitivity; Urinary retention; Gastric retention; Uncontrolled narrow-angle glaucoma; **ADRs:** blurred vision, constipation, dry mouth, dyspepsia, nausea; **Interactions:** CYP3A4 inhibitors ↑ levels; CYP3A4 inducers ↓ levels; **Dose:** *PO: Adults:* 5–10 mg once daily. *Hepatic impairment/severe renal impairment, concurrent CYP3A4 inhibitors*—5 mg/day; **Availability:** *Tabs:* 5, 10 mg; **Monitor:** Anticholinergic effects; **Notes:** Administer without regard to food. Do not crush tabs.

sotalol (Betapace, Betapace AF, Sorine) **Uses:** Life-threatening ventricular arrhythmias; **Betapace AF:** AF/AFl; **Class:** antiarrhythmics (class III); **Preg:** B; **CIs:** Hypersensitivity; Uncompensated HF; Asthma; Cardiogenic shock; QT_C prolongation; Sinus bradycardia; 2nd- or 3rd-degree AV block (unless pacemaker present); CrCl <40 ml/min (Betapace AF); **ADRs:** fatigue, weakness, dizziness, depression, bronchospasm, wheezing, ARRHYTHMIAS, ↓ HR, HF, QT_C prolongation, N/V/D, ED, itching, rash, paresthesia; **Interactions:** ↑ risk of QT_C prolongation with other QT_C-prolonging drugs; ↑ risk of bradycardia with digoxin, diltiazem, verapamil, or beta blockers; ↑ hypotension with antihypertensives, alcohol, or nitrates; May alter the effectiveness of insulins or oral hypoglycemic agents; **Dose:** *PO: Adults:* 80 mg bid; may ↑ gradually up to 240–320 mg/day (max: 640 mg/day (ventricular arrhythmias); 320 mg/day (AF/AFl). *Renal Impairment PO: Adults:* ↓ dose for CrCl <60 ml/min; Betapace AF contraindicated in CrCl <40 ml/min; **Availability (G):** *Tabs:* 80, 120, 160, 240 mg. *Tabs (Betapace AF):* 80, 120, 160 mg; **Monitor:** BP, HR, RR, ECG, CBC, electrolytes, BUN/SCr, I/Os, wt; **Notes:** Should be initiated in hospital setting.

spironolactone (Aldactone) **Uses:** Primary hyperaldosteronism; Edema associated with HF, cirrhosis, and nephrotic syndrome; HTN; Treatment of hypokalemia (caused by other diuretics); **Class:** potassium-sparing diuretics; **Preg:** C; **CIs:** Hypersensitivity; Anuria; Acute renal insufficiency; Hyperkalemia; **ADRs:** dizziness, HA, ↑ LFTs, N/V/D, edema, ↑ BUN, gynecomastia, rash, deepening of voice, hirsutism, ↑ K, ↓ Na, hyperchloremic metab acidosis, agranulocytosis, muscle cramps; **Interactions:** ↑ hypotension with alcohol, antihypertensive agents, or nitrates; ACEIs, indomethacin, K supplements, ARBs, or cyclosporine ↑ risk of hyperkalemia; ↓ lithium excretion;

Effects ↓ by NSAIDs and salicylates; ↑ effects of digoxin; **Dose:** *PO: Adults:* 25–400 mg/day in 1–2 divided doses. *HF*—12.5–25 mg/day. *PO: Peds: >1 mo Diuretic, HTN*—1.5–3.3 mg/kg/day in 1–4 divided doses (max: 100 mg/day). *Primary aldosteronism*—125–375 mg/m^2/day in 1–2 divided doses. *PO: Neonates:* 1–3 mg/kg/day divided q 12–24 hr. *Renal Impairment Adults and Peds:* ↓ dose for CrCl <50 ml/min; **Availability (G):** *Tabs:* 25, 50, 100 mg; **Monitor:** BP, electrolytes, BUN/SCr, LFTs, I/Os, wt; **Notes:** PO Administer in the morning with food.

streptokinase (Streptase) **Uses:** Acute MI; PE; DVT; Acute peripheral arterial thrombosis; Occluded arteriovenous cannulae; **Class:** plasminogen activators; **Preg:** C; **CIs:** Active bleeding; History of CVA; Recent (within 2 mo) intracranial or intraspinal injury/trauma; Intracranial neoplasm AVM, or aneurysm; Severe uncontrolled HTN; Hypersensitivity; Recent (within 10 days) major surgery, trauma, GI/GU bleeding; **ADRs:** INTRACRANIAL HEMORRHAGE, bronchospasm, reperfusion arrhythmias, ↓ BP, BLEEDING, ↑ LFTs, N/V, flushing, urticaria, allergic reactions including ANAPHYLAXIS; **Interactions:** Aspirin, clopidogrel, ticlopidine, dipyridamole, NSAIDs, GP IIb/IIIa inhibitors, warfarin, heparin, and LMWHs ↑ risk of bleeding; **Dose:** *IV: Adults: Acute MI*—1.5 million units continuous infusion over 60 min. *IV: Adults: Acute PE*—250,000 units LD, followed by 100,000 units/hr for 24 hr. *IV: Adults: Catheter occlusion*—250,000 units/2 ml NS instilled into catheter for 2 hr. *IV: Peds:* 3500–4000 units/kg over 30 min, followed by 1000–1500 units/kg/hr infusion. *Catheter occlusion*—Instill 10,000–25,000 units diluted in NS to a volume equal to catheter volume for 1 hr; **Availability:** *Inject:* 250,000, 750,000 units; **Monitor:** BP, HR, RR, ECG, cardiac enzymes, CBC, aPTT, INR, CP, bleeding, neurologic status; **Notes:** If local bleeding occurs, apply pressure to site. If severe or internal bleeding occurs, discontinue.

sucralfate (Carafate) **Uses:** Ulcer prophylaxis/treatment; GERD; Stomatitis; **Class:** GI protectants; **Preg:** B; **CIs:** Prior sensitivity to sucralfate; Renal failure; **ADRs:** <u>constipation</u>, bezoar formation, pruritus, rash; **Interactions:** ↓ absorption of phenytoin, digoxin, warfarin, ketoconazole, quinolones, quinidine, theophylline, or tetracycline; **Dose:** *PO: Adults: Ulcer prophylaxis*—1 g bid–qid. *Ulcer treatment*—1 g q 4–6 h or 2 g bid. *Stomatitis*—500 mg–1 g swish and spit/swallow qid. *Peds*—40–80 mg/kg/day divided q 6 h; **Availability (G):** *Tabs:* 1 g. *Susp:* 1 g/10 ml; **Monitor:** Abdominal pain, stool for blood; **Notes:** Give 1 hr ac and at bedtime. Aluminum salt is minimally absorbed but can accumulate in renal failure.

sulfasalazine (Azulfidine, Azulfidine EN-tabs) **Uses:** IBD, RA; **Class:** sulfonamides; **Preg:** B, D (at term); **CIs:** Hypersensitivity reactions to sulfonamides, salicylates, or sulfasalazine; GU/GI

S

obstruction; Porphyria; Pregnancy (at term); **ADRs:** HA, ↑ BUN/SCr, anorexia, N/V/D, ↑ LFTs, crystalluria, oligospermia, rash, photosensitivity, thrombocytopenia, anemia, urine discoloration, SERUM SICKNESS; **Interactions:** ↑ toxicity from oral hypoglycemic agents, phenytoin, methotrexate, zidovudine, or warfarin; ↑ risk of drug-induced hepatitis with other hepatotoxic agents; ↑ risk of crystalluria with methenamine; ↑ effects/toxicity of mercaptopurine or thioguanine; ↓ cyclosporine levels; **Dose:** *PO: Adults: IBD*—1 g tid–qid; MD 2 g/day. *PO: Peds: >2 yr Initial*—40–60 mg/kg/day in 3–6 divided doses. *Maintenance*—20–30 mg/kg/day divided qid. *PO: Adults: RA*—500 mg–1 g/day (as DR tabs) × 1 wk, then ↑ by 500 mg/day q wk up to 2 g/day in 2 divided doses; then after 12 wk, may ↑ to 3 g/day if needed. *PO: Peds: ≥6 yr:* 30–50 mg/kg/day in 2 divided doses (as DR tabs); then ↑ weekly to MD (max: 2 g/day). *Renal Impairment Adults and Peds:* ↓ dose for CrCl <30 ml/min; **Availability (G):** *Tabs:* 500 mg. *DR (EC) tabs:* 500 mg; **Monitor:** CBC, LFTs, BUN/SCr, abdominal pain and stool frequency (for IBD), range of motion, joint pain/swelling (for RA); **Notes:** Maintain UO of at least 1200–1500 ml/day to prevent crystalluria and stone formation. Do not crush EC tabs.

sulindac (Clinoril) **Uses:** OA; RA; Gout; Ankylosing spondylitis; Tendonitis/bursitis; **Class:** NSAIDs; **Preg:** C, D (3rd tri); **CIs:** Hypersensitivity to aspirin or NSAIDs; Active bleeding; Perioperative pain from CABG surgery; **ADRs:** HA, dizziness, tinnitus, edema, GI BLEEDING, N/V/D, ↑ LFTs, ↑ SCr, rash; **Interactions:** ↑ adverse GI effects with aspirin and corticosteroids; ↓ effects of aspirin, diuretics, or antihypertensives; ↑ risk of bleeding with drugs affecting platelet function; ↑ risk of nephrotoxicity with cyclosporine; ↑ levels of methotrexate, lithium, aminoglycosides, and vancomycin; **Dose:** *PO: Adults: OA, RA, ankylosing spondylitis*—150 bid. *Gout, bursitis/tendonitis*—200 mg bid; **Availability (G):** *Tabs:* 150 mg, 200 mg; **Monitor:** Pain, temp, S/S of GI upset/bleeding, BUN/SCr, LFTs, CBC; **Notes:** Avoid use in oliguria/anuria. Give with food.

S

sumatriptan (Imitrex) **Uses: PO, Subcut, Intranasal:** Acute treatment of migraines; **Subcut:** Acute treatment of cluster HAs; **Class:** 5-HT_1 agonists; **Preg:** C; **CIs:** Hypersensitivity; CAD or significant CV disease; Uncontrolled HTN; Use of other 5-HT_1 agonists or ergot-type drugs (dihydroergotamine) within 24 hr; Basilar or hemiplegic migraine; Concurrent or recent (within 2 wk) use of MAOI; CV risk factors (use only if CV status has been determined to be safe and 1st dose is administered under supervision); Severe hepatic impairment; **ADRs:** dizziness, drowsiness, CORONARY ARTERY VASOSPASM, MI/ISCHEMIA, VT/VF, nausea; **Interactions:** MAOI ↑ levels (concurrent or recent [within 2 wk] use contraindicated); Use with other 5-HT_1 agonists or ergot-type compounds may ↑ risk of vasospasm (avoid use within 24 hr of each other); Use with SSRIs or SNRIs may ↑ risk of serotonin syndrome; **Dose:** *PO: Adults:* 25–100 mg initially, may repeat in 2 hr (not to exceed 200 mg in 24 hr). *Subcut: Adults:* Up to 6 mg may be used, may repeat in 1 hr (not to exceed 12 mg in 24 hr). *Intranasal: Adults:* 5–20 mg in one nostril, may repeat in 2 hr (not to exceed 40 mg in 24 hr). *Hepatic Impairment PO: Adults:* Do not exceed single doses of 50 mg; **Availability:** *Tabs:* 25, 50, 100 mg. *Inject (STAT dose system):* 4 mg/0.5-ml, 6 mg/0.5-ml. *Nasal spray:* 5 mg/spray, 20 mg/spray; **Monitor:** BP, HR, HA pain; **Notes:** For acute treatment only, not for prophylaxis; give as soon as migraine symptoms occur.

sunitinib (Sutent) **Uses:** GI stromal tumor; Advanced renal cell carcinoma; **Class:** antineoplastics; **Preg:** D; **CIs:** Hypersensitivity; Pregnancy; **ADRs:** fatigue, dizziness, HA, HF, ↑ BP, peripheral edema, DVT, N/V/D, dyspepsia, stomatitis, altered taste, anorexia, constipation, ↑ lipase/amylase, ↑ LFTs, oral pain, alopecia, hand-foot syndrome, hair color change, rash, bleeding, skin discoloration, hypothyroidism, dehydration, ↓ PO_4, anemia, lymphopenia, neutropenia, ↓ platelets, ↑ uric acid, arthralgia, back pain, ↓↑ K, myalgia, fever; **Interactions:** CYP3A4 inhibitors↑ levels/toxicity; CYP3A4 inducers ↓ levels/effects; **Dose:** *PO: Adults:* 50 mg/day × 4 wk, then 2 wk off. *Concurrent CYP3A4 inhibitors*—↓ dose to a min of 37.5 mg/day. *Concurrent CYP3A4 inducers*—need to ↑ dose to a max of 87.5 mg/day; **Availability:** *Caps:* 12.5, 25, 50 mg; **Monitor:** LFTs, BUN/SCr, LVEF, BP, electrolytes, uric acid, amylase/lipase, CBC, platelets, S/S HF and bleeding; **Notes:** Give without regard to meals. ↓ dose if LVEF <50% or >20% reduction from baseline.

tacrine (Cognex) **Uses:** Dementia associated with AD; **Class:** cholinergics; **Preg:** C; **CIs:** Hypersensitivity to tacrine or other acridines; Jaundice associated with previous tacrine therapy; Risk of GI bleeding; **ADRs:** dizziness, HA, ↓ HR, GI BLEEDING, anorexia, N/V/D, ↑ LFTs, dyspepsia; **Interactions:** ↑ theophylline levels/toxicity; ↑ effects of succinylcholine and cholinesterase inhibitors; ↑ effects of bethanechol; Fluvoxamine and cimetidine ↑ levels/ADRs; NSAIDs ↑ risk of GI bleeding; **Dose:** *PO: Adults:* 10 mg qid × 4 wk. If ALT unchanged, ↑ to 20 mg qid; may ↑ q 4 wk up to 160 mg/day; **Availability:** *Caps:* 10, 20, 30, 40 mg; **Monitor:** Cognitive function, LFTs; **Notes:** If ALT levels are >3 to <5 × ULN, ↓ dose by 40 mg/day and resume titration when ALT returns to normal; should be discontinued if ALT levels are >5 × ULN. Give on an empty stomach.

tacrolimus (Prograf, Protopic) **Uses:** Prevention of organ rejection in patients who have undergone liver, kidney, or heart transplantation; **Topical:** Atopic dermatitis in non-immunocompromised patients resistant to conventional therapies; **Class:** immunosuppressants; **Preg:** C; **CIs:** Hypersensitivity; Malignant or pre-malignant skin conditions;

ADRs: SEIZURES, dizziness, HA, insomnia, tremor, anxiety, depression, hallucinations, psychoses, somnolence, abnormal vision, amblyopia, tinnitus, cough, pleural effusion, asthma, HTN, edema, QT_C prolongation, GI BLEEDING, abdominal pain, anorexia, ascites, constipation, dyspepsia, ↑ LFTs, N/V/D, ↑ appetite, cholestatic jaundice, dysphagia, flatulence, ↑ BUN/SCr, pruritus, rash, alopecia, ↑ infection risk, hirsutism, sweating, photosensitivity, ↑ BG, ↑↓ K, hyperlipidemia, ↓ Mg, ↑↓ PO_4, ↑ uric acid, ↓ Ca, ↓ Na, metab acidosis, metab alkalosis, anemia, leukocytosis, leukopenia, thrombocytopenia, coagulation defects, arthralgia, paresthesia, ANAPHYLAXIS, fever, ↑ risk of lymphoma/skin CA; **Interactions:** CYP3A4 inhibitors may ↑ levels/toxicity; CYP3A4 inducers may ↓ levels/effects; ↑ risk of nephrotoxicity with other nephrotoxic drugs (e.g., amphotericin, aminoglycosides, trimethoprim/sulfamethoxazole, vancomycin, acyclovir, cisplatin, NSAIDS); Voriconazole may ↑ levels/toxicity; ↓ tacrolimus dose by 66%; Antacids ↓ absorption; separate by ≥2 hr; **Dose:** *PO: Adults: Kidney transplant*—0.2 mg/kg/day divided q 12 hr; titrate to achieve therapeutic levels. *Liver transplant*—0.1–0.15 mg/kg/day divided q 12 hr; titrate to achieve therapeutic levels. *Heart transplant*—0.075 mg/kg/day divided q 12 hr; titrate to achieve therapeutic levels. *IV: Adults and Peds: Liver or kidney transplant*—0.03–0.05 mg/kg/day as continuous infusion. *Heart transplant*—0.01 mg/kg/day as continuous infusion. *PO: Peds: Liver transplant*—0.15–0.2 mg/kg/day in 2 divided doses; titrate to achieve therapeutic levels. *Topical: Adults and Peds: ≥2 yr:* 0.03%–0.1% oint bid; **Availability:** *Cap:* 0.5, 1, 5 mg. *Inject:* 5 mg/ml. *Oint:* 0.03%, 0.1%; **Monitor:** BP, S/S infection, BUN/SCr, electrolytes, uric acid, lipid panel, CBC, LFTs, tacrolimus levels, S/S organ rejection, skin lesions (for dermatitis); **Notes:** Levels vary per transplant and time post-transplant; range: 5–20 ng/ml. Should start no sooner than 6 hr after surgery. Discontinue oint when the S/S of atopic dermatitis subside; instruct patients to limit sun exposure (for top).

tadalafil (Cialis) **Uses:** ED; **Class:** PDE-5 inhibitors; **Preg:** B; **CIs:** Hypersensitivity; Concurrent use of nitrates; Severe hepatic impairment; Uncontrolled HTN (BP >170/110 mmHg), hypotension (BP <90/50 mmHg), angina during intercourse, HF, or CAD, Life-threatening arrhythmias, stroke, or MI within 6 mo; **ADRs:** HA, hearing loss, nasal congestion, abnormal vision, ↓ BP, dyspepsia, priapism, flushing, back pain, myalgia; **Interactions:** Nitrates and alpha-adrenergic blockers may cause serious, life-threatening hypotension; CYP3A4 inhibitors may ↑ levels/toxicity; CYP3A4 inducers may ↓ levels/effects; **Dose:** *PO: Adults: As-needed regimen*—5–20 mg ≥30 min before sexual activity (max: one dose/day). *Once-daily regimen*— 2.5–5 mg daily. *Concurrent use of strong CYP3A4 inhibitors*—As-needed regimen: max dose of 10 mg (not to be given more frequently than q 72 hr); once-daily regimen: max dose of 2.5 mg/day. *Renal Impairment PO: Adults:* ↓ dose if CrCl <50 ml/min. *Hepatic Impairment PO: Adults: Mild-to-moderate hepatic* *impairment*—10 mg; **Availability:** *Tabs:* 5, 10, 20 mg; **Monitor:** Response, ADRs; **Notes:** Give without regard to meals; duration may last up to 36 hr. Patients should be on stable dose of alpha-blocker therapy before starting therapy with tadalafil.

tamoxifen (Soltamox) **Uses:** Breast CA treatment/prevention; Treatment of ductal carcinoma *in situ* following breast surgery and radiation; McCune-Albright syndrome with precocious puberty in girls 2–10 yr; **Class:** antiestrogens; **Preg:** D; **CIs:** Hypersensitivity; Concurrent warfarin therapy with history of DVT; Pregnancy/lactation; ↓ bone marrow reserve; **ADRs:** ↑ LFTs, depression, HA, weakness, blurred vision, PE, STROKE, edema, N/V, UTERINE MALIGNANCIES, vag bleeding, ↑ Ca, leukopenia, thrombocytopenia, hot flashes, bone pain, tumor flare; **Interactions:** Estrogens and aminoglutethimide may ↓ effecs; Levels ↑ by bromocriptine; ↑ anticoagulant effects of warfarin; ↑ risk of thromboembolic events with antineoplastics; **Dose:** *PO: Adults: Breast CA treatment*—10–20 mg bid. *PO: Adults: Breast CA prevention/ Ductal carcinoma in situ*—20 mg/day × 5 yr. *PO: Peds: [girls] 2–10 yr:* 20 mg/day for up to one year; **Availability (G):** *Tabs:* 10, 20 mg. *EC tabs:* {20 mg}. *Oral soln:* 10 mg/5 ml; **Monitor:** CBC, platelets, Ca, LFTs, mammogram, bone pain, S/S vag bleeding; **Notes:** Gynecologic exams should be performed regularly.

telmisartan (Micardis) **Uses:** HTN; **Class:** ARBs; **Preg:** C (1st tri), D (2nd and 3rd tri); **CIs:** Hypersensitivity; Pregnancy/lactation; Obstructive biliary disorders or hepatic impairment; **ADRs:** dizziness, fatigue, HA, ↓ BP, sinusitis, ↑ K, abdominal pain, diarrhea, dyspepsia, ↑ SCr, back pain, myalgia, ANGIOEDEMA; **Interactions:** ↑ effects with other antihypertensives; ↑ risk of hyperkalemia with ACEIs, K supplements, K salt substitutes, K-sparing diuretics, or NSAIDs; NSAIDs may ↓ effectiveness; May ↑ digoxin levels; **Dose:** *PO: Adults:* 20–80 mg/ day; **Availability:** *Tabs:* 20, 40, 80 mg; **Monitor:** BP, HR, wt, edema, BUN/SCr, K; **Notes:** Can be used in patients intolerant to ACEI (due to cough); just as likely as ACEI to cause ↑ K and ↑ SCr.

T

temazepam (Restoril) **Uses:** Short-term management of insomnia; **Class:** BZs; **Preg:** X; **CIs:** Prior sensitivity to other BZs; Acute narrow-angle glaucoma; Sleep apnea; Severe hepatic/renal/ pulmonary impairment; **ADRs:** sedation, HA, ataxia, slurred speech, amnesia, confusion, mental depression, blurred vision, resp depression, APNEA, CARDIAC ARREST, ↓ HR, ↓ BP, constipation, N/V/D, rash, physical/psychological dependence, tolerance; **Interactions:** ↑ CNS depression with alcohol, antihistamines, antidepressants, opioid analgesics, clozapine, and other sedative/hypnotics; ↓ sedative effects when used with theophylline; CYP3A4 inhibitors may ↑ levels/effects; **Dose:** *PO: Adults:* 15–30 mg at bedtime. *PO: Geriatric Patients:* 7.5 mg at bedtime; **Availability (G):** *Caps:* 7.5, 15, 30 mg; **Monitor:** Sleep patterns, HR, BP, RR, S/S CNS depression; **Notes:** Do not discontinue abruptly.

tenecteplase (TNKase) **Uses:** Acute MI; **Class:** plasminogen activators; **Preg:** C; **CIs:** Active bleeding; History of CVA; Recent (within 2 mo) intracranial or intraspinal injury/trauma; Intracranial neoplasm, AVM, or aneurysm; Severe uncontrolled HTN; Hypersensitivity; Recent (within 10 days) major surgery, trauma, GI/GU bleeding; Concurrent anticoagulant therapy; **ADRs:** INTRACRANIAL HEMORRHAGE, reperfusion arrhythmias, ↓ BP, BLEEDING, N/V, flushing, urticaria, allergic reactions including ANAPHYLAXIS; **Interactions:** Aspirin, clopidogrel, ticlopidine, dipyridamole, NSAIDs, GP IIb/IIIa inhibitors, warfarin, heparin, and LMWHs ↑ risk of bleeding; **Dose:** *IV: Adults: <60 kg:* 30 mg. *IV: Adults: ≥60 kg and <70 kg:* 35 mg. *IV: Adults: ≥70 kg and <80 kg:* 40 mg. *IV: Adults: ≥80 kg and <90 kg:* 45 mg. *IV: Adults: ≥90 kg:* 50 mg; **Availability:** *Inject:* 50 mg; **Monitor:** BP, HR, RR, ECG, cardiac enzymes, CBC, aPTT, INR, CP, bleeding, neurologic status; **Notes:** If local bleeding occurs, apply pressure to site. If severe or internal bleeding occurs, discontinue.

tenofovir disoproxil fumarate (Viread) **Uses:** HIV infection; **Class:** NRTIs; **Preg:** B; **CIs:** Hypersensitivity; Concurrent chronic hepatitis B; Obesity, women, prolonged nucleoside exposure (↑ risk for lactic acidosis/hepatomegaly); **ADRs:** HA, weakness, HEPATOMEGALY, <u>N/V/D</u>, abdominal pain, anorexia, flatulence, renal impairment, LACTIC ACIDOSIS, ↓ PO_4; **Interactions:** ↑ levels of didanosine (give 2 hrs before or 1 hr after didanosine); Levels ↑ by cidofovir, acyclovir, ganciclovir, or valganciclovir; ↑ renal toxicity with other nephrotoxic agents; Combination with atazanavir may ↓ virologic response/resistance to atazanavir (ritonavir may be added to boost levels); Combination with abacavir and lamivudine may cause virologic nonresponse and should be avoided; **Dose:** *PO: Adults:* 300 mg once daily; **Availability:** *Tabs:* 300 mg; **Monitor:** Viral load, CD4 count, CBC, BUN/SCr, LFTs, PO_4, S/S lactic acidosis; **Notes:** Give with a meal. Lactic acidosis may occur with hepatic toxicity causing hepatic steatosis and may be fatal, especially in women.

T

terazosin (Hytrin) **Uses:** HTN; BPH; **Class:** peripherally acting antiadrenergics; **Preg:** C; **CIs:** Hypersensitivity; Concurrent use with PDE-5 inhibitors (sildenafil, tadalafil, or vardenafil); **ADRs:** <u>dizziness</u>, <u>HA</u>, drowsiness, blurred vision, <u>first-dose orthostatic hypotension</u>, edema, palpitations, diarrhea, dry mouth, nausea; **Interactions:** ↑ effects with other antihypertensives and PDE-5 inhibitors; **Dose:** *PO: Adults: HTN*—1 mg at bedtime; may ↑ slowly as needed up to 20 mg/day. *BPH*—1 mg at bedtime; may ↑ up to 10 mg/day (max: 20 mg/day);

Availability (G): *Caps:* 1, 2, 5, 10 mg; **Monitor:** BP (sitting, standing), HR, PSA, S/S BPH, I/Os, wt, edema; **Notes:** First-dose orthostatic hypotension most frequently occurs 30 min–2 hr after initial dose; give 1st dose at bedtime.

terbinafine (Lamisil, Lamisil AT) **Uses:** **PO:** Onychomycosis, tinea capitis; **Topical:** Cutaneous fungal infections, including tinea pedis, tinea cruris, and tinea corporis; **Class:** antifungals; **Preg:** B; **CIs:** Hypersensitivity; Liver disease; Renal impairment (CrCl ≤50 ml/min); **ADRs:** HA, cough, HF, HEPATOTOXICITY, anorexia, N/V/D, stomach pain, altered taste, ↑ LFTs, taste disturbance, SJS, TEN, itching, rash, neutropenia, pancytopenia, pyrexia; **Interactions:** May ↑ levels of CYP2D6 substrates; Alcohol or other hepatotoxic agents ↑ risk of hepatotoxicity; Rifampin and other drugs that induce hepatic drug-metabolizing enzymes may ↓ effects; Cimetidine and other drugs that inhibit hepatic drug-metabolizing enzymes may ↑ effects; **Dose:** *PO: Adults:* 250 mg/day × 6 wk for fingernail infection or 12 wk for toenail infection. *PO: Peds: ≥4 yr and ≥35 kg:* 250 mg/day × 6 wk. *PO: Peds: ≥4 yr and 25–35 kg:* 187.5 mg/day × 6 wk. *PO: Peds: ≥4 yr and <25 kg:* 125 mg/day × 6 wk. *Topical: Adults and Peds: ≥12 yr:* Apply bid × 1 wk for tinea pedis. Apply daily × 1 wk for tinea cruris or tinea corporis; **Availability (G):** *Tabs:* 250 mg. *Granules:* 125-, 187.5-mg packets. *Cream/Gel/Spray:* 1%; **Monitor:** CBC, LFTs, BUN/SCr, S/S infection; **Notes:** Discontinue if rash or symptomatic ↑ LFTs occurs. Avoid occlusive dressings with top use; may stain fabric, skin, or hair. Granules may be sprinkled on soft, nonacidic food.

terbutaline **Uses:** Management of reversible airway disease due to asthma or COPD; Tocolytic agent; **Class:** adrenergics; **Preg:** B; **CIs:** Hypersensitivity to adrenergic amines; Tachycardia; HTN; HF; Diabetes; Glaucoma; **ADRs:** nervousness, restlessness, tremor, HA, insomnia, PARADOXICAL BRONCHOSPASM, angina, arrhythmias, HTN, ↑ HR, N/V, ↓ K, hyperglycemia; **Interactions:** Concurrent use with other adrenergics ↑ adrenergic side effects; Use with MAOIs may lead to hypertensive crisis; Beta blockers may negate therapeutic effect; **Dose:** *PO: Adults and Peds: >15 yr Bronchodilation*—2.5–5 mg tid, given q 6 hr (max: 15 mg/24 hr). *Tocolysis*—2.5 mg q 4–6 hr until delivery. *PO: Peds: 12–15 yr:* 2.5 mg tid (given q 6 hr). *Subcut: Adults: Bronchodilation*—250 mcg; may repeat in 15–30 min (max: 500 mcg/4 hr). *Tocolysis*—250 mcg q 1 hr until contractions stop. *IV: Adults: Tocolysis*—10 mcg/min infusion; increase by 5 mcg/min q 10 min until contractions stop (max: 80 mcg/min). After contractions have stopped for 30 min, ↓ infusion rate to lowest effective amount for 4–8 hr; **Availability (G):** *Tabs:* 2.5, 5 mg. *Inject:* 1 mg/ml; **Monitor:** RR, HR, BP, PFTs, fetal HR (tocolysis), K, glucose, S/S bronchospasm; **Notes:** Give with meals to ↓ gastric irritation. May give IV undiluted.

testosterone (Depo-Testosterone, Delatestryl, Testopel) **Uses:** Hypogonadism in androgen-deficient men, Delayed puberty in men; Androgen-responsive inoperable breast CA (enanthate only); **Class:** androgens; **Preg:** X; **CIs:** Hypersensitivity; Pregnancy/lactation; Male patients with breast or prostate CA; **ADRs:** deepening of voice, edema, cholestatic jaundice, drug-induced hepatitis, ↑ LFTs, N/V, change in libido, ED, oligospermia, priapism, prostatic enlargement, gynecomastia, hirsutism, ↑ cholesterol, ↑ Ca, ↑ K, ↑ PO_4, male pattern baldness, pain at implantation site; **Interactions:** ↑ effects of warfarin, oral hypoglycemic agents, and insulin; Corticosteroids ↑ risk of edema; **Dose:** *IM: Adults: Female inoperable breast CA*—200–400 mg q 2–4 wk (enanthate only). *IM: Adults: Hypogonadism*—50–400 mg q 2–4 wk (cypionate/enanthate). *IM: Peds: Delayed male puberty*—40–50 mg/m^2/dose q 4 wk for up to 6 mo (cypionate/enanthate). *Subcut pellets for implantation: Adults and Peds: Delayed male puberty/hypogonadism*—150–450 mg q 3–6 mo; **Availability:** *Pellets:* 75 mg. *Depot inject (in oil as enanthate):* 200 mg/ml. *Depot inject (in oil as cypionate):* 100 mg/ml, 200 mg/ml; **Monitor:** LFTs, PSA, cholesterol, CBC, electrolytes, wt, I/Os, bone age (in peds), pubertal signs; **Notes:** Administer IM deep into gluteal muscle; pellets should be implanted subcut by health care professional.

tetracycline (Achromycin, Sumycin) **Uses:** Various infections caused by unusual organisms, including *Mycoplasma*, *Chlamydia*, *Rickettsia*, and *Borrelia burgdorferi*; Gonorrhea and syphilis in penicillin-allergic patients; Prevention of exacerbations of chronic bronchitis; Acne, *H. pylori* (with other drugs); **Class:** tetracyclines; **Preg:** D; **CIs:** Hypersensitivity; Pregnancy, lactation, or peds <8 yr—risk of permanent staining of teeth in infant/ped (for pregnancy, risk is ↑ during last half of pregnancy); **ADRs:** bulging fontanelles, dizziness, vestibular reactions, PSEUDOMEMBRANOUS COLITIS, N/V/D, esophagitis, ↑ LFTs, photosensitivity, rash, pigmentation of skin and mucous membranes, hypersensitivity reactions, superinfection; **Interactions:** Use with antacids, bismuth subsalicylate, or drugs containing Ca, aluminum, Mg, iron, or zinc may ↓ absorption; May ↑ effects of warfarin; May ↓ effectiveness of estrogen-containing oral contraceptives; Phenobarbital, carbamazepine, or phenytoin may ↓ levels/effects; ↑ effects of warfarin; Ca in foods or dairy products may ↓ absorption; **Dose:** *PO: Adults:* 250–500 mg bid–qid. *H. pylori*—500 mg bid–qid with ≥1 other antibiotic and either PPI or H_2 antagonist. *PO: Peds: ≥8 yr:* 6.25–12.5 mg/kg q 6 hr or 12.5–25 mg/kg q 12 hr. *Renal Impairment PO: Adults and Peds:* ↓ dose for CrCl <80 ml/min; **Availability (G):** *Caps:* 250, 500 mg; **Monitor:** BP, HR, temp, sputum, U/A, CBC, LFTs, acne lesions; **Notes:** Do not administer within 1–4 hr of other meds. Give ≥1 hr ac or ≥2 hr after pc (may be taken with food if GI irritation occurs). Advise patient to use sunscreen.

thalidomide (Thalomid) Uses: Cutaneous manifestations of ENL; Prevention and suppression of recurrent ENL; Multiple myeloma; **Class:** immunosuppressants; **Preg:** X; **CIs:** Pregnancy; Peripheral neuropathy; Women with childbearing potential and sexually mature men (unless specific conditions are met); Lactation; Hypersensitivity; **ADRs:** dizziness, drowsiness, ↓ HR, edema, orthostatic hypotension, thromboembolic events (↑ risk with dexamethasone in multiple myeloma), constipation, rash, photosensitivity, neutropenia, peripheral neuropathy, SEVERE BIRTH DEFECTS, hypersensitivity reactions, ↑ HIV viral load; **Interactions:** ↑ CNS depression with barbiturates, sedative/hypnotics, alcohol, chlorpromazine, reserpine, or other CNS depressants; Concurrent use of agents that may cause peripheral neuropathy ↑ risk of peripheral neuropathy; **Dose:** *PO: Adults:* 100–400 mg/day. *PO: Adults: Multiple myeloma*—200 mg daily in 28-day treatment cycles. Dexamethasone 40 mg is administered on Days 1–4, 9–12, 17–20; **Availability:** *Caps:* 50, 100, 150, 200 mg; **Monitor:** BP, HR, WBC, S/S peripheral neuropathy/VTE; **Notes:** Give with water, preferably at bedtime and at least 1 hr after the evening meal. Taper gradually in decrements of 50 mg q 2–4 wk.

theophylline (Elixophyllin, Quibron-T, Theochron, Theo-24, Uniphyl) Uses: Reversible airway obstruction caused by asthma or COPD; Neonatal apnea/bradycardia; **Class:** xanthines; **Preg:** C; **CIs:** Hypersensitivity to aminophylline or theophylline; Cardiac arrhythmias; **ADRs:** SEIZURES, anxiety, HA, insomnia, irritability, ARRHYTHMIAS, ↑ HR, angina, N/V, anorexia, tremor; **Interactions:** Additive CV and CNS side effects with adrenergics (sympathomimetic); CYP1A2 inhibitors and CYP3A4 inhibitors may ↑ levels/toxicity; CYP1A2 inducers and CYP3A4 inducers may ↓ levels/effects; **Dose: All doses expressed as theophylline (not aminophylline)** *PO: Adults: Non-smokers* 5 mg/kg LD, then 10 mg/kg/day divided q 8–12 hr (max: 900 mg/day). *PO: Adults: HF, Cor Pulmonale, or Liver Dysfunction:* 5 mg/kg LD, then 5 mg/kg/day divided q 8–12 hr (max: 400 mg/day). *PO: Peds: 12–16 yr, Non-smokers:* 5 mg/kg LD, then 13 mg/kg/day divided q 8–12 hr. *PO: Peds: 9–12 yr, Adolescents, and Adult Smokers: <50 yr:* 5 mg/kg LD, then 16 mg/kg/day divided q 8–12 hr. *PO: Peds: 1–9 yr:* 5 mg/kg LD, then 20–24 mg/kg/day divided q 8–12 hr. *PO: Infants 6 mo–1 yr:* 5 mg/kg LD, then 12–18 mg/kg/day divided q 6–8 hr. *PO: Infants 6 wk–6 mo:* 5 mg/kg LD, then 10 mg/kg/day divided q 6–8 hr. *PO: Neonates up to 6 wk:* 4 mg/kg LD, then 4 mg/kg/day divided q 12 hr. *IV: Adults and Peds:* See aminophylline monograph for IV doses; **Availability:** *SR tabs:* 300 mg. *ER tabs:* 100, 200, 300, 450 mg. *CR tabs:* 400, 600 mg. *ER caps (24 hr):* 100, 200, 300, 400 mg. *Elixir:* 80 mg/15 ml. *Inject:* 0.8 mg/ml, 1.6 mg/ml, 2 mg/ml, 3.2 mg/ml, 4 mg/ml; **Monitor:** BP, HR, RR, ECG, lung sounds, CP, PFTs, ABGs, theophylline level; **Notes:** Peak levels should be evaluated 30 min after a IV LD, 12–24 hr after initiation

T

of a continuous infusion and 1–2 hr after oral forms. Therapeutic levels: 10–15 mcg/ml (asthma); 6–13 mcg/ml (neonatal apnea). ↑ risk of toxicity with levels >20 mcg/ml. Tachycardia, arrhythmias, or seizures may be 1st sign of toxicity.

thiamine (vitamin B_1) **Uses:** Thiamine deficiencies (beriberi); Prevention of Wernicke's encephalopathy; Dietary supplement in patients with GI disease, alcoholism, or cirrhosis; **Class:** water soluble vitamins; **Preg:** A; **CIs:** Hypersensitivity; **ADRs:** restlessness, weakness, pulmonary edema, resp distress, VASCULAR COLLAPSE, ↓ BP, vasodilation, GI bleeding, nausea, cyanosis, pruritus, sweating, tingling, urticaria, ANGIOEDEMA; **Interactions:** None significant; **Dose:** *PO: Adults: Thiamine deficiency*—5–10 mg tid. *IM, IV: Adults: Thiamine deficiency*—5–30 mg tid. *Alcohol withdrawal syndrome*—100 mg/day IM/IV for several days, then 50–100 mg/day PO *Wernicke's encephalopathy*—100 mg IV initially, then 50–100 mg/day IV/IM until eating balanced diet. *PO: Peds: Thiamine deficiency*—10–50 mg/day in divided doses. *IM, IV: Peds: Thiamine deficiency*—10–25 mg/day; **Availability (G):** *Tabs:* 50, 100, 250, 500 mg. *Inject:* 100 mg/ml; **Monitor:** S/S thiamine deficiency, thiamine level; **Notes:** Infusing slowly (over 30 min) may ↓ infusion-related reactions. Give before parenteral glucose solutions in Wernicke's encephalopathy to prevent precipitation of HF.

thyroid (Armour thyroid, Thyrar, Thyroid Strong, Westhroid) **Uses:** Thyroid supplementation in hypothyroidism; Euthyroid goiters and thyroid CA; Diagnostic agent; **Class:** thyroid preparations; **Preg:** A; **CIs:** Hypersensitivity; Recent MI; Hyperthyroidism; Hypersensitivity to beef (Thyrar product); Severe renal insufficiency; Uncorrected adrenocortical disorders; **ADRs:** insomnia, irritability, HA, arrhythmias, ↑ HR, angina pectoris, abdominal cramps, N/V/D, hyperhidrosis, hyperthyroidism, menstrual irregularities, wt loss, heat intolerance, accelerated bone maturation in peds; **Interactions:** Bile acid sequestrants ↓ absorption; ↑ effects from warfarin; ↑ requirement for insulin or oral hypoglycemic agents; Estrogens may ↑ thyroid replacement requirements; ↑ CV effects with adrenergics (sympathomimetics); **Dose:** *PO: Adults and Peds: Hypothyroidism*—60 mg/day; ↑ q 4 wk by 30 mg to 60–120 mg/day. *Myxedema/hypothyroidism with CV disease*—15 mg/day then ↑ 30 mg/day q 2 wk, then ↑ by 30–60 mg q 2 wk to 60–120 mg/day. *PO: Geriatric Patients:* 7.5–15 mg/day initially; may double dose q 6–8 wk until desired effect; **Availability:** *Tabs:* 15, 30, 60, 90, 120, 180, 240, 300 mg; **Monitor:** HR, BP, wt, TFTs, glucose, S/S hyperthyroidism; **Notes:** Give before breakfast to prevent insomnia.

tiagabine (Gabitril) **Uses:** Partial seizures; **Class:** anticonvulsants; **Preg:** C; **CIs:** Hypersensitivity; **ADRs:** dizziness, drowsiness, nervousness, weakness, cognitive impairment, confusion, ↑ LFTs, hallucinations, HA, mental depression, personality disorder, abnormal vision, ear pain, tinnitus, dyspnea, epistaxis, CP, edema, HTN, ↑ HR, syncope, abdominal pain, gingivitis, nausea, stomatitis, dysmenorrhea, dysuria, metrorrhagia, urinary incontinence, alopecia, dry skin, rash, sweating, ↑ wt/loss, arthralgia, neck pain, ataxia, tremors, allergic reactions, chills, lymphadenopathy; **Interactions:** Carbamazepine, phenytoin, primidone, and phenobarbital induce metabolism and ↓ levels; dose adjustments may be required; **Dose:** *PO: Adults: >18 yr:* 4 mg once daily × 1 wk; ↑ by 4–8 mg/day q wk, up to 56 mg/day in 2–4 divided doses. *PO: Peds: 12–18 yr:* 4 mg once daily × 1 wk; ↑ by 4 mg/day q wk, then ↑ by 4–8 mg/day q wk, up to 32 mg/day in 2–4 divided doses; **Availability:** *Tabs:* 2, 4, 12, 16, 20 mg; **Monitor:** Seizure frequency, CBC, BUN/SCr, LFTs; **Notes:** Abrupt discontinuation may ↑ seizure frequency. Give with food.

ticarcillin/clavulanate (Timentin) **Uses:** Intra-abdominal infections, skin/skin structure infections, gynecologic infections, septicemia, bone/joint infections, UTIs, or resp tract infections due to susceptible organisms (e.g., *S. aureus*, *E. coli*, *Citrobacter*, *Enterobacter*, *B. fragilis*, *H. flu*, *Klebsiella*, *Pseudomonas*); **Class:** extended spectrum penicillins; **Preg:** B; **CIs:** Hypersensitivity (cross-sensitivity to other beta-lactam antibiotics may exist); **ADRs:** SEIZURES, HA, PSEUDOMEMBRANOUS COLITIS, N/V/D, ↑ LFTs, ↑ BUN/SCr, rash, urticaria, pruritis, thrombocytopenia, phlebitis, allergic reactions including ANAPHYLAXIS, SERUM SICKNESS; **Interactions:** Probenecid ↓ excretion and ↑ levels; **Dose:** *IV: Adults:* 3.1 g q 4–6 hr. *IV: Peds:* ≥ *3 mo <60 kg*—50 mg ticarcillin/kg q 4–6 hr. ≥ *60 kg*—3 g ticarcillin q 4–6 hr. *Renal Impairment IV: Adults:* ↓ dose if CrCl ≤60 ml/min; **Availability:** *Inject:* 3.1 g (3 g ticarcillin/100 mg clavulanic acid); **Monitor:** BP, HR, temp, sputum, U/A, CBC, LFTs, BUN/SCr; **Notes:** Use with caution in patients with beta-lactam allergy (do not use if history of anaphylaxis or hives). Na content per 1 gram = 4.5 mEq; K content per 1 gram= 0.15 mEq.

ticlopidine (Ticlid) **Uses:** Prevention of stroke in patients unable to tolerate aspirin; Prevention of coronary stent thrombosis; **Class:** platelet aggregation inhibitors; **Preg:** B; **CIs:** Hypersensitivity; Bleeding disorders or active bleeding; Severe liver disease; **ADRs:** dizziness, HA, weakness, epistaxis, tinnitus, N/V/D, ↑ LFTs, anorexia, GI fullness, GI pain, hematuria, rash, pruritus, urticaria, AGRANULOCYTOSIS, APLASTIC ANEMIA, INTRACEREBRAL BLEEDING, NEUTROPENIA, bleeding, thrombocytopenia, ↑ cholesterol, ↑ TGs; **Interactions:** Aspirin potentiates the effect of ticlopidine on platelets; ↑ bleeding with heparins, warfarin, tirofiban, eptifibatide, clopidogrel, or thrombolytic agents; Cimetidine ↓ metabolism/↑ toxicity; Ticlopidine ↓ metabolism of theophylline and ↑ toxicity; **Dose:** *PO: Adults:* 250 mg bid; **Availability:** *Tabs:* 250 mg; **Monitor:** CBC, LFTs, cholesterol, TGs, bleeding time, S/S bleeding; **Notes:** Take with food to ↑ absorption.

T

tigecycline (Tygacil) **Uses:** Complicated skin/skin structure infections or intra-abdominal infections due to susceptible organisms (e.g., *S. aureus* (MSSA, MRSA), *E. coli*, *B. fragilis*, *E. faecalis* [vanco-sensitive], *Citrobacter*, *Enterobacter*, *Klebsiella*); **Class:** glycylcycline; **Preg:** D; **CIs:** Hypersensitivity; Peds <18 yr; Pregnancy; **ADRs:** HA, PSEUDOMEMBRANOUS COLITIS, N/V/D, ↑ LFTs, ↑ BUN/SCr, ↑ BG, ↓ K, inject site reactions, allergic reactions; **Interactions:** ↓ effects of hormonal contraceptives; May ↑ effects of warfarin; **Dose:** *IV: Adults:* 100 mg initially, then 50 mg q 12 hr. *Hepatic Impairment IV: Adults: >18 yr Severe hepatic impairment*—100 mg initially, then 25 mg q 12 hr; **Availability:** *Inject:* 50 mg; **Monitor:** BP, HR, temp, CBC, cultures/sensitivity, BUN/SCr, LFTs, electrolytes, S/S infection; **Notes:** Give IV at a concentration of <1 mg/ml over 30–60 min.

timolol (Betimol, Istalol, Timolol GFS, Timoptic, Timoptic-XE) **Uses:** HTN; Post-MI; Migraine prophylaxis; **Ophth:** Glaucoma; **Class:** beta blockers; **Preg:** C; **CIs:** Hypersensitivity; Decompensated HF; Pulmonary edema; Cardiogenic shock; Bradycardia or ≥2nd-degree heart block (in absence of pacemaker); **ADRs:** fatigue, weakness, depression, dizziness, drowsiness, nightmares, blurred vision, bronchospasm, BRADYCARDIA, HF, PULMONARY EDEMA, ↓ BP, N/V/D, ED, ↓ libido, ↑ BG, ↓ BG; **Interactions:** ↑ risk of bradycardia with digoxin, diltiazem, verapamil, or clonidine; ↑ effects with other antihypertensives; ↑ risk of hypertensive crisis if concurrent clonidine discontinued; May alter the effectiveness of insulins or oral hypoglycemic agents; May ↓ the effects of $beta_1$ agonists (e.g., dopamine or dobutamine); **Dose:** *PO: Adults: HTN*—10 mg bid initially; may ↑ q 7 days up to 60 mg/day. *Post-MI*—10 mg bid, starting 1–4 wk after MI. *Migraine prophylaxis*—10 mg bid (max: 30 mg/day). *Ophth Adults:* 1 gtt bid of 0.25% soln; may ↑ to 1 gtt bid of 0.5% soln if inadequate response. *Istalol (0.5%)*—1 gtt daily in AM. *Gel-forming soln (0.25% or 0.5%)*—1 gtt daily; **Availability (G):** *Tabs:* 5, 10, 20 mg. *Ophth gel-forming soln (Timolol GFS or Timoptic-XE):* 0.25%, 0.5%. *Ophth soln (Betimol, Istalol, Timoptic):* 0.25%, 0.5%; **Monitor:** BP, HR, ECG, S/S HF, edema, wt, S/S angina, BG (in DM), migraine frequency/intensity; **Notes:** Abrupt withdrawal may cause life-threatening arrhythmias, hypertensive crises, or myocardial ischemia. May mask S/S of hypoglycemia (esp. tachycardia) in DM.

T

tinzaparin (Innohep) **Uses:** Treatment of DVT with or without PE; **Class:** antithrombotics, LMWH; **Preg:** B; **CIs:** Hypersensitivity to bisulfites (contains metabisulfite), benzyl alcohol, or pork products; Active bleeding; History of heparin-induced thrombocytopenia; Spinal or epidural anesthesia; **ADRs:** ↑ LFTs, BLEEDING, thrombocytopenia, pain at injection site; **Interactions:** ↑ risk of bleeding with antiplatelets, thrombolytics, or other anticoagulants; **Dose:** *Subcut: Adults:* 175 anti-Xa units/kg/day × 6 days and until therapeutic anticoagulation achieved with warfarin; **Availability:** *Inject:* 20,000 anti-Xa units/ml; **Monitor:** BUN/SCr, CBC, LFTs, bleeding; **Notes:** Do not administer IM or IV. If on warfarin, PT/INR should be drawn just prior to dose of tinzaparin.

tiotropium (Spiriva) **Uses:** Bronchospasm due to COPD; **Class:** anticholinergics; **Preg:** C; **CIs:** Hypersensitivity to tiotropium or atropine derivatives; Concurrent ipratropium; Angle-closure glaucoma, prostatic hyperplasia, bladder neck obstruction; **ADRs:** glaucoma, paradoxical bronchospasm, ↑ HR, dry mouth, constipation, urinary difficulty, urinary retention, ANGIOEDEMA; **Interactions:** Ipratropium ↑ anticholinergic effects; **Dose:** *Inhaln: Adults:* 18 mcg once daily; **Availability:** *Caps for inhaln:* 18 mcg; **Monitor:** RR, HR, SOB, bronchospasm relief; **Notes:** Should be given only via the Handihaler; tiny amounts of powder may be left in caps after use. Not for treatment of acute bronchospasm.

tipranavir (Aptivus) **Uses:** Advanced HIV disease (must be used with ritonavir); **Class:** protease inhibitors; **Preg:** C; **CIs:** Hypersensitivity; Moderate-to-severe hepatic impairment (Child-Pugh Class B and C); Concurrent use of amiodarone, flecainide, propafenone, quinidine, ergot derivatives, midazolam, pimozide, or triazolam; Known sulfonamide allergy; Hemophilia (may ↑ risk of bleeding); **ADRs:** INTRACRANIAL HEMORRHAGE, fatigue, HA, HEPATOTOXICITY, abdominal pain, N/V/D, rash (↑ in women), hyperglycemia, ↑ cholesterol, ↑ TGs, allergic reactions, fat redistribution, fever, immune reconstitution syndrome; **Interactions:** ↑ levels/toxicity from amiodarone, flecainide, propafenone, quinidine, ergot derivatives; Hormonal contraceptives ↑ risk of rash; ↓ effects of hormonal contraceptives; **Dose:** *PO: Adults:* 500 mg bid with ritonavir 200 mg; **Availability:** *Caps:* 250 mg; **Monitor:** CBC, CD4 count, viral load, glucose, LFTs, TGs, S/S bleeding; **Notes:** Should be discontinued if symptomatic ↑ of AST and ALT of 5–10 × ULN and BR ↑ 2.5 × ULN. Give with ritonavir with meals.

T

tirofiban (Aggrastat) **Uses:** ACS (unstable angina/non–ST-segment elevation MI), including patients who will be managed medically and those who will undergo PCI; **Class:** glycoprotein IIb/IIIa inhibitors; **Preg:** B; **CIs:** Hypersensitivity; Active bleeding or history of bleeding within previous 30 days; Aortic dissection; Pericarditis; Severe uncontrolled HTN (SBP >180 mmHg and/or DBP >110 mmHg); Major surgery in previous 30 days; History of any stroke in previous 30 days or any history of hemorrhagic stroke; Intracranial neoplasm, AVM, or aneurysm; Concurrent use of another glycoprotein IIb/IIIa receptor inhibitor; History of thrombocytopenia with previous tirofiban use; **ADRs:** BLEEDING, thrombocytopenia; **Interactions:** ↑ risk of bleeding with anticoagulants, thrombolytics, or other antiplatelet agents; **Dose:** *IV: Adults:* 0.4 mcg/kg/min × 30 min, then 0.1 mcg/kg/min, continued throughout angiography and for 12–24 hr after procedure. *Renal Impairment IV: Adults:* ↓ dose if CrCl <30 ml/min; **Availability:** *Inject:* 50 mcg/ml, 250 mcg/ml; **Monitor:** BP, HR, CBC, BUN/SCr, ACT, aPTT, bleeding; **Notes: High Alert:** Accidental overdose of antiplatelet medications has resulted in patient harm or death from internal hemorrhage or intracranial bleeding. Have second practitioner independently check original order, dose calculations, and infusion pump settings. Usually used concurrently with aspirin and heparin; heparin usually discontinued after PCI. If platelets ↓ to <90,000, discontinue tirofiban and heparin.

tizanidine (Zanaflex) **Uses:** Increased muscle tone associated with spasticity due to MS or spinal cord injury; **Class:** adrenergics; **Preg:** C; **CIs:** Hypersensitivity; Hypotension; Severe hepatic dysfunction; **ADRs:** dizziness, sedation, weakness, dyskinesia, hallucinations, nervousness, blurred vision, pharyngitis, rhinitis, ↓ BP, ↓ HR, abdominal pain, N/V/D, dry mouth, dyspepsia, constipation, ↑ LFTs, urinary frequency, rash, skin ulcers, sweating, back pain, myasthenia, paresthesia, fever, speech disorder; **Interactions:** Effects ↑ by hormonal contraceptives or alcohol; ↑ hypotension with alpha$_2$-adrenergic agonist antihypertensives; ↑ CNS depression with alcohol, CNS depressants, sedative/hypnotics, antihistamines, and opioid analgesics; Concurrent CYP1A2 inhbitors (ciprofloxacin, fluvoxamine, and others) may ↑ levels/hypotension and sedation; **Dose:** *PO: Adults:* 4 mg q 6–8 hr initially (max: 3 doses/day); ↑ by 2–4 mg/dose up to 8 mg/dose or 24 mg/day (max: 36 mg/day). *Hepatic/Renal Impairment Adults:* ↓ dose; **Availability (G):** *Tabs:* 2, 4 mg. *Caps:* 2, 4, 6 mg; **Monitor:** Muscle spasticity, BP, HR, LFTs, BUN/SCr; **Notes:** Give without regard to meals.

tobramycin (Nebcin, TOBI, Tobrex) **Uses:** Treatment of serious infections due to Gram (–) organisms (e.g., *P. aeruginosa*, *E. coli*, *Serratia*, *Acinetobacter*); **Inhaln:** Management of cystic fibrosis patients with *P. aeruginosa*; **Class:** aminoglycosides; **Preg:** D; **CIs:** Hypersensitivity to aminoglycosides; **ADRs:** vertigo, ototoxicity (vestibular and cochlear), nephrotoxicity; **Interactions:** May ↑ effects of neuromuscular blockers; ↑ risk of ototoxicity with loop diuretics; ↑ risk of nephrotoxicity with other nephrotoxic drugs (e.g., amphotericin, vancomycin, acyclovir, cisplatin); **Dose:** *IM, IV: Adults:* 3–6 mg/kg/day divided q 8 hr, or 4–7 mg/kg once daily. *IM, IV: Peds: >5 yr:* 6–7.5 mg/kg/day divided q 8 hr, up to 13 mg/kg/day divided q 6–8 hr in cystic fibrosis. *IM, IV: Peds: 1 mo–5 yr:* 7.5 mg/kg/day divided q 8 hr, up to 13 mg/kg/day divided q 6–8 hr in cystic fibrosis. *IM, IV: Neonates:* 2.5 mg/kg/dose q 8–24 hr. *Inhaln: Adults and Peds: ≥6 yr:* 300 mg bid × 28 days, then off for 28 days, then repeat cycle. *Ophth: Adults and Peds: ≥2 months Oint*—0.5 in. ribbon into affected eye bid–tid. *Soln*—1–2 gtt into affected eye q 4 hr bid–tid. *Renal Impairment IM, IV: Adults: CrCl*<60 ml/min—↓ frequency of administration or dose by levels; **Availability (G):** *Inject:* 10 mg/ml, 40 mg/ml.

Ophth soln/oint (TOBI): 0.3%. *Neb soln:* 60 mg/ml; **Monitor:** HR, BP, temp, cultures/sensitivity, CBC, BUN/SCr, I/Os, hearing; **Notes:** Use cautiously in renal dysfunction. Monitor blood levels (peak 8–10 mcg/ml; trough <1 mcg/ml). Keep patient well hydrated, if possible.

topiramate (Topamax) **Uses:** Seizures including: Partial-onset, Primary generalized tonic-clonic, Seizures due to Lennox-Gastaut syndrome; Migraine prophylaxis; **Class:** anticonvulsants; **Preg:** C; **CIs:** Hypersensitivity; Disease states predisposing to metab acidosis; Dehydration; **ADRs:** INCREASED SEIZURES, dizziness, drowsiness, fatigue, impaired concentration/memory, nervousness, psychomotor slowing, speech problems, sedation, abnormal vision, diplopia, nystagmus, acute myopia/secondary angle-closure glaucoma, nausea, anorexia, dry mouth, kidney stones, oligohydrosis (↑ in peds), hyperchloremic metab acidosis, leukopenia, wt loss, hyperthermia (↑ in peds), ataxia, paresthesia, tremor, SUICIDE ATTEMPT; **Interactions:** Levels/effects ↓ by phenytoin, carbamazepine, or valproic acid; ↑ levels/effects of phenytoin or amitriptyline; ↓ levels/effects of hormonal contraceptives, risperidone, lithium, or valproic acid; ↑ CNS depression with alcohol and CNS depressants; Acetazolamide ↑ risk of kidney stones; Valproic acid may ↑ risk of hyperammonemia/encephalopathy; **Dose:** *PO: Adults and Peds: ≥10 yr Seizures (monotherapy)*—50 mg/day initially, gradually ↑ over 6 wk to 400 mg/day in 2 divided doses. *PO: Peds: 2–16 yr:* 1–3 mg/kg/day × 1 wk then ↑ q 1–2 wk to 5–9 mg/kg/day. *PO: Adults and Peds: ≥ 17 yr Seizures (adjunctive therapy)*—25–50 mg/day ↑ by 25–50 mg/day q week up to 200–400 mg/day in 2 divided doses. *PO: Adults: Migraine prophylaxis*—25 mg at night initially, ↑ by 25 mg/day q wk to 100 mg/day in 2 divided doses. *Renal Impairment Adults and Peds:* ↓ dose by 50% for CrCl <70 ml/min; **Availability:** *Sprinkle caps:* 15, 25 mg. *Tabs:* 25, 50, 100, 200 mg; **Monitor:** Seizure frequency, migraine frequency/intensity, CBC, electrolytes, acid/base status, BUN/SCr, ammonia level (with VPA); **Notes:** Give tabs without regard to meals. Swallow, sprinkle/food mixture immediately without chewing. Gradually taper to prevent seizures and status epilepticus.

topotecan (Hycamtin) **Uses:** Metastatic ovarian CA; Small-cell lung CA; Stage IV-B cervical CA; **Class:** enzyme inhibitors; **Preg:** D; **CIs:** Hypersensitivity; Pregnancy or lactation; Pre-existing severe myelosuppression; **ADRs:** HA, fatigue, weakness, dyspnea, abdominal pain, N/V/D, anorexia, constipation, ↑ LFTs, stomatitis, alopecia, anemia, leukopenia, thrombocytopenia, arthralgia; **Interactions:** Neutropenia is prolonged by filgrastim (do not use until 24 hr after topotecan); ↑ myelosuppression with other antineoplastics or radiation therapy; ↓ antibody response/↑ adverse reactions from live-virus vaccines; **Dose:** *PO: Adults:* 2.3 mg/m²/day × 5 days q 21 days (round PO dose to nearest 0.25 mg). *IV: Adults: Ovarian and small-cell lung CA*—1.5 mg/m²/day × 5 days starting on Day 1 of a 21-day course. *Cervical CA*—75 mg/m² on Days

1, 2, and 3, followed by cisplatin on Day 1 and repeated every 21 days. *Renal Impairment PO: Adults: Ovarian and small-cell lung CA CrCl 30–49 mL/min—* 1.8 mg/m^2/day starting on day 1 of a 21-day course. *IV: Adults: CrCl 20–39 ml/min*—0.75mg/m^2/day for 5 days starting on day 1 of a 21-day course. *Cervical CA*—Standard doses only if SCr is ≤1.5 mg/dl. Do not administer if serum creatinine is >1.5 mg/dl; **Availability:** *Caps:* 0.25, 1 mg. *Inject:* 4 mg; **Monitor:** HR, RR, BP, CBC, platelets, LFTs, S/S bleeding; **Notes:** Baseline neutrophils ≥1500 cells/mm^3 and platelets of ≥100,000 cells/mm^3 are required before 1st dose. Neutropenic nadir occurs in 11 days, for 7 days. Thrombocytopenic nadir occurs in 15 days, for 5 days. Nadir of anemia occurs in 15 days. Subsequent doses should not be given until neutrophils = >1000 cells/mm^3, platelets = >100,000 cells/mm^3, and Hgb = 9.0 mg/dl. If severe neutropenia occurs, subsequent doses should be reduced by 0.25 mg/m^2 or filgrastim may be given 24 hr after topotecan. Do not open or crush caps.

torsemide (Demadex) Uses: Edema due to HF, hepatic disease, or renal impairment; HTN; **Class:** loop diuretics; **Preg:** B; **CIs:** Hypersensitivity (cross-sensitivity with thiazides and sulfonamides may occur); Hepatic coma; Anuria; Severe electrolyte depletion; **ADRs:** dizziness, HA, hearing loss, tinnitus, ↓ BP, N/V/D, photosensitivity, rash, ↑ BG, ↑ uric acid, dehydration, ↓ Ca, ↓ K, ↓ Mg, ↓ Na, hypovolemia, metab alkalosis, muscle cramps, azotemia; **Interactions:** ↑ effects with other antihypertensives; May ↑ lithium levels; ↑ risk of ototoxicity with aminoglycosides; NSAIDs may ↓ effectiveness; **Dose:** *PO, IV: Adults: HF*—10–20 mg/day (max: 200 mg/day). *Renal failure*—20 mg/day (max: 200 mg/day). *Cirrhosis*—5–10 mg/day (with aldosterone antagonist or K-sparing diuretic) (max: 40 mg/day). *HTN*—2.5–5 mg/day, may ↑ to 10 mg/day after 4–6 wk; **Availability (G):** *Tabs:* 5, 10, 20, 100 mg. *Inject:* 10 mg/ml; **Monitor:** BP, HR, electrolytes, BUN/SCr, BG, uric acid, weight, I/Os, edema; **Notes:** 10–20 mg torsemide = 40 mg furosemide. Give in AM to prevent disruption of sleep.

tramadol (Ultram, Ultram ER) Uses: Moderate-to-severe pain; **Class:** nonopioid analgesics; **Preg:** C; **CIs:** Prior sensitivity to tramadol or opioids; Acute intoxication with alcohol, sedative/hypnotics, centrally acting analgesics, opioid analgesics, or psychotropic agents; Opioid-dependent patients; *ER formulation*—Severe renal failure (CrCl <30 mL/min) or severe hepatic impairment (Child-Pugh Class C); MAOI use within 2 wk; **ADRs:** SEIZURES, dizziness, HA, somnolence, anxiety, CNS stimulation, confusion, coordination disturbance, euphoria, malaise, nervousness, sleep disorder, weakness, visual disturbances, vasodilation, constipation, N/V/D, abdominal pain, anorexia, dry mouth, dyspepsia, flatulence, menopausal symptoms, urinary retention/frequency, pruritus, sweating, hypertonia, physical/psychological dependence, tolerance; **Interactions:** ↑ CNS depression with CNS depressants, alcohol, antihistamines, sedative/hypnotics, opioid analgesics, anesthetics, or psychotropic agents; ↑ seizures with high doses of penicillins, cephalosporins, phenothiazines, opioid analgesics, or antidepressants; Carbamazepine ↑ metabolism/ ↓ effects; Concurrent MAOI use ↑ risk of ADRs; **Dose:** *PO: Adults: ≥ 18 yr Rapid titration*—50–100 mg q 4–6 hr (max: 400 mg/day or 300 mg in elderly). *Gradual titration*—25 mg/day; ↑ by 25 mg/day q 3 days to 100 mg/day, then ↑ by 50 mg/day q 3 days up to 200 mg/day *or* ER 100–300 mg/day. *Renal Impairment PO: Adults: CrCl <30 ml/min;* max 200 mg/day (IR only). *Hepatic Impairment PO: Adults:* 50 mg q 12 hr (IR only); **Availability (G):** *Tabs:* 50 mg. *ER tabs:* 100, 200, 300 mg; **Monitor:** Pain relief, RR, HR, BP, BUN/SCr, LFTs; **Notes:** Give without regard to meals. Do not crush extended-release tabs. Taper gradually to prevent withdrawal.

trandolapril (Mavik) Uses: HTN; HF post-MI; **Class:** ACEIs; **Preg:** C (1st tri), D (2nd and 3rd tri); **CIs:** Previous sensitivity/ intolerance to ACEIs; **ADRs:** dizziness, cough, ↓ BP, ↑ SCr, ↑ K, ANGIOEDEMA; **Interactions:** ↑ effects with other antihypertensives; ↑ risk of hyperkalemia with ARBs, K supplements, K salt substitutes, K-sparing diuretics, or NSAIDs; NSAIDs may ↓ effectiveness; ↑ lithium levels; **Dose:** *PO: Adults: HTN/HF post-MI*—1–4 mg/day. *Renal Impairment PO: Adults:* ↓ dose if CrCl <30 ml/min. *Hepatic Impairment PO: Adults:* Start with 0.5 mg/day; **Availability (G):** *Tabs:* 1, 2, 4 mg; **Monitor:** BP, HR, wt, edema, BUN/SCr, K; **Notes:** Correct volume depletion. Advise patient on S/S angioedema and avoidance of K salt substitutes.

tranylcypromine (Parnate) Uses: Treatment of major depressive episode without melancholia; **Class:** MAOIs; **Preg:** C; **CIs:** Hypersensitivity; Liver disease; Cerebrovascular disease; CV disease; HTN; Pheochromocytoma; History of HA; Concurrent use of meperidine, SSRI antidepressants, CNS depressants, bupropion, buspirone, sympathomimetics, MAOIs, dextromethorphan, alcohol, general anesthetics, or antihistamines; Foods high in tyramine; Suicidal tendency; **ADRs:** SEIZURES, confusion, dizziness, HA, hallucinations, insomnia, abnormal thinking, nausea, abdominal pain, CP, orthostatic hypotension, dry mouth, HYPERTENSIVE CRISIS, edema, ↑ HR, ↑ LFTs, sexual dysfunction, urinary retention, AGRANULOCYTOSIS, leukopenia, thrombocytopenia, alopecia, rash, muscle spasm; **Interactions:** Serotonin syndrome with cyclobenzaprine, anorexiants, TCAs, or SSRI antidepressants; Hypertensive crisis may occur with amphetamines, methyldopa, buspirone, levodopa, dopamine, epinephrine, norepinephrine, reserpine, methylphenidate, or vasoconstrictors; Hyper/hypotension, coma, seizures, resp depression, and death may occur with meperidine (avoid use within 2–3 wk); ↑ hypotension with antihypertensives, spinal anesthesia, opioids, or barbiturates; ↑ hypoglycemia with insulins or oral hypoglycemic agents; Risk of seizures may be ↑ with tramadol; **Dose:** *PO: Adults:* 30 mg/day in 2 divided doses (morning and afternoon); after 2 wk ↑ by 10 mg/day, q 1–3 wk, up to 60 mg/day; **Availability:** *Tabs:* 10 mg; **Monitor:** Mental status, mood, LFTs, CBC, BP; **Notes:** Instruct patient to avoid tyramine-containing foods, tryptophan, and caffeine. Do not give in the evening due to psychomotor stimulating effects. Abrupt discontinuation may precipitate withdrawal.

trastuzumab (Herceptin) Uses: Metastatic breast tumors that display overexpression of the human EGRF 2 (HER2); **Class:** monoclonal antibodies; **Preg:** B; **CIs:** Pre-existing pulmonary/cardiac dysfunction; Hypersensitivity to trastuzumab or Chinese hamster ovary cell proteins; **ADRs:** dizziness, HA, insomnia, weakness, depression, dyspnea, cough, pharyngitis, rhinitis, sinusitis, CARDIOTOXICITY, ↑ HR, <u>abdominal pain</u>, <u>anorexia</u>, <u>N/V/D</u>, <u>rash</u>, acne, herpes simplex edema, anemia, leukopenia, <u>back/bone pain</u>, arthralgia, neuropathy, paresthesia, peripheral neuritis, HYPERSENSITIVITY REACTIONS, <u>chills</u>, <u>fever</u>, <u>infection</u>, flu-like syndrome; **Interactions:** Concurrent anthracycline therapy ↑ risk of cardiotoxicity; Levels ↑ by paclitaxel; **Dose:** *IV: Adults:* 4 mg/kg × 1, then 2 mg/kg q wk; **Availability:** *Inject:* 440 mg; **Monitor:** HR, RR, BP, LVEF, CBC, S/S cardiac/pulmonary toxicity; **Notes:** Pretreatment with acetaminophen, diphenhydramine, and/or meperidine may help ↓ infusion-related reactions. Do not give with D5W. Do not give IV push or bolus. Discontinue if HF develops.

trazodone (Desyrel) Uses: Major depression; **Class:** antidepressants; **Preg:** C; **CIs:** Hypersensitivity; Recovery period after MI; Concurrent MAOI therapy; Seizure disorder; Suicidal behavior; **ADRs:** <u>drowsiness</u>, confusion, dizziness, fatigue, hallucinations, HA, insomnia, nightmares, slurred speech, syncope, weakness, blurred vision, tinnitus, ↓ <u>BP</u>, arrhythmias, CP, HTN, ↑ HR, <u>dry mouth</u>, altered taste, constipation, N/V/D, excess salivation, flatulence, hematuria, ED, priapism, urinary frequency, rash, anemia, leukopenia, myalgia, tremor; **Interactions:** ↑ digoxin or phenytoin levels; ↑ CNS depression with CNS depressants, alcohol, opioid analgesics, and sedative/hypnotics; ↑ hypotension with antihypertensives, alcohol, or nitrates; Fluoxetine ↑ levels/toxicity; CYP3A4 inhibitors ↑ levels/toxicity; CYP3A4 inducers ↓ levels/effects; Do not use within 14 days of MAOIs; ↑ PT with warfarin; **Dose:** *PO: Adults: Depression*—150 mg/day divided tid; ↑ by 50 mg/day q 3–4 days until desired response (max: 600 mg/day). *Insomnia*—25–100 mg at bedtime (max: 200 mg/day). *PO: Geriatric Patients:* 25–50 mg/day; may ↑ q 3–4 days to 75–150 mg/day; **Availability (G):** *Tabs:* 50, 100, 150, 300 mg; **Monitor:** BP, HR, ECG, mood, CBC; **Notes:** Administer with or immediately after meals to minimize nausea and dizziness.

triamcinolone (inhalation/intranasal) (Azmacort, Nasacort AQ, Tri-Nasal) Uses: Inhaln: Maintenance treatment of asthma (prophylactic therapy); **Intranasal:** Seasonal and perennial allergic rhinitis; **Class:** corticosteroids; **Preg:** C; **CIs:** Hypersensitivity; Acute asthma attack/status asthmaticus; Active untreated infections; **ADRs:** HA, dizziness, cataracts, dysphonia, epistaxis, nasal irritation, nasal stuffiness, oropharyngeal fungal infections, pharyngitis, rhinorrhea, sinusitis, sneezing, tearing eyes, nausea, bronchospasm, cough, wheezing, adrenal suppression (↑ dose, long-term therapy only), ↓ growth (peds); **Interactions:** None known; **Dose:** *Inhaln: Adults and Peds: >12 yr:* 2 inhaln tid–qid or 4 inhalations bid (max: 16 inhaln/day). *Inhaln: Peds 6–12 yr:* 1–2 inhalations tid–qid or 2–4 inhaln bid (max: 12 inhaln/day). *Intranasal: Adults and Peds: >12 yr Tri-Nasal*—2 sprays in each nostril/day (max: 4 sprays in each nostril/day). *Nasacort AQ*—2 sprays in each nostril/day. *Intranasal: Peds: 6–11 yr Nasacort AQ*—1 spray in each nostril once daily (max: 2 sprays in each nostril/day); **Availability:** *Inhaln aerosol:* 75 mcg/inhaln. *Nasal spray (Nasacort AQ):* 55 mcg/spray. *Nasal spray (Tri-Nasal):* 50 mcg/spray; **Monitor:** RR, lung sounds, PFTs, growth rate (in peds), S/S asthma/allergies; **Notes:** Prime nasal spray/MDI canister prior to 1st use; clear nasal passages before nasal spray use. Rinse mouth with water or mouthwash after MDI use. Decrease dose to lowest amount required to control symptoms. Not for acute asthma attacks.

triamcinolone (systemic/topical) (Aristospan, Kenalog, Triderm, Triesence) **Uses:** Treatment of: Inflammatory, Allergic, Hematologic, Neoplastic, Autoimmune disorders; Replacement therapy in adrenal insufficiency; *Topical:* Inflammation and pruritis associated with various allergic/immunologic skin problems; **Class:** corticosteroids; **Preg:** C; **CIs:** Active untreated infections; **ADRs:** depression, euphoria, personality changes, restlessness, cataracts, ↑ BP, PEPTIC ULCERATION, anorexia, N/V, acne, hirsutism, petechiae, allergic contact dermatitis, atrophy, burning sensation, dryness, folliculitis, irritation, ↓ wound healing, adrenal suppression, ↑ BG, fluid retention (long-term high doses), ↓ K, THROMBOEMBOLISM, ↑ wt, muscle wasting, osteoporosis, muscle pain, cushingoid appearance, infection; **Interactions:** Additive hypokalemia with thiazide and loop diuretics, or amphotericin B; May ↑ requirement for insulins or oral hypoglycemic agents; Phenytoin, phenobarbital, and rifampin may ↓ levels; ↑ risk of adverse GI effects with NSAIDs; **Dose:** *PO: Adults and Peds: Adrenocortical insufficiency*—4–12 mg/day. *Dermatologic/rheumatic/asthmatic disorders*—8–16 mg/day. *IM: Adults: Acetonide*—2.5–60 mg/day. *IM: Peds: Acetonide/hexacetonide*—0.03–0.2 mg/kg q 1–7 days. *Intra-articular: Adults and Peds: >12 yr:* 2.5–40 mg (acetonide); 2–20 mg (hexacetonide). *Intra-articular: Peds: 6–12 yr:* 2.5–15 mg. *Topical: Adults:* Apply tid–qid. *Topical: Peds:* Apply daily–bid; **Availability (G):** *Tabs:* 4 mg. *Inject (acetonide):* 10 mg/ml, 40 mg/ml. *Injection (hexacetonide):* 5 mg/ml, 20 mg/ml. *Cream/Oint:*

T

0.025%, 0.1%, 0.5%. *Lotion:* 0.025%, 0.1%. *Spray:* 0.2 mg/2 sec spray; **Monitor:** Systemic therapy: S/S adrenal insufficiency, wt/ht (peds), edema, electrolytes, BG, pain. Top therapy: skin condition (inflammation, erythema, pruritis); **Notes:** Do not give injection IV. Give PO with food. Use lowest possible dose to treat condition.

triamterene (Dyrenium) Uses: Counteracts K loss from other diuretics; Edema/HTN; **Class:** K-sparing diuretics; **Preg:** C; **CIs:** Hypersensitivity; Hyperkalemia; Hepatic dysfunction; Renal insufficiency (avoid use if CrCl <10 ml/min); History of gout or kidney stones; **ADRs:** dizziness, arrhythmias, N/V, ED, bluish urine, nephrolithiasis, photosensitivity, ↑ <u>K</u>, ↓ Na, blood dyscrasias, muscle cramps, allergic reactions; **Interactions:** ↑ hypotension with alcohol, other antihypertensive agents, or nitrates; ACEIs, indomethacin, ARBs, K supplements, or cyclosporine ↑ risk of hyperkalemia; ↓ lithium excretion; Effects ↓ by NSAIDs; ↓ effects of folic acid; ↑ toxicity from amantadine; **Dose:** *PO: Adults:* 25–100 mg/day (max: 300 mg/day). *PO: Peds:* 2–4 mg/kg/day in divided doses daily or every other day (max: 6 mg/kg/day or 300 mg/day). *Hepatic Impairment Adults and Peds:* ↓ dose for cirrhosis; **Availability:** *Caps:* 50, 100 mg; **Monitor:** K, Na, CBC, BUN/SCr, I/Os, wt, BP; **Notes:** Administer in AM to avoid interrupting sleep pattern from urination. Instruct patient to avoid salt substitutes and foods that contain high levels of K or Na and to use sunscreen.

triazolam (Halcion) Uses: Short-term management of insomnia; **Class:** BZs; **Preg:** X; **CIs:** Prior sensitivity to other BZs; Pre-existing CNS depression; Uncontrolled severe pain; Suicidal tendency; **ADRs:** abnormal thinking, behavior changes, <u>dizziness</u>, <u>excessive sedation</u>, <u>hangover</u>, <u>HA</u>, anterograde amnesia, confusion, hallucinations, lethargy, mental depression, paradoxical excitation, blurred vision, constipation, diarrhea, N/V, rash, physical/psychological dependence, tolerance; **Interactions:** Cimetidine, erythromycin, fluconazole, itraconazole, ketoconazole, indinavir, nelfinavir, ritonavir, or saquinavir ↓ metabolism/ ↑ effects, ↑ CNS depression with alcohol, antidepressants, antihistamines, and opioid analgesics; ↓ effects of levodopa; ↑ toxicity of zidovudine; Isoniazid ↓ excretion/↑ effects; Sedative effects ↓ by theophylline; **Dose:** *PO: Adults:* 0.125–0.25 mg (up to 0.5 mg) at bedtime. *PO: Geriatric Patients or Debilitated Patients:* 0.125 mg at bedtime; **Availability (G):** *Tabs:* 0.125, 0.25 mg; **Monitor:** Sleep patterns, HR, BP, RR, S/S CNS depression; **Notes:** Do not discontinue abruptly.

T

trimethoprim/sulfamethoxazole (Bactrim, Bactrim DS, Septra, Septra DS, SMZ-TMP, Sulfatrim, Sulfatrim DS) Uses: Treatment of: Bronchitis, *Shigella* enteritis, OM, PCP, UTIs, Traveler's diarrhea; Prevention of PCP; **Class:** folate antagonists, sulfonamides; **Preg:** C, D (term); **CIs:** Hypersensitivity to sulfonamides or trimethoprim; Megaloblastic anemia secondary to folate deficiency; Severe hepatic or renal impairment (CrCl <15 ml/min); Pregnancy/lactation; Infants <2 mo; **ADRs:** fatigue, hallucinations, HA, insomnia, mental depression, PSEUDOMEMBRANOUS COLITIS, N/V/D, ↑ LFTs, stomatitis, cholestatic jaundice, crystalluria, SJS, TEN, rash, photosensitivity, AGRANULOCYTOSIS, APLASTIC ANEMIA, hemolytic anemia, leukopenia, megaloblastic anemia, thrombocytopenia, phlebitis at IV site, fever; **Interactions:** ↑ levels of and exaggerate folic acid deficiency caused by phenytoin; ↑ effects of sulfonylurea oral hypoglycemics, phenytoin, and warfarin; ↑ toxicity of methotrexate; ↑ nephrotoxicity of cyclosporine; **Dose:** *PO, IV: Adults and Peds: >2 mo Mild-to-moderate infections*—8–10 mg TMP/kg/day divided q 6–12 hr. *Serious infection/PCP*—15–20 mg TMP/kg/day divided q 6–8 hr. *PO: Adults: UTI/chronic bronchitis*—1 double-strength tab (160 mg TMP/800 mg SMZ) q 12 hr. *PO: Adults: PCP prophylaxis*—1 double-strength tab (160 mg TMP/800 mg SMZ) daily or 3×/week. *PO: Peds: >1 mo PCP prophylaxis*—150 mg TMP/m²/day divided q 12 hr on 3 consecutive days/wk (max: 320 mg TMP/1600 mg SMZ/day) *or* 150 mg TMP/m²/day as single daily dose on 3 consecutive days/wk *or* 150 mg TMP/m²/day divided q 12 hr × 7 days/wk *or* 150 mg TMP/m²/day divided q 12 hr on 3 alternative days/wk. *Renal Impairment Adults and Peds:* ↓ dose if CrCl = 15–30 ml/min; do not use if CrCl <15 ml/min; **Availability (G):** *Tabs:* 80 mg TMP/400 mg SMZ (single strength), 160 mg TMP/800 mg SMZ (double strength). *Oral susp:* 40 mg TMP/200 mg SMZ per 5 ml. *Inject:* 16 mg TMP/80 mg SMZ per ml; **Monitor:** BP, HR, RR, temp, CBC, cultures/sensitivity, LFTs, BUN/SCr, I/Os, S/S rash; **Notes:** Maintain UO of at least 1200–1500 ml daily to prevent crystalluria and stone formation.

urokinase (Abbokinase) **Uses:** PE; DVT; MI; Catheter clearance; **Class:** thrombolytics; **Preg:** B; **CIs:** Active bleeding; CVA; Recent (within 2 mo) intracranial or intraspinal surgery or trauma; Intracranial neoplasm, AVM, or aneurysm; Severe uncontrolled HTN; Hypersensitivity; **ADRs:** INTRACRANIAL HEMORRHAGE, epistaxis, bronchospasm, hemoptysis, ↓ BP, N/V, ecchymoses, flushing, BLEEDING, phlebitis, musculoskeletal pain, fever; **Interactions:** Aspirin, NSAIDs, warfarin, heparin, LMWH, abciximab, eptifibatide, tirofiban, clopidogrel, ticlopidine, or dipyridamole ↑ bleeding risk; Effects ↓ by antifibrinolytic agents; **Dose:** *IV: Adults: DVT/PE*—4400 units/kg load, f/b 4400 units/kg/hr × 12 hr. *MI*—750,000 units intracoronary over 2 hr. *Catheter clearance*—5,000–10,000 units in each lumen, dwell 1–4 hr, then aspirate *or* 200 units/kg/hr IV infusion in each lumen × 12–48 hr; **Availability:** *Inject:* 250,000 units; **Monitor:** BP, HR, CBC with platelets, aPTT, UA, S/S bleeding; **Notes:** Do not shake reconstituted soln; use immediately after mixing; may use <0.45 micron filter.

valacyclovir (Valtrex) **Uses:** Initial and recurrent genital herpes; Herpes zoster (shingles); Herpes labialis (cold sores); **Class:** purine analogues; **Preg:** B; **CIs:** Hypersensitivity to acyclovir or valacyclovir; **ADRs:** SEIZURES, HA, anorexia, N/V/D, ↑ LFTs, ↑ BUN/SCr, crystalluria, rash, THROMBOTIC THROMBOCYTOPENIC PURPURA/ HEMOLYTIC UREMIC SYNDROME (high doses in immunosuppressed patients); **Interactions:** Probenecid ↑ levels; Concurrent use of other nephrotoxic drugs ↑ risk of renal dysfunction; **Dose:** *PO: Adults: Zoster (shingles)* 1 g tid × 7 days. *Genital herpes*—Initial episode: 1 g bid × 10 days; recurrence: 500 mg bid × 3 days; chronic suppressive therapy: 1 g daily (500 mg daily if <9 recurrences/yr; 500 mg bid if HIV-infected); reduction of transmission: 500 mg daily (source partner). *Herpes labialis*—2 g bid × 1 day. *Renal Impairment PO: Adults:* ↓ dose if CrCl <50 ml/min; **Availability:** *Tabs:* 500 mg, 1 g; **Monitor:** BUN/SCr, CBC, lesions; **Notes:** Give without regard to meals. Start ASAP after herpes simplex symptoms appear and within 72 hr of herpes zoster outbreak.

valganciclovir (Valcyte) **Uses:** CMV prevention/treatment; **Class:** antivirals; **Preg:** C; **CIs:** Prior sensitivity to valganciclovir or ganciclovir; ANC <500/mm^3; Platelet count <25,000/mm^3; Hgb <8 g/dl; **ADRs:** SEIZURES, HA, insomnia, agitation, dizziness, hallucinations, psychosis, retinal detachment, abdominal pain, N/V/D, ↑ BUN/SCr, APLASTIC ANEMIA, NEUTROPENIA, THROMBOCYTOPENIA, anemia, granulocytopenia, paresthesia, peripheral neuropathy, fever; **Interactions:** Probenecid ↑ levels; Concurrent use of other nephrotoxic drugs ↑ risk of renal dysfunction; ↑ risk of immunosuppression with other immunosuppressive drugs; ↑ levels/toxicity of didanosine; **Dose:** *PO: Adults: CMV retinitis*—900 mg bid × 21 days, then 900 mg/day. *CMV prevention post–transplant*—900 mg/day beginning within 10 days after transplant and continuing until 100 days post-transplant. *Renal Impairment PO: Adults:* ↓ dose if CrCl <60 ml/min; **Availability:** *Tabs:* 450 mg; **Monitor:** BUN/SCr. CBC, retinal exam, S/S bleeding and infection; **Notes:** Take with meals. Do not crush tabs. Do not use in dialysis patients (CrCl <10 ml/min).

V

valproic acid and derivatives (Depakote, Depakote ER, Depacon, Depakene) **Uses:** Monotherapy and adjunctive therapy for simple and complex absence or partial seizures; **Divalproex sodium only:** Manic episodes associated with bipolar disorder, Prevention of migraine; **Class:** anticonvulsants; **Preg:** D; **CIs:** Hypersensitivity; Hepatic impairment; Known/suspected urea cycle disorders (may result in fatal hyperammonemic encephalopathy); Pregnancy/lactation; Peds <2 yr (↑ risk for potentially fatal hepatotoxicity); **ADRs:** agitation, dizziness, HA, insomnia, sedation, confusion, depression, peripheral edema, visual disturbances, HEPATOTOXICITY, PANCREATITIS, abdominal pain, anorexia, diarrhea, indigestion, N/V, ↑ appetite, alopecia, rash, ↑ wt, leukopenia, thrombocytopenia, HYPERAMMONEMIA, HYPOTHERMIA, tremor, ataxia; **Interactions:** ↑ risk of bleeding with warfarin; Blood levels/toxicity ↑ by aspirin or felbamate; ↑ CNS depression with CNS depressants, including alcohol, antihistamines, antidepressants, opioid analgesics, and sedative/hypnotics; MAOIs and antidepressants may ↓ seizure threshold and ↓ effectiveness of valproate; Carbamazepine, phenobarbital, phenytoin, or rifampin may ↓ levels/effects; May ↑ levels/toxicity of carbamazepine, diazepam, amitriptyline, nortriptyline, ethosuximide, lamotrigine, phenobarbital, phenytoin, or zidovudine; Use with topiramate may ↑ risk of hyperammonemia; Carbapenems may ↓ blood levels; **Dose: Regular-release and DR formulations usually given in 2–4 divided doses daily; ER formulation (Depakote ER) usually given once daily.** *PO: Adults and Peds: ≥10 yr Complex partial seizures*—10–15 mg/kg/day; ↑ by 5–10 mg/kg q wk until therapeutic response achieved (max: 60 mg/kg/day). *PO: Adults and Peds: >2 yr (≥10 yr for Depakote ER) Simple and complex absence seizures*—15 mg/kg/day; ↑ by 5–10 mg/kg q wk until therapeutic response achieved (max: 60 mg/kg/day). *IV: Adults and Peds:* Same daily dose as PO; switch to PO as soon as possible. *Rect: Adults and Peds:* Dilute syrup 1:1 with water for use as a retention enema. Give 17–20 mg/kg load, maintenance 10–15 mg/kg/dose q 8 hr. *PO: Adults: Mania associated with bipolar disorder (Depakote)*—750 mg/day in divided doses initially, titrated rapidly to desired clinical effect or trough plasma levels of 85–125 mcg/ml (max: 60 mg/kg/day). *Depakote ER*—25 mg/kg once daily initially; titrated rapidly to desired clinical effect of trough plasma levels of 85–125 mcg/ml (max: 60 mg/kg/day). *PO: Adults and Peds: ≥16 yr Migraine prevention (Depakote only)*—250 mg bid (max: 1000 mg/day). *Depakote ER*—500 mg/day × 1 wk, then ↑ to 1000 mg/day; **Availability (G):** *Valproic Acid (generic available) Caps:* 250 mg. *Syrup:* 250 mg/5 ml. *Valproate Sodium Inject:* 100 mg/ml. *Divalproex Sodium DR tabs (Depakote):* 125, 250, 500 mg. *Caps (sprinkle):* 125 mg. *ER tabs (Depakote ER):* 250, 500 mg; **Monitor:** CBC, LFTs, amylase, lipase, serum ammonia, valproate levels, seizure frequency, mood (bipolar disorder), migraine frequency; **Notes:** Therapeutic levels for epilepsy: 50–100 mcg/ml; for mania: 85–125 mcg/ml. Give with meals to minimize GI irritation. ER and DR tabs should be swallowed whole, do not break or chew. Do not give tabs with milk or carbonated beverages. Sprinkles may be swallowed whole or opened and capsule contents sprinkled on a teaspoonful of soft, cool food; do not chew sprinkle/food mixture.

valsartan (Diovan) Uses: HTN; HF; Patients with LV dysfunction post-MI; **Class:** ARBs; **Preg:** C (1st tri), D (2nd and 3rd tri); **CIs:** Hypersensitivity; Pregnancy/lactation; **ADRs:** <u>dizziness</u>, fatigue, HA, ↓ BP, edema, ↑ LFTs, ↑ K, abdominal pain, diarrhea, nausea, ↑ SCr, arthralgia, back pain; **Interactions:** ↑ effects with other antihypertensives; ↑ risk of hyperkalemia with ACEIs, K supplements, K salt substitutes, K-sparing diuretics, or NSAIDs; NSAIDs may ↓ effectiveness; **Dose:** *PO: Adults: HTN*—80–160 mg/day (max: 320 mg/day). *HF*—40–160 mg bid (max: 320 mg/day). *Post-MI*—20–160 mg bid; **Availability:** *Tabs:* 40, 80, 160, 320 mg; **Monitor:** BP, HR, wt, edema, BUN/SCr, K; **Notes:** Can be used in patients intolerant to ACEI (due to cough); just as likely as ACEI to cause ↑ K and ↑ SCr.

vancomycin (Vancocin) **Uses:** **IV:** Treatment of Gram-positive infections including MRSA; **PO:** *C. difficile* pseudomembranous colitis; **Class:** antibiotics; **Preg:** C; **CIs:** Hypersensitivity; **ADRs:** ototoxicity, ↓ BP, N/V, nephrotoxicity, rash, eosinophilia, phlebitis, fever, "red man" syndrome, superinfection; **Interactions:** ↑ ototoxicity and nephrotoxicity with aspirin, aminoglycosides, cyclosporine, cisplatin, and loop diuretics; **Dose:** *IV: Adults:* 2–3 g/day in 2–4 divided doses; adjust dose based on trough concentrations. *IV: Peds: >1 mo:* 10–15 mg/kg q 6 hr. *CNS infection*—15 mg/kg q 6 hr (max: 1 g/dose). *IV: Neonates:* 10–20 mg/kg q 8–24 hr. *IT: Adults:* Up to 20 mg/day. *IT: Peds:* 5–20 mg/day. *IT: Neonates:* 5–10 mg/day. *PO: Adults:* 125–500 mg q 6 hr. *PO: Peds:* 10 mg/kg q 6 hr. *Renal Impairment IV: Adults: CrCl<50 ml/min*—↓ frequency of administration/dose or dose by levels; **Availability (G):** *Caps:* 125, 250 mg. *Inject:* 500 mg, 1, 5, 10 g; **Monitor:** BUN/SCr, trough levels (5–20 mcg/ml), CBC, cultures, hearing, S/S infection; **Notes:** Give over 60 min; if red-man syndrome occurs (↓ BP, maculopapular rash on face/neck/upper extremities/trunk) ↓ infusion rate (may also treat with antihistamines and/or corticosteroids).

vardenafil (Levitra) **Uses:** ED; **Class:** PDE-5 inhibitors; **Preg:** B; **CIs:** Hypersensitivity; Concurrent use of nitrates; Uncontrolled HTN (BP >170/110 mmHg), hypotension (BP <90/50 mmHg), angina during intercourse, HF, or CAD; Life-threatening arrhythmias, stroke, or MI within 6 mo; **ADRs:** HA, hearing loss, nasal congestion, abnormal vision, ↓ BP, dyspepsia, priapism, flushing, back pain, myalgia; **Interactions:** CYP3A4 inhibitors may ↑ levels/toxicity, CYP3A4 inducers may ↓ levels/effects; Nitrates and alpha-adrenergic blockers may cause serious, life-threatening hypotension; **Dose:** *PO: Adults:* 5–20 mg 1 hr prior to sexual activity (max: one dose/day). *Concurrent use of alpha-blockers (with Viagra)*—Initial dose: 5 mg/24 hr. *Concurrent use of atazanavir, clarithromycin, indinavir, itraconazole/ketoconazole 400 mg/day, ritonavir, or saquinavir*—Initial dose: 2.5 mg/24 hr. *Concurrent use of erythromycin or itraconazole/ketoconazole 200 mg/day*—Initial dose of 5 mg/24 hr. *Hepatic Impairment PO: Adults: Moderate hepatic impairment*—5–10 mg; **Availability:** *Tabs:* 2.5, 5, 10, 20 mg; **Monitor:** Response, ADRs; **Notes:** Give without regard to meals. Patients should be on stable dose of alpha-blocker therapy before starting therapy with vardenafil.

V

varenicline (Chantix) **Uses:** Smoking cessation; **Class:** nicotine agonists; **Preg:** C; **CIs:** Hypersensitivity; Renal impairment; Psychiatric illness; **ADRs:** ↓ attention span, anxiety, depression, insomnia, irritability, dizziness, restlessness, abnormal dreams, agitation, aggression, disorientation, dissociation, HA, psychomotor hyperactivity, gingivitis, N/V/D, ↑ appetite, constipation, dyspepsia, dysphagia, enterocolitis, flatulence, ↑ LFTs; **Interactions:** Smoking cessation ↓ metabolism/↑ effects of theophylline, warfarin, and insulin; **Dose:** *PO: Adults:* 0.5 mg/day × 3 days, followed by 0.5 mg bid × 4 days, then 1 mg bid. *Renal Impairment PO: Adults: Renal*—↓ dose for CrCl <30 ml/min; **Availability:** *Tabs:* 0.5, 1 mg; **Monitor:** LFTs, BUN/SCr, changes in mood/behavior; **Notes:** Start 1 wk prior to smoking cessation. Give with food and full glass of water. Nausea may require ↓ dose.

vasopressin (Pitressin) Uses: Diabetes insipidus; GI hemorrhage; Vasodilatory shock; **Class:** antidiuretic hormones; **Preg:** C; **CIs:** HF; CAD; HTN; Renal impairment; **ADRs:** dizziness, HA, MI, angina, CP, abdominal cramps, flatulence, heartburn, N/V/D, perioral blanching, sweating, trembling, fever; **Interactions:** Antidiuretic effect ↓ by alcohol, lithium, demeclocycline, heparin, or norepinephrine; Antidiuretic effect ↑ by carbamazepine, chlorpropamide, clofibrate, TCAs, or fludrocortisone; Vasopressor effect ↑ by ganglionic blocking agents; **Dose:** *IM, Subcut: Adults and Peds: Diabetes Insipidus*—2.5–10 units bid–qid prn. *Continuous infusion*—0.0005 units/kg/hr titrate q 30 min to max of 0.01 units/kg/hr. *GI hemorrhage*—0.2–0.4 units/min. *IV: Adults: Pulseless arrest (ACLS guidelines)*—40 units × 1. *Septic shock*—0.01–0.04 units/min continuous infusion; **Availability (G):** *Inject:* 20 units/ml; **Monitor:** BP, HR, ECG, I/Os, wt, urine osmolality, urine specific gravity, electrolytes; **Notes:** High doses may lead to water intoxication.

venlafaxine (Effexor, Effexor XR) Uses: Major depressive disorder; GAD (XR only); SAD (XR only); Panic disorder (XR only); **Class:** SNRIs; **Preg:** C; **CIs:** Hypersensitivity; Concurrent MAOI therapy; **ADRs:** SEIZURES, SUICIDAL THOUGHTS (↑ in peds), abnormal dreams, anxiety, dizziness, HA, insomnia, nervousness, weakness, drowsiness, rhinitis, visual disturbances, CP, HTN, ↑ HR, abdominal pain, altered taste, anorexia, constipation, dry mouth, dyspepsia, N/V/D, ↓ wt, sexual dysfunction, urinary frequency, urinary retention, ecchymoses, itching, rash, paresthesia, chills, yawning; **Interactions:** ↑ risk of toxicity with MAOIs (discontinue for ≥2 wk); ↑ CNS depression with other CNS depressants including alcohol, antihistamines, opioids, and sedative/hypnotics; ↑ risk of serotonin syndrome with SSRIs, sibutramine, and triptans; CYP2D6 inhibitors and CYP3A4 inhibitors may ↑ levels/effects; **Dose:** *PO: Adults: Depression*—IR: 75 mg/day in 2–3 divided doses; may ↑ by 75 mg/day q 4 days, up to 225 mg/day (max: 375 mg/day in 3 divided doses); XR: 37.5–75 mg daily × 4–7 days; may ↑ q 4 days up to 225 mg/day. *GAD, SAD*—XR: 37.5–75 mg/day × 4–7 days; may ↑ q 4 days up to 225 mg/day. *Panic disorder*—37.5 mg/day × 1 wk; may ↑ by

V

75 mg/day at 1-wk intervals (max: 225 mg/day). *Renal Impairment PO: Adults:* ↓ dose if CrCl ≤70 ml/min. *Hepatic Impairment PO: Adults: Moderate hepatic impairment*—↓ dose by 50%; **Availability (G):** *Tabs:* 25, 37.5, 50, 75, 100 mg. *ER caps:* 37.5, 75, 150 mg; **Monitor:** BP, HR, mood, mental status, wt, LFTs, BUN/SCr; **Notes:** Give with food. ER caps should be swallowed whole; do not crush, break, or chew. May open caps and sprinkle on applesauce. Therapy for >6 months should be gradually tapered upon discontinuation.

verapamil (Calan, Calan SR, Covera-HS, Isoptin SR, Verelan, Verelan PM) **Uses:** HTN; Angina (chronic, stable, or vasospastic); Supraventricular tachyarrhythmias (AF, AFl, or PSVT) (to control ventricular rate); **Class:** Ca channel blockers; **Preg:** C; **CIs:** Hypersensitivity; 2nd/3rd-degree heart block or sick sinus syndrome (in absence of pacemaker); Severe LV dysfunction or cardiogenic shock; BP <90 mmHg; AF or AFl and a bypass tract (e.g., WPW syndrome); **ADRs:** dizziness, HA, weakness, dyspnea, HF, ↓ HR, edema, ↓ BP, syncope, <u>constipation</u>, nausea, flushing, gingival hyperplasia; **Interactions:** ↑ effects with other antihypertensives; CYP3A4 inhibitors may ↑ levels/toxicity; CYP3A4 inducers may ↓ levels/effects; May ↑ levels/toxicity of CYP3A4 substrates; NSAIDs may ↓ effectiveness; May ↑ digoxin levels/toxicity; ↑ risk of bradycardia with digoxin, beta-blockers, or clonidine; **Dose:** *PO: Adults: Angina*—80–120 mg tid (IR) (max: 480 mg/day). *HTN*—80 mg tid (IR) (max: 320 mg/day) *or* 120–360 mg/day (SR) in 1–2 divided doses *or* 120–400 mg daily (ER). *PO: Peds: 1–5 yr:* 4–8 mg/kg/day in 3 divided doses. *PO: Peds: >5 yr:* 80 mg q 6–8 hr. *IV: Adults: Supraventricular arrhythmias*—2.5–5 mg; may repeat with 5–10 mg after 15–30 min (max total dose: 20 mg). *IV: Peds: 1–15 yr:* 0.1–0.3 mg/kg (max: 5 mg/dose); may repeat in 15 min (max repeat dose: 10 mg). *IV: Peds: <1 yr:* 0.1–0.2 mg/kg; may repeat q 30 min prn. *Renal Impairment Adults and Peds:* ↓ dose if CrCl <10 ml/min. *Hepatic Impairment Adults and Peds:* ↓ dose in cirrhosis; **Availability (G):** *Tabs:* 40, 80, 120 mg. *ER tabs:* 120, 180, 240 mg. *ER caps:* 100, 200, 300 mg. *SR caps:* 120, 180, 240, 360 mg. *Inject:* 2.5 mg/ml; **Monitor:** BP, HR, ECG, peripheral edema, S/S angina, S/S HF; **Notes:** Instruct patient to avoid grapefruit juice (may ↑ effects). Do not open, crush, break, or chew SR/ER caps/tabs.

vinBLAStine (Velban) **Uses:** Chemotherapy of malignancies including: Lymphomas; Nonseminomatous testicular carcinoma, Advanced breast CA; **Class:** vinca alkaloids; **Preg:** D; **CIs:** Hypersensitivity; Pregnancy/lactation; Active infection; Decreased bone marrow reserve; **ADRs:** SEIZURES, depression, neurotoxicity, weakness, BRONCHOSPASM, ↑ BP, <u>constipation</u>, <u>N/V</u>, anorexia, diarrhea, stomatitis, gonadal suppression, alopecia, dermatitis, vesiculation, <u>anemia</u>, <u>leukopenia</u>, <u>thrombocytopenia</u>, <u>phlebitis at IV site</u>, ↑ uric acid, paresthesia; **Interactions:** Additive bone marrow depression with other antineoplastics or radiation therapy; ↑ risk of bronchospasm in patients previously treated with mitomycin; May ↓ antibody response/↑ risk of ADRs to live-virus vaccines; May ↓ phenytoin levels; **Dose:** *IV: Adults and Peds:* 4–20 mg/m² q 7–10 days *or* 1.5–2 mg/m²/day continuous infusion × 5 days *or* 0.1–0.5 mg/kg/wk. *IV: Hepatic Impairment Adults and Peds:* ↓ dose by 50% if serum bilirubin >3 mg/dl; **Availability (G):** Soln for *inject:* 1 mg/ml. *Powder for inject:* 10 mg; **Monitor:** BP, HR, RR, neuro status, S/S bronchospasm/bleeding, I/Os, CBC (with diff), LFTs, uric acid; **Notes:** Refer to individual protocols. **High Alert:** Fatalities have occurred with chemotherapeutic agents. Before administering, clarify all ambiguous orders; double-check single, daily, and course-of-therapy dose limits; have second practitioner independently double-check original order, dose calculations, and infusion pump settings. Do not administer subcut, IM, or IT. IT administration is fatal. Vinblastine must be dispensed in an overwrap stating, "For IV use only." Overwrap should remain in place until immediately before administration. Nadir of leukopenia occurs in 5–10 days and recovery usually occurs in 7–14 days. Do not confuse with vincristine.

vinCRIStine (Vincasar PFS) **Uses:** Treatment of malignancies including: Lymphomas, Leukemias, Neuroblastoma, Rhabdomyosarcoma, Wilms' tumor; **Class:** vinca alkaloids; **Preg:** D; **CIs:** Hypersensitivity; Pregnancy/lactation; Active infection; Decreased bone marrow reserve; **ADRs:** agitation, insomnia, depression, bronchospasm, <u>constipation</u>, <u>N/V</u>, abdominal cramps, anorexia, ileus, stomatitis, gonadal suppression, nocturia, oliguria, urinary retention, <u>alopecia</u>, anemia, leukopenia, thrombocytopenia, <u>phlebitis at IV site</u>, tissue necrosis (from extravasation), ↑ uric acid, <u>ascending peripheral neuropathy</u>, <u>paresthesia</u>; **Interactions:** ↑ risk of bronchospasm in patients previously treated with mitomycin; May ↓ phenytoin levels; May ↓ antibody response/↑ risk of ADRs to live-virus vaccines; **Dose:** *IV: Adults:* 0.4–1.4 mg/m² once weekly (max: 2 mg/dose). *IV: Peds: >10 kg:* 1–2 mg/m² once weekly (max: 2 mg/dose). *IV: Peds: <10 kg:* 0.05 mg/kg once weekly. *IV: Hepatic Impairment Adults and Peds:* ↓ dose by 50% if serum bilirubin >3 mg/dl; **Availability (G):** *Inject:* 1 mg/ml; **Monitor:** BP, HR, RR, neuro status, S/S neuropathy, I/Os, CBC (with diff), LFTs, uric acid; **Notes:** Refer to individual protocols; **High Alert:** Fatalities have occurred with chemotherapeutic agents. Before administering, clarify all ambiguous orders; double-check single, daily, and course-of-therapy dose limits; have second practitioner independently double-check original order, dose calculations, and infusion pump settings. Do not administer subcut, IM, or IT. IT administration is fatal. Vincristine must be dispensed in an overwrap stating "For IV use only." Overwrap should remain in place until immediately before administration. Do not confuse with vinblastine.

vinorelbine (Navelbine) **Uses:** Inoperable non–small-cell CA of the lung (alone or with cisplatin); **Class:** vinca alkaloids; **Preg:** D;

CIs: Hypersensitivity; Pregnancy/lactation; Active infection; ↓ bone marrow reserve; Peds (safe use not established); **ADRs:** fatigue, shortness of breath, CP, constipation, N/V, abdominal pain, anorexia, diarrhea, ↑ LFTs (transient), alopecia, rash, anemia, neutropenia, thrombocytopenia, irritation at IV site, skin reactions, phlebitis, jaw pain, myalgia, peripheral neuropathy, pain in tumor-containing tissue; **Interactions:** ↑ bone marrow depression with other antineoplastics or radiation therapy; Concurrent use with cisplatin ↑ risk and severity of bone marrow depression; Concurrent use with mitomycin or chest radiation ↑ risk of pulmonary reactions; **Dose:** *IV: Adults: As single agent*—30 mg/m^2 once weekly. *With cisplatin*—25–30 mg/m^2 once weekly. *Hepatic Impairment IV: Adults:* ↓ dose if bilirubin >2 mg/dl; **Availability (G):** *Inject:* 10 mg/ml; **Monitor:** BP, HR, RR, S/S bronchospasm/paresthesia, neuro status, CBC (with diff), LFTs, uric acid, I/Os; **Notes: High Alert:** Fatalities have occurred with chemotherapeutic agents. Before administering, clarify all ambiguous orders; double-check single, daily, and course-of-therapy dose limits; have second practitioner independently double-check original order, dose calculations, and infusion pump settings. The nadir of granulocytopenia usually occurs within 7–10 days and recovery occurs within 7–15 days. If granulocyte count is <1500/mm^3, dose reduction or temporary interruption of vinorelbine may be warranted. If repeated episodes of fever and/or sepsis occur during granulocytopenia, future dose of vinorelbine should be modified.

vitamin E (alpha tocopherol, Aquasol E, Liqui-E) Uses: PO: Dietary supplement; Used in low-birth-weight infants to prevent and treat hemolysis due to vitamin E deficiency; **Topical:** Treatment of irritated, chapped, or dry skin; **Class:** fat soluble vitamins; **Preg:** A (doses within RDA), C (doses >RDA); **CIs:** Hypersensitivity to ingredients in preparations (parabens, propylene, glycol); **ADRs:** fatigue, HA, weakness, blurred vision, NECROTIZING ENTEROCOLITIS (low-birth-weight infants), cramps, diarrhea, nausea, rash; **Interactions:** Cholestyramine, colestipol, orlistat, mineral oil, and sucralfate ↓ absorption; May ↓ hematologic response to iron supplements; May ↑ risk of bleeding with warfarin; **Dose:** *PO: Adults: Vitamin E deficiency*—Treatment: 60–75 units/day; Prevention: 30 units/day. *PO: Peds: Vitamin E deficiency*—Treatment: 1 unit/kg/day. *PO: Neonates Vitamin E deficiency*—Treatment: 25–50 units/day; Prevention: 5 units/day in low-birth-weight infants or 5 units/L formula for full-term neonates. *Topical: Adults and Peds:* Apply prn; **Availability:** *Caps:* 100 units, 200 units, 400 units, 600 units, 1000 units. *Oral soln:* 15 units/0.3 ml. *Tabs:* 100 units, 200 units, 400 units, 500 units. *Oint:* 30 units/g. *Cream:* 30 units/g, 50 units/g, 100 units/g; *Oral/top oil:* 100 units/0.25 ml; **Monitor:** S/S vitamin E deficiency; **Notes:** Give with or after meals.

voriconazole (VFEND) **Uses:** Invasive aspergillosis; Candidemia and other Candidal infections (intra-abdominal abscesses, peritonitis, kidney); Esophageal candidiasis; Serious fungal infections caused by *Scedosporium apiospermum* or *Fusarium solani*; **Class:** antifungals; **Preg:** D; **CIs:** Concurrent use of rifampin, carbamazepine, phenobarbital, ritonavir (high dose), rifabutin, or St. John's wort (↓ antifungal activity); Concurrent use of sirolimus, pimozide, quinidine, ergot derivatives (↑ risk of toxicity of these agents); Tabs contain lactose and should be avoided in patients with galactose intolerance, Lapp lactase deficiency, or glucose-galactose malabsorption; Renal impairment (CrCl <50 ml/min) (IV form should be avoided, use oral form only); Pregnancy or lactation (use only if benefits justify risk); Peds <12 yr (safety not established); **ADRs:** dizziness, hallucinations, HA, visual disturbances, QT_C prolongation, peripheral edema, HEPATOTOXICITY, abdominal pain, N/V/D, photosensitivity, rash, ↓ K, allergic reactions including SJS, chills, fever, infusion reactions; **Interactions:** Carbamazepine, ritonavir, phenobarbital, St. John's wort, rifabutin, and rifampin ↓ levels/effect (contraindicated); Efavirenz ↓ levels/effects; voriconazole also ↑ levels/toxicity of efavirenz; Dihydroergotamine, ergotamine, pimozide, rifabutin, quinidine, and sirolimus ↑ levels/toxicity (contraindicated); May ↑ levels/toxicity of CYP3A4 substrates; Phenytoin ↓ levels; voriconazole also ↑ phenytoin levels/toxicity; **Dose:** *IV: Adults and Peds:* ≥*12 yr LD*—6 mg/kg q 12 hr × 2 doses, then maintenance dose of 4 mg/kg q 12 hr. Switch to oral dosing when possible. *Concomitant use of phenytoin*—↑ voriconazole MD to 5 mg/kg q 12 hr. *PO: Adults and Peds:* ≥*12 yr <40 kg*: 100 mg q 12 hr (may ↑ to 150 mg q 12 hr if inadequate response); ≥40 kg: 200 mg q 12 hr (may ↑ to 300 mg q 12 hr if inadequate response). *Concomitant use of efavirenz*—↑ voriconazole dose to 400 mg q 12 hr and ↓ efavirenz dose to 300 mg PO daily. *Concomitant use of phenytoin*—↑ voriconazole MD to 400 mg q 12 hr (if ≥40 kg) or 200 mg q 12 hr (if <40 kg). *Hepatic Impairment IV: Adults and Peds:* ≥*12 yr Mild-to-moderate hepatic impairment*—Use standard LD, decrease MD by 50%. *Renal Impairment IV: Adults and Peds:* ≥*12 yr:* If CrCl <50 ml/min, IV should not be used; use PO instead; **Availability:** *Tabs:* 50, 200 mg. *Oral susp:* 40 mg/ml. *Inject:* 200 mg; **Monitor:** ECG (QT_C prolongation), electrolytes, BUN/SCr, LFTs, visual changes; **Notes:** Administer PO 1 hr ac or pc. Infuse IV over 1–2 hr at a rate not to exceed 3 mg/kg/hr; IV formulation contains vehicle that accumulates in renal insufficiency (IV should not be used if CrCl <50 ml/min; use PO instead).

warfarin (Coumadin) **Uses:** Prophylaxis and treatment of: DVT, PE, AF with embolization; Prevention of clot formation and embolization after prosthetic valve placement and post-MI; **Class:** anticoagulants; **Preg:** X; **CIs:** Active bleeding/patients at high risk for bleeding; Severe liver or kidney disease; **ADRs:** cramps, nausea, dermal necrosis, BLEEDING, fever; **Interactions:** Abciximab, acetaminophen (>1.3 g/day × 1 wk) androgens, capecitabine, cefoperazone, cefotetan, chloral hydrate, chloramphenicol, clopidogrel, disulfiram, fluconazole, FQs, itraconazole, metronidazole, thrombolytics, eptifibatide, tirofiban, ticlopidine, sulfonamides, quinidine, quinine, NSAIDs, valproates, and aspirin ↑ risk of bleeding; Chronic alcohol, barbiturates, and estrogen-containing contraceptives ↓ anticoagulant response; Acute alcohol ingestion ↑ effects; foods high in vitamin K ↓ anticoagulant effects; **Dose:** *PO: Adults:* 2.5–10 mg/day × 2–4 days, then dose according to INR. *PO: Peds: >1 mo:* 0.05–0.34 mg/kg/day × 2–4 days, then dose according to INR. *IV: Adults:* 2–5 mg/day; **Availability (G):** *Tabs:* 1, 2, 2.5, 3, 4, 5, 6, 7.5, 10 mg. *Inject:* 5 mg; **Monitor:** PT/INR, CBC, LFTs, S/S bleeding; **Notes:** Elderly may require lower starting doses. Goal INR = 2–3.5 (depends on indication); takes 3–5 days to affect INR.

zafirlukast (Accolate) **Uses:** Asthma; **Class:** leukotriene antagonists; **Preg:** B; **CIs:** Hypersensitivity; **ADRs:** HA, dizziness, N/V/D, ↑ LFTs, back pain, myalgia, fever, infection, pain; **Interactions:** ↑ levels by aspirin; ↓ levels by erythromycin and theophylline; ↑ effects/bleeding with warfarin; **Dose:** *PO: Adults:* 20 mg bid. *PO: Peds:* 10 mg bid; **Availability:** *Tabs:* 10, 20 mg; **Monitor:** RR, peak flow, LFTs; **Notes:** Give on an empty stomach.

zaleplon (Sonata) **Uses:** Insomnia; **Class:** sedative/hypnotics; **Preg:** C; **CIs:** Sensitivity to zaleplon or tartrazine; **ADRs:** abnormal thinking, behavior changes, amnesia, dizziness, drowsiness, hallucinations, HA, sleep driving, weakness, abnormal vision, abdominal pain, anorexia, nausea, dysmenorrhea, rash, peripheral edema, photosensitivity, paresthesia, tremor, physical/psychological dependence; **Interactions:** Cimetidine may ↑ levels/toxicity (↓ zaleplon dose by 50%); ↑ CNS depression with alcohol, BZs, opioids, and other sedatives/hypnotics; **Dose:** *PO: Adults: <65 yr:* 10 mg (range: 5–20 mg) at bedtime. *PO: Geriatric Patients or Patients <50 kg:* 5 mg at bedtime. *Hepatic Impairment PO: Adults:* 5 mg at bedtime; **Availability:** *Caps:* 5, 10 mg; **Monitor:** Mental status, sleep patterns, abnormal behaviors; **Notes:** Schedule IV controlled substance. Give immediately prior to sleep. Prolonged use (>10 days) may result in physical/psychological dependence. High-fat meals ↓ absorption.

zanamivir (Relenza) **Uses:** Treatment/prevention of influenza; **Class:** antiviral; **Preg:** C; **CIs:** Hypersensitivity; Asthma/COPD; Peds <5 yr (prophylaxis); <7 yr (treatment); **ADRs:** delirium, hallucination, HA, self-injurious behavior, bronchospasm, cough, N/V/D, throat pain; **Interactions:** Do not give within 2 wk of influenza vaccine nasal spray; **Dose:** *Inhaln: Adults and Peds: ≥7 yr Treatment*—10 mg bid × 5 days. *Inhaln: Adults and Peds: ≥ 5 yr Prophylaxis*—10 mg/day × 10 days (4 wk for community outbreak); **Availability:** *Powder for inhaln:* 5-mg/blister;

Monitor: S/S influenza, mental status; **Notes:** Give within 2 days of symptom onset (treatment) or exposure (prophylaxis).

zidovudine (AZT, Retrovir) **Uses:** HIV (treatment, post-exposure prophylaxis, and ↓ maternal/fetal transmission); **Class:** NRTIs; **Preg:** C; **CIs:** Prior sensitivity to AZT; **ADRs:** HA, malaise, dizziness, syncope, abdominal pain, N/V/D, anorexia, ↑ LFTs, dyspepsia, oral mucosa/nail pigmentation, gynecomastia, anemia, granulocytopenia, pure red-cell aplasia, back pain, myopathy, tremor; **Interactions:** ↑ bone marrow depression with bone marrow–depressants, antineoplastics, or ganciclovir; ↑ neurotoxicity with acyclovir; Toxicity ↑ by probenecid or fluconazole; levels ↓ by clarithromycin; **Dose:** *PO: Adults and Peds: >13 yr:* 100 mg q 4 hr or 200 mg tid or 300 mg bid. *PO: Peds: 3 mo–12 yr:* 90–180 mg/m² q 6 hr (max: 200 mg q 6 hr). *IV: Adults and Peds: >12 yr:* 1 mg/kg infused over 1 hr q 4 hr. *IV: Peds:* 120 mg/m² q 6 hr (max: 160 mg/dose). *PO: Adults: >14-wk Pregnant:* 100 mg 5 × daily until onset of labor. *IV: Adults: during Labor and Delivery:* 2 mg/kg over 1 hr, then continuous infusion of 1 mg/kg/hr until umbilical cord is clamped. *IV: Infants:* 1.5 mg/kg q 6 hr until PO. *PO: Infants:* 2 mg/kg q 6 hr, within 12 hr of birth × 6 wk. *Renal*—↓ dose for CrCl <15 ml/min. *Hepatic*—↓ dose by 50% for cirrhosis; **Availability:** *Caps:* 100 mg. *Tabs:* 300 mg. *Oral syrup:* 50 mg/5 ml. *Inject:* 10 mg/ml; **Monitor:** CBC with platelets, LFTs, viral load, CD4 count, S/S opportunistic infections; **Notes:** Stress importance of compliance. Give IV only if NPO. Consider dose reduction for hematologic toxicity.

zinc sulfate (Orazinc, Zincate) **Uses:** Zinc supplementation; **Class:** trace metals; **Preg:** C; **CIs:** Prior sensitivity; Renal failure; **ADRs:** gastric irritation, N/V; **Interactions:** ↓ absorption of tetracyclines or FQs; **Dose:** *PO: Adults:* 110–220 mg zinc sulfate tid. *PO: Peds:* 0.5–1 mg elemental zinc/kg/day. *IV: Adults:* 2.5–6 mg/day. *IV: Peds:* 100 mcg/kg/day. *IV: Neonates ≤ 3 kg:* 300 mcg/kg/day; **Availability (G):** *Tabs:* 110 mg. *Caps:* 220 mg. *Inject:* 1, 5 mg/ml; **Monitor:** S/S zinc deficiency; serum zinc levels; **Notes:** Give with food.

ziprasidone (Geodon) **Uses:** Schizophrenia; Bipolar mania; **Class:** antipsychotics; **Preg:** C; **CIs:** History of QT_C prolongation, arrhythmias, recent MI, or uncompensated HF; Concurrent use of QT_C-prolonging agents; Dementia-related behavioral disorders; Renal/hepatic impairment; **ADRs:** seizures, dizziness, drowsiness, ↑ wt, extrapyramidal reactions, syncope, tardive dyskinesia, cough/runny nose, PROLONGED QT_C INTERVAL, orthostatic hypotension, constipation, N/V/D, dysphagia, rash, urticaria; **Interactions:** Concurrent use of dofetilide, class Ia and III antiarrhythmics, pimozide, sotalol, thioridazine, chlorpromazine, pentamadine, mefloquine, dolasetron, tacrolimus, droperidol, and moxifloxacin will prolong the QT_C interval; ↑ CNS depression with

Z

alcohol, antidepressants, antihistamines, opioid analgesics, or sedative/hypnotics; Levels/effects ↓ by carbamazepine; Levels/effects ↑ by ketoconazole; **Dose:** *PO: Adults: Schizophrenia*—20–80 mg bid. *Mania*—40–80 mg bid. *IM: Adults:* 10–20 mg q 2–4 hr prn up to 40 mg/day; **Availability:** *Caps:* 20, 40, 60, 80 mg. *Inject:* 20 mg; **Monitor:** Mental status, BP, QT_C interval, electrolytes, wt, BMI, EPS; **Notes:** Correct hypokalemia and hypomagnesemia prior to therapy. Give with food.

zoledronic acid (Reclast, Zometa) **Uses:** **Zometa:** Hypercalcemia of malignancy, Multiple myeloma and bone metastases from solid tumors; **Reclast:** Osteoporosis, Paget's disease; **Class:** biphosphonates; **Preg:** D; **CIs:** Hypersensitivity to zoledronic acid or other biphosphonates; Severe renal insufficiency (CrCl <35 ml/min); Hypocalcemia; **ADRs:** agitation, anxiety, confusion, HA, insomnia, wt loss, ↓ BP, alopecia, leg edema, abdominal pain, constipation, N/V/D, ↑ BUN/SCr, pruritus, rash, ↓ PO_4, ↓ Ca, ↓ K, ↓ Mg, musculoskeletal pain, osteonecrosis (of jaw), flu-like syndrome; **Interactions:** Loop diuretics or aminoglycosides ↑ risk of hypocalcemia; ↑ risk of GI effects with NSAIDs; **Dose:** *IV: Adults: Hypercalcemia of malignancy*—4 mg × 1, may repeat in 7 days. *Multiple myeloma and bone metastases*—4 mg q 3–4 wk. *Osteoporosis*—5 mg yearly. *Paget's disease*—5 mg. *Renal Impairment Adults:* ↓ dose if CrCl ≤60 ml/min; **Availability:** *Inject:* 4 mg/5 ml (Zometa). *Infusion:* 5 mg/100 ml (Reclast); **Monitor:** BMD, S/S Paget's (bone pain, HA), Ca, alk phos (for Paget's), BUN/SCr, dental exam (for osteonecrosis); **Notes:** Adequately hydrate and do not give diuretics prior to therapy; give over at least 15 min. May give acetaminophen prior to infusion and for 72 hr after infusion to ↓ infusion reaction.

zolmitriptan (Zomig, Zomig-ZMT) **Uses:** Acute treatment migraines; **Class:** 5-HT_1 agonists; **Preg:** C; **CIs:** Hypersensitivity; CAD or significant CV disease; Uncontrolled HTN; Use of other 5-HT_1 agonists or ergot-type drugs (dihydroergotamine) within 24 hr; Basilar or hemiplegic migraine; Concurrent or recent (within 2 wk) use of MAOI; CV risk factors (use only if CV status has been determined to be safe and 1st dose is administered under supervision); Symptomatic WPW syndrome or other arrhythmias; **ADRs:** dizziness, drowsiness, CORONARY ARTERY VASOSPASM, MI/ISCHEMIA, VT/VF, nausea; **Interactions:** MAOIs ↑ levels (concurrent or recent (within 2 wk) use contraindicated); Use with other 5-HT_1 agonists or ergot-type compounds may ↑ risk of vasospasm (avoid use within 24 hr of each other); Use with SSRIs or SNRIs may ↑ risk of serotonin syndrome; Propranolol and hormonal contraceptives ↑ levels; **Dose:** *PO: Adults:* ≤2.5 mg initially, may repeat in 2 hr (max: 10 mg in 24 hr). *Intranasal: Adults:* 5 mg, may repeat in 2 hr (max: 10 mg in 24 hr); **Availability:** *Tabs:* 2.5, 5 mg. *ODTs:* 2.5, 5 mg. *Nasal spray:* 5 mg/spray; **Monitor:** BP, HR, HA pain; **Notes:** For acute treatment only, not for prophylaxis; give as soon as migraine symptoms occur.

zolpidem (Ambien, Ambien CR) **Uses:** Insomnia; **Class:** sedative/hypnotics; **Preg:** C; **CIs:** Sleep apnea; Previous history of sedative/hypnotic abuse; **ADRs:** abnormal thinking, anxiety, depression, behavior changes, daytime drowsiness, dizziness, HA, hallucinations, sleep driving, ↑ BP, N/V/D, rash, physical/psychological dependence; **Interactions:** ↑ CNS depression with alcohol, BZs, opioids, and other sedative/hypnotics; CYP3A4 inhibitors may ↑ levels/toxicity; CYP3A4 inducers may ↓ levels/effects; **Dose:** *PO: Adults: Tabs*—10 mg at bedtime. *ER tabs*—12.5 mg at bedtime. *PO: Geriatric Patients, Debilitated Patients, or Patients with Hepatic Impairment Tabs*—5 mg at bedtime. *ER tabs*—6.25 mg at bedtime; **Availability (G):** *Tabs:* 5, 10 mg. *ER tabs:* 6.25, 12.5 mg; **Monitor:** Mental status, sleep patterns, abnormal behaviors; **Notes:** Do not give with food. Give immediately prior to sleep. Do not crush or chew ER tabs. Prolonged use (>7–10 days) may lead to physical/psychological dependence.

zonisamide (Zonegran) **Uses:** Partial seizures; **Class:** anticonvulsants; **Preg:** C; **CIs:** Prior sensitivity to zonisamide or sulfonamides; **ADRs:** <u>dizziness</u>, <u>drowsiness</u>, ataxia, HA, depression, psychomotor slowing, diplopia, <u>anorexia</u>, N/V/D, ↑ BUN/SCr, oligohydrosis (peds), SJS/TEN, rash, hyperthermia (peds), paresthesia; **Interactions:** ↑ CNS depression with alcohol, antidepressants, BZs, antihistamines, and opioids; CYP3A4 inhibitors may ↑ levels; CYP3A4 inducers may ↓ levels; **Dose:** *PO: Adults and Peds: >16 yr:* 100 mg/day × 2 wk; may then ↑ dose by 100 mg/day q 2 wk (max: 600 mg/day); **Availability:** *Caps:* 25, 50, 100 mg; **Monitor:** Seizure activity, mental status, S/S rash, BUN/SCr; **Notes:** Discontinue if rash occurs. Titrate slower in renal/hepatic disease.

zoster vaccine (Zostavax) **Uses:** Shingles prevention; **Class:** vaccines/immunizing agents; **Preg:** C; **CIs:** Sensitivity to gelatin, neomycin, or other vaccine components; Primary/acquired immunodeficiency states; Concurrent immunosupressive medications; Active untreated TB; Pregnancy; **ADRs:** swelling, redness, fever, tenderness; **Interactions:** Concurrent immunosupressants ↓ response and ↑ toxicity; **Dose:** *Subcut: Adults: ≥60 yr:* 0.65 ml; **Availability:** *Inject:* 19,400 PFU/0.65 ml; **Monitor:** fever, rash; **Notes:** Pregnancy should be avoided within 3 mo of vaccination.

Z

Appendix A: Commonly Used Antidotes for Drug Overdoses

The following table provides a list of drugs or drug classes that have specific antidotes available for the treatment of an acute overdosage. This information is meant for quick reference only and all ingestions should be managed with additional supportive care measures as directed by a local poison control center.

DRUG/ DRUG CLASS	ANTIDOTE	DOSE
acetaminophen	acetylcysteine	140 mg/kg PO × 1 dose followed by 70 mg/kg q 4 hr × 17 doses *or* 150 mg/kg IV over 60 min, then 50 mg/kg IV over 4 hr, then 100 mg/kg IV over next 16 hr
anticholinergics	physostigmine	Peds: 0.02 mg/kg up to 0.5 mg IV over 5 min; may repeat × 1 Adults: 1–2 mg IV over 2 min; may repeat × 1
benzodiazepines	flumazenil	0.2 mg IV over 30 sec; may repeat doses in 0.2–0.3-mg increments up to a total cumulative dose of 3 mg
beta-blockers	atropine	Peds: 0.02 mg/kg IV q 5 min (max dose: 0.5–1 mg) Adults: 0.5–1 mg IV q 5 min (max dose: 3 mg or 0.04 mg/kg)
	glucagon	5–10 mg IV over 1 min then 1–10 mg/hr infusion
	insulin	1 unit/kg IV bolus then 0.1–1 unit/kg/hr infusion
calcium channel blockers	calcium chloride or calcium gluconate	Peds: 10–30 mg/kg IV over 5 min Adults: 1–2 g IV over 5 min, then 2 g/hr IV infusion, titrate to maintain BP

DRUG/ DRUG CLASS	ANTIDOTE	DOSE
digoxin	digoxin immune Fab	Serum digoxin level (ng/ml) × body weight (kg) divided by 100 = number of vials to be given
heparin	protamine	1 mg protamine per 100 units heparin; give IV over 1–3 min at max rate of 5 mg/min
insulin	dextrose 25%–50%	Peds <6 mo: 0.25–0.5 g/kg IV Peds >6 mo: 0.5–1 g/kg IV Adults: 25 g IV
iron	deferoxamine	1 g IM/IV, then 500 mg IM/IV q 4 hr × 2 doses; if severe case, may continue 500 mg IM/IV q 4–12 hr (ig IV dose given at rate not to exceed 15 mg/kg/hr; 500 mg IV dose given at rate not to exceed 125 mg/hr) (max: 6 g/24 hr)
methotrexate	leucovorin	10–100 mg/m² IV/IM/PO q 6 hr until serum MTX level <0.01 micromole/L.
nondepolarizing neuromuscular blocking agents	atropine + neostigmine	Atropine: 1–1.5 mg IV 30–60 sec prior to neostigmine dose below Peds: 0.5 mg slow IV Adults: 1–3 mg slow IV
opiates	naloxone	0.4–2 mg IV/IM/ET; may repeat doses up to total cumulative dose of 10 mg
warfarin	phytonadione	Peds: 1–5 mg SQ/PO. Adults: 1–10 mg SQ/PO. if severe bleeding, may give IV over 30 min

Reference: Poisondex® online. www.thomsonhc.com. Accessed August 19, 2008.

Appendix B: Controlled Substances Schedules

Schedules are determined by the Drug Enforcement Agency (DEA), an arm of the United States Justice Department, and are based on the potential for abuse and dependence liability (physical and psychological) of the medication. Some states may have stricter prescription regulations. Physicians, dentists, podiatrists, and veterinarians may prescribe controlled substances. Nurse practitioners and physician's assistants may prescribe controlled substances with certain limitations.

Schedule I (C-I)

Potential for abuse is so high as to be unacceptable. May be used for research with appropriate limitations. Examples are LSD and heroin.

Schedule II (C-II)

High potential for abuse and extreme liability for physical and psychological dependence (amphetamines, opioid analgesics, dronabinol, certain barbiturates). Outpatient prescriptions must be in writing. In emergencies, telephone orders may be acceptable if a written prescription is provided within 72 hr. No refills are allowed.

Schedule III (C-III)

Intermediate potential for abuse (less than C-II) and intermediate liability for physical and psychological dependence (certain nonbarbiturate sedatives, certain nonamphetamine CNS stimulants, and certain opioid analgesics). Outpatient prescriptions can be refilled 5 times within 6 mo from date of issue if authorized by prescriber. Telephone orders are acceptable.

Schedule IV (C-IV)

Less abuse potential than Schedule III with minimal liability for physical or psychological dependence (certain sedative/hypnotics, certain antianxiety agents, some barbiturates, benzodiazepines, chloral hydrate, pentazocine, and propoxyphene). Outpatient prescriptions can be refilled 6 times within 6 mo from date of issue if authorized by prescriber. Telephone orders are acceptable.

Schedule V (C-V)

Minimal abuse potential. Number of outpatient refills determined by prescriber. Some products (cough suppressants with small amounts of codeine, diphenoxylate/atropine) may be available without prescription to patients >18 yr of age.

Appendix C: Critical Care Drug Infusions

DRUG	CONCENTRATION/ DILUENT	DOSE
Amiodarone	Intermittent: 150 mg/100 ml (1.5 mg/ml) Continuous: 900 mg/500 ml Concentration range: 1–6 mg/ml (if >2 mg/ml, infuse through central line) D5W or NS	Intermittent: Infuse over 10 min Continuous: 0.5–1 mg/min
Argatroban	250 mg/250 ml (1 mg/ml) D5W or NS	2–10 mcg/kg/min
Cisatracurium	200 mg/250 ml (0.8 mg/ml) D5W or NS	0.5–10 mcg/kg/min
Diltiazem	150 mg/150 ml (1 mg/ml) D5W or NS	5–15 mg/hr
Dobutamine	250–1000 mg/250–500 ml (0.25–4 mg/ml)D5W or NS	2.5–20 mcg/kg/min
Dopamine	200–800 mg/250–500 ml (0.8–3.2 mg/ml)D5W or NS	0.5–20 mcg/kg/min
Epinephrine	1–2 mg/250 ml (4–8 mcg/ml) D5W or NS	1–10 mcg/min
Esmolol	2500 mg/250 ml (10 mg/ml) D5W or NS	50–300 mcg/kg/min
Fentanyl	8 mg/250 ml (32 mcg/ml) D5W or NS	25–100 mcg/hr
Furosemide	10 mg/ml as undiluted drug	10–160 mg/hr
Heparin	25,000 units/250–500 ml (50–100 units/ml) D5W or NS	Based on heparin protocol
Insulin	100 units/100 ml (1 unit/ml) NS	Initial: 0.1 unit/kg/hr; titrate to serum glucose
Labetalol	5 mg/ml as undiluted drug	0.5–6 mg/min
Lepirudin	50 mg/250 ml (0.2 mg/ml) D5W or NS	Initial: 0.15 mg/kg/hr; titrate to achieve goal aPTT (max rate: 0.21 mg/kg/hr)
Lorazepam	2 mg/ml as undiluted drug	1–4 mg/hr
Milrinone	40 mg/200 ml (200 mcg/ml) D5W or NS	0.375–0.75 mcg/kg/min

(continued)

DRUG	CONCENTRATION/ DILUENT	DOSE
Morphine	250 mg/250 ml (1 mg/ml) D5W or NS	0.8–10 mg/hr
Nicardipine	20–40 mg/200 ml (0.1–0.2 mg/ml) D5W or NS	5–15 mg/hr
Nitroglycerin	100 mg/250 ml (400 mcg/ml) D5W or NS	5–200 mcg/min
Nitroprusside	50 mg/250 ml (200 mcg/ml) D5W	0.5–10 mcg/kg/min
Norepinephrine	16 mg/250 ml (64 mcg/ml) D5W	2–12 mcg/min
Phenylephrine	200 mg/250 ml (800 mcg/ml) D5W or NS	50–400 mcg/min
Propofol	1000 mg/100 ml (10 mg/ml; 10,000 mcg/ml) as undiluted drug	5–80 mcg/kg/min
Vasopressin	100 units/250 ml (0.4 units/ml) D5W or NS	0.04 units/min (septic shock)
Vecuronium	10–20 mg/100 ml (0.1–0.2 mg/ml) D5W or NS	0.8–1.2 mcg/kg/min

Appendix D: Cytochrome P450 Drug Interactions

CYP1A2

SUBSTRATES	INHIBITORS	INDUCERS
Alosetron	Cimetidine	Carbamazepine
Amitriptyline	Ciprofloxacin	Cigarette smoke
Clozapine	Fluvoxamine	Phenobarbital
Cyclobenzaprine	Ketoconazole	Rifampin
Desipramine	Lidocaine	
Diazepam	Mexiletine	
Fluvoxamine		
Imipramine		
Mexiletine		
Mirtazapine		
Olanzapine		
Propranolol		
Ropinirole		
Theophylline		
(R)-Warfarin		

CYP2C9

SUBSTRATES	INHIBITORS	INDUCERS
Celecoxib	Amiodarone	Carbamazepine
Glimepiride	Delavirdine	Phenobarbital
Glipizide	Efavirenz	Phenytoin
Losartan	Fluconazole	Rifampin
Montelukast	Fluvastatin	
Nateglinide	Ketoconazole	
Phenytoin	Sulfamethoxazole	
Sulfamethoxazole	Zafirlukast	
Voriconazole		
(S)-Warfarin		

CYP2C19

SUBSTRATES	INHIBITORS	INDUCERS
Citalopram	Delavirdine	Carbamazepine
Diazepam	Efavirenz	Phenytoin
Escitalopram	Esomeprazole	Rifampin
Esomeprazole	Fluoxetine	
Imipramine	Fluvoxamine	
Lansoprazole	Lansoprazole	
Nelfinavir	Omeprazole	
Omeprazole	Rabeprazole	
Pantoprazole	Sertraline	
Phenytoin	Ticlopidine	
Rabeprazole		
Voriconazole		

CYP2D6

SUBSTRATES	INHIBITORS	INDUCERS
Amitriptyline	Amiodarone	None
Aripiprazole	Cimetidine	
Atomoxetine	Clozapine	
Codeine	Delavirdine	
Desipramine	Desipramine	
Dextromethorphan	Fluoxetine	
Flecainide	Haloperidol	
Fluoxetine	Lidocaine	
Haloperidol	Methadone	
Imipramine	Paroxetine	
Lidocaine	Pimozide	
Metoprolol	Quinidine	
Mexiletine	Ritonavir	
Mirtazapine	Sertraline	
Nefazodone	Ticlopidine	
Nortriptyline		
Oxycodone		
Paroxetine		
Propafenone		
Propranolol		
Risperidone		

CYP2D6 *(cont'd)*

SUBSTRATES	INHIBITORS	INDUCERS
Ritonavir		
Tramadol		
Venlafaxine		

CYP3A

SUBSTRATES	INHIBITORS	INDUCERS
Alprazolam	Amiodarone	Carbamazepine
Amiodarone	Aprepitant	Efavirenz
Aprepitant	Cimetidine	Nevirapine
Aripiprazole	Clarithromycin	Phenobarbital
Atorvastatin	Cyclosporine	Phenytoin
Buspirone	Delavirdine	Rifabutin
Calcium channel blockers	Diltiazem	Rifampin
Carbamazepine	Efavirenz	St. John's wort
Cilostazol	Erythromycin	
Citalopram	Fluconazole	
Clarithromycin	Grapefruit juice	
Clonazepam	Imatinib	
Cyclosporine	Indinavir	
Dapsone	Itraconazole	
Delavirdine	Ketoconazole	
Diazepam	Metronidazole	
Disopyramide	Nefazodone	
Efavirenz	Nelfinavir	
Ergot derivatives	Quinidine	
Erlotinib	Ritonavir	
Erythromycin	Saquinavir	
Escitalopram	Sertraline	
Estrogens	Verapamil	
Fentanyl	Voriconazole	
Geftinib		
Glucocorticoids		
Imatinib		
Indinavir		

(continued)

CYP3A *(cont'd)*

SUBSTRATES	INHIBITORS	INDUCERS
Irinotecan		
Itraconazole		
Ketoconazole		
Lansoprazole		
Lidocaine		
Losartan		
Lovastatin		
Methadone		
Midazolam		
Mirtazapine		
Montelukast		
Nateglinide		
Nefazodone		
Nelfinavir		
Nevirapine		
Ondansetron		
Paclitaxel		
Pimozide		
Protease inhibitors		
Quetiapine		
Quinidine		
Repaglinide		
Rifabutin		
Sibutramine		
Sildenafil		
Simvastatin		
Sirolimus		
Tacrolimus		
Tadalafil		
Tamoxifen		
Theophylline		
Tiagabine		
Ticlopidine		
Vardenafil		
(R)-Warfarin		
Zolpidem		
Zonisamide		

Appendix E: Formulas Helpful for Calculating Doses

Calculation of Creatinine Clearance (CrCl) in Adults from Serum Creatinine

$$\text{Men: CrCl} = \frac{\text{IBW (kg)} \times (140 - \text{age})}{72 \times \text{serum creatinine (mg/dl)}}$$

$$\text{Women: CrCl} = 0.85 \times \text{calculation for men}$$

Calculation of Body Surface Area (BSA) in Adults and Children

Dubois method:
$\text{BSA (m}^2\text{)} = \text{wt (kg)}^{0.425} \times \text{ht (cm)}^{0.725} \times 0.007184$

Mosteller method:

$$\text{BSA (m}^2\text{)} = \sqrt{\frac{\text{ht (cm)} \times \text{wt (kg)}}{3600}}$$

Body Mass Index
$\text{BMI} = \text{wt (kg)} \div \text{ht}^2 \text{ (m}^2\text{)}$

Appendix F: Equianalgesic Dosing Guidelines

Opioid Analgesics Starting Oral Dose Commonly Used for Severe Pain

NAME	EQUIANALGESIC DOSE	
	ORAL	PARENTERAL
a. Morphine-like agonists		
morphine	30 mg	10 mg
hydromorphone (Dilaudid)	7.5 mg	1.5 mg
oxycodone	20 mg	—
methadone	10 mg	5 mg
levorphanol (Levodromoran)	4 mg (acute)	2 mg (acute)
	1 mg (chronic)	1 mg (chronic)
oxymorphone (Opana)	10 mg	1 mg
meperidine (Demerol)	300 mg	75 mg
b. Mixed agonists-antagonists		
nalbuphine (Nubain)	—	10 mg
butorphanol (Stadol)	—	2 mg
pentazocine (Talwin)	50 mg	30 mg
c. Partial agonist		
buprenorphine (Buprenex)	—	0.4 mg

Starting dose should be lower for older adults.

These are standard parenteral doses for acute pain in adults and can also be used to convert doses for IV infusions and repeated small IV boluses. For single IV boluses, use half the IM dose. IV doses for children >6 mos. = parenteral equianalgesic dose times weight (kg)/100.

Modified from *American Pain Society, Principles of Analgesic Use in the Treatment of Acute Pain and Cancer Pain,* ed.5. American Pain Society, 2003.

Fentanyl Transdermal Dose Based on Daily Morphine Dose

ORAL 24-HR MORPHINE (mg/day)	IM 24-HR MORPHINE (mg/day)	FENTANYL TRANSDERMAL (mcg/hr)
60–134	10–22	25
135–224	23–37	50
225–314	38–52	75
315–404	53–67	100
405–494	68–82	125
495–584	83–97	150
585–674	98–112	175
675–764	113–127	200
765–854	128–142	225
855–944	143–157	250
945–1034	158–172	275
1035–1124	173–187	300

A 10-mg IM or 60-mg oral dose of morphine every 4 hr for 24 hr (total of 60 mg/day IM or 360 mg/day oral) was considered approximately equivalent to fentanyl transdermal 100 mcg/hr.

Appendix G: Insulins and Insulin Therapy

The goal of therapy for diabetic patients is to provide insulin coverage that most closely resembles endogenous insulin production and results in the best glycemic control without hypoglycemia. Although daytime control of hyperglycemia may be accomplished with bolus doses of rapid-acting insulin analogs, elevations in fasting glucose may remain a problem. If fasting blood glucose levels remain elevated, the basal insulin dose (intermediate or long-acting) may have to be adjusted.

Most insulins used today are recombinant DNA human insulins. Produced through genetic engineering, synthetic human insulin is "manufactured" by yeast or nonpathogenic *E. coli*. In recent years, pharmaceutical companies have developed several new types and formulations of insulin.

Different insulins are distinguished by how quickly they are absorbed, the time and length of peak activity, and overall duration of action. Onset, peak, and duration of action times are approximate and vary according to individual factors such as injection site, blood supply, concurrent illnesses, lifestyle, and exercise level. These factors can vary from patient to patient and can vary in any patient from day to day.

There are 4 kinds of insulins: rapid-acting, short-acting, intermediate-acting, and long-acting. Premixed combinations of these different types of insulins are also available.

Rapid-Acting Insulins

Rapid-acting insulins are analogs of regular insulin. An analog is a chemical structure very similar to another but differing in one component. Humalog (lispro), Apidra (glulisine), and Novolog (aspart) are rapid-acting insulin analogs. The amino acid sequences of these analogs are nearly identical to human insulin. They differ in the positioning of certain proteins, which allow them to enter the bloodstream rapidly—within 10 minutes of subcutaneous injection. This closely mimics the body's own insulin response and allows greater flexibility in eating schedules for diabetic patients. Also, because these insulins leave the bloodstream quickly, the risk of hypoglycemic episodes several hours after the meal is lessened. The onset of rapid-acting insulins is 15–30 minutes, their peak effect occursin 1–2 hours and their 1-2 hours and their duration is 3-4 hours. Rapid-acting insulin solutions are clear.

Short-Acting Insulin

Regular insulin is a short-acting insulin and is available commercially as Humulin R or Novolin R. The onset of regular insulin is 0.5-1 hour; its peak activity occurs 2-3 hours after subcutaneous injection and its duration of action is 6-8 hours. This time/action profile makes rigid meal scheduling necessary, as the patient must estimate that a meal will occur within 45 minutes of injection. Short-acting insulin solutions are clear. Regular insulin is the only insulin that can be given intravenously.

Intermediate-Acting Insulins

Intermediate-acting insulins contain protamine, which delays onset, peak, and duration of action to provide basal insulin coverage. Basal insulins are given to control blood glucose levels throughout the day when not eating. Commercially, intermediate-acting insulins are available as Humulin N or Novolin N. (The "N" stands for NPH). Action starts between 2 and 4 hours after injecting. Peak activity occurs between 6 and 12 hours. Duration of action lasts 18–24 hours. The addition of protamine causes the cloudy appearance of intermediate-acting insulins and results in the formulation being a suspension rather than a solution. This is why these insulins must be gently mixed before administering. Intermediate-acting insulins can be mixed with short or rapid-acting insulins to provide both basal and bolus coverage.

Long-Acting Insulins

Long-acting insulins have the most delayed onset and the longest duration of all insulins. Products include Lantus (glargine) and Levemir (detemir). Peaks are not as prominent in long-acting insulins. In fact, insulin glargine has no real peak action because it forms slowing dissolving crystals in the subcutaneous tissue. The onset of action of insulin glargine is 3–4 hours after subcutaneous injection and the duration of action lasts 24 hours. Insulin detemir has a similar onset of action; however, its duration of action is dose dependent at lower dosages (0.2 units/kg), the duration of action is approximately 14 hours, while at higher dosages (70.6 units/kg), it is nearly 24 hours. Even though insulin glargine and insulin detemir are clear solutions, neither can be diluted or mixed with any other insulin or solution. Mixing insulin glargine or insulin detemir with other insulin products can alter the onset of action and time to peak effect. If bolus insulin is to be given at the same time as insulin glargine or insulin detemir, two separate syringes and injection sites must be used.

Combination Insulins

Various combinations of premixed insulins are available, containing fixed proportions of two different insulins, usually a short and an intermediate-acting insulin. Typically the intermediate-acting insulin makes up 70% to 75% of the mixture, with rapid- or short-acting insulin making up the remainder. Onset, peak, and duration vary according to each specific product. Brand names of these products include Humulin 70/30 or Novolin 70/30 (70% NPH, 30% regular), Humulin 50/50 (50% NPH, 50% regular) Humalog Mix 75/25 (75% insulin lispro protamine suspension, 25% insulin lispro), Humalog Mix 50/50 (50% insulin lispro-protamine suspension, 50% insulin lispro) or Novolog Mix 70/30 (70% insulin aspart protamine suspension, 30% insulin aspart).

BRAND NAME	GENERIC NAME	TYPE OF INSULIN	ONSET/PEAK/ DURATION
Apidra	insulin glulisine	Rapid-acting	15–30 min/ 1–2 hr/3–4 hr
Humalog	insulin lispro	Rapid-acting	15–30 min/ 1–2 hr/3–4 hr
Novolog	insulin aspart	Rapid-acting	15–30 min/ 1–2 hr/3–4 hr
Humulin R/ Novolin R	regular insulin	Short-acting	0.5–1 hr/ 2–3 hr/6–8 hr
Humulin N/ Novolin N	NPH	Intermediate-acting	2–4 hr/6–12 hr/ 18–24 hr
Levemir	insulin detemir	Long-acting	minimal peak; lasts up to 24 hr
Lantus	insulin glargine	Long-acting	no peak; lasts up to 24 hr

Appendix H: Measurement Conversion Table

Metric System Equivalents

1 gram (g) = 1000 milligrams (mg)
1000 grams = 1 kilogram (kg)
0.001 milligram = 1 microgram (mcg)
1 liter (L) = 1000 milliliters (ml)
1 milliliter = 1 cubic centimeter (cc)
1 meter = 100 centimeters (cm)
1 meter = 1000 millimeters (mm)

Conversion Equivalents

Volume
1 milliliter = 15 drops (gtt)
5 milliliters = 1 teaspoon (tsp)
15 milliliters = 1 tablespoon (T)
30 milliliters = 1 ounce (oz)
473 milliliters = 1 pint (pt)
946 milliliters = 2 pints = 1 quart (qt)

Weight
1 kilogram = 2.2 pounds (lb)
1 gram (g) = 1000 milligrams = 15 grains (gr)
0.6 gram = 600 milligrams = 10 grains
0.5 gram = 500 milligrams = 7.5 grains
0.3 gram = 300 milligrams = 5 grains
0.06 gram = 60 milligrams = 1 grain

Length
2.54 centimeters = 1 inch

Centigrade/Fahrenheit Conversions

$C = (F - 32) \times 5/9$
$F = (C \times 9/5) + 32$

Appendix I: Pediatric Intravenous Medication Quick Reference Chart

Risk of fluid overload in infants and children is always a consideration when administering IV medications. The following table provides maximum concentrations—the smallest amount of fluid necessary for diluting specific medications—and the maximum rate at which the medications should be given.

DRUG	MAXIMUM CONCENTRATION	MAXIMUM RATE
acyclovir	10 mg/ml	Give over 1 hr
amphotericin B	0.1 mg/ml (peripherally)	Give over 2–6 hr
	0.5 mg/ml (centrally)	
ampicillin	100 mg/ml	10 mg/kg/min
azithromycin	2 mg/ml	Give over 1 hr
calcium chloride	100 mg/ml	100 mg/min
calcium gluconate	100 mg/ml	100 mg/min
cefazolin	138 mg/ml (IVP)	Give over 3–5 min
	20 mg/ml (intermittent infusion)	Give over 10–60 min
cefotaxime	<200 mg/ml (IVP)	Give over 3–5 min
	60 mg/ml (intermittent infusion)	Give over 10–30 min
cefoxitin	180 mg/ml (IVP)	Give over 3–5 min
	40 mg/ml (intermittent infusion)	Give over 15–40 min
ceftazidime	200 mg/ml (IVP)	Give over 3–5 min
	40 mg/ml (intermittent infusion)	Give over 10–30 min
ceftriaxone	40 mg/ml	Give over 10–30 min
cefuroxime	100 mg/ml (IVP)	Give over 3–5 min
	30 mg/ml (intermittent infusion)	Give over 15–60 min
digoxin	100 mcg/ml	Give over 5 min
diphenhydramine	50 mg/ml	25 mg/min
fluconazole	2 mg/ml	Give over 1–2 hr
fosphenytoin	25 mg/ml	3 mg/kg/min
furosemide	10 mg/ml	0.5 mg/kg/min
gentamicin	40 mg/ml	Give over 30 min
magnesium sulfate	60 mg/ml	1 mEq/kg/hr (125 mg/kg/hr)
metronidazole	8 mg/ml	Give over 1 hr
morphine	5 mg/ml	Give over 4–5 min
ondansetron	2 mg/ml	Give over 2–15 min
pentobarbital	50 mg/ml	Give over 10–30 min
phenobarbital	130 mg/ml	2 mg/kg/min
phenytoin	50 mg/ml	3 mg/kg/min

DRUG	MAXIMUM CONCENTRATION	MAXIMUM RATE
phytonadione	10 mg/ml	Give over 15–30 min
piperacillin/ tazobactam	20 mg/ml	Give over 30 min
potassium chloride	80 mEq/L (peripherally) 200 mEq/L (centrally)	1 mEq/kg/hr
ticarcillin/clavulanate	100 mg/ml	Give over 10–60 min.
tobramycin	40 mg/ml	Give over 30 min
trimethoprim/ sulfamethoxazole	1 ml drug per 10 ml diluent	Give over 1–1.5 hr
valproate sodium	50 mg/ml	2–6 mg/kg/min
vancomycin	5 mg/ml	Give over 60 min

Source: Phelps SJ and Hak EB: Pediatric Injectable Drugs, 7th Edition. American Society of Heath-System Pharmacists, Bethesda, MD 2004.

Appendix J: Pregnancy Categories

Category A

Adequate, well-controlled studies in pregnant women have not shown an increased risk of fetal abnormalities.

Category B

Animal studies have revealed no evidence of harm to the fetus; however, there are no adequate and well-controlled studies in pregnant women.

or

Animal studies have shown an adverse effect, but adequate and well-controlled studies in pregnant women have failed to demonstrate a risk to the fetus.

Category C

Animal studies have shown an adverse effect and there are no adequate and well-controlled studies in pregnant women.

or

No animal studies have been conducted and there are no adequate and well-controlled studies in pregnant women.

Category D

Studies, adequate well-controlled or observational, in pregnant women have demonstrated a risk to the fetus. However, the benefits of therapy may outweigh the potential risk.

Category X

Studies, adequate well-controlled or observational, in animals or pregnant women have demonstrated positive evidence of fetal abnormalities. The use of the product is contraindicated in women who are or may become pregnant.

Note: The designation UK is used when the pregnancy category is unknown.

Appendix K: Routine Pediatric and Adult Immunizations

Immunization recommendations change frequently. For the latest recommendations see http://www.cdc.gov/nip.

Routine Pediatric Immunizations (0–18 yr)

GENERIC NAME (BRAND NAMES)	ROUTE/DOSAGE	CONTRAINDICATIONS/ PRECAUTIONS	ADVERSE REACTIONS/ SIDE EFFECTS	NOTES
DTaP diphtheria toxoid, tetanus toxoid, and acellular pertussis vaccine (Daptacel, Infanrix, Tripedia)	0.5 ml IM at 2, 4, 6, and 15–18 mo; booster at 4–6 yr (4th dose in series may be given at 12 mo).	Acute infection, immunosuppressive therapy, previous CNS damage or convulsions.	Redness, tenderness, induration at site; fever; malaise; myalgia; urticaria; hypotension; neurologic reactions; allergic reactions (all less than with DTwP).	Individual components may be given as separate injections if unusual reactions occur.
Tetanus toxoid, **reduced** diphtheria toxoid and acellularm pertussis vaccine (absorbedHDTap, Adacell, Boostrix)	0.5 ml IM to replace 1 dose of DTaP at from age 10–18 (Boostrix) or 11–18 (Adacel).	Previous reactions to DTaP, progressive neurological disease or recent (within 7 days) CNS pathology.	Fatigue, headache, gastrointestinal symptoms, pain at injection site.	Pertussis protection in addition to diphtheria and tetanus designed to protect against older children becoming ill with pertussis and passing it on to very young unprotected children in whom the disease has heightened morbidity.

(continued)

Routine Pediatric Immunizations (0–18 yr) *(cont'd)*

GENERIC NAME (BRAND NAMES)	ROUTE/DOSAGE	CONTRAINDICATIONS/ PRECAUTIONS	ADVERSE REACTIONS/ SIDE EFFECTS	NOTES
Polio vaccine, inactivated (IPV, IPOL, Poliovax)	0.5 ml subcut at 2, 4, and 6–18 mo with a booster at 4–6 yr.	Hypersensitivity to neomycin, streptomycin, or polymyxin B; acute febrile illness.	Erythema, induration, pain at injection site; fever.	Oral polio vaccine (OPV) is no longer recommended for use in the United States.
Measles, mumps, and rubella vaccines (M-M-R II)	Single dose 0.5 ml subcut at 12–15 mo with a booster at 4–6 yr or 11–12 yr.	Allergy to egg, gelatin, or neomycin; active infection; immunosuppression.	Burning, stinging, pain at injection site; arthritis/arthralgia (40%); fever; encephalitis; allergic reactions.	If unusual reactions occur, individual components may be given as separate injections.
Hemophilus b conjugate vaccine (PedvaxHIB, ActHIB, HibTITER)	0.5 ml IM at 2, 4, and 6 mo (6 mo dose not needed for PedvaxHIB), with a booster at 12–15 mo.	If co-administered with other immunizations, consider contraindications of all products.	Induration, erythema, tenderness at injection site; fever.	
Hepatitis B vaccine (Engerix-B, Recombivax HB)	10 mcg IM Engerix-B or 5 mcg IM Recombivax HB 1st dose at 0–2 mo, 2nd dose at 1–4 mo, and 3rd dose at 6–18 mo (1st and 2nd dose about 1 mo apart). Dose is same for patients up to 20 yrs old.	Hypersensitivity to yeast.	Local soreness.	Children who have not been vaccinated as infants should complete the series by 12 yr.

Routine Pediatric Immunizations (0–18 yr) *(cont'd)*

GENERIC NAME (BRAND NAMES)	ROUTE/DOSAGE	CONTRAINDICATIONS/ PRECAUTIONS	ADVERSE REACTIONS/ SIDE EFFECTS	NOTES
	Infants born to HBsAg-positive mothers: Administer 0.5 ml of hepatitis B immune globulin within 12 hours of birth and 1st dose of 5 mcg Recombivax or 10 mcg of Engerix B IM and 2nd dose at 1–2 mo, 3rd dose at 6 mo. *Children up to 10 yr:* 2.5 mcg Recombivax HB or 10 mcg Engerix-B IM as 3-dose series; 2nd dose 1 mo after 1st dose, 3rd dose 4 mo after 1st dose, and 2 mo after 2nd dose. *Children up to 11–19 yr:* 5 mcg Recombivax HB or 10 mcg Engerix-B as 3-dose series; 2nd dose 1 mo after			

(continued)

Routine Pediatric Immunizations (0–18 yr) *(cont'd)*

GENERIC NAME (BRAND NAMES)	ROUTE/DOSAGE	CONTRAINDICATIONS/ PRECAUTIONS	ADVERSE REACTIONS/ SIDE EFFECTS	NOTES
	1st dose, 3rd dose 4 mo after 1st dose, and 2 mo after 2nd dose. In children 11–15 yr, may also be given as 2 doses of 10 mcg/ml (Recombivax HB) 4–6 mo apart.			
Meningococcal polysaccharide diphtheria toxoid conjugate vaccine (Menactra)	0.5 ml IM single dose at 11–12 yr or before entry to high school (15 yr).	Hypersensitivity to any components.	Fatigue, malaise, anorexia, pain at injection site.	Goal is to decrease invasive meningococcal disease. Routine vaccination with meningococcal vaccine also is recommended for college freshmen living in dormitories and other high risk populations (military recruits, travelers to areas in which meningococcal disease prevalent); other high risk patients may elect to receive vaccine.

Routine Pediatric Immunizations (0–18 yr) *(cont'd)*

GENERIC NAME (BRAND NAMES)	ROUTE/DOSAGE	CONTRAINDICATIONS/ PRECAUTIONS	ADVERSE REACTIONS/ SIDE EFFECTS	NOTES
Varicella vaccine (Varivax)	0.5 ml IM single dose at 12–18 mo; those without a history of chickenpox should be vaccinated by the 11–12 yr visit; children around age 13 yr should receive 2 doses 1 mo apart.	Allergy to gelatin or neomycin; active infection; immunosuppression, including HIV.	Local soreness, fever.	Given to children who have not been vaccinated or have not had chickenpox. Salicylates should be avoided for 6 wk following vaccination.
Hepatitis A vaccine (Havrix, Vaqta)	*Children 2–18 yr:* 0.5 ml IM (pediatric formulation), repeated 6–12 mo later (pediatric dose form).	Acute febrile illness.	Local reactions, headache.	Recommended for children in areas with high rates of hepatitis A and other high-risk groups.
Pneumococcal 7-valent conjugate vaccine (Prevnar)	*Infants:* 0.5 ml IM for 4 doses at 2, 4, 6, and 12–15 mo. *Older infants and children starting at 7–11 mo of age:* Three doses of 0.5 ml IM, 2 doses at least 4 wk apart, 3rd dose after 1 yr birthday.	Hypersensitivity to all components including diphtheria toxoid; moderate to severe febrile illness; thrombocytopenia or coagulation disorder. Use cautiously in patients receiving anticoagulants; safe use in children <6 wk not established.	Erythema induration, tenderness, nodule formation at injection site, fever.	Antineoplastics, corticosteroids, radiation therapy, and immunosuppressants decrease antibody response; product is a suspension, shake before use.

(continued)

Routine Pediatric Immunizations (0–18 yr) *(cont'd)*

GENERIC NAME (BRAND NAMES)	ROUTE/DOSAGE	CONTRAINDICATIONS/ PRECAUTIONS	ADVERSE REACTIONS/ SIDE EFFECTS	NOTES
	Starting at 12–23 mo of age: Two doses of 0.5 ml IM at least 2 mo apart. *Starting 2–6 yr:* Single dose 0.5 ml IM.			
Influenza vaccine *(injection:* Fluarix, Fluvirin, Fluzone; *intranasal:* FluMist)	***Injection:*** *Children 6–35 mo:* 0.25 ml IM 1–2 doses (2 doses at least 1 mo apart for initial season) followed by single dose annually. *Children 3–8 yr:* 0.5 ml IM 1–2 doses (2 doses at least 1 mo apart for initial season) followed by single dose annually. *Children ≥9 yr:* 0.5 IM single dose annually.	Hypersensitivity to eggs/egg products. Hypersensitivity to thimerosal (injection only). Fluvirin should be used in children >4 yr only. Avoid use in patients with acute neurologic compromise. FluMist should be avoided in patients receiving salicylates or who are immunocompromised.	*Injection:* local soreness, fever myalgia, possible neurologic toxicity. *Intranasal:* upper respiratory congestion, malaise.	Immunosupression may decrease antibody response to injection and increase the risk of viral transmission with intranasal route.

Routine Pediatric Immunizations (0–18 yr) *(cont'd)*

GENERIC NAME (BRAND NAMES)	ROUTE/DOSAGE	CONTRAINDICATIONS/ PRECAUTIONS	ADVERSE REACTIONS/ SIDE EFFECTS	NOTES
	Nasal (Flumist): *Children 5–8 yr:* If not previously immunized with FluMist—2 doses of 0.5 ml intranasally (given as one 0.25-ml dose in each nostril) at least 2 mo apart, then one dose annually. If previously immunized with FluMist, 1 dose of 0.5 ml intranasally (given as one 0.25-ml dose in each nostril) annually. *Children ≥9 yr:* 1 dose of 0.5 ml intranasally (given as one 0.25 ml dose in each nostril) annually.			

Routine Adult Immunizations

GENERIC NAME (BRAND NAMES)	INDICATIONS	DOSAGE/ROUTE	CONTRAINDICATIONS	ADVERSE REACTIONS/ SIDE EFFECTS
Hepatitis A vaccine (Havrix, Vaqta)	High-risk patients, some health care workers, food handlers, clotting disorders, travel to endemic areas, chronic liver disease.	1 ml IM, followed by 1 ml IM 6–18 mo later (adult dose form).	Hypersensitivity to alum or 2-phenoxyethanol.	Local soreness, headache.
Hepatitis B vaccine (Engerix-B, Recombivax HB)	High-risk patients, health care workers, all unvaccinated adolescents.	3 doses of 1 ml IM, given at 0, 1–2, and 4–6 mo.	Anaphylactic allergy to yeast.	Local soreness.
Influenza vaccine (*Injection:* Fluzone, Fluvirin; *intranasal* FluMist)	All adults	*Injection:* 0.5 ml IM annually. *Intranasal for adults <50 yr:* Single 0.5 ml dose given as 0.25 ml in each nostril annually.	Hypersensitivity to eggs/egg products. Hypersensitivity to thimerosal (injection only). Avoid use in patients with acute neurologic compromise. FluMist should be avoided in patients receiving salicylates or who are immunocompromised.	*Injection:* local soreness, fever myalgia, possible neurologic toxicity. *Intranasal:* upper respiratory congestion, malaise. Immunosuppression may decrease antibody response to injection and increase the risk of viral transmission with intranasal route.
Measles, mumps, and rubella vaccines (M-M-R II)	Adults with unreliable history of MMR illness or immunization, occupational exposure.	0.5 ml subcut, single dose in those with unreliable history, 2 doses 1 mo apart	Allergy to egg, gelatin, or neomycin; active infection; immunosuppression;	Burning, stinging, pain at injection site; arthritis/ arthralgia; fever;

(continued)

Routine Adult Immunizations *(cont'd)*

GENERIC NAME (BRAND NAMES)	INDICATIONS	DOSAGE/ROUTE	CONTRAINDICATIONS	ADVERSE REACTIONS/ SIDE EFFECTS
		for those with occupational exposure.	pregnancy; also avoid becoming pregnant for 4 wk after immunization.	encephalitis; allergic reactions.
Meningococcal polysaccharide diphtheria toxoid conjugate vaccine (Menactra)	0.5 ml IM single dose at 11–12 yr or before entry to high school (15 yr).	Hypersensitivity to any components	Fatigue, malaise, anorexia, pain at injection site	Recommended for college freshmen living in dormitories and other high-risk populations(military recruits, travelers to areas in which meningococcal disease prevalent); other high-risk patients may elect to receive vaccine.
Pneumococcal vaccine, (polyvalent Pneumovax 23)	Everyone >65 yr, high-risk patients with chronic illnesses including HIV and other high-risk patients.	0.5 ml IM, high-risk patients (asplenics) should have a booster after 6 yr.	Safety in first trimester of pregnancy not established.	Local soreness.
Tetanus toxoid, **reduced** diphtheria toxoid and acellular pertussis vaccine (absorbedDTaP, Adacell)	0.5 ml IM to replace 1 dose of DTaP	Previous reactions to DTaP, progressive neurological disease or recent (within 7 days) CNS pathology	Fatigue, headache, gastrointestinal symptoms, pain at injection site	Pertussis protection in addition to diphtheria and tetanus designed to protect against those

(continued)

Routine Adult Immunizations *(cont'd)*

GENERIC NAME (BRAND NAMES)	INDICATIONS	DOSAGE/ROUTE	CONTRAINDICATIONS	ADVERSE REACTIONS/ SIDE EFFECTS
				becoming ill with pertussis from passing it on to very young unprotected children in whom the disease has heightened morbidity.
Tetanus-diphtheria (Adult Td)	All adults.	*Unimmunized:* 2 doses of 0.5 ml IM 1–2 mo apart, then a 3rd dose 6–12 mo later; *immunized:* booster every 10 yr.	Neurologic or severe hypersensitivity reaction to prior dose.	Local pain and swelling.
Varicella vaccine (Varivax)	Any adult without a history of chickenpox or herpes zoster.	0.5 ml subcut; repeated 4–8 wk later.	Allergy to gelatin or neomycin; active infection; immunosuppression including HIV; pregnancy; family history of immunodeficiency; blood/ blood product in past 5 mo.	Salicylates should be avoided for 6 wk following vaccination.

Less commonly used vaccines are not included.
SOURCE: Adapted from the recommendations of the National Immunization Program: http://www.cdc.gov/nip.

Index

D

E

H

I

N

O

P

Q

R

S